To Rosa,
for her courage
and love for life

Inflammatory Bowel Disease and Familial Adenomatous Polyposis

Clinical Management and Patients' Quality of Life

Gian Gaetano Delaini (Ed.)

Inflammatory Bowel Disease and Familial Adenomatous Polyposis

Clinical Management and Patients' Quality of Life

Foreword by
S.M. Goldberg

Springer

Gian Gaetano Delaini
Department of Surgery and Gastroenterology
University of Verona
Verona, Italy

Library of Congress Control Number: 2006924375

ISBN-10 88-470-0433-0 Springer Milan Berlin Heidelberg New York
ISBN-13 978-88-470-0433-7 Springer Milan Berlin Heidelberg New York

Springer is a part of Springer Science+Business Media
springer.com

Printed in Italy

Cover design: estudio Calamar, Barcelona, Spain
Typesetting: Compostudio, Cernusco s/N (MI), Italy
Printing: Printer Trento, Gardolo (TN), Italy

Foreword

There are many excellent textbooks on gastroenterology and surgery that cover the subject of inflammatory bowel disease and familial adenomatous polyposis. However, Professor Delaini has chosen authors in this book for their special interest, experience and expertise in their assigned topics. Even a superficial look at the chapter titles will reveal that certain disease processes occurring proximal to or outside the large intestine are covered in this text, yet all within the domain of the "abdominal" or colorectal surgeon. Medical management of the patient with inflammatory bowel disease and familial adenomatous polyposis is also included.

Inflammatory bowel disease surgery has undergone major progress in the last 25 years. There are new operations available for most patients with inflammatory bowel disease that alleviate suffering in Crohn's disease and offer curative therapy in ulcerative colitis while permitting ever-increasing opportunities for nearly normal intestinal and sexual function.

The objective of the editor in producing this volume has been essentially threefold: first, to assemble the current methods of treatment for these conditions; second, to present a thoughtful approach to management of complications associated with these therapies; and third, to explore newer therapies that are being tried for these diseases in which aetiologies are unknown.

To these ends, the editor has enlisted a group of authors who are already distinguished for their contributions in their respective fields. As a result, they have been able to bring readers up to date with the latest advances in their chosen field of excellence.

I have no doubt of the great value of this volume, and I offer my warmest congratulations to Professor Delaini and his collaborators on a very timely publication, which will assuredly earn them the deep gratitude of their colleagues who have to deal on a daily basis with patients suffering from these maladies.

Stanley M. Goldberg

Contents

Contents

Contributors

DONATO F. ALTOMARE
Coloproctological Unit
Department of Emergency and
Organ Transplantation
General Surgery and
Liver Transplantation Unit
University of Bari
Bari, Italy

SHAMIM ABSAR
Department of Colorectal Surgery
and Surgical Pathology
Stepping Hill Hospital
Trafford Healthcare Trust
Manchester, UK

LUCIANO ALESSANDRONI
Department of Surgery
S. Camillo Hospital
Rome, Italy

GIAMPAOLO ANGELINI
Unit of Digestive Endoscopy
Policlinico "G.B. Rossi"
University of Verona
Verona, Italy

CORRADO R. ASTERIA
Department of Clinical Physiopathology
University of Florence
Florence, Italy

OMER AZIZ
Department of Biosurgery and
Surgical Technology
Imperial College London
St. Mary's Hospital
London, UK

GORAN I. BARISIC
Institute for Digestive Diseases
Belgrade, Serbia-Montenegro

MICHELA BAROLLO
Department of General Surgery
University of Padua
Padua, Italy

DAVID C.C. BARTOLO
Colorectal Unit
Western General Hospital
Edinburgh, Scotland, UK

PIERO BAZZI
Unit of General Surgery
Policlinico S. Orsola-Malpighi
University of Bologna
Bologna, Italy

GABRIELE BAZZOCCHI
Unit of Visceral Disorder and
Autonomic Dysfunction
Montecatone Rehabilitation Institute
University of Bologna
Imola, Italy

LUIGI BENINI
Department of Biomedical and
Surgical Sciences
Division of Gastroenterology
Policlinico G.B. Rossi
Verona, Italy

LAURA BERNARDONI
Unit of Digestive Endoscopy
Policlinico "G.B. Rossi"
University of Verona
Verona, Italy

RICCARDO BERTOLINI
Department of Surgery
S. Camillo Hospital
Rome, Italy

FRANCESCO BIANCO
Department of Emergency Surgery
"S.G. Moscati" Hospital
Avellino, Italy

FABRIZIO BONFANTE
Department of Internal Medicine
Endoscopic Unit
Desenzano, Italy

Fiorenzo Botti
2nd Unit of General Surgery
IRCCS Maggiore Hospital
Foundation, Mangiagalli e Regina Elena
Milan, Italy

Maria Luisa Brandi
Departmentof Internal Medicine
University of Florence
Florence, Italy

Piero Brosolo
Unit of Gastroenterology
Hospital "S. Bonifacio"
Verona, Italy

Luca Campana
Section of Anal Physiology and Ultrasound
Coloproctology Service
Department of Surgery
Regional Hospital
Treviso, Italy

Massimo Campieri
Department of Internal Medicine and Gastroenterology
University of Bologna
Bologna, Italy

Alberto Carrara
2nd Unit of General Surgery
IRCCS Maggiore Hospital
Foundation Mangiagalli and Regina Elena
Milan, Italy

Giuseppe Casula
Department of General Surgery
University of Cagliari
Cagliari, Italy

Gianluca Colucci
Department of General Surgery and Gastroenterology
University of Verona
Verona, Italy

Michele Comberlato
Gastroenterology Unit
Central Hospital
Bolzano Italy

Ettore Contessini-Avesani
2nd Unit of General Surgery
IRCCS Maggiore Hospital
Foundation Mangiagalli and Regina Elena
Milan, Italy

Maurizio Coscia
Unit of General Surgery
Policlinico S. Orsola-Malpighi
University of Bologna
Bologna, Italy

Emanuela Dapunt
Department of Surgery
Hospital of Brunico
Brunico, Italy

Annibale D'Annibale
Department of Surgery
Camposampiero Hospital
Padua, Italy

Hans Dejaco
Department of Surgery
Hospital of Brunico
Brunico, Italy

Gian Gaetano Delaini
Department of General Surgery and Gastroenterology
University of Verona
Verona, Italy

Herbert M. Dal Corso
Department of General Surgery
Santa Croce e Carle Hospital
Cuneo, Italy

Fosca De Iorio
Department of Biomedical and Surgical Sciences
Division of Gastroenterology
Policlinico G.B. Rossi
Verona, Italy

Annalisa de Leone
Unit of Gastroenterology and Digestive Endoscopy
2nd University of Naples
Naples, Italy

Renata D'Incà
Department of Gastroenterology
University of Padua
Padua, Italy

Crescenzo Di Stazio
1st Division of General Surgery
2nd University of Naples
Naples, Italy

Vincenzo D'Onofrio
Department of Gastroenterology
"S.G. Moscati" Hospital
Avellino, Italy

Iris Dotan
Department of Gastroenterology and Liver Diseases
Inflammatory Bowel Disease Service
Tel Aviv Sourasky Medical Center
Tel Aviv, Israel

Adam Dziki
Department of General and Colorectal Surgery
Medical University
Lodz, Poland

Andrea Ederle
Unit of Gastroenterology
Hospital "S. Bonifacio"
Verona, Italy

Ilaria Esposito
Unit of Gastroenterology and Digestive Endoscopy
2nd University of Naples
Naples, Italy

Alberto Fantin
Unit of Gastroenterology
Hospital "S. Bonifacio"
Verona, Italy

Monica Fontana
Department of General Surgery and Gastroenterology
University of Verona
Verona, Italy

Bjørn Fortling
B-K Medical Engineer
Herlev, Denmark

Alessandro Franchi
Department of Human Pathology and Oncology
University of Florence
Florence, Italy

Luca Frulloni
Department of Gastroenterology
Policlinico "G.B. Rossi"
University of Verona
Verona, Italy

Susan Galandiuk
Section of Colon and Rectal Surgery
Department of Surgery
University of Louisville
School of Medicine
Louisville, USA

Lorenzo Gentilini
Unit of General Surgery
Policlinico S. Orsola-Malpighi
University of Bologna
Bologna, Italy

Elisa Gilardoni
2nd Unit of General Surgery
IRCCS Maggiore Hospital
Foundation Mangiagalli and Regina Elena
Milan, Italy

Paolo Gionchetti
Department of Internal Medicine and Gastroenterology
University of Bologna
Bologna, Italy

Veronica Girardi
Department of Radiology
Policlinico G.B. Rossi
Verona, Italy

Maria C. Giuffrida
Department of General Surgery
Santa Croce e Carle Hospital
Cuneo, Italy

Antonio Giuliani
1st Division of Surgery
2nd University of Naples
Naples, Italy

Ilaria Guadagni
1st Division of General Surgery
2nd University of Naples
Naples, Italy

Anke Gutweniger
Department of Surgery
Hospital of Brunico
Brunico, Italy

NAJIB HABOUBI
Department of Surgical Pathology
Trafford Healthcare Trust
Manchester, UK

ZAMIR HALPERN
Department of Gastroenterology and Liver Diseases
Tel Aviv Sourasky Medical Center
Tel Aviv, Israel

LEIF HULTÉN
Department of Surgery
Colorectal Unit
Sahlgrenska University Hospital
Göteborg, Sweden

PAOLO INTURRI
Unit of Gastroenterology
Civil Hospital "S. Bonifacio"
Verona, Italy

SIEGFRIED JESACHER
Department of Surgery
Hospital of Brunico
Brunico, Italy

YEHUDA KARIV
Unit of Colon and Rectal Surgery
Department of Surgery B
Tel Aviv Sourasky Medical Center
Tel Aviv, Israel

MIKE KEIGHLEY
Department of Surgery
Queen Elizabeth Hospital
Edgbaston, UK

ANIL KESHAVA
Department of Colorectal Surgery
Western General Hospital
Edinburg, UK

ALFRED KÖNIGSRAINER
Department of General, Visceral and Transplantation Surgery
Tübingen University Hospital
Tübingen, Germany

INGMAR KÖNIGSRAINER
Department of General, Visceral and Transplantation Surgery
Tübingen University Hospital
Tübingen, Germany

ZORAN V. KRIVOKAPIC
Institute for Digestive Diseases
Belgrade, Serbia-Montenegro

MARINO LANDRA
Department of General Surgery
Santa Croce e Carle Hospital
Cuneo, Italy

RUTH LADURNER
Department of General, Visceral and Transplantation Surgery
Tübingen University Hospital
Tübingen, Germany

SILVIO LAURETI
Unit of General Surgery
Policlinico S. Orsola-Malpighi
University of Bologna
Bologna, Italy

FEDERICA LIPANJE
Department of Rehabilitation
Brunico Hospital
Brunico, Italy

BARBARA MAHLKNECHT
Department of Surgery
Hospital of Brunico
Brunico, Italy

MAURIZIO MAINENTE
Department of Surgery and Gastroenterology
University of Verona
Verona, Italy

ROBERTO MALAGÒ
Department of Radiology
Policlinico G.B. Rossi
Verona, Italy

RICCARDO MANFREDI
Department of Radiology
Policlinico G.B. Rossi
Verona, Italy

RAIMUND MARGREITER
Department of General and Transplantation Surgery
Medical University Innsbruck
Innsbruck, Austria

Hansjorg Marsoner
Department of Surgery
Hospital of Brunico
Brunico, Italy

Federico Martin
Surgery Unit
Central Hospital
Bolzano, Italy

Emilio Morpurgo
Department of Surgery
Camposampiero Hospital
Padua, Italy

Claudia Morselli
Department of Internal Medicine and Gastroenterology
University of Bologna
Bologna, Italy

Gabriella Nesi
Department of Human Pathology and Oncology
University of Florence
Florence, Italy

Monika Niederkofler
Department of Surgery
Hospital of Brunico
Brunico, Italy

Filippo Nifosì
Department of General Surgery and Gastroenterology
University of Verona
Verona, Italy

Patrick O'Connolly
Department of Surgical Pathology and Gastrointestinal Surgery
Hope Hospital
Manchester, UK

Barbara Oreggia
II Unit of General Surgery
IRCCS Maggiore Hospital
Foundation, Mangiagalli e Regina Elena
Milan, Italy

Tom Öresland
Department of Surgery
Colorectal Unit
Sahlgrenska University Hospital
Göteborg, Sweden

Daniele Ortolani
Department of Surgery and Gastroenterology
University of Verona
Verona, Italy

Umberto Pandini
Department of Surgery
Hospital of Brunico
Brunico, Italy

Mario Pescatori
Coloproctology Unit
Villa Flaminia Hospital
Rome, Italy

Lucia Picariello
Department of Internal Medicine
University of Florence
Florence, Italy

Filippo Pierangeli
Unit of General Surgery
Policlinico S. Orsola-Malpighi
University of Bologna
Bologna, Italy

Walter Piubello
Department of Internal Medicine
Endoscopic Unit
Desenzano, Italy

Gilberto Poggioli
Unit of General Surgery
Policlinico S. Orsola-Malpighi
University of Bologna
Bologna, Italy

Roberto Pozzi Mucelli
Department of Radiology
Policlinico "G.B. Rossi"
Verona, Italy

Monica Preto
Unit of Gastroenterology
Hospital "S. Bonifacio"
Verona, Italy

Micha Rabau
Unit of Colon and Rectal Surgery
Department of Surgery B
Tel Aviv Sourasky Medical Center
Tel Aviv, Israel

GABRIELE RIEGLER
Unit of Gastroenterology and Digestive Endoscopy
2nd University of Naples
Naples, Italy

FERNANDO RIZZELLO
Department of Internal Medicine and Gastroenterology
University of Bologna
Bologna, Italy

JOAN ROBERT-YAP
Unit of Proctology
Department of Surgery
University Hospital of Geneva
Geneva, Switzerland

CHIARA ROCHA
2nd Unit of General Surgery
IRCCS Maggiore Hospital
Foundation Mangiagalli and Regina Elena
Milan, Italy

BRUNO ROCHE
Unit of Proctology
Department of Surgery
University Hospital of Geneva
Geneva, Switzerland

GIOVANNI ROMANO
Department of Emergency Surgery
"S.G. Moscati" Hospital
Avellino, Italy

EMIL SALMO
Department of Surgical Pathology
Trafford Healthcare Trust
Manchester, UK

BEATRICE SALVIOLI
Department of Internal Medicine and Gastroenterology
S. Orsola-Malpighi Hospital
University of Bologna
Bologna, Italy

GIULIO A. SANTORO
Section of Anal Physiology and Ultrasound
Coloproctology Service
Department of Surgery
Regional Hospital
Treviso, Italy

MARCO SCAGLIA
Department of Surgery
S. Luigi Gonzaga Hospital
Orbassano, Turin, Italy

CHIARA SCATTOLINI
Department of Gastroenterology
Policlinico "G.B. Rossi"
University of Verona
Verona, Italy

CLAUDIA SCHULZ
Department of General, Visceral and Transplantation Surgery
Tübingen University Hospital
Tübingen, Germany

GUIDO SCIAUDONE
1st Division of General Surgery
2nd University of Naples
Naples, Italy

DIEGO SEGRE
Department of General Surgery
Santa Croce e Carle Hospital
Cuneo, Italy

FRANCESCO SELVAGGI
1st Division of General Surgery
2nd University of Naples
Naples, Italy

TOMÁŠ SKŘIČKA
Bakeš Memorial Hospital
Brno, Czech Republic

MARIANNE STARCK
Department of Surgery
Malmö University Hospital
Malmö, Sweden

WOLFGANG STEURER
Department of General, Visceral and Transplantation Surgery
Tübingen University Hospital
Tübingen, Germany

GIACOMO C. STURNIOLO
Department of Gastroenterology
University of Padua
Padua, Italy

Naika Tacchella
Department of Biomedical and Surgical Sciences
Division of Gastroenterology
Policlinico "G.B. Rossi"
Verona, Italy

Rosy Tambasco
Department of Internal Medicine and Gastroenterology
University of Bologna
Bologna, Italy

Morena Tebaldi
Department of Internal Medicine
Endoscopic Unit
Desenzano, Italy

Roberto Tersigni
Department of Surgery
S. Camillo Hospital
Rome, Italy

Marco Testoni
Department of Radiology
Policlinico "G.B. Rossi"
Verona, Italy

Paris Tekkis
Department of Biosurgery and Surgical Technology
Imperial College London
St. Mary's Hospital
London, UK

Walter Thaler
Department of Surgery
Hospital of Brunico
Brunico, Italy

Francesco Tonelli
Department of Clinical Physiopathology
University of Florence
Florence, Italy

Hagit Tulchinsky
Unit of Colon and Rectal Surgery
Department of Surgery B
Tel Aviv Sourasky Medical Center
Tel Aviv, Israel

Federica Ugolini
Unit of General Surgery
S. Orsola-Malpighi Hospital
University of Bologna
Bologna, Italy

Rosa Valanzano
Department of Clinical Physiopathology
University of Florence
Florence, Italy

Italo Vantini
Department of Biomedical and Surgical Sciences
Division of Gastroenterology
Policlinico "G.B. Rossi"
Verona, Italy

Alex Wiegele
Department of Surgery
Hospital of Brunico
Brunico, Italy

Luigi Zorcolo
Department of General Surgery
University of Cagliari
Cagliari, Italy

Section I

General Approach

MRI in Inflammatory Small-Bowel Diseases

Riccardo Manfredi, Roberto Malagò, Marco Testoni, Veronica Girardi, Roberto Pozzi Mucelli

Introduction

In clinical practice, imaging techniques are used at the initial presentation to establish a diagnosis and to assess the exact location, extent, and severity of disease [1]. These modalities are also used as follow-up, during and after treatment, to determine the optimal choice and dose of medication (e.g., systemically or topically active) [2, 3]. With the advent of new medication such as infliximab, an immunomodulatory drug with considerable side effects, follow-up to determine if medication is becoming increasingly important.

In Crohn's disease, formation of perianal fistulas and/or abscesses can be seen in a large percentage of patients. Nowadays, there is a tendency towards imaging of these fistulae, given that in Crohn's disease fistulae can be very extensive and complex, rendering the conventional gold standard (i.e., examination under anesthesia) not wholly accurate [4]. As misclassification of fistulae can lead to severe, irreversible complications (e.g., fecal incontinence) or recurrent disease, the American Gastroenterology Association (AGA) has recently stated the importance of preoperative imaging. Another reason for performing imaging studies is the increasing use of infliximab, which has been associated not only with external closure of perianal fistulae but also with the persistence of tracks as can be visualized with MRI [5, 6].

The earliest change caused by the disease occurs in the submucosa and consists of lymphoid hyperplasia and lymphedema. Radiologic findings at this (early) stage include subtle elevations and aphthoid ulcers. As the disease progresses, it extends transmurally to the serosa (transmural stage) and beyond to the mesentery and adjacent organs (extramural stage). Aphthoid ulcers develop into linear ulcers and fissures to produce an ulcero-nodular or "cobblestone" appearance. The bowel wall is thickened by a combination of fibrosis and inflammatory infiltrates. Bowel obstruction, strictures, abscesses or phlegmon, fistulae, and sinus tracts are common complications of advanced disease [1, 2].

Abdominal MRI

The diagnosis of Crohn's disease should include assessment of the presence, severity, and extent of disease, inflammatory lesion activity, and the presence of extra-intestinal complications to aid in treatment planning, which largely depends on imaging findings, particularly those of cross-sectional imaging. Endoscopy and barium studies are the principal tools for diagnosis and evaluation of Crohn's disease; however, they are limited in their capability to demonstrate the transmural or extramural extent of disease or extra-intestinal complications.

With MRI, both inflammatory changes of the bowel wall and the extramural complications of Crohn's disease can be assessed. The non-invasiveness of this technique, as well as its lack of ionizing radiation, has prompted many groups to perform systematic studies of MRI for evaluation of Crohn's disease.

Computed tomography (CT) is currently the cross-sectional imaging modality of choice at most institutions; however, magnetic resonance (MR) imaging has also proved highly effective in this setting. The role of cross-sectional imaging in the diagnosis of Crohn's disease has expanded with recent advances in CT and MR imaging technology, which allow rapid acquisition of high-resolution images of the intestines during a breath-hold examination. Both imaging modalities provide information that is crucial in the diagnosis of Crohn's disease and in treatment planning [7–16].

Intraluminal Contrast Media

Adequate distension of the bowel lumen is mandatory in MRI, as it facilitates demonstration of morphological changes caused by Crohn's disease and allows identification of subtle abnormalities. Collapsed bowel loops can hide lesions or mimic disease by mimicking pathologically thickened bowel wall in collapsed segments [17]. Moreover, collapsed normal bowel loops can exhibit enhancement that is similar to diseased segments, after administration of an intravenous contrast medium [18].

Various kinds of intraluminal contrast agents have been proposed for MR imaging [7, 18–26] and are classified as positive, negative, or biphasic. Positive agents produce high intraluminal signal, and negative agents produce little or no intraluminal signal regardless of the applied pulse sequence. Biphasic contrast agents may produce either a high or low signal depending on the pulse sequence used, usually demonstrating low signal intensity on T1-weighted MR images and high signal intensity on T2-weighted images. Negative or biphasic contrast agents seem to be more suitable for assessing the small bowel [7, 19]. Polyethylene glycol has been proposed by several authors as a suitable biphasic contrast medium; it is not absorbable, remains unmodified in the small bowel, is easily prepared and administered, and provides adequate bowel distension. Furthermore, transit time is fast, allowing for small-bowel distension within 30 min. However, undesirable side effects (e.g., motion artifacts or severe diarrhea) can occur due to the prokinetic action of the solution. Theoretically, water would be a perfect biphasic contrast medium, but in many patients, the water is reabsorbed before it has reached the terminal ileum. Moreover, it does not optimally distend the bowel (Fig. 1).

An anti-peristaltic agent is injected to minimize potential artifacts caused by bowel movement or contraction. Although many authors reporting on MR enteroclysis administer anti-peristaltic drugs to reduce motion artifacts, reflex atony is induced by high flow rates, theoretically allowing images (almost) to be free of motion artifacts.

Sequences

Technological advances, including the use of respiration-suspended sequences, improved coils, fat suppressions, and intravenous gadolinium, have extend-

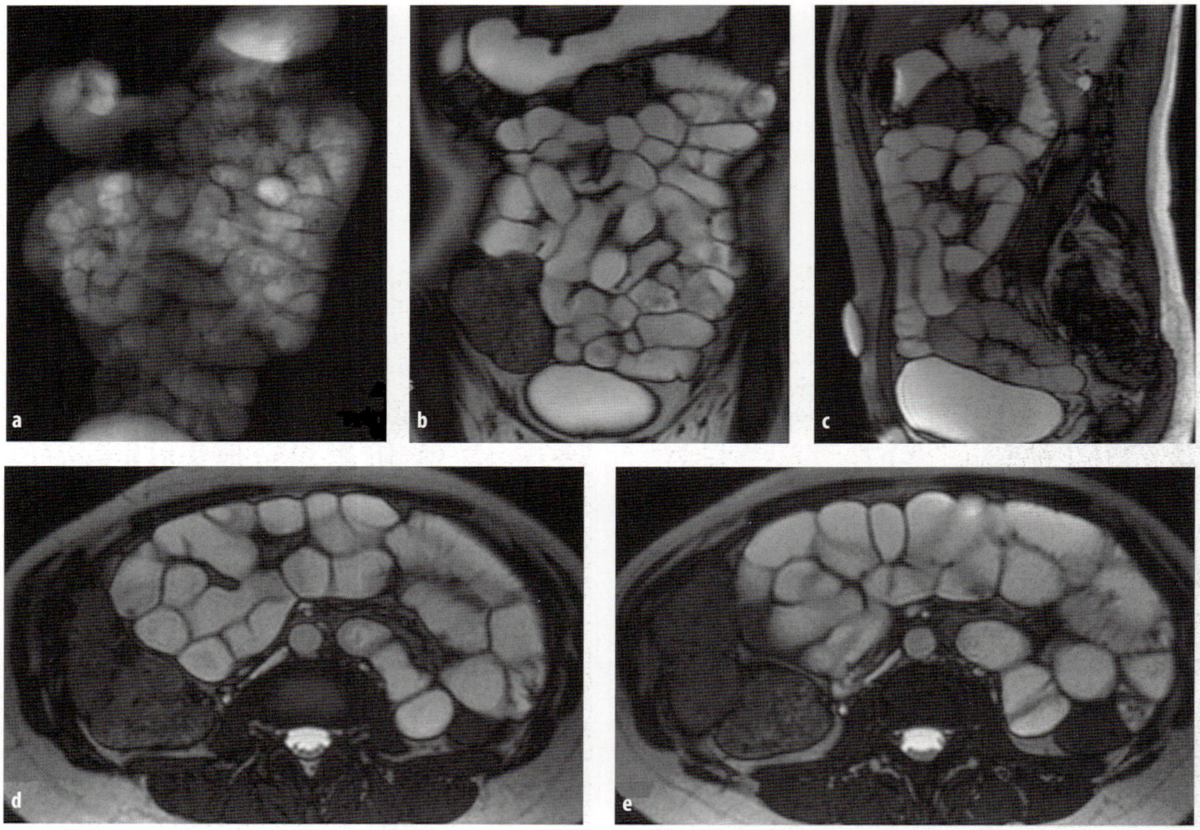

Fig. 1. Coronal T2W Hal Fourier RARE image (**a**) and fat-suppressed true-FISP images along the coronal (**b**), sagittal (**c**), and axial (**d**, **e**) planes show good distension of bowel loops after oral administration of biphasic contrast media (PEG), thus permitting the distinguishing of the jejunal and ileal loops

ed the role of MRI in the evaluation of the gastrointestinal tract. Various MR sequences for evaluating the gastrointestinal tract have been advocated by different authors. However, no sole sequence can be used for comprehensive imaging of Crohn's disease, as each sequence has its specific advantages and limitations. Therefore, it is essential to use a comprehensive examination protocol in which disadvantages of one sequence can be compensated by the advantages of the others.

Fast Spin Echo T2-Weighted Sequence

Half-Fourier acquisition single shot turbo spin echo (HASTE) demonstrate lack of magnetic susceptibility artifacts and lack of artifacts from bowel peristalsis theoretically making the HASTE sequence ideal for imaging bowel. A limitation of HASTE is its sensitivity to intraluminal flow voids, while another disadvantage is that no information on mesenteries can be obtained due to K-space filtering effects (Fig. 1).

True-FISP Sequence

Another sequence promoted for the evaluation of Crohn's disease is the true fast imaging with steady-state precession (true-FISP) sequence, which is a completely refocused steady-state gradient echo sequence (also called balanced fast-field echo (Fig. 1). Motion-related artifacts are minimal due to the short acquisition time, while at the same time insensitivity to intraluminal flow voids is observed due to the balanced and symmetric gradient design. The bowel wall is well visualized due to good differentiation in contrast (via positive or biphasic contrast agent) between the hypointense bowel wall and the hyperintense bowel lumen (Fig. 1). The true-FISP sequence is particularly good for obtaining information about extra-intestinal complications; the mesenteries are very well visualized and lymph nodes are very conspicuous with this technique. The black boundary artifact encountered with the true-FISP sequence, at fat-water interfaces, may hamper the perception of subtle thickening of the bowel wall.

Gadolinium-Enhanced T1-Weighted Sequence

Many study groups have focused on gadolinium-enhanced T1-weighted images for assessment of disease [27-30], as both localization and severity of inflammation can be appraised with this sequence. Inflamed bowel segments show pathological enhancement after administration of intravenous gadolinium. When combining T1-weighted sequences with fat suppression and use of intravenous gadolinium-chelates, very good differentiation in contrast is obtained between the pathologically enhancing bowel wall and the dark bowel lumen and suppressed perivisceral fat (Fig. 2). The marked increase in signal intensity of inflamed bowel after administration of

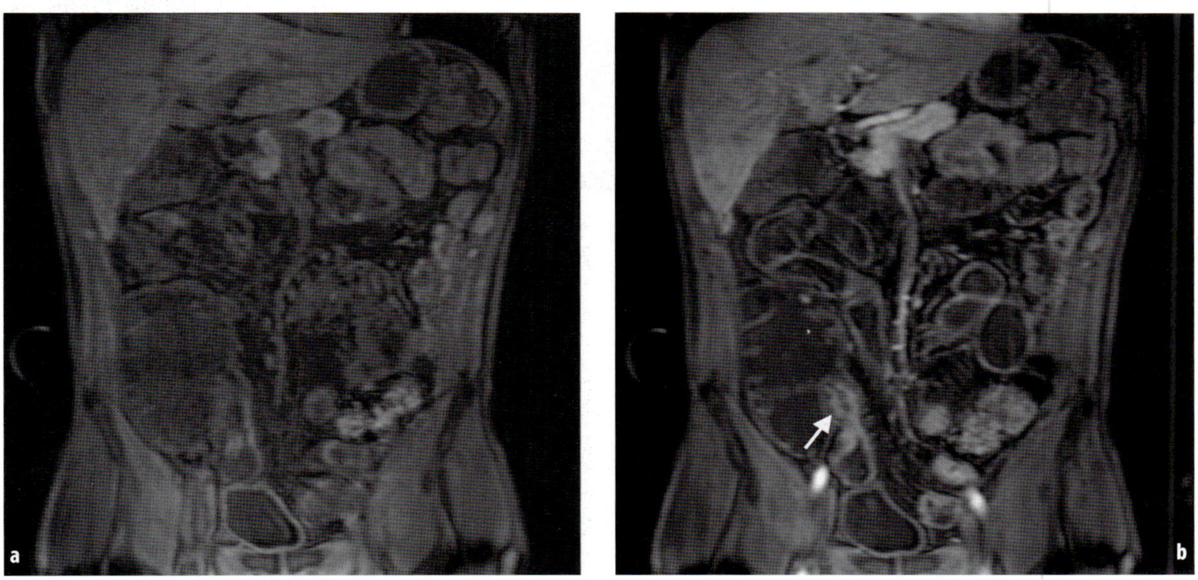

Fig. 2. Coronal fat suppressed T1-weighted spoiled gradient echo sequence acquired before (**a**) and 30 s following intravenous administration of gadolinium chelate (**b**), demonstrating marked parietal enhancement of the distal ileal loop (*arrow*)

intravenous gadolinium is due to increased tissue perfusion and vascular permeability (Fig. 2).

MR Enteroclisis Findings

Early lesions of Crohn's disease such as blunting, flattening, thickening, distortion and straightening of the valvulae conniventes and tiny aphthae were clearly shown at conventional enteroclysis, but they were not consistently depicted with MR enteroclysis due to its inadequate spatial resolution. The valvulae conniventes were shown to their best advantage and distortion of the mucosal folds was easily detected with MR enteroclysis.

The characteristic discrete longitudinal or transverse ulcers of Crohn's disease could be shown at MR enteroclysis, provided there was satisfactory distention of the bowel. MR enteroclysis was less sensitive than conventional enteroclysis in the detection of linear ulcers due to low spatial resolution and lack of compression techniques. Thin high-signal-intensity lines within the bowel wall on true FISP MR images represented linear ulcers. Cobblestoning was caused mostly by a combination of longitudinal and transverse ulceration and was easily shown with MR enteroclysis. The true FISP sequence was superior to HASTE in showing linear ulcers, cobblestoning, and intramural tracts, while the three-dimensional gradient echo sequence was less satisfactory in depicting such lesions smaller than 3 mm in diameter.

Bowel-wall thickening was clearly shown with all MR enteroclysis sequences (Figs. 2, 3). The thickened wall had moderate signal intensity on true FISP images and could be easily differentiated from the black boundary artifact. Bowel-wall thickness and length of small-bowel involvement could be measured on MR enteroclysis images. Narrowing of the lumen and associated prestenotic dilatation were easily recognized on MR enteroclysis images obtained with all sequences (Figs. 2, 3). Asymmetric involvement, pseudo-diverticula formation, and skip or multiple lesions were easily depicted via MR enteroclysis.

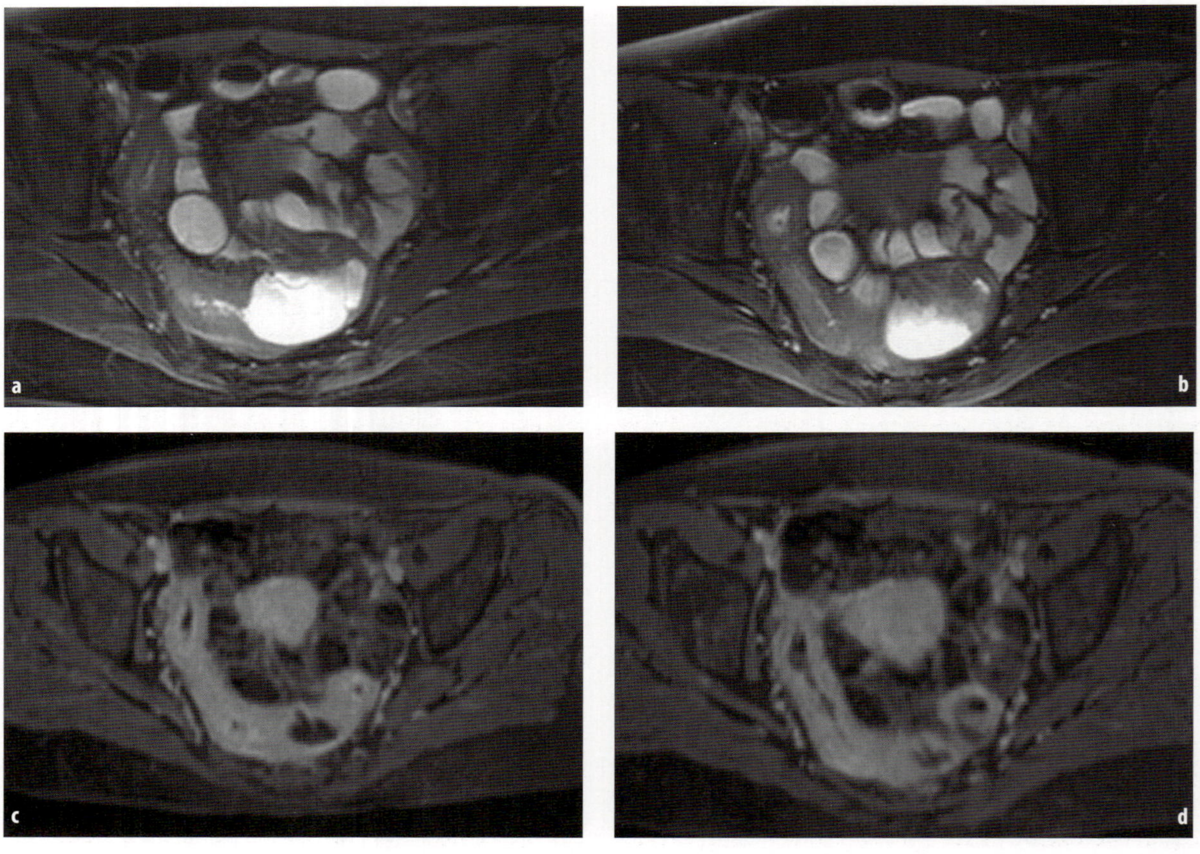

Fig. 3. A 57-year-old female with active Crohn's disease. **a, b** Axial fat-suppressed true-FISP images show severe thickening of the terminal ileum with luminal stenosis and fibro-fatty proliferation. **c, d** After Gadolinium administration fat suppressed T1-weighted spoiled gradient echo images show enhancement of the bowel wall due to Crohn's disease activity

Quantification of Dynamic Contrast-Enhanced MRI (DCE)

DCE-MRI imaging techniques are still evolving and methods of image analysis remain mostly qualitative, variable, and nonstandard, making these techniques unsuitable for comparisons between different institutions or different study protocols. In the attempt to standardize and make this analysis quantitative, a number of pharmacokinetic multicompartment models have been proposed that would serve to infer "absolute" physiological quantities from the data gathered with the dynamic scan.

When the contrast agent is injected, it equilibrates with the blood plasma and is rapidly delivered to the different tissues. The blood plasma (the central compartment) and the extra-vascular, extra-cellular space of the inflamed tissue lesion (the peripheral compartment) are connected by linear exchange processes in both directions. The measurement of microvessel permeability is possible by assessment of the rate at which a contrast agent transfers from the blood pool to the extra-vascular extra-cellular space. Similarly, the transfer of the contrast agent back to the blood can be expressed as the reflux coefficient. In addition, the measurement of increased blood volume is possible by permitting calculation of fractional plasma volume [31]. This method offers the great advantage of being quantitative, i.e., not measurement-dependent but pathology-dependent, so that the results from different studies/sites can be directly compared.

Clinical scoring (such as the Crohn's disease activity index [32], biologic indexes [33], endoscopy, and imaging studies have all been used to monitor activity, but no established gold standard exists. Assessment of activity is usually made using a combination of clinical symptoms, physical findings, laboratory investigations, endoscopy, and imaging tests. The assessment of biologic activity, based on the positivity for three of four acute phase reactants (WBC, erythrocyte sedimentation rate, and C-reactive protein), has been found to be a sensitive determinant of activity, especially when supported by endoscopic or imaging findings.

Extra-Mural Manifestations and Complications

MR enteroclysis had a clear advantage over conventional enteroclysis in the demonstration of extramural manifestations or complications of Crohn's disease. The extent of fibro-fatty proliferation and its composition, mostly fatty or mostly fibrotic, could be assessed with MR enteroclysis, especially when true FISP images were obtained (Fig. 3). The so-called comb sign (Fig. 4), corresponding to increased mesenteric vascularity, could be ideally seen on true FISP images close to the mesenteric border of a small-bowel segment in the form of short, parallel, low-signal-intensity linear structures perpendicular to the intestinal long axis. The comb sign could be seen on three-dimensional FLASH images as high-signal-intensity linear elements.

Small mesenteric lymph nodes were easily detected by their low signal intensity within the high-signal-intensity mesenteric fat on true FISP images (Fig. 5). Their presence was not as obvious with other MR enteroclysis sequences due to short T2 filtering effects on HASTE images and to saturation of mesenteric fat signal on three-dimensional FLASH images. Sinus tracts and fistulae were disclosed by the high-signal intensity of their fluid content on true FISP and HASTE images, but they could be missed on the three-dimensional FLASH images due to limited contrast with surrounding tissues. All fistulae shown at conventional enteroclysis were also depicted at MR enteroclysis, while only half of the sinus tracts were detected at MR enteroclysis, even in retrospect in our series. Abscesses could be recognized by their fluid content and contrast enhancement of the wall. There were strong indications that disease activity can be appreciated with MR enteroclysis (Fig. 6) [34, 35].

Conclusions

MR imaging is an emerging technique in this field and is expected to play a role similar to that of CT. The clinical efficacy of MR imaging has been investigated, and favorable results have been reported as described in this article. High soft-tissue contrast, static and dynamic imaging capabilities, and the absence of ionizing radiation exposure represent the advantages of MR imaging over CT. On the other hand, MR imaging is more time consuming, less readily available, and more expensive [36–39]. Advantages of CT over MR imaging include greater availability, shorter examination times, flexibility in choosing imaging thickness and planes after data acquisition with multidetector row CT, and higher spatial resolution. Precise indications for MR imaging in the diagnosis of Crohn's disease and its use as a complement to CT or other imaging procedures need further investigation. Clinical management decisions might be influenced by the presence of unsuspected additional lesions that were seen only on CT or MR imaging, as reported by Fishman et al. and Turetschek et al., with management changes occurring in 28 and 62% of cases, respectively. Cross-sectional imaging should be included or even performed as a primary examination in the clinical eval-

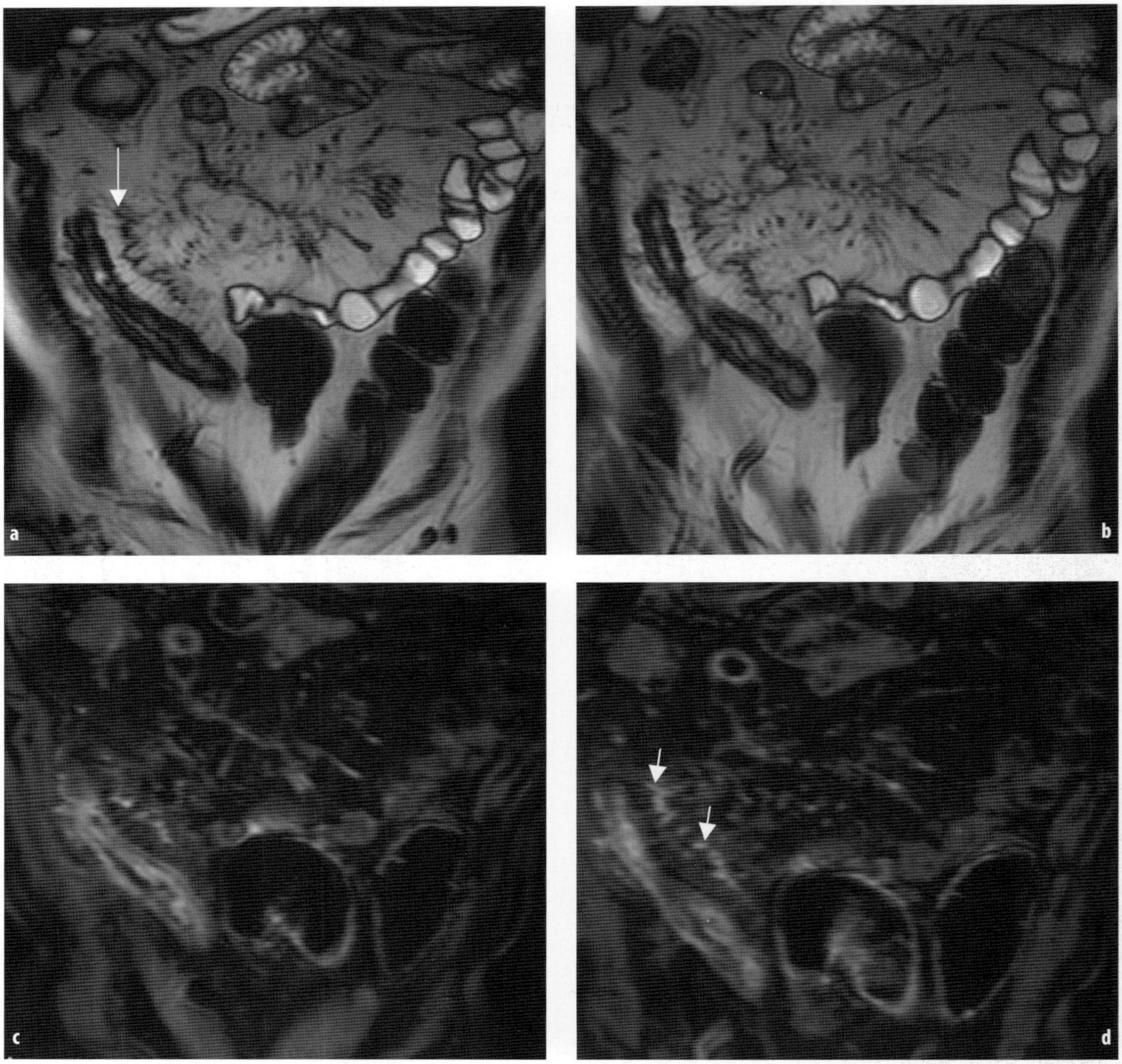

Fig. 4. A 27-year-old man with active Crohn's disease. **a, b** On coronal true FISP images Mesenteric vessels (vasa resta) are clearly detectable depicting the so-called "comb sign" which corresponds to hypertrophied mesenteric vascularisation perpendicular to the axis of the affected bowel loop (*arrow*). **c, d** Contrast enhanced T1-weighted gradient echo images, confirm disease activity (*arrows*)

uation of Crohn's disease, along with conventional imaging and clinical and laboratory tests. Cross-sectional imaging should be used to evaluate for the presence of entities that indicate elective gastrointestinal surgery–e.g., marked prestenotic dilatation (severe stenosis), skip lesions, fistulae, perforations, abscesses.

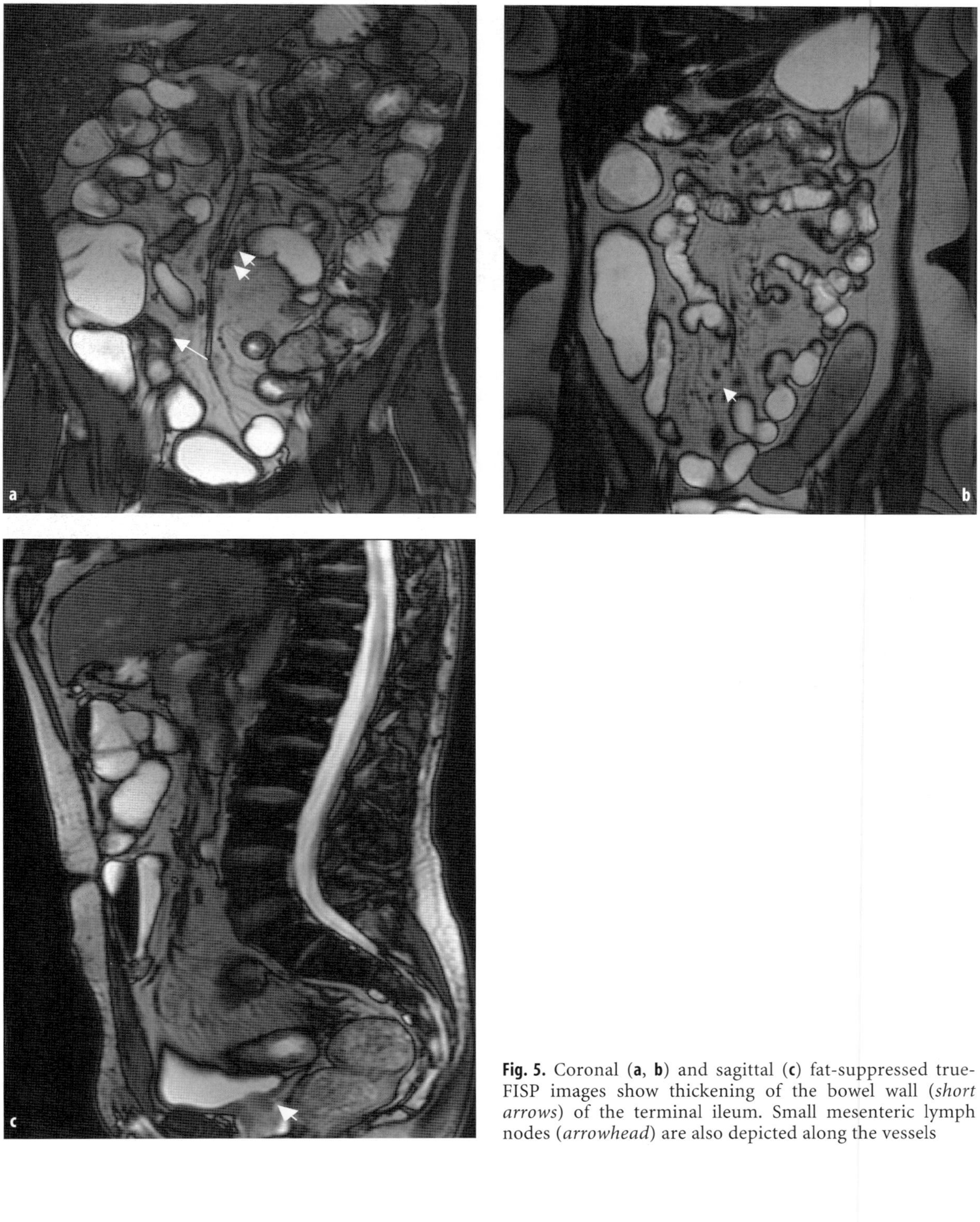

Fig. 5. Coronal (**a**, **b**) and sagittal (**c**) fat-suppressed true-FISP images show thickening of the bowel wall (*short arrows*) of the terminal ileum. Small mesenteric lymph nodes (*arrowhead*) are also depicted along the vessels

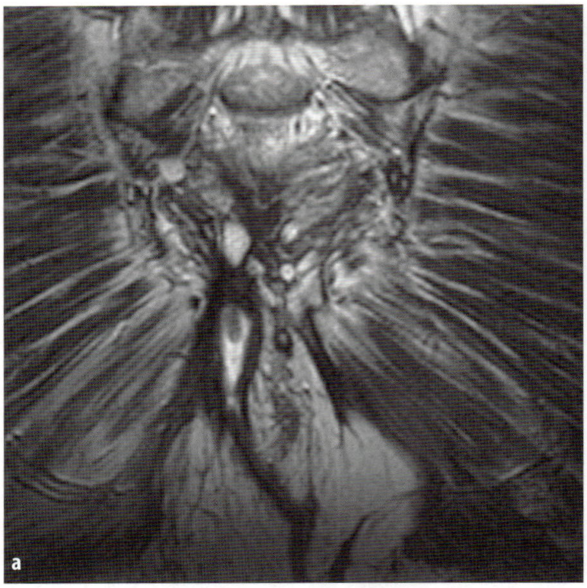

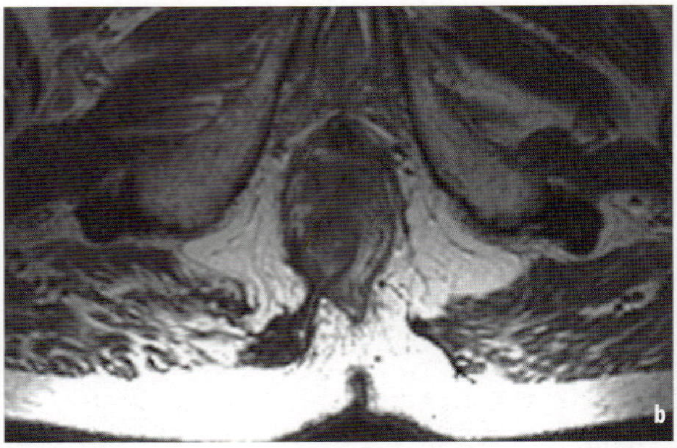

Fig. 6. Perirectal fistulas. (**a**) Coronal T2-weighted rapid acquisition with relaxation enhancement (RARE) shows a trans-sphincteric fistula extending into the fatty tissue of the right ischiorectal fossa and crossing the right elevator ani muscle. (**b**) Axial T1-weighted spin-echo image shows a fistulous tract crossing the anal sphincter and extending into the adipose tissue of the right ischiorectal fossas

References

1. Masselli G, Brizi MG, Menchini L et al (2005) Magnetic Resonance Enteroclysis imaging of Crohn's. Radiol Med 110(3):221–233
2. Broglia L, Gigante P, Papi C et al (2003) Magnetic Resonance enteroclysis imaging in Crohn's disease. Radiol Med 106(1–2):28–35
3. Laghi A, Passariello R (2003) Magnetic Resonance in the study of the small bowel. Radiol Med 106(1–2):1–15
4. Halligan S, Buchanan G (2003) MR imaging of fistula-in-ano. Eur J Radiol 47:98–107
5. Bell SJ, Halligan S, Windsor AC et al (2003) Response of fistulating Crohn's disease to infliximab treatment assessed by magnetic resonance imaging. Aliment Pharmacol Ther 17:387–393
6. Van Assche G, Vanbeckevoort D, Bielen D et al. (2003) Magnetic resonance imaging of the effects of infliximab on perianal fistulizing Crohn's disease. Am J Gastroenterol 98:332–339
7. Gourtsoyiannis N, Papanikolaou N, Grammatikakis J, Prassopoulos P (2002) MR enteroclysis: technical considerations and clinical applications. Eur Radiol 12:2651–2658
8. Low RN, Sebrechts CP, Politoske DA et al (2002) Crohn's disease with endoscopic correlation: singleshot fast spin-echo and gadolinium-enhanced fat-suppressed spoiled gradient-echo MR imaging. Radiology 222:652–660
9. Low RN, Francis IR, Politoske et al (2000) Crohn's disease evaluation: comparison of contrast-enhanced MR imaging and single-phase helical CT scanning. J Magn Reson Imaging 11:127–135
10. Mako EK, Mester AR, Tarjan Z et al (2000) Enteroclysis and spiral CT examination in diagnosis and evaluation of small bowel Crohn's disease. Eur J Radiol 35:168–175
11. Raptopoulos V, Schwartz RK, McNicholas MM et al (1997) Multiplanar helical CT enterography in patients with Crohn's disease. AJR Am J Roentgenol 169:1545–1550
12. Rollandi GA, Curone PF, Biscaldi E et al (1999) Spiral CT of the abdomen after distension of small bowel loops with transparent enema in patients with Crohn's disease. Abdom Imaging 24:544–549
13. Turetschek K, Schober E, Wunderbaldinger P et al (2002) Findings at helical CT-enteroclysis in symptomatic patients with Crohn's disease: correlation with endoscopic and surgical findings. J Comput Assist Tomogr 26:488–492
14. Umschaden HW, Szolar D, Gasser J et al (2002) Small-bowel disease: comparison of MR enteroclysis images with conventional enteroclysis and surgical findings. Radiology 215:717–725
15. Lee J, Marcos HB, Semelka RC (1998) MR imaging of the small bowel using the HASTE sequence. AJR Am J Roentgenol 170:1457–1463
16. Prassopoulos P, Papanikolaou N, Grammatikakis J et al (2001) MR enteroclysis imaging of Crohn's disease. Radiographics 21:S161–S172
17. Debatin JF, Patak MA (1999) MRI of the small and large bowel. Eur Radiol 9:1523–1534
18. Low RN, Francis IR (1997) MR imaging of the gastrointestinal tract with i.v., gadolinium and diluted barium oral contrast media compared with unenhanced MR imaging and CT. AJR Am J Roentgenol 169:1051–1059
19. Umschaden HW, Gasser J (2003) MR enteroclysis. Radiol Clin North Am 41:231–248
20. Giovagnoni A, Fabbri A, Maccioni F (2002) Oral contrast agents in MRI of the gastrointestinal tract. Abdom Imaging 27:367–375
21. Papanikolaou N, Prassopoulos P, Grammatikakis J et al (2002) Optimization of a contrast medium suitable for conventional enteroclysis, MR enteroclysis, and

virtual MR enteroscopy. Abdom Imaging 27:517–522
22. Maccioni F, Viscido A, Marini M, Caprilli R (2002) MRI evaluation of Crohn's disease of the small and large bowel with the use of negative superparamagnetic oral contrast agents. Abdom Imaging 27:384–393
23. Holzknecht N, Helmberger T, von Ritter C et al (1998). Breathhold MRI of the small bowel in Crohn's disease after enteroclysis with oral magnetic particles. Radiologe 38:29–36
24. Mattrey RF, Trambert MA, Brown JJ et al (1994) Perflubron as an oral contrast agent for MR imaging: results of a phase III clinical trial. Radiology 191:841–848
25. Rieber A, Aschoff A, Nussle K et al (2000) MRI in the diagnosis of small bowel disease: use of positive and negative oral contrast media in combination with enteroclysis. Eur Radiol 10:1377–1382
26. Kivelitz D, Gehl HB, Heuck A et al (1999) Ferric ammonium citrate as a positive bowel contrast agent for MR imaging of the upper abdomen: safety and diagnostic efficacy. Acta Radiol 40:429–435
27. Marcos HB, Semelka RC (2000) Evaluation of Crohn's disease using halffourier RARE and gadolinium-enhanced SGE sequences: initial results. Magn Reson Imaging 18:263–268
28. Low RN, Francis IR, Politoske D, Bennett M (2000) Crohn's disease evaluation: comparison of contrast-enhanced MR imaging and single-phase helical CT scanning. J Magn Reson Imaging 11:127–135
29. Shoenut JP, Semelka RC, Silverman R (1993) Magnetic resonance imaging in inflammatory bowel disease. J Clin Gastroenterol 17:73–78
30. Shoenut JP, Semelka RC, Magro CM (1994). Comparison of magnetic resonance imaging and endoscopy in distinguishing the type and severity of inflammatory bowel disease. J Clin Gastroenterol 19:31–35
31. Daldrup H, Shames DM, Wendland M et al (1998) Correlation of dynamic contrast-enhanced MR imaging with histologic tumor grade: comparison of macromolecular and small-molecular contrast media. AJR 171:941–949
32. Best WR, Becktel JM, Singleton JW, Kern F (1976) Development of a Crohn's disease activity index: National Cooperative Crohn's Disease Study. Gastroenterology 70:439–444
33. Maccioni F, Viscido A, Broglia L et al (2000) Evaluation of Crohn's disease activity with magnetic resonance imaging. Abdom Imaging 25:219–228
34. Horsthuis K, Lavini Mphil C, Stoker J (2005) MRI in Crohn's disease. J Magn Reson Imaging 22(1):1–12
35. Schunk K, Kern A, Oberholzer K et al (2000) Hydro-MRI in Crohn's disease: appraisal of disease activity. Invest Radiol 35:431–437
36. Lomas DJ, Graves MJ (1999) Small bowel MRI using water as a contrast medium. Br J Radiol 72:994–997
37. Prassopoulos P, PapanikolaouN, Grammatikakis J et al (2001) MR Enteroclysis Imaging of Crohn's Disease. Radiographics 21:S161–S172
38. Furukawa A, Saotome T, Yamasaki M et al (2004) Cross-sectional imaging in Crohn's disease. Radiographics 24(3):689–702
39. Koh DM, Miao Y, Chinn RJ et al (2001) MR imaging evaluation of the activity of Crohn's disease. AJR 177(6):1325–1332

SECTION II

Inflammatory Bowel Disease

IBD: Epidemiology and Risk Factors

Gabriele Riegler, Annalisa de Leone

Descriptive Epidemiology

Inflammatory bowel diseases (IBD) are a collection of diseases affecting the bowel, the most common of which are ulcerative colitis and Crohn's disease. Whereas UC is characterised by a continuous distribution of mucosal/submucosal inflammation within the colon, CD may result in focal areas of disease in any part of the gastrointestinal tract from the mouth to the anus; the inflammation is transmural and almost inevitably progresses over time, often leading to structuring or fistulising complications. Extra-intestinal complications affecting eyes, skin and joints occur in both illnesses. Although inflammatory bowel disease is not common or highly fatal, it is important to public health because its highest incidence is early in life, its therapy involves major surgery including a curative colectomy for ulcerative colitis, and having the disease increases the risk of developing colon cancer.

There are literally hundreds of articles describing the incidence of ulcerative colitis and Crohn's disease in many regions of the world. In general, the highest incidence rates and prevalence for both diseases have been reported in northern Europe [1–8], the United Kingdom [9–11], and North America [12–15], which are the geographic regions that have been historically associated with IBD. However, reports of increasing incidence and prevalence from other areas of the world such as southern or central Europe [16–18], Asia [19–22], Africa [23], and Latin America [24] underscore the fact that the occurrence of IBD is a dynamic process. Incidence of UC, especially, is rising in several areas previously thought to have low incidence including Japan [21], South Korea [25], Singapore [22], northern India [26] and Latin America [24]. In most of these areas, however, CD remains rare.

In North America, incidence rates range from 2.2 to 14.3 cases/100 000 person-years for UC and from 3.1 to 14.6 cases/100 000 person-years for CD. Prevalence ranges from 37 to 246 cases/100 000 persons for UC and from 26 to 199 cases/100 000 persons for CD [12–14].

The Multicenter European Collaborative Study on Inflammatory Bowel Disease (EC-IBD) reported blended incidence rates between 8.7 and 11.8 cases/100 000 person-years for UC and between 3.9 and 7.0 cases/100 000 person-years for CD [6]. The EC-IBD quantified the north–south gradient of incidence in Europe: the incidence rates for UC and for CD were respectively 40 and 80% higher in northern regions.

City	Period	Incidence x100000
Milan	1988-1992	8.8
Florence	1991-1993	9
Reggio Emilia*	1991-1993	8.7
Modena	1989-1992	3.4
Bologna	1989-1992	3.4
Avellino	1989-1992	5.14
L'Aquila	1989-1992	8.5
Messina	1989-1992	7.11
Palermo	1991-1993	10.5

*age > 15 years

Fig. 1. UC incidence rates in Italy ([27])

City	Period	Incidence x100000
Milan	1991-1993	3.4
Florence	1990-1992	3.4
Reggio Emilia	1991-1993	4.3*
Modena	1989-1992	2.4
Bologna	1989-1992	2.4
Avellino	1989-1992	2.30
L'Aquila	1989-1992	2.4
Messina	1989-1992	1.9
Palermo	1991-1993	6.6*

*age > 15 years

Fig. 2. CD incidence rates in Italy ([27])

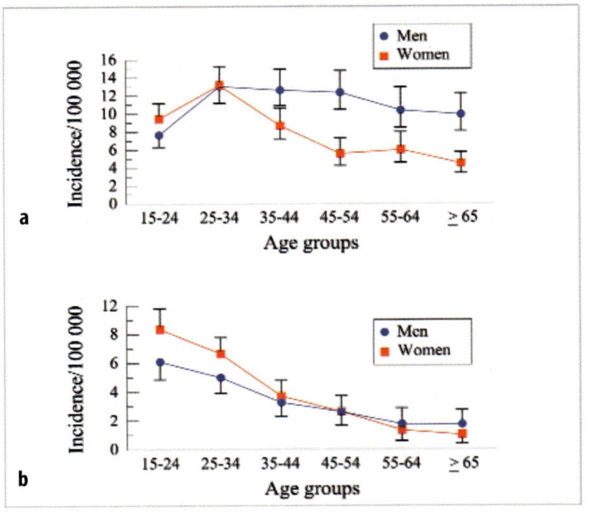

Fig. 3. a Male and female incidence in different age groups for UC. **b** Male and female incidence in different age groups for CD ([6])

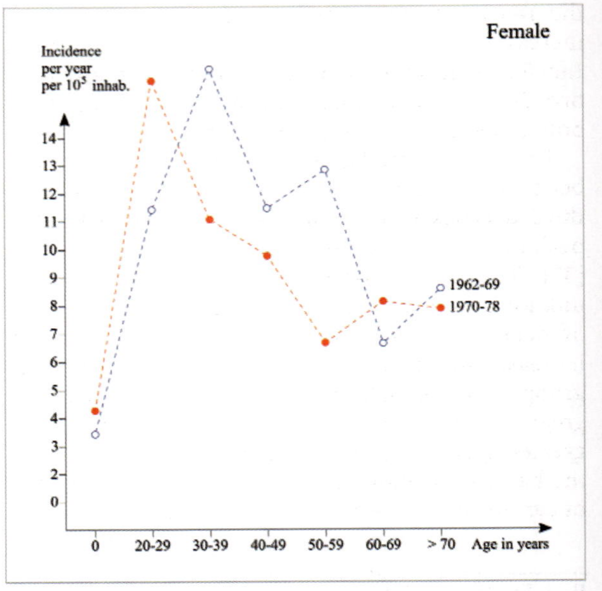

Fig. 4. Female annual incidence for UC ([32])

The last study from northern England [11] suggested that the prevalence of IBD in 1995 was 243/100 000 persons for UC and 144/100 000 persons for CD. Italy, until some years ago, was considered among the countries with low incidence. In Italy, incidence rates are of 5.2 cases/100 000 person-years for UC and 2.3 cases/100 000 person-years for CD (Figs. 1, 2) [27].

The northern European studies based on population grounds have shown that there is no increase in overall mortality in IBD [28]. Only in CD has there been an increased mortality observed in the first few years after diagnosis in young patients. In some studies, this was observed primarily in the females. The Italian studies data confirm other European studies [29–31].

In general, there is a slight female predominance in Crohn's disease, especially among women in late adolescence and early adulthood, which suggests that hormonal factors may play a role in disease expression. On the other hand, if there is a slight gender predominance regarding UC, it rests with males [15]. For UC, different patterns of incidence were observed for men and women aged 35 and over, with

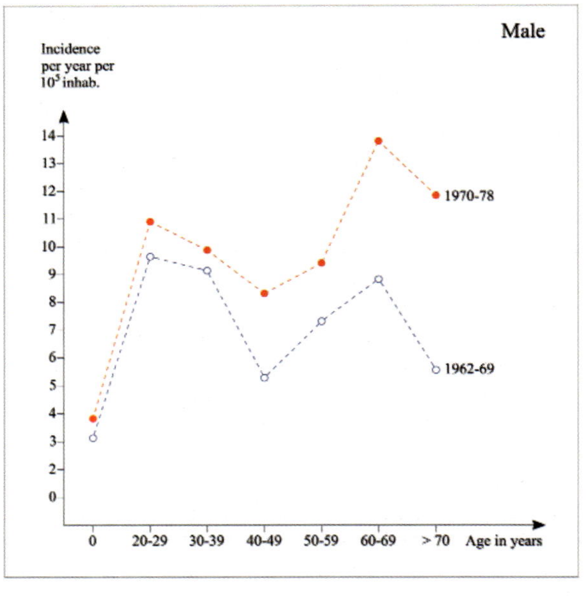

Fig. 5. Male annual incidence for UC ([32]

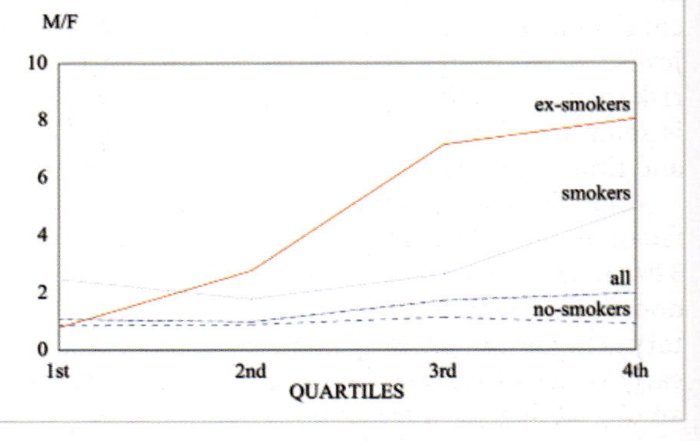

Fig. 6. Ratio of males to females according to smoking habits and age quartiles ([33])

the rates for men remaining fairly constant with increasing age, whereas those for women decreased. Incidence rates for CD were generally lower and were broadly similar for men and women, with rates for both sexes declining with increasing age (Fig. 3) [6].

For UC, a bimodal age distribution for men has been observed: incidence peak in the second and third decades in life followed by a second smaller peak in later decades (over 60 years of age; Figs. 4, 5) [32]. The reason for this bimodal pattern is still unknown. In fact, our study confirms the prevalence of males and the M/F ratio tends to significantly increase with age. The correlation between the age groups and the M/F ratio could be explained by a greater tendency to smoke in men and therefore by a greater, gradual prevalence among them of giving up the habit in relation to, for example, the occurrence of cardiovascular problems (Fig. 6) [33].

Risk Factors

The etiology and pathogenesis of IBD probably involve an interaction between genetic and environmental factors; the precise mechanism for the beginning of the intestinal inflammation remains unclear. There is increasing evidence that both environmental and host genetic factors are important in determining not only disease susceptibility, but also disease clinical course and response to therapy. Many factors have been suggested including family history of IBD, cigarette smoking, appendectomy, oral contraceptive agents, diet, breastfeeding, perinatal or early childhood infections, hygienic factors and physical activity.

Evidence for genetic factors includes epidemiological data showing differences in IBD among different races and ethnic groups, familial aggregation and high concordance for the IBD type in monozygotic vs. dizygotic twins [34–35]. The incidence is highest among whites, somewhat lower among blacks and lowest among Asians, although it is increasing among the latter [36]. Among Caucasians, the most consistent observation has been that the Ashkenazi Jewish population has been shown to be at higher risk than other ethnic groups (ratio 4:1) and this risk is maintained irrespective of geographical location and time period [37].

A family history is the single greatest known risk factor for the development of IBD. Between 6 and 32% of patients with IBD have an affected first or second-degree relative and the prevalence of family history is highest in Jewish patients and in patients with early onset of disease [38–39]. The risk is greatest among siblings, whereas it is lower among offsprings and second-degree relatives; the relative risk to a sibling of a patient with CD is 13–36% and for UC 7–17%. Therefore, a positive family history is more common in CD than in UC and relatives of patients with CD have a higher risk of developing IBD than those of patients with UC, suggesting a stronger genetic influence for CD [40–42].

Three twin studies have examined the relative genetic and environmental contributions to IBD by studying a total of 322 twin pairs. Combining these results produces CD concordance rates of 37 and 7% for monozygotic and dizygotic twins respectively, with equivalent results for UC of 10 and 3%. The genetic contribution is clearly less strong in UC than in CD, but the discordance between monozygotic and dizygotic prevalence rates again argues for a genetic contribution to UC. However, genes alone are not sufficient to cause the disease and complex environmental triggers are required for disease expression [43–45].

In genetic terms, the IBD are "complex" because classical Mendelian inheritance attributable to a single gene locus is not exhibited. The model which appears most pertinent at the present time suggests that CD and UC may be related heterogeneous polygenic disorders, sharing some but not all susceptibility loci. The disease phenotype is likely to be determined by the interaction between allelic variants at a number of loci and the interaction between genetic and environmental factors [46].

Recently the candidate genes have been selected on the basis of their location within an area of replicated linkage in multiplex IBD pedigrees (Fig. 7). The first susceptibility locus was identified in the pericentromeric region of chromosome 16 (IBD_1) [47]. The importance of this locus has been confirmed by various groups, including the GISC [48] and the International IBD Genetics Consortium [49]. In 2001, three independent studies reported the identification of the IBD_1 gene as NOD-2 [50–52]. Three coding region variants of this gene are associated with CD but not with UC. Patients carrying one high-risk allele have a 1.5–3-fold increased risk of developing CD, whereas those carrying two high-risk alleles have a 14–44-fold increased risk of developing CD [53]. The NOD_2 gene has recently been renamed $CARD_{15}$ (caspase recruitment domain gene) and is involved in the regulation of innate immune response and apoptosis; the leucine-rich repeat (LLR) domain of the gene appears to function as a sensor for bacterial products such as lipopolysaccharides (LPS; Fig. 8). Recently several genetic studies have been carried out in order to relate NOD_2/$CARD_{15}$ variants to specific clinical features of patients. The studies have generally correlated NOD_2 mutations with younger age at onset, ileal localisation and fibrostenotic behaviour of CD [54–57].

It has now been 23 years since the association of

Loci	Chromosomes	Genes
IBD1	16q12	NOD_2
IBD2	12q13	?
IBD3	6p13	HLA, TNF?
IBD4	14q11	?
IBD5	5q31-33	?
IBD6	19p	?
IBD7	1q	?
IBD*n*	3, x	?

Fig. 7. Significant areas of replicated linkage

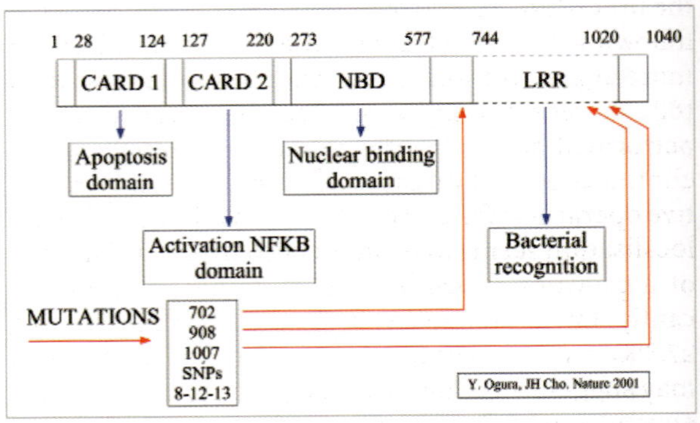

Fig. 8. Schematic representation of the $NOD_2/CARD_{15}$ [51]

non-smoking with UC was first identified by Harries et al. in 1982 [58], which was followed within 2 years by the observation that patients with CD were more often smokers [59]. This remarkable finding of "opposite associations" for smoking with IBD has been the subject of intense scrutiny in the hope that it may help identify important pathogenic mechanisms responsible for the two conditions and perhaps provide the key to alternative therapeutic options.

In 1989, Calkins reviewed the available studies on the association with IBD. A meta-analysis showed an increased risk of ulcerative colitis among lifelong non-smokers and ex-smokers compared with current smokers (OR 1.64) [60]. The M/F ratio, at diagnosis of UC, increases progressively with age in relation to the ex-smoker's habit compared with the M/F ratio that remains constant in non-smoking patients [33]. Moreover, it appears that ex-smokers are 70% more likely than those who never smoked to develop UC. In contrast to UC, several studies have implicated cigarette smoking as a risk factor for CD and the same meta-analysis suggests that in smokers the risk of having the disease is double in comparison to non-smokers. This association may not apply to all ethnic groups or geographic regions, a recent multicentre study performed in Israel has stressed the lack of association between smoking and CD and a negative association for UC [61]. Passive cigarette smoking has also been linked to IBD risk, but results have been conflicting. For UC the effect of passive smoking in childhood was comparable with that of active smoking in adulthood [62]. However, another study demonstrated that passive smoking exposure and maternal smoking at birth were significantly associated with development of either subtype of IBD; in CD the association had a dose-response relationship [63].

Cigarette smoking may also influence the clinical course of IBD. Active smokers were half as likely to be hospitalised for UC as non-smokers, whereas ex-smokers had higher hospitalisation and colectomy rates [64]. In another study, approximately 45% of UC patients who resumed smoking noted improvement in symptoms [65]. Moreover, significantly fewer smokers developed pouchitis compared with non-smokers among patients who had a restorative proctocolectomy for UC [66], and smoking is associated with decreased risk of primary sclerosing cholangitis (PSC) [67].

Patients with CD who smoke (>10 cigarettes/day, >150 cigarettes/year) are more likely to have ileal than colonic or ileocolonic involvement and fistulising or stenosing than inflammatory disease [68-70]. Most of the studies show severe symptoms, more frequent relapses, higher recurrence rate after surgery and more frequent treatments with steroids and immunosuppressors in smokers compared with non-smokers [71-73]. Young women with CD who continued to smoke, suffered more bowel and systemic symptoms in addition to more emotional dysfunction than female non-smokers [74].

More recently the role of the appendix in IBD epidemiology has become the subject of increasing interest. Appendectomy appears to be protective for the development of UC; important factors associated with a lower incidence of UC include an appendectomy before the age of 20 and appendectomy for appendicitis or mesenteric lymphadenitis [75–77]. Similar to the effect of cigarette smoking, an appendectomy also influences the clinical course of UC. In fact, patients who developed UC after appendectomy were diagnosed at an older age, showed few recurrent symptoms and were significantly less likely to require colectomy [78–79].

On the other hand, many studies have suggested that appendectomy is associated with future risk of CD even after excluding a diagnosis within 1 year of the procedure; moreover, patients who developed CD following a surgery for perforated appendicitis had a more aggressive form, requiring intestinal resection [80]. A recent study suggested that appendectomy performed before CD diagnosis can predict a worse clinical course of disease and a higher risk of resective operations for these patients. In addition, disease localisation seems to be influenced by the occurrence of a previous appendectomy, resulting in a significantly lower frequency of Crohn's colitis (9.8 *vs.* 27.3%, OR 0.3) compared with controls. This fact may suggest some hints on the pathogenic role of the appendix in CD; it could be hypothesised that an etiopathogenic process may be phenotypically expressed in the form of appendicitis avoiding the expression of CD in the colon, similar to the protective role of appendectomy regarding the development of UC. In addiction, the occurrence of an appendectomy before CD diagnosis seems to show a negative association with articular manifestations [81].

Several case-control and cohort studies have suggested an increased risk of IBD in women who take oral contraceptives. In some studies, a positive association between oral contraceptives use and risk of CD was confined to women who were current smokers (OR 2.64) [62], whereas the opposite finding has been reported in other studies in which the elevated risk was found only among non-smokers (OR 3.1 *vs.* 0.91) [82]. There was no association between oral contraceptive use and UC (OR 0.70). Therefore, there is no evidence suggesting that women predisposed to the development of UC should be advised to avoid oral contraceptive use [83]. However, a 1995 meta-analysis demonstrated an elevated risk both for UC (OR 1.29) and CD (OR 1.44) [84]. Since this meta-analysis, other studies have been published with the same pattern of results: an overall weak association for both diseases but non-sufficiently compelling to infer a causal association [85-86]. The mechanism for this association is not definitively known, but it is thought that the thrombogenic properties of oral contraceptives, in the setting of a process of multifocal, microvascular gastrointestinal infarction, might play a role [87].

Because dietary agents are, next to bacterial antigens, the most common type of luminal antigen, it is logical to surmise that diet might play a role in the expression of IBD. Furthermore, differences in diet might explain the significant differences in IBD risk across geographic regions and the increase in IBD incidence in migrant populations. However, numerous studies have investigated dietary factors in IBD, and the methodological problems related to studies of this kind (type of population studied, recall bias, measure) have brought contradictive results. The most consistent association noted in dietary studies has been the link between increased sugar intake and CD [88]. A population-based case-control study from The Netherlands implicated chocolate and cola drink consumption as possible risk factors for IBD [89]. Finally, high intake of dietary fibre, fruit or vegetables may be protective against the development of IBD, but results vary from study to study [90–91].

It has been proposed that the expression of IBD may be influenced by events in early childhood such as mode of feeding, domestic hygiene or perinatal infections. Although several studies have suggested an inverse association between breastfeeding and IBD [86, 92, 93], in most cases the odds ratios were not statistically significant and other studies have not demonstrated such an association [94-95]. In general, the association has been stronger for CD than for UC.

Perinatal infections, either in the infant or the mother, might influence the expression of IBD. It has been proposed that perinatal or childhood paramyxoviral infection might result in persistent infection of the vascular endothelium of the mesentery, resulting in a chronic granulomatous vasculitis (CD) [96]. However, other studies have not been able to confirm these findings [97]. The same investigators who initially proposed persistent measles infection as a cause of CD suggested that attenuated live measles virus vaccine might lead to IBD [98], but several case-control studies in different locales have not demonstrated significant differences in vaccination rates among IBD cases and unaffected controls [99]. Based on the available evidence, it would be difficult to conclude that measles vaccination is a risk factor for IBD. A study of IBD from central Sweden noted that IBD patients with an infection or serious illness, mother or child, had a fourfold increased risk for IBD. In the same study, infants from families of low socioeconomic status were 3 times more likely later to develop IBD [100]. On the other hand, some have suggested that the absence of infections might be a risk for IBD; CD, but not UC, is more common in those who lived in houses with a hot water tap during childhood [101]. In addition, toothpaste has been proposed as a risk factor for CD; it contains such microparticles that could serve as a proxy measure of hygienic conditions or have an impact on the microbiological intestinal flora [102]. However, no observational studies have shown such an association implicating toothpaste as an independent risk factor. Finally, Klein et al. have investigated the physical activity levels of patients with IBD and controls for the period prior to onset of the disease: IBD patients were over-represented in the low-activity group *vs.* controls [103].

References

1. Langholz E, Munkholm P, Nielsen OH et al (1991) Incidence and prevalence of ulcerative colitis in Copenhagen county from 1962 to 1987. Scand J Gastroenterol 26:1247–1256
2. Munkholm P, Langholz E, Nielsen OH et al (1992) Incidence and prevalence of Crohn's disease in Copenhagen county, 1962–1987: a sixfold increase incidence. Scand J Gastroenterol 27:609–614
3. Gower-Rousseau C, Salomez JL, Marti R et al (1994) Incidence of inflammatory bowel disease in northern France. Gut 35:1433–1438
4. Moum B, Vatn MH, Ekbom A et al (1996) Incidence of Crohn's disease in four counties in southeastern Norway, 1990–93: a prospective population study. Scand J Gastroenterol 31:355–361
5. Moum B, Vatn MH, Ekbom A et al (1996) Incidence of ulcerative colitis and indeterminate colitis in four counties of southeastern Norway, 1990–93: a prospective population study. Scand J Gastroenterol 31:362–366
6. Shivanada S, Lennard-Jones J, Logan R et al (1996) Incidence of inflammatory bowel disease across Europe: Is there a difference between north and south? Results of the European Collaborative Study on Inflammatory Bowel Disease (EC-IBD). Gut 39:690–697
7. Lapidus A, Bernell O, Hellers G et al (1997) Incidence of Crohn's disease in Stockholm County 1955–1989. Gut 41:480–486
8. Russel MG, Dorant E, Volovics A et al (1998) High incidence of inflammatory bowel disease in The Netherlands: a result of a prospective study. Dis Colon Rectum 41:33–40
9. Montgomery SM, Morris DL, Thompson NP et al (1998) Prevalence of inflammatory bowel disease in British 26 year olds: national longitudinal birth cohort. BMJ 316:1058–1059
10. Yapp TR, Stenson R, Thomas GAO et al (2000) Crohn's disease incidence in Cardiff from 1930: an update for 1991–1995. Eur J Gastroenterol Hepatol 12:907–911
11. Rubin GP, Hungin APS, Kelly PJ et al (2000) Inflammatory bowel disease: epidemiology and management in an English general practice population. Aliment Pharmacol Ther 14:1553–1559
12. Stowe SP, Redmond SR, Stormont JM et al (1990) An epidemiologic study of inflammatory bowel disease in Rochester, New York: hospital incidence. Gastroenterology 98:104–110
13. Loftus EV Jr, Silverstein MD, Sandborn WJ et al (1998) Crohn's disease in Olmsted County, Minnesota, 1940–1993: incidence, prevalence and survival. Gastroenterology 114:1161–1168
14. Bernstein CN, Blanchard JF, Rawstorne P et al (1999) Epidemiology of Crohn's disease and ulcerative colitis in a central Canadian province: a population-based study. Am J Epidemiol 149:916–924
15. Loftus EV Jr, Silverstein MD, Sandborn WJ et al (2000) Ulcerative colitis in Olmsted County, Minnesota, 1940–1993: incidence, prevalence and survival. Gut 46:336–343
16. Vucelic B, Korac B, Sentic M et al (1991) Epidemiology of Crohn's disease in Zagreb, Yugoslavia: a ten-year prospective study. Int J Epidemiol 20:216–220
17. Vucelic B, Korac B, Sentic M et al (1991) Ulcerative colitis in Zagreb, Yugoslavia: incidence and prevalence 1980–1989. Int J Epidemiol 20:1043–1047
18. Mate-Jimenez J, Munoz S, Vicent D, Pajares JM (1994) Incidence and prevalence of ulcerative colitis and Crohn's disease in urban and rural areas of Spain from 1981 to 1988. J Clin Gastroenterol 18:27–31
19. Fireman Z, Grossman A, Lilos P, Eshchar Y et al (1989) Epidemiology of Crohn's disease in the Jewish population of central Israel, 1970–1980. Am J Gastroenterol 84:255–258
20. Grossman A, Fireman Z, Lilos P et al (1989) Epidemiology of ulcerative colitis in the Jewish population of central Israel, 1970–1980. Hepatogastroenterology 36:193–197
21. Morita N, Toki S, Hirohashi T et al (1995) Incidence and prevalence of inflammatory bowel disease in Japan: nationwide epidemiological survey during the year 1991. J Gastroenterol 30:1–4
22. Lee YM, Fock KM, See SJ et al (2000) Racial differences in the prevalence of ulcerative colitis and Crohn's disease in Singapore. J Gastroenterol Hepatol 15:622–625
23. Wright JP, Froggat J, O'Keefe EA et al (1986) The epidemiology of inflammatory bowel disease in Cape Town 1980–1984. S Afr Med J 70:10–15
24. Linares de la Cal JA, Canton C, Hermida C et al (1999) Estimated incidence of inflammatory bowel disease in Argentina and Panama (1987–1993). Rev Esp Enferm Dig 91:277–286
25. Yang SK, Hong WS, Min YI et al (2000) Incidence and prevalence of ulcerative colitis in the Songpa-Kangdong District, Seoul, Korea, 1986–1997. J Gastroenterol Hepatol 15:1037–1042
26. Sood A, Midha V, Sood N et al (2003) Incidence and prevalence of ulcerative colitis in Punjab, North India. Gut 52:1587–1590
27. Tragnone A, Corrao G, Miglio F et al (1996) Incidence of inflammatory bowel disease in Italy: a nationwide population-based study. Int J Epidemiol 25:1044–1052
28. Ekbom A, Helmick CG, Zack M et al (1992) Survival and causes of death in patients with inflammatory bowel disease: a population-based study. Gastroenterology 103:954–960
29. Palli D, Trallori G, Saieva C et al (1998) General and specific mortality of a population based cohort of patients with inflammatory bowel disease. Gut 42:175–179
30. Davoli M, Prantera G, Berto E et al (1997) Mortality among patients with ulcerative colitis: Rome 1970–1989. Eur J Epidemiol 13:189–194
31. Cottone M, Magliocco A, Rosselli M et al (1996) Mortality in patients with Crohn's disease. Scand J Gastroenterol 31:372–375
32. Binder V, Both H, Hansen PK et al (1982) Incidence and prevalence of ulcerative colitis and Crohn's disease in the county of Copenhagen, 1962–1978. Gastroenterology 83:563–568
33. Riegler G, Tartaglione MT, Carratù R et al (2000) Age-related clinical severity at diagnosis in 1705 patients with ulcerative colitis: a study by GISC (Italian Colon-Rectum Study Group). Dig Dis Sci 45:462–465
34. Yang H, Rotter JI (2000) The genetic background of inflammatory bowel disease. Hepatogastroenterology

47:5–14
35. Ahmad T, Satsangi J, McGovern D, Jewell DP (2001) Review article: the genetics of inflammatory bowel disease. Aliment Pharmacol Ther 15:731–748
36. Sandler R (1994) Epidemiology of inflammatory bowel disease. In: Targan S, Shanahan F (eds) Inflammatory bowel disease: from bench to beside. Williams, Baltimore, MD, USA, pp 5–30
37. Roth MP, Petersen GM, McElree C et al (1989) Geographic origins of Jewish patients with inflammatory bowel disease. Gastroenterology 97:900–904
38. Farmer RG, Michener WM, Mortimer EA (1980) Studies of family history among patients with inflammatory bowel disease. Clin Gastroenterol 9:271–277
39. Yang H, McElree C, Roth MP et al (1993) Familial empirical risks for inflammatory bowel disease: differences between Jews and non-Jews. Gut 34:517–524
40. Orholm M, Munkolm P, Langholz E et al (1991) Familial occurrence of inflammatory bowel disease. N Engl J Med 324:84–88
41. Satsangi J, Rosenberg WMC, Jewell DP (1994) The prevalence of inflammatory bowel disease in relatives of patients with Crohn's disease. Eur J Gastroenterol Hepatol 6:413–416
42. Peeters M, Nevens H, Baert F et al (1996) Familial aggregation in Crohn's disease: increased age adjusted risk and concordance in clinical characteristics. Gastroenterology 111:597–603
43. Tysk C, Lindberg E, Jarnerot G, Floderus-Myrhed B (1988) Ulcerative colitis and Crohn's disease in an unselected population of monozygotic and dizygotic twins: a study of heritability and the influence of smoking. Gut 29:990–996
44. Orholm M, Binder V, Sorensen T, Kyvik K (1996) Inflammatory bowel disease in a Danish twin register. Gut 39:A187
45. Thompson NP, Driscoll R, Pounder RE, Wakefield AJ (1996) Genetics versus environment in inflammatory bowel disease: results of a British twin study. BMJ 312:95–96
46. Satsangi J, Parkes M, Jewell DP (1997) The genetics of inflammatory bowel disease: recent progress. In: McLeod RS, Martin F, Sutherland LR et al (eds) Inflammatory bowel diseases. Kluwer, Lancaster, pp 21–28
47. Hugot JP, Laurent-Puig P, Gower-Rousseau C et al (1996) Mapping of a susceptibility locus for Crohn's disease on chromosome 16. Nature 379:821–823
48. Annese V, Latiano A, Bovio P et al (1999) Genetic analysis in Italian families with inflammatory bowel disease supports linkage to the IBD1 locus: a GISC study. Eur J Hum Genet 7:567–573
49. The IBD International Genetics Consortium (2001) International collaboration provides convincing linkage replication in complex disease through analysis of a large pooled data set: Crohn's disease and chromosome 16. Am J Hum Genet 68:1165–1171
50. Hugot JP, Chamaillard M, Zouali H et al (2001) Association of NOD2 leucine-rich repeat variants with susceptibility to Crohn's disease. Nature 411:599–603
51. Ogura Y, Bonen DK, Inohara N et al (2001) A frameshift mutation in NOD2 associated with susceptibility to Crohn's disease. Nature 411:603–606
52. Hampe J, Cuthbert A, Croucher PJP et al (2001) Association between insertion mutation in NOD2 gene and Crohn's disease in German and British populations. Lancet 357:1925–1928
53. Lesage S, Zouali H, Cezard JP et al (2002) Card15/Nod2 mutational analysis and genotype–phenotype correlation in 612 patients with inflammatory bowel disease. Am J Hum Genet 70:845–857
54. Cuthbert AP, Fisher SA, Mirza MM et al (2002) The contribution of NOD2 gene mutations to the risk and site of disease of disease in inflammatory bowel disease. Gastroenterology 122:867–874
55. Radlmar M, Torok HP, Martin K, Folwaczny C (2002) The c-insertion mutation of the NOD2 gene is associated with fistulizing and fibrostenotic phenotypes in Crohn's disease. Gastroenterology 122:2091–2092
56. Abreu MT, Taylor KD, Lin YC et al (2002) Mutations in NOD2 are associated with fibrostenosing disease in patients with Crohn's disease. Gastroenterology 123:679–688
57. Louis E, Hugot JP, Colombel JF et al (2002) NOD2/CARD15 mutations in Crohn's disease are associated with young age at diagnosis and ileal location. Gastroenterology 122:M1405
58. Harries AD, Baird A, Rhodes J (1982) Non-smoking: a feature of ulcerative colitis. BMJ 284:706
59. Sommerville KW, Logan RF, Edmond M, Langman MJ (1984) Smoking and Crohn's disease. BMJ 289:954–956
60. Calkins BM (1989) A meta-analysis of the role of smoking in inflammatory bowel disease. Dig Dis Sci 34:1841–1854
61. Reif S, Lavy A, Keter D et al (2000) Lack of association between smoking and Crohn's disease but the usual association between ulcerative colitis in Jewish patients in Israel: a multicenter study. Am J Gastroenterol 95:474–478
62. Sandler RS, Sandler DP, McDonnel CW, Wurzelmann JI (1992) Childhood exposure to environmental tobacco smoke and the risk of ulcerative colitis. Am J Epidemiol 135:603–608
63. Lashner BA, Shaheen NJ, Hanauer SB, Kirschner BS (1993) Passive smoking is associated with an increased risk of developing inflammatory bowel disease in children. Am J Gastroenterol 88:1093–1099
64. Boyko EJ, Perera DR, Koepsell TD et al (1988) Effects of cigarette smoking on the clinical course of ulcerative colitis. Scand J Gastroenterol 23:1147–1152
65. Rudra T, Motley R, Rhodes J (1989) Does smoking improve colitis? Scand J Gastroenterol Suppl 170:61–63
66. Merret MN, Mortensen N, Kettlewell M, Jewell DO (1996) Smoking may prevent pouchitis in patients with restorative proctocolectomy for ulcerative colitis. Gut 38:362–364
67. van Erpecum KJ, Smits SJ, van de Meeberg PC et al (1996) Risk of primary sclerosing cholangitis is associated with non-smoking behaviour. Gastroenterology 110:1503–1506
68. Lindberg E, Jarnerot G, Huitfeldt B (1992) Smoking in Crohn's disease: effect on localisation and clinical course. Gut 33:779–782
69. Russel MG, Volovics A, Schoon EJ et al (1998) Inflammatory bowel disease: Is there any relation between

smoking status and disease presentation? Inflamm Bowel Dis 4:182–186
70. Picco MF, Bayless TM (2003) Tobacco consumption and disease duration are associated with fistulizing and stricturing behaviours in the first 8 years of Crohn's disease. Am J Gastroenterol 98:363–368
71. Sutherland LR, Ramcharan S, Bryant H, Fick G (1990) Effect of cigarette smoking on recurrence of Crohn's disease. Gastroenterology 98:1123–1128
72. Cottone M, Rosselli M, Orlando A et al (1994) Smoking habits and recurrence in Crohn's disease. Gastroenterology 106:643–648
73. Cosnes J, Carbonnel F, Carrat F et al (1999) Effects of current and former cigarette smoking on the clinical course of Crohn's disease. Aliment Pharmacol Ther 13:1403–1411
74. Russel MG, Nieman FH, Bergers JM, Stockbrugger RW (1996) Cigarette smoking and quality of life in patients with inflammatory bowel disease. Eur J Gastroenterol Hepatol 8:1075–1081
75. Rutgeerts P, D'Haens G, Hiele M et al (1994) Appendectomy protects against ulcerative colitis. Gastroenterology 106:1251–1253
76. Parrello T, Pavia M, Angelillo G et al (1997) Appendicectomy is an independent protective factor for ulcerative colitis: results of a multicenter case control study. Ital J Gastroenterol Hepatol 29:208–213
77. Andersson RE, Olaison G, Tysk C, Ekbom A (2001) Appendectomy and protection against ulcerative colitis. N Engl J Med 344:808–814
78. Naganuma M, Iizuka B, Torii A et al (2001) Appendectomy protects against the development of ulcerative colitis and reduces its recurrence: results of a multicenter case-controlled study in Japan. Am J Gastroenterol 96:1123–1126
79. Cosnes J, Carbonnel F, Beaugerie L et al (2002) Effects of appendicectomy on the course of ulcerative colitis. Gut 51:803–807
80. Andersson RE, Olaison G, Tysk C, Ekbom A (2003) Appendectomy is followed by increased risk of Crohn's disease. Gastroenterology 124:40–46
81. Riegler G, Caserta L, Esposito I et al (2005) Worse clinical course of disease in Crohn's patients with previous appendectomy. Eur J Gastroenterol Hepatol 17:623–627
82. Katschinski B, Fingerle D, Scherbaum B, Goebell H (1993) Oral contraceptive use and cigarette smoking in Crohn's disease. Dig Dis Sci 38:1596–1600
83. Lashner BA, Kane SV, Hanauer SB (1990) Lack of association between oral contraceptive use and ulcerative colitis. Gastroenterology 99:1032–1036
84. Godet PG, May GR, Sutherland LR (1995) Meta-analysis of the role of oral contraceptive agents in inflammatory bowel disease. Gut 37:668–673
85. Boyko EJ, Theis MK, Vaughan TL, Nicol-Blades B (1994) Increased risk of inflammatory bowel disease associated with oral contraceptive use. Am J Epidemiol 140:268–278
86. Corrao G, Tragnone A, Caprilli R et al (1998) Risk of inflammatory bowel disease attributable to smoking, oral contraception and breastfeeding in Italy: a nationwide case-control study. Int J Epidemiol 27:397–404
87. Wakefield AJ, Sawyerr AM, Hudson M et al (1991) Smoking, the oral contraceptive pill and Crohn's disease. Dig Dis Sci 36:1147–1150
88. Riordan AM, Ruxton CH, Hunter JO (1998) A review of associations between Crohn's disease and consumption of sugars. Eur J Clin Nutr 52:229–338
89. Russel MG, Engels LG, Muris JW et al (1998) "Modern life" in the epidemiology of inflammatory bowel disease: a case-control study with special emphasis on nutritional factors. Eur J Gastroenterol Hepatol 10:243–249
90. Reif S, Klein I, Lubin F et al (1997) Pre-illness dietary factors in inflammatory bowel disease. Gut 40:754–760
91. Persson PG, Ahlbom A, Hellers G (1992) Diet and inflammatory bowel disease: a case-control study. Epidemiology 3:47–52
92. Koletzko S, Sherman P, Corey M et al (1989) Role of infant feeding practices in development of Crohn's disease in childhood. BMJ 298:1617–1618
93. Rigas A, Rigas B, Glassman M et al (1993) Breastfeeding and maternal smoking in the etiology of Crohn's disease and ulcerative colitis in childhood. Ann Epidemiol 3:387–392
94. Thompson NP, Montgomery SM, Wadsworth ME et al (2000) Early determinants of inflammatory bowel disease: use of two national longitudinal birth cohorts. Eur J Gastroenterol Hepatol 12:25–30
95. Ekbom A, Adami HO, Helmick CG et al (1990) Perinatal risk factors for inflammatory bowel disease: a case-control study. Am J Epidemiol 132:1111–1119
96. Thompson NP, Pounder RE, Wakefield AJ (1995) Perinatal and childhood risk factors for inflammatory bowel disease: a case-control study. Eur J Gastroenterol Hepatol 7:385–390
97. Wakefield AJ, Ekbom A, Dhillon AP et al (1995) Crohn's disease: pathogenesis and persistent measles virus infection. Gastroenterology 108:911–916
98. Pardi DS, Tremaine WJ, Sandborn WJ et al (1999) Perinatal exposure to measles virus is not associated with the development of inflammatory bowel disease. Inflamm Bowel Dis 5:104–106
99. Thompson NP, Montgomery SM, Pounder RE, Wakefield AJ (1995) Is measles vaccination a risk factor for inflammatory bowel disease? Lancet 345:1071–1074
100. Davis RL, Kramarz P, Bohlke K et al (2001) Measles-mumps-rubella and other measles-containing vaccines do not increase the risk for inflammatory bowel disease: a case-control study from the Vaccine Safety Datalink Project. Arch Pediatr Adolesc Med 155:354–359
101. Gent AE, Hellier MD, Grace RH et al (1994) Inflammatory bowel disease and domestic hygiene in infancy. Lancet 343:766–767
102. Sullivan SN (1990) hypothesis revisited: toothpaste and the cause of Crohn's disease. Lancet 336:1096–1097
103. Klein I, Reif S, Farbstein H et al (1998) Preillness non dietary factors and habits in inflammatory bowel disease. Ital J Gastroenterol Hepatol 30:247–251

Inflammatory Bowel Disease: the Pathologists Approach to the Clinical Problem

Emil Salmo, Shamim Absar, Najib Haboubi

Introduction

Inflammatory bowel disease (IBD), comprising ulcerative colitis (UC) and Crohn's disease (CD) are idiopathic relapsing, lifelong chronic conditions of the gastrointestinal tract which may also affect extra-intestinal organs and tissues with sometimes devastating effects on the patient's quality of life. They share many common features; however, they may differ in their clinical manifestations and the way they affect the bowel. The questions that remain unanswered refer to whether they are two completely different diseases or two manifestations of one disease process with a very wide spectrum. If they are two separate entities, would the presence of one disease process preclude the presence of the other in the same patient?

UC mainly affects the large intestine starting distally, usually in the rectum, and spreads proximally in a continuous fashion. This is in contrast to CD, which classically affects the small bowel, but in the colon the involvement is classically discontinuous. However, CD can involve any part of the gastrointestinal tract from the mouth to the anus and both diseases can exhibit extra-intestinal manifestations affecting the skin, joints and the eyes. This chapter will briefly discuss the epidemiology, genetics, pathogenesis, and pathology of IBD but will mainly address the pathologist's approach in reporting these conditions.

Epidemiology and Pathogenesis

CD and UC are diseases commonly occurring with increasing frequency in Western countries and are traditionally considered a disorder of the industrialised world [1]. The incidence of UC is approximately 10–20 per 100 000 per year, while that of a CD is between 5–10 per 100 000 per year, and the incidence of the latter is on the increase. It is estimated that up to 240 000 are affected by IBD in the UK [2]. It is interesting to realise that the incidence of UC and CD has seen an increase in certain parts of Asia and the Middle East, but it remains uncommon in Africa and South America [3].

Several studies have demonstrated that first-degree relatives of an affected patient have up to 10 times an increased risk of IBD. The same investigators showed that the risk of UC in first-degree relatives is higher if the disease had been diagnosed before the age of 20. However, hereditary factors are shown to have stronger association with CD rather than UC [4], and it has been shown that monozygotic rather than dizygotic twins are more susceptible to CD [5].

The disease commonly starts in the third decade with a peak incidence between the ages of 10 and 40; however, several studies have demonstrated that children and young patients below the age of 21 can also be affected. There is a second incidence peak seen in the elderly [6, 7, 2]. In young females, the disease usually runs a milder course with fewer complications in contrast to young males where the disease tends to be more active with more complications and more extra-intestinal manifestations. Growth impairment is a particular problem in the paediatric age group in which up to 35% may continue to have permanent growth retardation [8]. Many reports have indicated that the incidence of ulcerative colitis is more common in certain ethnic groups, like for instance the Jewish population living in Western Europe and North America, so therefore their family members are at an increased risk of developing the disease [9, 10].

The etiologies of both diseases remain unknown; however, several factors are thought to contribute to their pathogenesis. Some of those factors are thought to result from abnormal activation of the mucosal immune system driven by the intraluminal flora. This consequently leads to an aberrant response facilitated by abnormalities within the intestinal mucosal epithelium and the immune system [1]. The role of the intestinal flora in IBD has been established in animals. If gene-knockout mice that normally develop IBD are made germ-free, the disease will disappear [11]. Some other environmental factors have also been implicated in the pathogenesis, the most consistent of which is the use of non-steroidal anti-inflammatory drugs [12]. These classes of drugs can exacerbate the disease and their use has been associated with an increased incidence of emergency admissions to the hospital for colitis due to IBD. Interestingly, some studies have demonstrated that an early appendectomy is associated with a reduced incidence of UC, and that those patients who had genuine appendicitis or lymphadenitis rather than non-specific abdominal pain and were less than 20 years old at the time of surgery had lower risk of developing UC [13].

Stress has also been implicated in the causation of IBD. Significant association between acute daily stressful events and bowel symptoms in patients with CD has been shown and these patients have a greater risk of active disease [14, 15]. Stress-related IBD was also demonstrated in one study where Bedouin Arabs developed UC when moving from their rural life style into government housing [16]. Smoking has been shown to be associated with an increase susceptibility to CD together with rapid disease progression and immune suppression. In contrast, smoking has been demonstrated to have a protective effect against the development of UC through unknown mechanisms [17].

Genetic factors have been shown to play an important part in the causation of both UC and CD and they have a stronger link to the latter. The relative risk to a sibling of a patient with Crohn's disease is 13–36% and for ulcerative colitis it is 7–17% [18]. Additionally, it is estimated that between 6 and 32% of patients with inflammatory bowel disease have an affected first or second-degree relative [19].

Numerous candidate genes have been analysed in inflammatory bowel disease, especially genes related to the HLA system [20]. A gene, located on chromosome 16, named NOD2 (encodes a protein which has a nucleotide-binding oligomerisation domain) with a locus designated IBD1, has recently been shown to be linked with CD [21, 22], and it has been shown that persons who are homozygous for variant NOD2 may have a 20-fold increase tendency for CD with a predominantly ileal involvement [23]. Additionally, it has been shown that possession of the DRB1*103 and DRB1*12 alleles are associated with UC and DR3 DQ2 haplotype is predictive of extensive disease but not of the need for surgery [24]. Interestingly, patients with CD have greater concentration of NOD2 mRNA in the Paneth cells which are found most frequently in the ileum; hence, CD commonly affects this region [20].

Recommended Approach to Diagnosis

Ulcerative colitis and Crohn's disease have, in many cases, quite distinguishing histopathological features with typical investigative findings and clinical features; however, this is not universal and in many cases these features might overlap. Common histological changes might be absent or the changes may lack the characteristic features, therefore the findings usually need to be analysed more meticulously in the all-important clinical pathological conferences (CPCs). Despite all the efforts, there are cases where it is not possible to give a definite diagnosis and which might need further investigation [25, 26–29].

In previous reports [30, 31], our group has maintained that, in addition to good biopsy samples, there are three important factors which help in reaching a more accurate histopathological diagnosis and making appropriate clinical decisions. These are:

1. Adequate information for histopathologist
2. Standard definition of histological terms
3. Maintenance of communication between clinician and histopathologist

It is very important for the clinician to remember that the pathologist's aim is to come to a diagnosis with the help of information derived from other different subspecialties and therefore coordination is essential. Similarly it is important for the pathologist to follow a clear and standard reporting system that is understood by the clinicians and all members of the IBD team who must work in absolute harmony and understanding in dealing with these diseases [32–41].

The diagnosis of IBD is confirmed by clinical evaluation and a combination of biochemical, endoscopic, radiological, histological and sometimes nuclear medical investigations as stated earlier. It is inappropriate to expect the pathologists to make a diagnosis of IBD in general and specifically to differentiate UC from CD without providing enough information regarding clinical suspicion, endoscopic findings and previous investigations.

Information required by the pathologist:

1. History and clinical examination: a summary of history with the symptoms, their duration, recent travel, medication, smoking and family history. The presence of intestinal manifestations—for example diarrhoea, mucous, blood etc.—their duration and a brief clinical examination finding is indispensable.
2. Investigations (laboratory and radiological): abnormal routine investigations such as blood count, CRP, liver function tests and the results of microscopical examination of stool and culture help in coming to a diagnosis. Infections and conditions that mimic IBD can be excluded based on

this information as sometimes inflammation such as clostridium and other infections can be easily diagnosed. Previous positive and negative radiological investigations help in reaffirming diagnosis and identifying subtle changes in light of the investigative findings. It is important to realise that sometimes there is super imposition of infection on IBD. Indeed some of the flare-up cases of IBD reported lately are due to superimposed CMV infection [42].

3. Endoscopies (sigmoidoscopy/colonoscopy): the diagnosis of IBD is greatly dependent upon the presence of visible endoscopic changes such as vascular pattern, mucosal viability and ulcerations and/or presence of polyps. The signs of involvement and whether it is continuous or discontinuance and other findings are of significant help. In certain cases, visual microscopic appearance, as in pseudo-membranous colitis, gives a better idea of the colonic disease than histological examination. In our unit, we regard the endoscopic changes of such importance that we routinely receive a copy of the endoscopy report with the request form for the histological examination. It is also important to realise that normal endoscopy is not synonymous with normal structure. We therefore recommend that 'normal' looking areas between abnormal ones be biopsied in patients suspected of IBD.
4. Others: the use of different treatments, the stage of the disease, its duration and if there are any previous biopsies, as their interpretations are greatly helpful to the pathologist in correlating the findings.

A clear and definitive diagnosis makes it easy for the clinician to understand and interpret the results and to manage the patient appropriately. Standard histological terms should be used in reporting as it not only makes it easier to understand them but also helps in the exchange of information between different members of the team involved in the management of the patient as well as for research and auditing purposes [43].

Pattern of Disease

In ulcerative colitis, the classical teaching is that the inflammation is always continuous with the rectum being primarily involved. Topographically, UC is classified as distal colitis referring to colitis confined to the rectum, recto-sigmoid, left sided when the disease extends to the splenic flexure, extensive colitis if the disease extends to the hepatic flexure. Pan-colitis is a term used when the inflammatory process involves the entire colon. There are, however, two exceptions to the rule.

Firstly, there are various reports suggesting that UC can be associated with relatively uninvolved patches including rectal sparing, thus giving the false impression of discontinuous disease and therefore suggesting CD in a genuine case of UC [38]. This is especially true in the paediatric age group where it has been shown that children may present initially with relative or complete rectal sparing or even patchy disease. Thus, non-classical features of UC in the paediatric age group do not exclude its diagnosis [44]. The patchiness of inflammation has also been described and recognised in some cases of left-sided UC where there is an area of inflammation in the caecum ("caecal patch"), in the periappendiceal mucosa or involving the appendix [45]. Secondly, it is important to remember that some workers suggest that the mucosa in a long standing UC may go back to normal with or without treatment with 5-Amiosalicylic Acid [46, 35].

In CD, the inflammation is classically patchy, transmural and may affect any part of the gastrointestinal tract. It is usually defined by its location such as terminal ileitis, colonic, upper gastrointestinal etc., or by the pattern of the disease inflammation, which could be infiltrating or stricturing. These variables are combined in the Vienna classification, which veers from the original anatomic classification of CD. The Vienna classification is a simple and objective classification of Crohn's disease and encompasses different variables such as age at onset, location and disease behaviour [47]. Application of the Vienna classification has demonstrated that in CD the process changes with time and 80% of inflammatory diseases ultimately evolve into a stricturing or penetrating pattern and about 15% undergo a change in anatomical location (Table 1) [48]. A new classification is under consideration following the 2005 World Congress at Montreal and it is envisaged to be a combined clinical, molecular and serological classification for IBD [49].

Table 1. The Vienna classification of Crohn's disease [47, 48]

Age at diagnosis		
	A1	<40 years
	A2	>40 years
Location		
	L1	Terminal ileum
	L2	Colon
	L3	Ileocolon
	L4	Upper gastrointestinal
Behaviour		
	B1	Non-stricturing non-penetrating
	B2	Stricturing
	B3	Penetrating

The Impact of CPC on the Diagnosis

As we discussed earlier, CPCs are the best forum [50] for discussing cases, corroborating findings and coming to a definitive diagnosis. In many hospitals, however, CPCs are not held regularly. It has been shown that when discussing gastrointestinal cases at CPCs, in over 40% of cases there is a change of management following a change in diagnosis [50]. A recent study was carried out by our group with the use of a combined clinicopathological form with sufficient information, clinical investigations and endoscopic findings along with a pattern based report by the pathologist. We suggest using those forms in places where CPCs are not regularly held as the use of this form could significantly increase the range of accurate diagnoses of UC or CD. The study showed that without regular CPCs, but with the use of regular available information, only approximately 60% of cases of IBD are accurately diagnosed as CD or UC. However, the use of this form has raised the possibility of a definite diagnosis to approximately 77%, which is slightly inferior to the 82% of CPCs and we concluded that in the absence of regular CPCs, it definitely shows great potential and is the next best substitute [51]. A reproduction of the form, which contains most of the information the pathologist expects and is usually necessary for a definitive diagnosis, is shown in Fig. 1. Histological diagnosis of any condition, by and large, is greatly dependent on the availability of adequate and accurate clinical information, and this greatly holds true for the histological examination of tissues for IBD [52]. Providing adequate information in blank form is often difficult and lacks uniform application. We have tried to work around this problem via this form and we suggest that it, or a modified version, will be a simple way to overcome a lack of CPCs. It will also help the histopathologist in coming to a diagnosis or narrowing the list of differential diagnoses. This form also uses the standard definition of histological terms and gives a list of more likely diagnoses, which is essential not only in understanding and managing different patients, but is indispensable for proper auditing, research and the communication of findings between the pathologist and clinician across different specialty institutions [53, 43].

Macroscopic Features of IBD

In IBD, the gross appearance of the colon depends on the stage of the disease and the clinical severity [54]. In UC, the mucosa of the distal colon in early phases is red, friable, mucoid, with petechial haemorrhages. With the progression of the disease, broad-based ulceration of the mucosa develops, separating isolated islands of mucosa which could be inflamed or show features of regeneration. They may be seen to be protruding into the lumen to create the so-called pseudo-polyps commonly seen in this disease. We discourage the use of the term pseudo-polyp as a polyp is a mucosal protrusion and the surviving islands often undergo regenerative or inflammatory changes, and thus can be regarded as polyps. We therefore designate these polyps as either inflammatory, regenerative polyps or polypoid mucosal tags. These polyps are typically small and multiple; however, sometimes they can attain a large size mimicking carcinoma [55]. These polyps do not correlate with the disease severity and are not precancerous. Commonly, the ulcers are aligned along the long axis of the colon. In chronic cases or in cases where the disease has healed, the mucosa shows atrophy with flattening of the surface and becomes featureless. The serosa usually shows no abnormal features except in cases of toxic megacolon where the bowel wall is massively dilated and the wall is very thin and liable to perforate [54]. In this case, distinguishing UC from CD becomes difficult macroscopically or even, indeed, microscopically. In one study, the surgeons and pathologists failed to accurately differentiate UC from CD intra-operatively and on examining the gross appearance in the 198 patients entered in the study, they concluded that the distinction between the two conditions should not be made macroscopically [56]. In the same study, cobblestone mucosa was most common in Crohn's disease and inflammatory polyps were commonly seen in ulcerative colitis; however, there was considerable overlap, and a similar incidence of strictures and skip lesions occurring in both diseases.

In CD, every organ in the gastrointestinal tract can be involved from the mouth to the anus; however small intestinal involvement can occur between 25–50% of cases. The most distinguishing feature of CD is that it is a discontinuous disease and grossly demonstrated by a sharp demarcation between uninvolved and diseased segments commonly called 'skip lesions' [57]. The diseased bowel shows thickened, fibrotic, dull brown, granular and hyperaemic serosal surface that is sometimes covered by exudate. Fibrous adhesions between the small bowel loops are often present. The mesenteric fat usually wraps around the bowel (creeping fat), which has been shown to correlate with transmural inflammation [58]. The wall of the intestine is commonly thick and rubbery, which often leads to a narrow lumen that shows the characteristic radiological "string sign". The mucosa shows focal ulceration with oedema and loss of a normal appearance. Serpentine linear and

TRAFFORD HEALTHCARE NHS TRUST **DEPARTMENT OF HISTOPATHOLOGY**

Surname: Forename: Sex: D.o.B:
Consultant: GP: Source: Case Note No:
Pathologist: Lab Number: Copy For:

I Present Clinical Episode

Date of Onset: / ./ Duration: days
Main symptoms:
1) Diarrhoea Watery ĩ Bloody ĩ
2)

3)

4)

III Radiological Features
Procedure(s) : Findings :
1)

2)

Radiologist impression:

IV Lab and Microbiology
1- Stool test:
2- Stool culture:
3- Blood test:

II Endoscopy Findings
Procedure : Date: / /

Biopsy site(s):

Mucosal Features:

Extent of disease:

Pattern: Focal □ Segmental □ Continuous □ Skip □
Pancolitis □

Severity: Mild □ Moderate □ Extensive □.
Suspicion of neoplasia: □

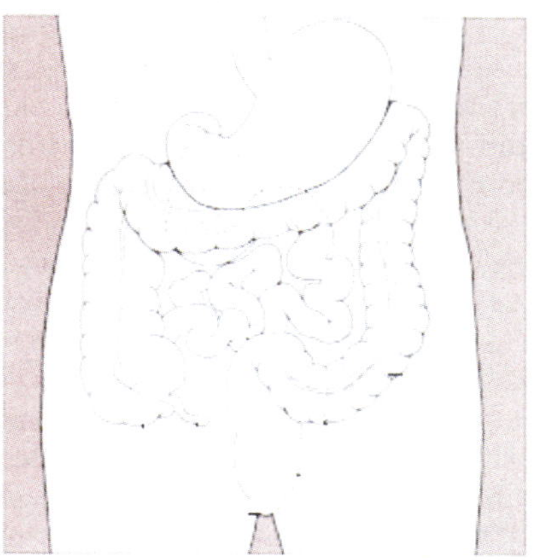

V Disease History
Total duration: ________ days/months.

Duration type: Persistent □ Remittent □ .

Previous Biopsy: Yes □ No □

Treatment:
- Surgery:

- Radiotherapy:

- Chemotherapy:

- Medicines:

- Others:

VI Additional information (if Appropriate)
□ Other disease(s) present
□ Previous GI surgery
□ Familial history

VII Clinical impression: ....
Differential Diagnoses :
i)
ii)
iii)

VIII Microscopy
Focal □ Continuous □ Discontinuous □

Activity: Absent □ Mild □ Moderate □ Severe □

Features of Chronicity : Present □ Absent □

Probable Diagnosis :
Crohn's Disease □ Ulcerative Colitis □
Infective Colitis □ Transient Colitis □
Microscopic / Collagenous / Lymphocytic Colitis □

Other Comments:..
....

Fig. 1. Trafford General Hospital gastrointestinal reporting proforma discontinuous ulcers develop along the long axis of the bowel with the intervening unremarkable mucosa sometimes connected by short transverse ulcers leading to the cobblestone appearance [57]. Fissures commonly develop which penetrate deeply to cause serositis. Thus sinuses and fistulas are common features of this disease [54]. Villiform inflammatory/hyperplastic polyps are sometimes seen in CD [59].

Microscopic Features of IBD

Changes in UC usually begin in the rectum and may extend proximally to involve a variable length of and sometimes, the entire colon (pancolitis). The mucosa shows intense and diffuse inflammatory cell infiltrate, crypt abscesses, mucin depletion and surface ulceration, especially in active colitis where it is characterised predominantly by cryptitis (neutrophils into crypt epithelium), and crypt abscesses (neutrophils within the crypt lumen) [54]. Superficial broad ulcerations occur and, when severe, can extend into the muscularis propria. Paneth cell metaplasia is also a feature. The inflammation is mainly mucosal and the infiltrate is mainly composed of mononuclear cells, including lymphocytes (many of which are activated T lymphocytes), plasma cells with occasional eosinophils and mast cells together with neutrophil polymorphs [60, 61]. There is marked mucin depletion of the crypts (goblet cell depletion), resulting from both atrophic and regenerative changes [54, 62].

It is important to realize that polymorph nuclear infiltrate in the crypts or the surface epithelium is associated with mucous depletion and this is indicative of the disease activity index and has no specific diagnostic attributes. Architectural distortion of crypts is the hallmark of IBD in which the surface attains villiform configuration with the crypts exhibiting irregularity with abnormal branching. The degree of architectural distortion is usually more severe in UC than in CD.

Architectural disarray, Paneth cell metaplasia, pseudo-pyloric metaplasia, villiform configuration of the surface epithelium, dense chronic inflammatory cell infiltrate of the deeper aspect of the lamina propria and the so-called 'ilealisation' of the colonic epithelium, constitute the cardinal features of chronicity in IBD but also can be seen to a variable degree in some other forms of chronic irritation and injury like in radiation, diversion, chronic ischemia.

Epithelioid granulomas together with multinucleated giant cells are characteristically not seen in UC. However, intramucosal leakage granulomas in close association with crypt rupture can be evident in this disease. On the other hand, isolated giant cells and well-defined epithelioid granulomas that are distant from the crypts in a biopsy showing features of chronicity are a strong indicator of a diagnosis of Crohn's disease [63]. The mucosa sometimes contains dilated blood vessels some of which may contain thrombi [64]. Features of endarteritis obliterans are seen in submucosal vessels and the muscularis mucosa may appear reduplicated [65]. In quiescent disease the mucosa may appear nearly normal with slight crypt distortion and presence of Paneth cells and very occasional neutrophils in the lamina propria [66]. As mentioned earlier, if the rectal biopsy appears normal, a diagnosis of UC is unlikely. However, subtle inflammatory changes can occur, especially if the patient is a child or if the disease has been treated with steroids [67, 68].

Colitis Indeterminate

The condition known now as colitis indeterminate or indeterminate colitis (IC) was first described by Ashley Price in 1978. He found that 9% of resected colon from patients with IBD in his series did not show enough diagnostic features to enable a definitive diagnosis of UC or CD and that 90% of these cases had undergone emergency surgery [69]. Subsequent publications confirmed the condition and quoted the incidence as being between 4–15%. There are, however, two areas of possible confusion in regards to this condition. The first is the terminology, as many synonyms have been given or substituted for IC like toxic dilatation, fulminant colitis and disintegrative colitis [70]. Although these entities may be descriptive, they have been associated with conditions other than IBD such as infection and occasionally ischaemia [71]. Therefore, it is inappropriate to use them synonymously with IC.

The second problem regards that of definition. Over the years, the term IC itself has undergone changes in definition and the term has been used liberally in different situations or institutions. When it was first described by Price, it only included surgical specimens of the colon that were mostly generated from emergency procedures. Therefore, strictly speaking, it was used as a condition which usually presents as an emergency and the pathologist is unable to distinguish between UC and CD after colectomy due to the overlap in pathological features. Since then, Kangas et al. have defined the condition as regarding "patients who had the clinical and the macroscopical features of either CD or UC both pre- and post-operatively and the histology remains indeterminate both pre- and post-operatively". This definition refers to mucosal biopsies and not to surgical resectates in conditions which are not necessarily presenting as an emergency, and is a significant variance from the original definition [72]. A third definition came from the Mayo Clinic which defines IC as "the unequivocal diagnosis of UC pre-operatively but inconclusive histology on examination of the pathologic specimens intra-operatively" [73]. Prior to that, Koultun et al. [74] defined the condition as "inflammatory colitis containing features in macroscopic and microscopic evaluation of the colon that were consistent with both CD and UC". To confuse the issue further, Price has subsequently redefined the condition as "the inability to make a confident diagnosis of the pattern of colitis despite examination of adequate surgical resectates or adequate mucosal biopsy series from the colon and rectum" [75]. It is possible, therefore, to see why the outcome of these condition(s) varies from series to series as they use different diagnostic criteria. In our unit, we use the original Price definition of 1978. It has been suggested that up to two thirds of patients diagnosed initially as IC will polarise after long-time follow-up into either UC or CD after careful appraisal of all available evidence and close clinicopathological correlation [76]. Often the history, clinical correlation and further investigations like rectal stump biopsy may show diagnostic features.

There is a strong clinical need to classify patients either as UC or CD since this affects the patient's management (pouch procedure is generally unsuitable for CD patients). Recent studies showed that about 20% of IC patients develop severe pouch complications and this incidence is between that of UC (8–10%) and CD (30–40%), and the overall literature suggests that IC patients have a similar outcome as those with UC [77, 78]. It is recommended, as said previously, that the term IC be reserved for colectomy specimens where the distinction between UC and CD is not possible, and that it not be used in endoscopic biopsies; however, in cases where the distinction is not possible, some use the term 'IBD not yet classified' [79].

Using the original Price definition macroscopically, the specimen usually shows total colitis, sometimes with macroscopic rectal sparing, and there is usually a varying degree of colonic dilatation. Microscopically, it shows severe disease with transmural inflammation, severe ulceration, fissuring or clefts, myocytolysis with intact islands of surviving mucosa showing minimal inflammation, intense congestion and a regular glandular pattern [69, 70, 72, 76, 80].

Pathological Considerations

The clinical history provided by the clinicians is of utmost importance to the histopathologist. It is particularly relevant in gastrointestinal pathology when assessing biopsies suspected of IBD. Due to the very many mimics of IBD, we regard IBD as strictly a clinicopathological diagnosis in which the clinician and the pathologist must shoulder the responsibility in the right cooperative environment. A great improvement in the diagnosis can be achieved by a positive interaction between the pathologist and the gastroenterologist. In addition, multiple colonic biopsies have been shown by many studies to be far superior in arriving at a diagnosis than a single biopsy. It is imperative to emphasise again that the final diagnosis usually depends on the collaboration of all data including pathologic, radiologic, clinical features and endoscopic [81].

Several studies have shown that the histological appearances are not alone sufficient in predicting the diagnosis in up to 30% of cases of UC and 60% of CD [82]. When reporting endoscopic biopsies for a suspected IBD, it is important to assess certain parameters in reaching the diagnosis such as mucosal architecture, lamina propria cellularity, neutrophil polymorph infiltration and epithelial changes.

Increase in intraepithelial lymphocytes, presence of thickened subepithelial collagen, and changes of mucosal prolapse should be excluded before reporting the biopsy as normal [53]. It is crucial that the reporting pathologist should be familiar with the normality in large bowel biopsies and changes accepted to be within normal limits. The normal surface of the large bowel is almost flat and in IBD the surface may be irregular and sometime attain a villiform architecture; however, normal crypt architecture does not entirely exclude the diagnosis of IBD [46, 83]. Most of the times, in a resected specimen, normal architecture can be found overlying a fragmented or duplicated muscularis mucosa which clearly indicates previous mucosal damage; thus, a clinical history, especially of IBD, is crucial in these types of biopsies for arriving at the correct diagnosis rather than reporting the biopsy as normal [84].

In UC, one of the most differentiating features from CD is that the inflammation is mainly mucosal but sometimes spills over into the submucosa, thus it is usually assessable by endoscopic biopsies [81]. The crypts in UC are classically infiltrated by neutrophil polymorphs in a uniform manner; therefore, any isolated involvement of crypts and spared mucosa is strongly suggestive of CD [84]. One has to keep in mind that neutrophil polymorph infiltration does not have to be an indication of inflammatory changes, because vigorous bowel preparation can lead to mild neutrophil polymorph infiltration within crypts, and also occasional polymorphs within otherwise normal lamina propria are not uncommon [85].

Diffuse crypt abscess is highly suggestive of UC

over CD; however, focal crypt abscess formation can occur in UC, CD and infectious colitis [54]. Focal erosions on a background of a relatively unremarkable mucosa should raise the possibility of CD [84]. Diverticular colitis should be kept in mind whenever sigmoid colitis resembling UC but with rectal sparing is seen [84].

In a normal large bowel, the crypts are straight, parallel and extend from above the muscularis mucosae into the surface. However, some normal variations are seen in the region of lymphoid follicles [85]. The average 1 mm length of muscularis mucosa should normally contain seven to eight crypts, which are usually closely packed [53]. In IBD, this number will be reduced to an average of three to five per 1 mm of muscularis mucosae and the crypts are usually short and irregular in shape [83]. However, increased spacing between crypts is normally seen in the caecum and distal rectum and should not be confused with inactive IBD.

Crypt branching is commonly seen in IBD; however, some focal crypt branching (less than 10% of all crypts) is not uncommon but two or more abnormally branching crypts within 2 mm of muscularis mucosae is regarded as abnormal [86]. Lamina propria should be assessed for changes in cellularity and the presence of granulomas. In normal lamina propria, inflammatory cells are more concentrated in the upper third than the lower third together with some lymphoid follicles, which may occupy the full thickness of the lamina propria. In contrast to IBD where basal plasmacytosis is common [83, 87].

Muciphages are commonly seen in large-bowel biopsies examined for IBD and some authors suggest that they reflect previous occult and clinically unimportant mucosal damage and that, in an otherwise normal colorectal mucosa, they have no diagnostic significance [88, 89]. Granulomas in intestinal biopsies are classically linked to CD; however, a well-formed epithelioid granuloma is a specific but non-sensitive feature of CD, being seen in up to 50% of cases and in as few as 18% of CD [90]. Mucin depletion is a non-specific feature of IBD, but the presence of severe mucin/goblet cell depletion occurs more in UC than CD [91].

Paneth cell metaplasia together with pseudopyloric metaplasia (cells of the ulcer-associated cell lineage) appears in epithelium, which has been subjected to chronic insults, but their diagnostic value is unclear. Paneth cells can be seen in colonic crypts in inflammatory bowel disease; however, one should be wary of the fact that Paneth cells can be a normal finding in biopsies from the caecum and ascending colon [92].

In UC, changes resembling features of a hyperplastic polyp is sometimes seen [93]. Artefacts such as effects of bowel preparation and trauma to the biopsy can produce certain changes which can be confused with features of IBD. Bowel preparation can produce a mild increase in the number of mitotic figures, causing surface degeneration with increased apoptotic bodies within the crypt epithelium. It can also lead to mild neutrophilic infiltrate within the glands together with some degree of goblet cell depletion [92, 94, 53].

In defining the accuracy of diagnosis in IBD, it has been shown that multiple colonic biopsies give the best diagnostic improvement and it has also been shown that, in the interpretation of large-bowel biopsies, there is no significant difference between expert and non-expert pathologists [29, 30].

A constellation of features such as the presence of granulomas, especially submucosal, focal or patchy inflammation and discontinuous crypt distortion helps in diagnosing CD. For UC, the symptoms are diffuse crypt distortion, diffuse cryptitis, basally concentrated chronic inflammatory cell infiltrate, reduced crypt numbers, severe architectural distortion, villous surface, severe diffuse transmucosal lamina propria inflammation and mucin depletion are highly suggestive of the disease [95, 53]. An appendiceal involvement is rare in cases of total colitis and more common as a skip lesion in distal colitis especially in UC [96, 97].

IBD and its Mimics

It is important to differentiate features of IBD from mimics, especially regarding whether they are features of chronicity or not. Those in which there are no histological features of chronicity could be seen in etiologies like infective, transient and antibiotic-related-type colitides. Those which may exhibit features of chronicity include ischemia, radiation and diversion colitides.

It is also important to realise that in the event of having a series of biopsies in a patient with active disease but no features of chronicity, we recommend another series of biopsies in 6-weeks time because most of the infective colitides or other causes of active disease will revert back to normal, whereas IBD in the early stage of evolution may not. It is also important to appreciate that patients with chronic IBD may not have histological features of chronicity; in this instance the pathologist should not exclude such a diagnosis.

Endoscopic biopsy plays an important role in the diagnosis of infective type colitis, because in a high number of cases the causative organism is not found [98]. This is called transient or self-limiting colitis. Diagnosis of infective colitis depends heavily on the absence of features seen in IBD, especially absence of architectural distortion and a diffuse increase in inflammatory cells. Architectural distortion, together with transmural increase in lamina propria cellularity and epithelial changes, are more common in IBD than infective type colitis. On the other hand, preservation of crypt architecture, superficial increase in lamina propria cellularity with neutrophil infiltration is suggestive of infective etiology [54]. Some forms of chronic intestinal infection, e.g. shigellosis, amoebiasis and yersinia may resemble features seen in IBD [99].

In the first attack of IBD, the distinction from infective-type colitis is difficult and features depend on the timing of diseases [61]. Florid neutrophilic infiltrate is characteristically seen in the first 2 weeks of infective colitis [100, 40]. Even poorly formed microgranulomas can be seen in certain infections like salmonella [101]. The most useful histological features of infective colitis on endoscopic biopsy are the predominance of acute over chronic inflammation, lack of crypt distortion and the occurrence of oedema and neutrophil polymorph infiltration within the lamina propria and the crypt epithelium rather than the lumen [102, 74].

Drugs, especially non-steroidal anti-inflammatory drugs (NSAIDs), have also been known to cause colitis, the features of which can be confused with IBD, and the elderly seem to be at a higher risk [102]. Thus a drug history is mandatory when investigating patients with suspected IBD. Non-steroidal anti-inflammatory drugs (NSAIDs) can cause small-intestinal ulceration together with mucosal inflammation and colonic ulcerations. Other drugs such as methyldopa and gold treatment can also be complicated by colitis [103–106]. Colitis associated with diverticular disease of the sigmoid is a well-recognised feature and can be mistaken for features of IBD. Mucosal biopsies from an area of inflammation associated with diverticular disease may show features of crypt distortion, basal plasmacytosis, cryptitis and even crypt abscesses [107]. CD-like changes in the sigmoid of a patient with diverticular disease are an idiosyncratic inflammatory response to the diverticulosis rather than to coexistent CD. Pathologists should be wary of making the diagnosis of sigmoid CD in the context of diverticular disease unless there is CD in other parts of the bowel [108].

Microscopic colitis (collagenous and lymphocytic) are characterised by distinct histological and clinical presentation and should not ideally be confused with changes seen in IBD. However, lymphocytic and collagenous colitis patterns of injury preceded the eventual clinical diagnosis of CD in one study [109].

Summary

1. IBD is a common disease of the industrialised world and getting more common in the developing world.
2. The best platform for diagnosing IBD is in the CPC. Short of that, use of the proforma is highly recommended.
3. The final diagnosis of IBD is the mutual responsibility of the clinician and the pathologist.
4. There are many histological mimics of IBD.
5. There is no histological feature that is seen in UC which is not present CD.

References

1. Podolsky DK (2002) Inflammatory bowel disease. N Engl J Med 8 347(6):417–429
2. Carter MJ, Lobo AJ, Travis SP (2004) British Society of Gastroenterology: guidelines for the management of inflammatory bowel disease in adults. Gut 53(Suppl 5):1–16
3. Al-Shamali MA, Kalaoui M, Patty I et al (2003) Ulcerative colitis in Kuwait: a review of 90 cases. Digestion 67(4):218–224
4. Orholm M, Munkholm P, Langholz E et al (1991) Familial occurrence of inflammatory bowel disease. N Engl J Med 324(2):84–88
5. Tysk C, Lindberg E, Jarnerot G et al (1988) Ulcerative colitis and Crohn's disease in an unselected population of monozygotic and dizygotic twins: a study of heritability and the influence of smoking. Gut 29(7):990–996
6. Mir-Madjlessi SH, Michener WM, Farmer RG (1986) Course and prognosis of idiopathic ulcerative proctosigmoiditis in young patients. J Pediatr Gastroenterol Nutr 5(4):571–575
7. Brocklehurst JC (1985) Colonic disease in the elderly. Clin Gastroenterol 14(4):725–747
8. Markowitz J, Grancher K, Rosa J et al (1993) Growth failure in pediatric inflammatory bowel disease. J Pediatr Gastroenterol Nutr 16(4):373–380
9. Lewkonia RM, McConnell RB (1976) Familial inflammatory bowel disease: heredity or environment? Gut 17(3):235–241
10. Roth MP, Petersen GM, McElree C et al (1989) Geographic origins of Jewish patients with inflammatory bowel disease. Gastroenterology 97(4):900–904
11. McKay DM (1999) Intestinal inflammation and the gut microflora. Can J Gastroenterol 13(6):509–516
12. Evans JM, McMahon AD, Murray FE et al (1997) Non-steroidal anti-inflammatory drugs are associated with emergency admission to hospital for colitis due to inflammatory bowel disease. Gut 4(5):619–622
13. Andersson RE, Olaison G, Tysk C, Ekbom A (2001) Appendectomy and protection against ulcerative colitis. N Engl J Med 344(11):808–814
14. Garrett VD, Brantley PJ, Jones GN et al (1991) The relation between daily stress and Crohn's disease. J Behav Med 14(1):87–96

15. Duffy LC, Zielezny MA, Marshall JR et al (1991) Relevance of major stress events as an indicator of disease activity prevalence in inflammatory bowel disease. Behav Med 17(3):101–110
16. Salem SN, Shubair KS (1967) Non-specific ulcerative colitis in Bedouin Arabs. Lancet 1(7488):473–475
17. Rubin DT, Hanauer SB (2000) Smoking and inflammatory bowel disease. Eur J Gastroenterol Hepatol 12(8):855–862
18. Ahmad T, Satsangi J, McGovern D et al (2001) The genetics of inflammatory bowel disease. Aliment Pharmacol Ther 15(6):731–748
19. Satsangi J, Rosenberg WMC, Jewell DP (1994) The prevalence of inflammatory bowel disease in relatives of patients with Crohn's disease. Eur J Gastroenterol Hepatol 6:413–416
20. Russell RK, Wilson DC, Satsangi J (2004) Unravelling the complex genetics of inflammatory bowel disease. Arch Dis Child 89(7):598–603
21. Hugot JP, Laurent-Puig P, Gower-Rousseau C et al (1996) Mapping of a susceptibility locus for Crohn's disease on chromosome 16. Nature 379(6568):821–823
22. Hugot JP, Chamaillard M, Zouali H et al (2001) Association of NOD2 leucine-rich repeat variants with susceptibility to Crohn's disease. Nature 411(6837):599–603
23. Ahmad T, Armuzzi A, Bunce M et al (2002) The molecular classification of the clinical manifestations of Crohn's disease. Gastroenterology 122(4):854–866
24. Satsangi J, Welsh KI, Bunce M et al (1996) Contribution of genes of the major histocompatibility complex to susceptibility and disease phenotype in inflammatory bowel disease. Lancet 347(9010):1212–1217
25. Riley SA, Mani V, Goodman MJ et al (1991) Microscopic activity in ulcerative colitis: What does it mean? 32:174–178
26. Shepherd NA (2002) Granuloma in the diagnosis of intestinal Crohn's disease: a myth exploded? Histopathology 41:166–168
27. Tanaka M, Riddell RH, Saito H et al (1999) Morphologic criteria applicable to biopsy specimens/an effective distinction of inflammatory bowel disease from other forms of colitis and of Crohn's disease from ulcerative colitis. Scand J Gastroenterology 1:56–67
28. Haboubi NY, Kamal F (2001) Non-specific colitis, is it a justifiable diagnosis? Colorectal Dis 3:263–265
29. Bentley E, Jenkins D, Campbell F et al (2002) How could pathologists improve the initial diagnosis of colitis? Evidence from an international workshop. J Clin Pathol 55(12):955–960
30. Haboubi NJ, Schofield PF (1994) Large bowel biopsies in colitis: a clinico-pathological correlation. J Royal Soc Med 87:16–17
31. Haboubi NY, Shaath NM, Safarani MN et al (2004) Improved diagnostic accuracy of inflammatory bowel disease: a clinicopathological collaborative approach. Tech Coloproctol 8:117–121
32. Fociani P, Carsana L, Zerbi P et al (2003) Histopathological differential diagnosis in inflammatory bowel diseases. Ann Ital Chir 74(6):641–649
33. Tamboli CP, Neut C, Desreumaux P et al (2004) Diagnosis in inflammatory bowel disease. Gut 53:1–4
34. Wada Y, Matsui T, Matake H et al (2003) Intractable ulcerative colitis caused by cytomegalovirus infection. Dis Colon Rectum 46:10:S59–S65
35. Kleer C, Appleman H (1988) Ulcerative colitis, patterns of involvement in colorectal biopsies and changes with time. Am J Surg Path 22(8):983–989
36. Gimes P, Du Boulay C, Smith CL et al (1986) Relationship between disease activity and colonoscopic findings in patients with colonic inflammatory bowel disease. Gut 27:92–95
37. Ectors N, Deiessen A, Gebose K (1998) Reversibilite des lesion histologiques. Acta Endoscopica 28:221–232
38. Bernstein C, Shanahan F, Anton P et al (1995) Patchiness of mucosal inflammation in treated ulcerative colitis. Gastrointest Endosc 42:232–237
39. Haboubi NJ, Kaftan S, Scofield PF (1992) Radiation colitis is another mimic of chronic inflammatory bowel disease. J Clin Pathol 45:272
40. Shepherd NA (1991) Pathological mimics of chronic inflammatory bowel disease. J Clin Pathol 44:726–733
41. Schumacher G, Kollberg B, Sandstedt B (1994) A prospective study of first attacks of inflammatory bowel disease and infectious colitis. Scand J Gastroenterol 29:318–332
42. Yoshihisa T, Tsuyoshi T (2004) Prevalence of cytomegalovirus infection in inflammatory bowel disease patients. Dis Colon Rectum 47:722–726
43. Shirandana S, Hordijk ML, Tenkute F et al (1991) Differential diagnosis of inflammatory bowel disease: a comparison of various diagnostic classifications. Scand J Gastroenterol 26:167–173
44. Glickman JN, Bousvaros A, Farraye FA et al (2004) Pediatric patients with untreated ulcerative colitis may present initially with unusual morphologic findings. Am J Surg Pathol 28(2):190–7
45. D'Haens G, Geboes K, Pters M et al (1997) Patchy cecal inflammation associated with distal ulcerative colitis: a prospective endoscopic study. Am J Gastroenterol 8:1275–1279
46. Odze R, Antonioli D, Peppercorn M et al (1993) Effect of topical 5-aminosalicylic acid (5-ASA) therapy on rectal mucosal biopsy morphology in chronic ulcerative colitis. Am J Surg Pathol 17(9):869–75
47. Gasche C, Scholmerich J, Brynskov J et al (2000) A simple classification of Crohn's disease: report of the Working Party for the World Congresses of Gastroenterology, Vienna 1998. Inflamm Bowel Dis 6(1):8–15
48. Fedorak RN (2004) Is it time to re-classify Crohn's disease? Best Pract Res Clin Gastroenterol 18(Suppl):99–106
49. Silverberg MS, Satsangi J, Ahmad T et al (2005) Toward an integrated clinical, molecular and serological classification of inflammatory bowel disease: report of the Working Party of the 2005 Montreal World Congress of Gastroenterology. Can J Gastroenterol 19(Suppl A):5–36
50. McBroom HM, Ramsay AD (1993) The clinicopathological meeting: a means of auditing diagnostic performance. Am J Surg Pathol 17:75–80
51. Absar S, Mason J, Anjum K Haboubi N (2006) A new combined endoscopy and histology form: an attempt to increase the rate of accurate pathological diagnosis in inflammatory bowel disease, a follow-up. Tech Coloproctol (in press)
52. Gebose K, Riddell R, Ost A et al (2000) A reproducible grading scale for histopathological assessment in

ulcerative colitis. Gut 47:404–410

53. Jenkins D, Balsitis M, Gallivan S et al (1997) Guidelines for the initial biopsy diagnosis of suspected chronic idiopathic inflammatory bowel disease. J Clin Pathol 50(2):93–105
54. Fenoglio-Preiser CM, Noffsinger AE, Lantz PE et al (1999) Gastrointestinal pathology, an atlas and text. 2nd edition, Lippincott, Philadelphia
55. Kelly JK, Langevin JM, Price LM et al (1986) Giant and symptomatic inflammatory polyps of the colon in idiopathic inflammatory bowel disease. Am J Surg Pathol 10(6):420–8
56. Palnaes Hansen C, Hegnhoj J, Moller A et al (1990) Ulcerative colitis and Crohn's disease of the colon. Is there a macroscopic difference? Ann Chir Gynaecol 79(2):78–81
57. Lockhart-Mummery He, Morson BC (1964) Crohn's disease of the large intestine. Gut 19:493–509
58. Sheehan AL, Warren BF, Gear MW et al (1992) Fat-wrapping in Crohn's disease: pathological basis and relevance to surgical practice. Br J Surg 79(9):955–958
59. Rozenbajgier C, Ruck P, Jenss H et al (1992) Filiform polyposis: a case report describing clinical, morphological, and immunohistochemical findings. Clin Investig 70(6):520–528
60. Bischoff SC, Wedemeyer J, Herrmann A et al (1996) Quantitative assessment of intestinal eosinophils and mast cells in inflammatory bowel disease. Histopathology 28(1):1–13
61. Haruta J, Kusugami K, Kuroiwa A et al (1992) Phenotypic and functional analysis of lamina propria mononuclear cells from colonoscopic biopsy specimens in patients with ulcerative colitis. Am J Gastroenterol 87(4):448–454
62. Renison DM, Forouhar FA, Levine JB et al (1983) Filiform polyposis of the colon presenting as massive hemorrhage: an uncommon complication of Crohn's disease. Am J Gastroenterol 78(7):413–416
63. Mahadeva U, Martin JP, Patel NK et al (2002) Granulomatous ulcerative colitis: a re-appraisal of the mucosal granuloma in the distinction of Crohn's disease from ulcerative colitis. Histopathology 41(1):50–55
64. L Dhillon AP, Anthony A, Sim R et al (1992) Mucosal capillary thrombi in rectal biopsies. Histopathology 21(2):127–133
65. Soundy VC, Davies SE, Warren BF (1998) The double muscularis mucosa in ulcerative colitis: Is it all new? Histopathology 32(5):484–5
66. Riddell RH, Goldman H, Ransohoff DF et al (1983) Dysplasia in inflammatory bowel disease: standardized classification with provisional clinical applications. Hum Pathol 14(11):931–968
67. Markowitz J, Kahn E, Grancher K et al (1993) Atypical rectosigmoid histology in children with newly diagnosed ulcerative Colitis. Am J Gastroenterol 88(12):2034–2037
68. Morson B (1970) Current concepts of colitis. Trans Med Soc Lond 86:159–176
69. Price AB (1978) Overlap in the spectrum of non-specific inflammatory bowel disease "Colitis indeterminate". J Clin Pathol 31:567–577
70. Meucci G, Bortoli A, riccioli FA et al (1999) Frequency and clinical evolution of indeterminate colitis: a retrospective multicentre stiudy in northern Italy. Eur J Gastroenterol Hepatol 11:909–913
71. Carr ND, Wells S, Haboubi NY et al (1986) Ischaemic dilatation of the colon. Ann R Coll Surg Engl 68:264–266
72. Kangas E, Matikainen M, Mattila J (1994) Is "indeterminate colitis" Crohn's disease in the long-term follow-up? Int Surg 79(2):120–123
73. McIntyre PB, Pemberton JH, Wolf BG et al (1995) Indeterminate colitis: long-term outcome in patients after ileal pouch-anal anastomosis. Dis Colon Rectum 38:51–54
74. Koultun WA, Schoetz DJ Jr, Roberts PL et al (1991) Indeterminate colitis predisposes to perineal complications after ileal pouch: anal anastomosis. Dis Colon Rectum 34:857–860
75. Price AB (1996) Indeterminate colitis-broadening the perspective. Curr Diagnos Pathol 3:35–44
76. Wells AD, Mcmillan I, Price AB et al (1991) Natural history of indeterminate colitis. Br J Surg 78:179–81
77. Marcello PW, Schoetz DJ Jr, Roberts PL et al (1997) Evolutionary changes in the pathologic diagnosis after the ileoanal pouch procedure. Dis Colon Rectum 40(3):263–269
78. Yu CS, Pemberton JH, Larson D (2000) Ileal pouch-anal anastomosis in patients with indeterminate colitis: long-term results. Dis Colon Rectum 43(11):1487–1496
79. Geboes K, Villanacci V (2005) Terminology for the diagnosis of colitis. J Clin Pathol 58(11):1133–1134
80. Haboubi NY (2001) Colitis indeterminate. Colorectal Dis 3:147–148
81. Fiocca R, Ceppa P (2003) Endoscopic biopsies. J Clin Pathol 56(5):321–322
82. Frei JV, Morson BC (1982) Medical audit of rectal biopsy diagnosis of inflammatory bowel disease. J Clin Pathol 35(3):341–344
83. Jenkins D, Goodall A, Drew K et al (1988) What is colitis? Statistical approach to distinguishing clinically important inflammatory change in rectal biopsy specimens. J Clin Pathol 41(1):72–79
84. Riddell R, Montgomery E (2004) Traps in the diagnosis of ulcerative colitis. Pathol Case Rev 9(3):87–92
85. Levine DS, Haggitt RC (1989) Normal histology of the colon. Am J Surg Pathol 13(11):966–84
86. Goodman MJ, Kirsner JB, Riddell RH (1977) Usefulness of rectal biopsy in inflammatory bowel disease. Gastroenterology 72(5):952–6)
87. O'Leary AD, Sweeney EC (1986) Lymphoglandular complexes of the colon: structure and distribution. Histopathology 10(3):267–83
88. Shepherd NA (2000) What is the significance of muciphages in colorectal biopsies? Muciphages and other mucosal accumulations in the colorectal mucosa. Histopathology 36(6):559–562
89. Bejarano PA, Aranda-Michel J, Fenoglio-Preiser C (2000) Histochemical and immunohistochemical characterization of foamy histiocytes (muciphages and xanthelasma) of the rectum. Am J Surg Pathol 24(7):1009–1015
90. Korelitz BI, Sommers SC (1977) Rectal biopsy in patients with Crohn's disease: normal mucosa on sigmoidoscopic examination. JAMA 237(25):2742–2744
91. Seldenrijk CA, Morson BC, Meuwissen SG et al (1991) Histopathological evaluation of colonic mucosal biop-

sy specimens in chronic inflammatory bowel disease: diagnostic implications. Gut 32(12):1514–1520
92. Goldman H, Antonioli DA (1982) Mucosal biopsy of the rectum, colon, and distal ileum. Hum Pathol 13(11):981–1012
93. Franzin G, Grigioni WF, Dina R et al (1983) Mucin secretion and morphological changes of the mucosa in non-neoplastic diseases of the colon. Histopathology 7(5):707–718
94. Saunders DR, Haggitt RC, Kimmey MB et al (1990) Morphological consequences of bisacodyl on normal human rectal mucosa: effect of a prostaglandin E1 analog on mucosal injury. Gastrointest Endosc 36(2):101–104
95. Surawicz CM (1987) Diagnosing colitis: biopsy is best. Gastroenterology 92(2):538–540
96. Scott IS, Sheaff M, Coumbe A et al (1998) Appendiceal inflammation in ulcerative colitis. Histopathology 33(2):168-173
97. Yang SK, Jung HY, Kang GH et al (1999) Appendiceal orifice inflammation as a skip lesion in ulcerative colitis: an analysis in relation to medical therapy and disease extent. Gastrointest Endosc 49(6):743-747
98. Kumar NB, Nostrant TT, Appelman HD (1982) The histopathologic spectrum of acute self-limited colitis (acute infectious-type colitis). Am J Surg Pathol 6(6):523–529
99. Dronfield MW, Fletcher J, Langman MJ (1974) Coincident salmonella infections and ulcerative colitis: problems of recognition and management. BMJ (898):99–100
100. Nostrant TT, Kumar NB, Appelman HD (1987) Histopathology differentiates acute self-limited colitis from ulcerative colitis. Gastroenterology 92(2):318–328
101. Day DW, Mandal BK, Morson BC (1978) The rectal biopsy appearances in Salmonella colitis. Histopathology 2(2):117–131
102. Gibson GR, Whitacre EB, Ricotti CA (1992) Colitis induced by non-steroidal anti-inflammatory drugs (NSAIDS): report of four cases and a review of the literature. Arch Intern Med 152(3):625–632
103. Lang J, Price AB, Levi AJ et al (1988) Diaphragm disease: pathology of disease of the small intestine induced by non-steroidal anti-inflammatory drugs. J Clin Pathol 41(5):516–526
104. Sheers R, Williams WR (1989) NSAIDs and gut damage. Lancet 2(8672):1154
105. Graham CF, Gallagher K, Jones JK (1981) Acute colitis with methyldopa. N Engl J Med 304(17):1044–1045
106. Martin DM, Goldman JA, Gilliam J et al (1981) Gold-induced eosinophilic enterocolitis: response to oral cromolyn sodium. Gastroenterology 80(6):1567–1570
107. Makapugay LM, Dean PJ (1996) Diverticular disease: associated chronic colitis. Am J Surg Pathol 20(1):94–102
108. Goldstein NS, Leon-Armin C, Mani A (2000) Crohn's colitis-like changes in sigmoid diverticulitis specimens are usually an idiosyncratic inflammatory response to the diverticulosis rather than Crohn's colitis. Am J Surg Pathol 24(5):668–675
109. Goldstein NS, Gyorfi T (1999) Focal lymphocytic colitis and collagenous colitis: patterns of Crohn's colitis? Am J Surg Pathol 23(9):1075–1081

Dysplasia in Inflammatory Bowel Disease: from Genetics to Treatment

Emil Salmo, Patrick O'Connolly, Najib Haboubi

Introduction

The potential development of colorectal carcinoma (CRC) as a complication of either ulcerative colitis (UC) or Crohn's disease (CD) is well recognised [1]. Patients with UC have a lifetime risk, between 6–10 times that of the general population of developing CRC, whereas patients with CD develop an increased life-time risk when more than 30% of the colon has become involved [2]. The development of neoplasia, in the form of either colonic epithelial dysplasia or adenocarcinoma, appears to be related to factors such as the severity and duration of the illness, the extent of colonic involvement and the overall responsiveness to medical intervention [3, 4]. Patients at higher risk are those with UC, extensive colitis, those with disease duration of more than 10 years, those with primary sclerosing cholangitis and patients with an early age of onset of colitis [5, 6]. The risk of developing CRC as a result of longstanding CD is less than the risk faced by patients with UC in which, regardless of the extent of the colitis, the latter has been estimated as a 2% risk at 10 years, 8% at 20 years and 18% at 30 years [7]. It is assumed that CRC in patients with inflammatory bowel disease (IBD) develops, in most instances, in the background of colonic epithelial dysplasia.

This chapter looks briefly into the various definitions and classifications, pathological observations, genetic changes, types and validity of various surveillance programmes and treatment options of dysplasia complicating IBD.

Definition and Classification of Dysplasia in Ulcerative Colitis

Dysplasia is defined as an unequivocal neoplastic change that is intraepithelial and within confinement of the gland basement membrane or as an unequivocal neoplastic alteration of the colonic epithelium. It may be a marker of carcinoma or may itself be malignant and associated with invasion into the underlying tissue [8].

It is important to realise that, for a very important and practical reason, diagnosing colonic dysplasia is one of the most challenging exercises that the surgical pathologist can go through. This is because the diagnosis of dysplasia is subjective and unless the pathologist sticks to rigid criteria, the diagnosis can be either missed or misdiagnosed. For that reason the Dysplasia Morphology Study Group proposed a broad three-tiered classification scheme for the evaluation of dysplasia. This was designed to alert the pathologist to the histopathological criteria and pitfalls of diagnosing dysplasia, and also to propose treatment and surveillance strategies. The classification consisted of three main categories including (1) negative for dysplasia, (2) positive for dysplasia, either low-grade or high-grade and (3) indefinite for dysplasia (probably negative, unknown or probably positive (Table 1) [8]. The importance of such classifications at that time was to advise a follow-up strategy, which is still used by some centres today. Whilst this classification was met with general acceptance from practicing pathologists in Europe and North America, it was soon discovered that our Japanese colleagues have a lower threshold for using the term cancer in cases in which the tumour has not invaded the muscularis mucosa and to which most European and North American colleagues have given it the term dysplasia. In other words the term cancer is used by one school of practice while the other school

Table 1. Classification of dysplasia [8]

Category	Recommended follow-up
Negative	Regular 1 year
Indefinite	
Probably negative	Regular 1 year
Unknown	Short interval
Probably positive	Short interval
Positive	
Low grade	Short interval or colectomy if there is a mass
High grade	Colectomy

prefers the term dysplasia. In most centres in Europe, the term cancer, in regards to the colon, is given only when there is invasion through the biological basement membrane of the colonic epithelium, i.e. the muscularis mucosa. Malignant tumours confined to the mucosa have practically no metastatic potential and therefore we prefer not to use such a term. In 1993, the Research Committee on Inflammatory Bowel Disease of the Ministry of Health and Welfare of Japan [9] proposed a variation of the classification of Riddell et al. (Table 2); however, it was not universally used. Riddell's classification of dysplasia remained unchanged until 2000 when a group of gastrointestinal pathologists from Europe, Japan and North America gathered in Vienna to propose a new classification to bridge the huge gap between the terminologies used by the various groups. The Vienna classification categorises epithelial dysplasia, found any where in the gastrointestinal tract including the colon, as negative for dysplasia, indefinite for dysplasia, low- and high-grade mucosal neoplasia and submucosal or deeper invasion by carcinoma (Table 3) [10]. Regarding this classification, high-grade mucosal neoplasia encompassed the following categories including dysplasia, non-invasive carcinoma and suspicious for invasive carcinoma. However, intramucosal carcinoma was included in category 5 (carcinoma) of the original Vienna classification but then later was moved into category 4 (high-grade dysplasia) in the revised Vienna classification [11]. Schlemper and Iwashita subsequently summarised the revised Vienna classification in a review article in 2004 [12]. We feel that the original classification of dysplasia by Riddell et al. has stood the test of time and we recommend using it in conjunction with the revised Vienna classification [11, 12].

Table 2. Histopathological classification of neoplastic epithelium in UC [9]

Category	Description
UC-I	Inflammatory
UC-II	Indefinite
UC-II a	Probably inflammatory
UC-II b	Probably neoplastic
UC-III	Neoplastic but non invasive
UC-IV	Carcinoma

Research Committee on IBD of the Ministry of Health and Welfare of Japan

Table 3. Classification of gastrointestinal neoplasia (Vienna classification) [10]

1. Negative for dysplasia/neoplasia
2. Indefinite for dysplasia/neoplasia
3. Non-invasive low-grade neoplasia (low-grade adenoma/dysplasia)
4. Non-invasive high-grade neoplasia (high-grade adenoma/dysplasia, non-invasive carcinoma, suspicious for invasion)
5. Invasive neoplasia (intramucosal carcinoma, submucosal carcinoma or beyond)[a]

[a] In the modified Vienna classification [11, 12], intramucosal carcinoma moved to category 4.

Morphological Features

According to Riddell et al. [8] dysplasia is strictly a histopathological diagnosis and is characterised microscopically by the following histological features:

1. architectural changes often resembling colonic adenoma.
2. Cellular atypia as characterised by nuclear stratification, loss of polarity, hyperchromasia and an increase in mitotic figures. High-grade epithelial dysplasia commonly shows a greater degree of glandular architectural abnormality (complex budding and branching), with enlarged hyperchromatic nuclei with prominent nucleoli and stratification (Fig. 1).
3. The above changes are sometimes associated with the so-called 'incomplete crypt maturation'. This is characterised by a marked reduction in the number of goblet cells (or their focal absence) rendering some of the crypts containing absorptive cells only and dystrophic goblet cells (upside down rotation of goblet cells/signet ring formation).

In practice, however, the distinction between reac-

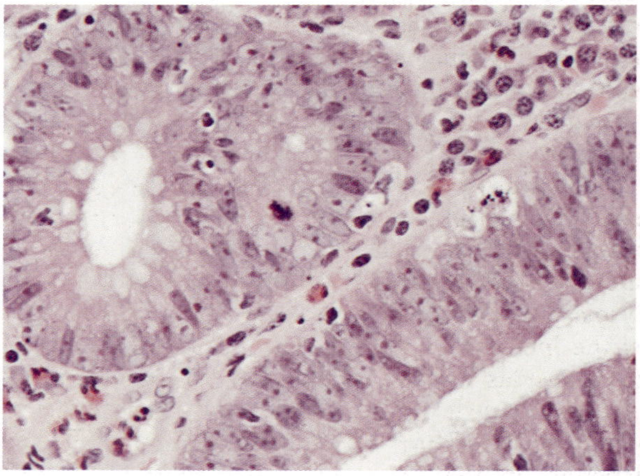

Fig. 1. Crypts showing high-grade dysplasia with nuclear stratification and pleomorphism together with numerous mitotic figures

tive and dysplastic epithelium is not always straight forward. While the dysplastic epithelium shows certain histological changes that distinguish it from normal epithelium, it is not always easy to differentiate dysplasia from the reactive type morphology seen in cases of inflammation or repair. In a reactive process, there are usually enlarged nuclei, nuclear pseudostratification but no loss of polarity and no nuclear coarse chromatin formation. They may both, however, show some degree of mucin loss together with increased density of the cytoplasm and high mitotic figures.

Macroscopically, dysplasia can be categorised as either flat or raised. The former is usually detected during random biopsies taken by conventional colonoscopy [13]. In contrast, the raised dysplastic areas are usually visible endoscopically and have been referred to as a dysplasia associated lesion or mass (DALM) [14]. Raised lesions can take many forms including plaques, polyps, velvety patches, clusters of polyps or nodular areas [13].

As mentioned earlier, the first problem encountered by the pathologist is the histologic recognition of dysplasia, and its distinction from that of a reparative process. As noted in several studies, there is a significant degree of intra- and interobserver variability in recognising dysplasia, particularly in the distinction between indefinite probably positive for dysplasia *vs.* low-grade dysplasia [15, 16]. This necessitates a well-accepted policy of diagnosing dysplasia by two different pathologists with one of them having a special interest in gastrointestinal pathology and dysplasia [16]. The distinction between high-grade dysplasia is less of an issue because the degree of concordance is better than with low-grade dysplasia [17]. The distinction between high and low-grade dysplasia bears significant consequences to the patient in some colorectal surgical units because the detection of high-grade dysplasia requires immediate intervention, which is usually colectomy, since it is associated with 40–70% of invasive carcinomas [18], while in some centres, low-grade dysplasia requires a less radical approach.

In contrast to high-grade dysplasia, some studies have shown that low-grade dysplastic change has a positive predictive value of 7–24% for development of cancer and 16–54% for progression to high-grade dysplasia in 5 years, and this has been demonstrated by the increase frequency of p53 mutation in low-grade dysplasia [19, 20]. However, there are no strict criteria for distinguishing between low and high-grade dysplasia, and the distinction between them depends on the subjective interpretation of the reporting pathologist. An active chronic colitis that shows marked reparative changes can be difficult if not impossible to differentiate from genuine dysplasia and, under such circumstances, a diagnosis of indefinite for dysplasia is warranted.

Mapping studies by Levine et al. [21] and Rutegard et al. [22] have shown that dysplasia may be localised to a small area within the colon, and may require extensive sampling beyond what is clinically or economically feasible, thus creating another hurdle in detecting the small foci of epithelial changes that may require surgical intervention.

Sporadic Adenomas vs. Dysplasia Associated Lesion/Mass (DALM)

Several different subtypes of DALMs in IBD have been described. These subtypes broadly fall into two forms, adenoma-like and non-adenoma like. This distinction is based primarily on their gross/endoscopic appearance. Non-adenoma-like lesions are usually large, sessile with a broad base, irregular masses or ill-defined nodules. To some, a biopsy finding of dysplasia in a non-adenoma-like DALM, either low or high-grade, is usually an indication for colectomy because of the high probability (between 30 to 80%) of an associated adenocarcinoma [14]. Adenoma-like DALM is present as an isolated, well-circumscribed and pedunculated adenoma-like polypoid dysplastic lesion, which is basically not unlike the appearance of a sporadic adenoma either endoscopically or macroscopically. In this instance, the clinical differential diagnosis includes an adenoma-like DALM in UC *vs.* a sporadic adenoma, a lesion that occurs coincidentally in a patient with underlying IBD.

The fact that sporadic adenomas can also arise within colons affected by IBD creates a problem in diagnosis and management. Sporadic adenoma arising in patients with IBD can sometimes be difficult if not impossible to differentiate from IBD-associated dysplasia (polypoid dysplasia). One can be confident that one is dealing with a sporadic adenoma if it is found in an area not affected by IBD (a right-sided adenoma in a patient with left-sided colitis). On the other hand, finding such a lesion in a colonic segment affected by IBD in a young age group is in favour of polypoid dysplasia rather than adenomas, as these tend to occur mostly in a middle age group or older. However, if the adenoma-like dysplastic lesion arises within an area involved by IBD, then this problem becomes much more difficult. It used to be recommended to 'judge the lesion by the company of the epithelium it keeps'. In other words, if the epithelium adjacent to the lesion is dysplastic, then the lesion is judged to be the same. We feel that is a feeble way of addressing the issue scientifically.

In an attempt to distinguish sporadic adenomas

from adenoma-like dysplastic lesions arising in IBD, studies have evaluated as to whether histologic features [23], molecular genetic studies or the location of the lesion can be used reliably to distinguish between them. Torres et al. [24] evaluated 89 polypoid adenomatous lesions from 59 patients with IBD, including 51 patients with UC and 8 patients with CD, and correlated the morphologic features of these adenoma-like lesions with clinical, endoscopic and follow-up data. If the lesion was located proximal to histologically diseased mucosa, lesions were classified as A, or probable sporadic adenomas. If they developed within an area of colitis associated with flat dysplasia or carcinoma, which was detected during follow-up, lesions were classified as B, or probable IBD-associated polypoid dysplasia. If they were located in an area of colitis, but with no flat dysplasia or carcinoma on the follow-up evaluation, the lesions were classified as C, or indeterminate type. In nine patients with probable sporadic adenomas (group A), follow-up information was available and none developed subsequent dysplasia or adenocarcinoma. In contrast, of the 31 patients with either indeterminate polyps or probable IBD-associated dysplastic lesions (groups B and C), in the follow-up information, 13 patients either had or developed flat dysplastic lesions or adenocarcinoma in adjacent mucosa (including five patients with probable IBD-associated dysplastic lesions who had flat dysplasia in adjacent mucosa at the onset). Using these categories, it was found that patients with probable IBD-associated dysplastic lesions were younger (median age 48 years) than those with probable sporadic adenomas (median age 63.5 years), were more likely to have active colitis and were more likely to have a longer duration of disease (median 11 *vs.* 5 years). Histologically, patients with probable IBD-associated dysplastic lesions more commonly had lamina propria mononuclear inflammation, lamina propria neutrophilia and most importantly, were significantly more likely to have an admixture of dysplastic and non-dysplastic crypts on the surface of the polyp (60 *vs.* 16%). Others suggest that superficial, or the so-called "top down", dysplasia is more specific for a subset of adenoma-like polyps. In such lesions, the dysplastic glands are usually located in the upper part of the polyp and confined to the surface, forming a band like array [13].

Genetics of Dysplasia

Although several other studies have evaluated immunohistochemical findings in these two groups of lesions (DALM *vs.* sporadic adenoma), none have been shown to be useful in this differential diagnosis [25, 26]. However, some investigators have suggested that IBD-associated adenoma-like DALMs has a higher degree of p53, and a lower degree of nuclear beta-catenin and bcl-2 staining in contrast to sporadic adenomas, thus p53 protein expression favours DALM, and expression of bcl-2 and nuclear B-catenin favours a sporadic adenoma (Table 4) [27, 28].

Table 4. Immunohistochemistry in DALM *vs.* sporadic adenoma

	DALM	Sporadic adenoma
P53	+	-
Bcl-2	-	+
B-catenin	-	+

One study of UC-associated dysplasia and carcinoma has shown that the tumour-suppressor gene APC is demonstrated infrequently and plays an unimportant role compared to sporadic colorectal cancers. It has been shown that the APC gene was mutated in more than 60% of sporadic adenomas and CRC [29], while it was mutated in approximately 6% of colitic cancers [30].

Mutation in K-ras has been reported in cases of ulcerative colitis with a villous and hypermucinous mucosal surface prior to the appearance of dysplasia and it was suggested that these particular cases should be followed-up more frequently as a potential risk lesion for cancer development [31]. However, the majority of the studies revealed a lower incidence of K-ras mutation in UC-associated cancer compared to sporadic ones [32]. In a study by Odze et al., there were no significant differences in the frequencies of loss of heterozygosity (LOH) of 3p, APC or p16 in the UC-associated adenoma-like lesions that occurred within areas of colitis compared to those that occurred in a background of normal mucosa. These data suggest that UC-associated flat dysplastic (non-adenoma-like) DALMs have a different molecular genotype than UC-associated adenoma-like lesions as well as non-UC sporadic adenomas, although the latter two lesions are pathogenetically similar, if not identical, to one another [33, 34]. The tumour-suppressor gene p53 is shown by many investigators to be altered in UC-associated dysplasia and carcinoma. Some use it to differentiate between reactive inflammatory epithelial changes and true dysplasia and others use it as a tool to discriminate between DALM and sporadic adenoma. Its positivity favours dysplasia over reactive change and DALM over a sporadic adenoma [35, 29].

Some authors reported clonal chromosomal alterations in 85% of colitic cancers, 86% of UC-associated dysplasia and 36% of non-neoplastic epithelium [36]. The high rate of chromosomal alterations in non-neoplastic epithelium in colitic cancer, compared to the very low rate in sporadic cancers, has lead to the suggestion that these changes appear early in the neoplastic pathway of colitis.

Microsatellite instability was reported in cases of high-grade dysplasia associated with IBD and also in cases of colorectal cancer in a range between 46 to 50% in some studies and 3% in others. [37, 38]. Mutation of the p16^{INK4a} promoter region (an inhibitor of the cyclin-dependent protein kinase 4 and 6) was not demonstrated in cases of sporadic colonic cancers. However, it has been shown to be present in 70% of dysplastic lesion and 100% of colitic cancers in IBD patients [39]. Expression of apoptosis-related proteins like Fas and Bcl-xl (both with negative or weak expression in sporadic tumours and positive in UC-associated neoplasia) is sometimes useful in distinguishing between IBD-dysplasia and sporadic adenoma, thus leaving the patient with local resection rather than colectomy [40].

Screening and Treatment Options of Patients with Dysplasia-Associated IBD

The evidence of the association of dysplasia with cancer in patients with IBD has been noticed since the first publication of Crohn and Rosenberg early in the 1900s [41–43]. The fact that dysplasia is commonly seen near areas of invasive carcinoma in up to 74% of resection specimens from IBD patients, has lead to the conclusion that this is a precursor to the invasive lesion [44]. The diagnosis of dysplasia in patients with IBD is a crucial step because in some centres it will leave the patient with either a colectomy or life-long surveillance to prevent the development of cancer [25].

The rationale behind screening in these groups of patients is based on the recognition that CRC in these groups follows the sequence of chronic inflammation with the subsequent development of dysplasia of the colonic epithelium, progressing to carcinoma. This is roughly the same argument used in detecting and treating adenomatous polyps, since they are known to be the classical precancerous lesions in the colon and rectum. The issue when the diagnosis of dysplasia is established is what to do or advise next. Classically, and according to the recommendations proposed by Riddell et al., the procedure is to follow up cases with low-grade dysplasia and operate on DALMs and high-grade dysplasia. This seems at a glance to be good simple advice; however, there have been a few studies that have shown some data that has made the decision more complex. Charles Bernstein says that "when low grade dysplasia is the preoperative diagnosis, cancer may already be present in the colon in 20% of these cases". He quoted the St Marks series by saying that in about 50% of the cases of CRC in UC, low-grade dysplasia is the only type of dysplasia seen in the colonic resections adjacent or away from the tumour. It is also important to know that dysplasia may not be seen in 25% of patients with CRC complicating IBD [45]. There is also mounting evidence showing that the story of natural progression from low-grade to high-grade dysplasia and then to full-blown cancer can not always be substantiated. Dysplasia has been recognised as a premalignant condition since the 1980s [46]. If dysplasia is detected by random biopsy, its presence may correlate with the presence of deposits of micro-invasive adenocarcinoma. The presence of dysplasia in colonic biopsies is a reliable histological marker which can be used to predict which patients are at risk of developing CRC before there is macroscopic evidence of disease [47]. Prior to enrolling in surveillance programmes, all patients should be counselled as to the possibility of requiring a prophylactic proctocolectomy with either a permanent end ileostomy or formation of an ileo-anal pouch in order to prevent the future development of CRC, if the presence of dysplasia is confirmed. It is interesting to realise that most of the rarely reported cases of carcinoma arising in the ileo-anal pouch are those that have carcinoma or dysplasia in the initial resectates [18].

The British Society of Gastroenterology and the Association of Coloproctology have suggested guidelines for the screening of asymptomatic colorectal cancer in patients with inflammatory bowel disease. These guidelines suggest that colonoscopy surveillance with four random biopsies every 10 cm should commence after the patient has endured the condition for a minimum of 8 years. The risk of CRC is relatively low during the first decade of the disease. As a result, the surveillance protocols recommend three yearly colonoscopies for the first 12 years, then biannual endoscopies for the next 10 years, followed indefinitely with annual colonoscopy [48]. This is at variance with the recommendation originally suggested by Riddell et al. in their classic paper in 1983 (see Table 1) In high risk groups such as those patients with positive family histories of CRC at a young age or primary sclerosing cholangitis, annual colonoscopy is recommended [49].

The overall sensitivity of direct colonoscopy for the detection of dysplasia is between 70–85%. Biopsy of any macroscopically visible lesion is advised along with four random biopsies at 10-cm intervals. In practice, the colonoscopy may be performed more frequently, depending upon the severity of the illness and the extent of colonic involvement.

Sampling error, where the endoscopist fails to take an adequate number of biopsies to exclude dysplasia or carcinoma [50], is also a known problem. The detection of high-grade dysplasia (HGD) in flat lesions is sufficient histological evidence for the recommendation for a prophylactic colectomy to be made. Multifocal low-grade dysplasia (LGD) should also be treated with a prophylactic proctocolectomy [51, 52]. Until recently there has been no consensus as to whether the detection of a single focus of low-grade dysplasia could be managed by accelerated colonoscopic surveillance prior to the detection of HGD and the recommendation of proctocolectomy. However, analysis of prospective studies assessing continued colonoscopic screening after detection of LGD has revealed that 53% of patients with LGD developed CRC at 5 years. Twenty-four percent of patients diagnosed with LGD after colonoscopy, who had elected to be treated with proctocolectomy, had unrecognised advanced CRC after histological analysis of the colectomy specimen with a rate of progression to advanced neoplasia that approached 53% [52]. In a separate study, the presence of dysplasia was found to have a sensitivity of 81% and specificity of 79% as a marker for the presence of a synchronous CRC. The positive predictive value of the detection of LGD was 70% [53]. In view of these results and other similar studies, detection of LGD is now widely accepted as an indication for prophylactic proctocolectomy with formation of an ileo-anal pouch or end ileostomy. However, many clinicians still pursue a more conservative approach in treating LGD rather than recommending surgery, since other studies have presented a less worrisome prognosis of LGD. Befrits et al. followed 60 patients with flat LGD and found that none developed cancer on follow-up [54].

Any raised non-adenomatous mass containing evidence of dysplasia on biopsy would also require a proctocolectomy. Some suggest that dysplasia detected in adenomatous lesions can be safely treated with endoscopic resection, preventing an unnecessary colectomy. Unfortunately colonoscopy with random biopsies of macroscopically normal looking mucosa is an inherently unreliable technique due to the sporadic nature of dysplasia, which often leads to a low detection rate of positive results [55]. Inaccuracies may occur at different stages of the screening process due to inadequate colonic biopsies: macroscopically visible lesions which remain undetected after colonoscopy due to operator technique. Errors that lead to misinterpretation will lead to false positive or negative biopsy results. One of the major criticisms of CRC surveillance programmes is the failure of routine biopsy to detect the neoplasia that is subsequently found after histological analysis of colectomy specimens after surgery for symptom control, in the interval prior to the next surveillance colonoscopy. The potential for areas of dysplasia to remain undetected after colonoscopy may be a factor contributing to the failure of screening to dramatically reduce the incidence of CRC developing as a complication of IBD. This limitation of colonoscopy needs to be discussed with patients willing to enter surveillance programmes, as the limited sensitivity of this test needs to be evaluated by each individual against the potential complications that arise as a result of colonoscopy. In UK practice, the development of an iatrogenic colonic perforation or haemorrhage requiring laparoscopy occurs in approximately 1:1 000 patients undergoing colonoscopy [56]. A full discussion of all of the possible advantages of surveillance must be held with the patient prior to them enrolling in the follow-up programme, in view of the potential physical and psychological complications. The most reliable method to date for predicting the risk of CRC is the presence of confirmed dysplasia from colonoscopic biopsies. However, as yet there have been no randomised controlled trials to compare the effectiveness of different surveillance programmes in improving survival from CRC in patients with IBD. There are few actual studies which compare outcomes of surveillance against no surveillance. This is partly due to the recognition that dysplasia is a pre-malignant condition and early detection of neoplasia with subsequent prophylactic proctocolectomy can reduce the number of deaths from CRC. This is a powerful argument supporting the implementation of surveillance programmes. The opposing argument focuses on the finding that surveillance has had little effect on reducing the mortality rate of IBD patients dying from CRC [57]. Histological analysis of specimens from prophylactic proctocolectomies performed after the detection of dysplasia often reveals the presence of unexpected early Dukes A or B cancers. Earlier detection may result in reduced morbidity and improved survival for the individual but this may be attributable to the lead time bias of earlier diagnosis. There is no clear evidence that screening has reduced the mortality rate of patients with IBD [58]. Attention has recently been focused on developing an alternative approach to improve the efficiency of surveillance programmes. The routine practice of obtaining four random biopsies at 10-cm intervals generates a vast number of biopsies for analysis, of which only a small proportion contain evidence of dysplasia. This is an expensive and highly laborious process with a low diagnostic yield for both the endoscopist and pathologist. There is great interest in developing new techniques which can target areas of macroscopically invisible dysplasia directly and obviate the need for random biopsies. Chromoendoscopy is the term given to the technique of endoscopically spraying the colonic mucosa with dyes such as 0.1% methylene blue or 0.4% indigo carmine to emphasise unusual mucosal irregularities [59]. This is an easily adapted procedure which can be performed by the application of dye to the colonic mucosa from a conventional colonoscope. The rational behind chromoendoscopy is based on the dyes not being absorbed by the mucosa but simply pooling in the mucosal pits allowing easier endoscopic identification of abnormal mucosa [60]. In Vivo studies in animal subjects have allowed analysis of patterns of dye uptake in colonic mucosa which has been repeatedly verified by histological analysis of the resected or biopsied specimens [61]. Clinical studies utilising chromoendoscopy have indicated that this improved endoscopic technique provides better improved detection rates of dysplastic lesions. The detection of flat lesions by routine colonoscopy is very difficult as the mucosal changes are very subtle. Intravital staining significantly improves the endoscopic detection of flat lesions [62]. These lesions are classified according to the pit pattern system which was developed in response to the enhanced images obtained from using magnifying endoscopes. Two separate prospective trials comparing the detection rates of neoplastic lesions by traditional random biopsy on routine colonoscopy followed by immediate repeat colonoscopy and targeted biopsy after mucosal staining both testify that detection of dysplasia is significantly improved by chromoendoscopy [63, 64]. This finding has significant implications for the screening of patients with IBD, as the improved detection rates will result in more patients undergoing prophylactic proctocolectomies at an earlier stage, which may inevitably include the detection of synchronous CRC at earlier stages. Pan-colonic chromoendoscopy also detects a large number of non-neoplastic lesions. To maximise the detection of dysplasia and minimise the biopsy of non-neoplastic tissue, the endoscopist must adhere to targeting biopsies of lesions with suspicious staining patterns as determined by the pit pattern system—grade III and IV lesions are likely to represent neoplastic change. In a recent article on chromoendoscopy, it was suggested that the so-called SURFACE guidelines in ulcerative colitis be followed [65].

1. Strict patient selection. Patients with histologically proven ulcerative colitis and at least an 8-year duration in clinical remission. Avoid patients with active disease.
2. Unmask the mucosal surface. Excellent bowel preparation is needed. Remove mucus and remaining fluid in the colon when necessary.
3. Reduce peristaltic waves. When drawing back the endoscope, a spasmolytic agent should be used (if necessary).
4. Full length staining of the colon. Perform full length staining of the colon (panchromoendoscopy) in ulcerative colitis rather than local staining.
5. Augmented detection with dyes. Intravital staining with 0.4% indigo carmine or 0.1% methylene blue should be used to unmask flat lesions more frequently than with conventional colonoscopy.
6. Crypt architecture analysis. All lesions should be analysed according to the pit pattern classification. Whereas pit pattern types I–II suggests the presence of non-malignant lesions, staining patterns III–V suggest the presence of intraepithelial neoplasias and carcinomas.
7. Endoscopic targeted biopsies. Perform targeted biopsies of all mucosal alterations, particularly of circumscript lesions with staining patterns indicative of intraepithelial neoplasias and carcinomas (pit patterns III–V).

The use of high resolution endoscopy and dye staining is 97% sensitive and 93% specific in predicting neoplasia [66]. Novel techniques that have been developed include ultra high-powered magnifying endoscopes which have 1 000 times greater magnification and are able to visualise cellular microstructures. The resultant images of In Vivo cells have such clarity that the possibility exists in the future of endoscopically generated virtual histology [69].

Other experimental techniques include Raman spectroscopy, fluorescence spectroscopy light scattering spectroscopy, optical coherence tomography and confocal laser microscopy. However, at this time, these techniques are still experimental [68]. It is possible that in the future these diagnostic techniques will be used with molecular markers to improve detection of neoplasia. The benefit of surveillance techniques utilising chromoendoscopy for the detection of dysplasia in patients with long-term IBD are enormous and as such are likely to initiate a radical change in current practice during this decade. There is wide support for offering patients with adenoma-like polypoid dysplasia a local resection if certain criteria are met. These include the absence of flat dysplasia in the multiple biopsies of the area adjacent to the lesion or the absence of flat or raised dysplasia in other parts of the colon, and the willingness of the patient to undergo continued surveillance [13]. Laser fluorescence spectroscopy for In Situ dysplasia diagnosis and faecal DNA testing are some of the techniques that have been indicated as being useful in the future [69]. A recent study had suggested that in longstanding extensive ulcerative colitis, the severity of colonic inflammation is an important determinant of the risk of colorectal neoplasia. Endoscopic and histological grading of inflammation could allow better risk stratification for surveillance programmes [70].

As we mentioned before, there seems to be no standard or universally agreed treatment for dysplasia. It was Blackstone et al. who advocated in a case study the importance of having a definitive radical surgery (total colectomy) in cases of dysplasia and demonstrated the horrid prognosis relating to the raised dysplastic lesions in patients with IBD [71]. Adenoma-like lesions that occur proximal to histological areas of colitis (i.e. right-sided lesion in a patient with left-sided UC), can easily be diagnosed as a sporadic adenoma because it is well known that dysplasia related to IBD develops only in areas involved by the inflammatory process. However, adenoma-like lesions that occur within areas affected by colitis are more difficult to distinguish from true polypoid dysplastic lesions related to the underlying colitis [24, 34]. Recent data, primarily based on the results of two follow-up studies, suggest that IBD patients with an adenoma-like DALM, regardless of whether it has been determined as representing a sporadic or an IBD-related lesion, may be treated adequately by polypectomy and continued surveillance if there is no evidence of flat dysplasia elsewhere in the patient or especially the base of the polyp [72–74]. Further studies may be needed to verify the above observations but for the time being it seems that this has momentarily alleviated the pressure on the pathologists to differentiate between DALM and sporadic adenoma.

Conclusions

- Definition of dysplasia is standard.
- Classifications are clear.
- Genetic studies are variable and may be useful in differentiating between lesions and helpful in choosing treatment modalities.
- Treatment varies according to condition of lesion.
- Not all CRC in IBD follow the logic of the low-grade dysplasia, high-grade dysplasia then carcinoma sequence.
- Modified chromoendoscopy is more sensitive than routine endoscopy in identifying dysplastic epithelium.

References

1. Ullman TA (2005) Preventing neoplastic progression in ulcerative colitis. J Clin Gastroenterol 39(4):S66–S69
2. Sjoqvist U (2004) Dysplasia in ulcerative colitis: clinical consequences? Langenbecks Arch Surg 389(5):354–360
3. Itzkowitz SH, Present DH (2005) Consensus conference: colorectal cancer screening and surveillance in inflammatory bowel disease. Inflamm Bowel Dis 11(3):314–321
4. Judge TA, Lewis JD, Lichtenstein GR (2002) Colonic dysplasia and cancer in inflammatory bowel disease. Gastrointest Endosc Clin N Am 12(3):495–523
5. Ekbom A, Helmick C, Zack M et al (1990) Ulcerative colitis and colorectal cancer: a population-based study. N Engl J Med 323(18):1228–1233
6. Sugita A, Sachar DB, Bodian C et al (1991) Colorectal cancer in ulcerative colitis: influence of anatomical extent and age at onset on colitis-cancer interval. Gut 32(2):167–169
7. Chambers WM, Warren BF, Jewell DP et al (2005) Cancer surveillance in ulcerative colitis. Br J Surg 92(8):928–936
8. Riddell RH, Goldman H, Ransohoff DF et al (1983) Dysplasia in inflammatory bowel disease: standardized classification with provisional clinical applications. Hum Pathol 14(11):931–968
9. Konishi F, Wakasa H, Kino I et al (1993) Histological classification of the neoplastic epithelium arising in ulcerative colitis (in Japanese with English abstract). Annual Report (for 1992) of the Research Committee of Inflammatory Bowel Disease Tokyo, Ministry of Health and Welfare of Japan, Tokyo, pp 153–156
10. Schlemper RJ, Riddell RH, Kato Y et al (2000) The Vienna classification of gastrointestinal epithelial neoplasia. Gut 47(2):251–155
11. Schlemper RJ, Kato Y, Stolte M (2000) Diagnostic criteria for gastrointestinal carcinomas in Japan and western countries: proposal for a new classification system of gastrointestinal epithelial neoplasia. J Gastroenterol Hepatol 15:49–57
12. Schlemper RJ, Iwashita I (2004) Classification of gastrointestinal epithelial neoplasia. Current Diagnos Pathol 10(2):128–139
13. Harpaz N (2004) Adenoma-like dysplastic polyps in inflammatory bowel disease. Pathol Case Rev9(4):135–141
14. Odze RD (1999) Adenomas and adenoma-like DALMs in chronic ulcerative colitis: a clinical, pathological, and molecular review. Am J Gastroenterol 94(7):1746–1750
15. Melville DM, Jass JR, Morson BC et al (1989) Observer study of the grading of dysplasia in ulcerative colitis: comparison with clinical outcome. Hum Pathol 20:1008–1014
16. Dixon MF, Brown LJR, Gilmour HM et al (1988) Observer variation in the assessment of dysplasia in ulcerative colitis. Histopathology 13:385–397
17. Hulten L, Willen R, Nilsson O et al (2002) Mucosal assessment for dysplasia and cancer in the ileal-pouch mucosa in patients operated on for ulcerative colitis: a 30-year follow-up study. Dis Colon Rectum 45(4):448–452
18. Raithel M, Weidenhiller M, Schwab D et al (2001) Pathobiology of dysplasia in chronic inflammatory bowel disease: current recommendation for surveillance of dysplasia. Z Gastroenterol 39(10):861–875
19. Yin J, Harpaz N, Tong Y et al (1993) p53 point mutations in dysplastic and cancerous ulcerative colitis lesions. Gastroenterology 104(6):1633–1639
20. Bernstein CN, Shanahan F, Weinstein WM (1994) Are we telling patients the truth about surveillance colonoscopy in ulcerative colitis? Lancet 8(343):71–74
21. Levine DS, Reid BJ, Haggitt RC et al (1991) Distribution of aneuploid cell populations in ulcerative colitis with dysplasia or cancer. Gastroenterology 101(5):1198–210

22. Rutegard J, Ahsgren L, Stenling R et al (1988) DNA content in ulcerative colitis: flow cytometric analysis in a patient series from a defined area. Dis Colon Rectum 31:710–715
23. Schneider A, Stolte M (1993) Differential diagnosis of adenomas and dysplastic lesions in patients with ulcerative colitis. Z Gastroenterol 31(11):653–656
24. Torres C, Antonioli D, Odze RD (1998) Polypoid dysplasia and adenomas in inflammatory bowel disease: a clinical, pathologic, and follow-up study of 89 polyps from 59 patients. Am J Surg Pathol 22(3):275–284
25. Fogt F, Wellmann A, Urbanski SJ et al (2001) Glut-1 expression in dysplastic and regenerative lesions of the colon. Int J Mol Med 7(6):615–619
26. Fogt F, Zimmerman RL, Poremba C et al (2002) Immunohistochemical screening of mismatch repair genes hMLH1, hMSH2, and hMSH6 in dysplastic lesions of the colon. Appl Immunohistochem Mol Morphol 10(1):57–61
27. Mueller E, Vieth M, Stolte M et al (1999) The differentiation of true adenomas from colitis-associated dysplasia in ulcerative colitis: a comparative immunohistochemical study. Hum Pathol 30(8):898–905
28. Walsh SV, Loda M, Torres CM et al (1999) P53 and beta catenin expression in chronic ulcerative colitis-associated polypoid dysplasia and sporadic adenomas: an immunohistochemical study. Am J Surg Pathol 23(8):963–969
29. Powell SM, Zilz N, Beazer-Barclay Y et al (1992) APC mutations occur early during colorectal tumorigenesis. Nature 359(6392):235–237
30. Tarmin L, Yin J, Harpaz N al (1995) Adenomatous polyposis coli gene mutations in ulcerative colitis-associated dysplasias and cancers versus sporadic colon neoplasms. Cancer Res 55(10):2035–2038
31. Andersen SN, Lovig T, Clausen OP et al (1999) Villous, hypermucinous mucosa in long standing ulcerative colitis shows high frequency of K-ras mutations. Gut 45(5):686–692
32. Chaubert P, Benhattar J, Saraga E et al (1994) K-ras mutations and p53 alterations in neoplastic and non neoplastic lesions associated with longstanding ulcerative colitis. Am J Pathol 144(4):767–775
33. Odze RD, Brown CA, Hartmann CJ et al (2000) Genetic alterations in chronic ulcerative colitis-associated adenoma-like DALMs is similar to non-colitic sporadic adenomas. Am J Surg Pathol 24:1209–1216
34. Fogt F, Urbanski SJ, Sanders ME et al (2000) Distinction between dysplasia-associated lesion or mass (DALM) and adenoma in patients with ulcerative colitis. Hum Pathol 31:288–291
35. Fujii S, Fujimori T, Kashida H (2002) Ulcerative colitis-associated neoplasia. Pathol Int 52(3):195–203
36. Willenbucher RF, Aust DE, Chang CG et al (1999) Genomic instability is an early event during the progression pathway of ulcerative-colitis-related neoplasia. Am J Pathol 154(6):1825–1830
37. Brentnall TA, Crispin DA, Bronner MP et al 1996) Microsatellite instability in non neoplastic mucosa from patients with chronic ulcerative colitis. Cancer Res 56(6):1237–1240
38. Cawkwell L, Sutherland F, Murgatroyd H et al (2000) Defective hMSH2/hMLH1 protein expression is seen infrequently in ulcerative colitis associated colorectal cancers. Gut 46(3):367–369
39. Hsieh CJ, Klump B, Holzmann K et al (1998) Hypermethylation of the p16INK4a promoter in colectomy specimens of patients with long-standing and extensive ulcerative colitis. Cancer Res 58(17):3942–3945
40. van der Woude CJ, Moshage H, Homan M et al (2005) Expression of apoptosis related proteins during malignant progression in chronic ulcerative colitis. J Clin Pathol 58(8):811–814
41. Crohn B, Rosenberg H (1925) The sigmoidoscopic picture of chronic ulcerative colitis. Am J Med Sci 170:220–228
42. Warren S, Sommers SC (1949) Pathogenesis of ulcerative colitis Am J Pathol 25:657–679
43. Morson BC, Pang LS (1967) Rectal biopsy as an aid to cancer control in ulcerative colitis. Gut 8(5):423–434
44. Connell WR, Talbot IC, Harpaz N et al (1994) Clinicopathological characteristics of colorectal carcinoma complicating ulcerative colitis. Gut 35(10):1419–1423
45. Bernstein CN (2005) The case of colectomy in patients with low-grade dysplasia in ulcerative colitis. World Gastroenterol News 10(2):12–13
46. Manning AP, Bulgim OR, Dixon MF et al (1987) Screening by colonoscopy for colonic epithelial dysplasia in inflammatory bowel disease. Gut 28(11):1489–1494
47. Nugent FW, Haggitt RC, Gilpin PA (1991) Cancer surveillance in ulcerative colitis. Gastroenterology 100(5):1241–1248
48. Eaden JA, Mayberry JF (2002) Guidelines for screening and surveillance of asymptomatic colorectal cancer in patients with inflammatory bowel disease. Gut 1(Suppl 5):10–12
49. Itzkowitz SH, Harpaz N (2004) Diagnosis and management of dysplasia in patients with inflammatory bowel diseases. Gastroenterology 126(6):1634–1648
50. Rubin CE, Haggitt RC, Burmer GC et al (1992) DNA aneuploidy in colonic biopsies predicts future development of dysplasia in ulcerative colitis. Gastroenterology 103(5):1611–1620
51. Rosenstock E, Farmer RG, Petras R et al (1985) Surveillance for colonic carcinoma in ulcerative colitis. Gastroenterology 89(6):1342–1346
52. Ullman T, Croog V, Harpaz N et al (2003) Progression of flat low-grade dysplasia to advanced neoplasia in patients with ulcerative colitis. Gastroenterology 125(5):1311–1319
53. Gorfine SR, Bauer JJ, Harris MT et al (2000) Dysplasia complicating chronic ulcerative colitis: Is immediate colectomy warranted? Dis Colon Rectum 43(11):1575–1581
54. Befrits R, Ljung T, Jaramillo E et al (2002) Low-grade dysplasia in extensive, long-standing inflammatory bowel disease: a follow-up study. Dis Colon Rectum 45(5):615–620
55. Rutter MD, Saunders BP, Schofield Get al (2004) Pan colonic indigo carmine dye spraying for the detection of dysplasia in ulcerative colitis. Gut 53(2):256–260
56. Bowles CJ, Leicester R, Romaya C et al (2004) A prospective study of colonoscopy practice in the UK today: are we adequately prepared for national colorectal cancer screening tomorrow? Gut 53(2):277–283

57. Mayer R, Wong WD, Rosenberger DA et al (1999) Colorectal cancer in inflammatory bowel disease: a continuing problem. Dis Colon Rectum 42(3):343–347
58. Mpofu C, Watson AJ, Rhodes J M (2004) Strategies for detecting colon cancer and/or dysplasia in patients with inflammatory bowel disease. Cochrane Database Syst Rev 2:CD000279
59. Herfarth H, Rogler G (2005) Inflammatory bowel disease. Endoscopy 37(1):42–47
60. Kiesslich R, Neurath MF (2004) Surveillance colonoscopy in ulcerative colitis: magnifying chromoendoscopy in the spotlight. Gut 53:165–167
61. Becker C, Fantini MC, Wirtz S et al (2005) In vivo imaging of colitis and colon cancer development in mice using high resolution chromoendoscopy. Gut 54(7):950–954
62. Kiesslich R, Fritsch J, Holtmann M et al (2003) Methylene blue aided chromoendoscopy for the detection of intraepithelial neoplasia and colon cancer in ulcerative colitis. Gastroenterology 124(4):880–888
63. Rutter MD, Saunders BP, Wilkinson KH et al (2004) Most dysplasia in ulcerative colitis is visible at colonoscopy. Gastrointest Endosc 60(3):334–339
64. Trecca A, Gai F, Di Lorenzo GP et al (2004) Conventional colonoscopy versus chromoendoscopy and magnifying endoscopy for the diagnosis of colorectal lesions: a comparative prospective study in 995 patients. Chir Ital 56(1):31–36
65. Kiesslich R, Neurath MF (2004) Potential of new endoscopic techniques: intravital staining and in vivo confocal endomicroscopy in the detection of premalignant lesions and early cancer in patients with ulcerative colitis. Acta Endoscop 34(2): 189-197
66. Hurlstone DP (2004) Further validation of high-magnification chromoscopic-colonoscopy for the detection of intraepithelial neoplasia and colon cancer in ulcerative colitis. Gastroenterology 126(1):376–378
67. Inoue H, Kudo SE, Shiokawa A (2004) Novel endoscopic imaging techniques toward in vivo observation of living cancer cells in the gastrointestinal tract. Dig Dis 22(4):334–337
68. Dekker E, Fockens P (2005) Advances in colonic imaging: new endoscopic imaging methods. Eur J Gastroenterol Hepatol 17(8):803–808
69. Ullman TA (2005) Colonoscopic surveillance in inflammatory bowel disease. Curr Opin Gastroenterol 21(5):585–588
70. Rutter M, Saunders B, Wilkinson K et al (2004) Severity of inflammation is a risk factor for colorectal neoplasia in ulcerative colitis. Gastroenterology 126(2):451–359
71. Blackstone MO, Riddell RH, Rogers BH et al (1981) Dysplasia-associated lesion or mass (DALM) detected by colonoscopy in long-standing ulcerative colitis: an indication for colectomy. Gastroenterology 80(2):366–374
72. Engelsgjerd M, Farraye FA, Odze RD (1999) Polypectomy may be adequate treatment for adenoma-like dysplastic lesions in chronic ulcerative colitis. Gastroenterology 117(6):1288–1294
73. Rubin PH (1999) Adenomas in ulcerative colitis: endoscopic polypectomy or colectomy? Inflamm Bowel Dis 5(4):304–305
74. Odze RD, Farraye FA, Hecht JL et al (2004) Long-term follow-up after polypectomy treatment for adenoma-like dysplastic lesions in ulcerative colitis. Clin Gastroenterol Hepatol 2(7):534–541

IBD: Cancer Risk and Surveillance

Gabriele Riegler, Ilaria Esposito

Introduction

Patients with inflammatory bowel disease (IBD) are at an increased risk for colorectal cancer (CRC) [1–4], but the quantisation of the risk of CRC in this specific population varies widely in different studies. However, CRC complicating ulcerative colitis (UC) and Crohn's disease (CD) only accounts for 1–2% of all cases of CRC in the general population. Most cases of CRC are either sporadic (65–85%) or familial (10–30%; Fig. 1) [3–4].

CRC is considered a serious complication of the disease and accounts for approximately 15% of all deaths in IBD patients [5]. The mortality in patients diagnosed with CRC who are also diagnosed with IBD is higher than for sporadic CRC [6]. However, much more is known about the risk in UC. The incidence of colorectal cancer in patients with ulcerative colitis is higher than in the general population. In a meta-analysis, the overall prevalence of CRC in any UC patient, based on 116 studies, was estimated to be 3.7%. The incidence rate corresponded to cumulative probabilities of 2% by 10 years, 8% by 20 years and 18% by 30 years [7].

The major risk factors for the development of CRC include young age at onset of IBD [1], extensive disease [8] and long disease duration [5]. It is biologically plausible that the excess cancer risk is secondary to chronic inflammation and it is recognised that duration of colitis is an important risk factor for CRC. Rutter et al. [9] showed for the first time that increasing severity of colonic inflammation is associated with an increase in the rate of colorectal neoplasia in UC. Patients with disease extending to the hepatic flexure or more proximally have the greatest risk of CRC [10–12]. Most studies have found that the risk of CRC increases after 15 to 20 years; approximately one decade later than in pancolitis in patients with colitis confined to the left colon [8]. Patients with ulcerative proctitis and proctosigmoiditis are probably not at increased risk for CRC [13]. An increased risk of CRC has been observed in patients with UC complicated by primary sclerosing cholangitis. In these cases, cancer was more likely to be in the right colon, suggesting a possible role of bile acids in oncogenesis [14].

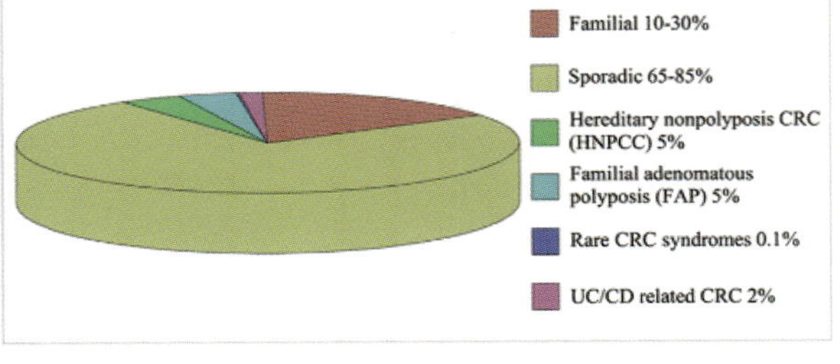

Fig. 1. Distribution of CRC

The evidence for other potential risk factors is scarce. Smoke [15], folate depletion [16–17] and a positive family history of colon cancer [18] may affect the occurrence of CRC. A hypothesis has been put forward according to which UC, CD and CRC occur in predisposed patients because of a mixture of genetic and environmental factors. One study has shown that relatives of patients with both IBD and CRC have an 80% increased risk of CRC [19]. In our study, there is no statistically significant difference between IBD and control cases of family members as far as prevalence of malignant colorectal, digestive extra-colonic or extra-digestive tract tumours [20]. Another recent study has investigated the prevalence of all malignancies in first-degree relatives of CD patients. The result showed a higher prevalence of breast cancer in female relatives, mainly in mothers, of CD patients compared with controls. The presence of breast cancer was not associated with any specific phenotype of the CD [21].

As in UC, Crohn's disease of the colon carries an increased risk of CRC. Ekbom et al. [1] found a relative risk of 5.6% for CRC among patients with CD, whereas in another Swedish patient cohort study, Persson et al. [22] did not find that the population relative risk increased. Similarly, Fireman et al. [23] from Israel and Jess et al. [24] in the Danish cohort, did not find an increased risk of CRC among their patients with CD. Although analyzing subgroups within the CD study meant that there were few cancers identified, when patients with CD of >10-year duration were analyzed, the relative risk for CRC was 4.8%. For those patients with at least 10 years of disease and no surgery within the first 10 years, the relative risk was 8.3%. Thus, even among this reportedly negative study, when variables such as disease duration and possibly disease extent (based on no surgery) are analysed, the relative risk increases [5]. In the study of Gillen et al. [25], however, it appears that the malignant potential in CD and UC is of the same order of magnitude. Cancer developed in inflamed areas in both diseases, and was thus located in the right colon in 49% of patients with CD compared with 36% with UC, reflecting the difference in inflammatory sites in the two cases. Adenocarcinomas develop only in affected segments of the small intestine, and are difficult to diagnose at an early stage because the radiological appearance is similar to that of stricturing CD.

Pathogenesis of CRC in IBD

The pathogenesis of CRC in IBD is poorly understood. However, several lines of evidence suggest that the pathobiology is different than sporadic CRC:

1. the mean age of developing CRC in the setting of IBD is lower than sporadic CRC (40–50 vs. 60 years).
2. Dysplasia in UC is preceded by a long history of chronic inflammation and can be found at distant sites from the cancer. In contrast, dysplasia in sporadic CRC is usually associated with a discrete polyp without inflammation.
3. Mutations in the ras protooncogene are present in 40–60% of sporadic CRC and are probably an early event; in contrast, these mutations are less frequently observed in cancer associated with UC, and are probably a late event [26–27].
4. Loss of heterozygosity for the p53 gene and src activation occur earlier in cancers associated with IBD than in sporadic CRC. Src activity in UC correlates with the degree of dysplasia [28].
5. Abnormalities of the p53 locus are absent in non-dysplastic mucosa of patients with sporadic CRC. In contrast, non-dysplastic mucosa in UC frequently has aneuploid DNA content and may show clones of cells with loss of heterozygosity of the p53 gene [29].

It is generally accepted that CRC in IBD is preceded by dysplasia, which is defined as unequivocal neoplastic epithelium and is currently the most important and best-defined marker of an increased risk of malignancy. Dysplasia is present in >70% of UC patients with carcinoma. Although it may occur in any portion of the colon, it typically parallels the location of cancer arising from chronically inflamed mucosa [30–32]. From an endoscopic viewpoint, dysplasia is characterised as flat (endoscopically invisible but detected in mucosal specimens) or raised (endoscopically visible), in which case "dysplasia associated lesions or mass" (DALM) is applied, a term that was coined by Blackstone et al. in 1981 [33]. In their study, 12 of 112 patients with long-standing UC were found to have a DALM, and of these, seven (58%) had carcinoma. Given the strong association with cancer, the presence of DALM constituted a strong indication for colectomy, which has become the standard therapy for this type of lesion. DALM are a heterogeneous population of tumours that may endoscopically appear as a plaque, mass (irregular, broad-based or strictured lesions), a discrete sessile nodule, or polyp. The cancer risk is not equal among these various subtypes. Unfortunately, most of the previous studies of UC associated DALMs failed to evaluate these lesions in relation to their gross appearance. For instance, there is one specific subtype of discrete DALM that endoscopically and histologically resembles a sporadic adenoma (isolated dysplastic nodule or polyp) and, as such, poses a difficult diagnostic challenge both to clinicians and to pathologists [34]. This is a critically important distinction, because an adenoma-like DALM is a tumour that arises as a result of UC and, thus, is an indication for colectomy, whereas an adenoma which is also by definition a "polypoid dysplastic lesion", the development of which is unrelated to the underlying chronic colitis (but coincidentally exists with it), is usually treated by polypectomy.

Since both UC and sporadic adenomas (SA) are not uncommon disorders, it is not surprising that gastroenterologists regularly encounter patients who have both conditions. Sporadic adenomas coexist with UC if they are located next (proximal) to the colitis because UC-related dysplasia does not develop from non-inflamed epithelium. UC associated adenoma-like DALMs were classified as lesions that were located within histologically proven areas of colitis and were associated with either synchronous or metachronous flat dysplasia or adenocarcinoma [35].

A number of clinical, histologic and molecular features have been studied to help make a distinction between DALM and SA:

1. patients with non-adenoma-like DALM are more likely to be younger and have a longer duration of disease, more extensive disease, and larger lesions [36].
2. Lesions that appear endoscopically as adenomas (pedunculated or sessile) rather than having other characteristics (such as flat, ulcerated, or plaque-

like appearance), even if found within an area of histologic colitis, may have a favourable prognosis with endoscopic removal and close follow-up [35, 37, 38].

In addition to the clinical and histologic features described above, several molecular markers have been proposed for distinguishing DALM from SA. Two of these are beta catenin and p53 [39–40]. Beta catenin is a cell membrane protein that accumulates more frequently in the nuclei of cells within sporadic colon cancer as compared to DALM. Mutations with p53 (a tumour suppressor gene) occur more frequently in DALM than sporadic adenomas. Several studies have provided evidence that p53 polymorphism at codon 72 (Arg and Pro alleles) may be associated with a high risk of malignancies. A recent study investigated Arg72Pro polymorphism in UC and found that p53 Pro homozygosis was more frequent in patients who had a continuous disease and, therefore, may also favour the progression from dysplasia to colon cancer [41].

The predictive value of dysplasia has been studied in UC. Although dysplasia is a marker for future or concurrent malignancy, it can also regress or remain stable for long periods. Most patients with dysplasia do not have cancer and dysplasia is absent in the colonic regions distant from the malignancy in 25–30% of patients [42-43].

The association between dysplasia and CRC in CD appears to be similar to that in UC. Dysplasia is present in 83% of patients diagnosed with CRC, and dysplasia distant from the cancer is found in 23–70%. In contrast, dysplasia is much less common in colectomy specimens of patients with CD than without CRC, and has occurred in only 2% of the specimens in one series [44–45].

Interpretation of biopsy samples may be confounded by interobserver variation in the recognition and grading of dysplasia. A uniform terminology for dysplasia in IBD has been proposed [29]. The classification categories histology as:

1. negative.
2. Indefinite (with subgroups of probably negative, unknown, and probably positive.
3. Positive (with subgroups of low grade and high-grade dysplasia).

Dysplasia may be difficult to distinguish from inflammation and regeneration on histologic sections. As a result, the presence of dysplasia should be confirmed by an experienced pathologist. The criteria for dysplasia stress the uniform clonal nature of dysplastic changes, which affects equally all parts of the crypt and surface epithelium. In contrast, regenerative changes are usually most prominent at the base of the crypts and show evidence of maturation as they migrate toward the crypt surface.

Other architectural and cytological abnormalities seen in regards to dysplastic epithelium include [29]: increased epithelium proliferation and mitoses; increased epithelial height; branching of crypts; back-to-back glandular formation; variation in the size and shape of nuclei; increased nuclear/cytoplasmatic ratio; altered nuclear polarity globet cells.

Surveillance

Dysplastic epithelium may be a marker for coexisting malignancy, and provides the rationale for surveillance. The optimal surveillance strategy remains controversial [45]. Surveillance colonoscopy in IBD is advocated for early diagnosis of neoplasia, but is imperfect because some patients develop cancer despite surveillance. In effect, a few reports have shown conflicting results and these studies suggest that surveillance leads to the detection of early-stage cancer in only a minority of patients and a significant number of patients develop cancer at an advanced stage despite surveillance.

The American Gastroenterological Association (AGA) recommends that colonoscopic surveillance should begin after 8 years in patients with pancolitis and 15 years in patients with colitis involving the left colon. Colonoscopy should be repeated every 1–2 years.

The American College of Gastroenterology (ACG) recommends annual surveillance colonoscopy beginning after 8–10 years of disease. Multiple biopsies should be obtained at regular intervals. The finding of definite dysplasia is an indication for colectomy. Patients whose biopsies are indefinite for dysplasia should undergo repeat surveillance colonoscopy at a shorter interval.

The American Society for Gastrointestinal Endoscopy (ASGE) recommends that patients with UC who have pancolitis should begin surveillance colonoscopy after 8 years of disease. Four biopsies should be obtained every 10 cm from the cecum to the rectum. In addiction, any suspicious lesions or masses should be biopsied. Colonoscopy should be repeated every 1–3 years. The finding of carcinoma or high-grade dysplasia is an indication for colectomy. Colectomy is also indicated for any degree of dysplasia associated with lesion or mass. However, in patients in whom colectomy is not feasible or is unacceptable, frequent surveillance, every 3–6 months, is considered an acceptable alternative. For patients with left-sided colitis, the ASGE recommends that surveillance should begin after 15 years of disease. Surveillance is not indicated in ulcerative proctitis. In CD, the risk of colorectal cancer is increased only in regard to Crohn's colitis. Surveillance colonoscopy and biopsy for dysplasia should be offered to patients with longstanding disease. Furthermore, a reduction in mortality due to surveillance has not yet been established.

On the other hand, prophylactic colectomy is a method to prevent the development of CRC in IBD. The development of the stapling of the ileal pouch-anal anastomosis with preservation of the anal transitional zone is an important advancement in surgical treatment, but remains controversial because of concerns about the potential risk of dysplasia and cancer. The risk factor for carcinoma is inflammation in the small intestinal and rectal mucosa. Pouchitis is the most frequent late complication and clearly related to a worse outcome. The etiology of pouchitis remains unknown. Possible causes are fecal stasis resulting in bacterial overgrowth and infection [46], microbial imbalance [47], production of volatile fatty acids, ischemia [48], oxygen-free radical injury [49], nitric oxide [50] and deprivation of short chain fatty acids [51]. Penna et al. [52] reported a strong correlation between primary sclerosing cholangitis and pouchitis, suggesting a common link in their pathogenesis. Teixeira et al. [53] showed that pouchitis was more frequent in patients with extra-intestinal manifestations. Acute pouchitis was more frequent than chronic pouchitis described by others.

Conclusion

In conclusion, patients with UC who undergo an ileal anal pouch operation also require surveillance. More recent research has focused on the chemoprevention of CRC in IBD using aminosalicylate (5-ASA) preparations. Several retrospective correlative studies have suggested that the long-term use of 5-ASA in IBD patients may significantly reduce the risk of development of CRC. Moody et al. [54] demonstrated that patients with UC who did not comply with 5-ASA therapies were significantly more likely to develop CRC than their counterparts. Eaden et al. [55] found that regular 5-ASA therapy reduces cancer risk by 75% in IBD patients. Mesalazine at a dose of 1.2 g/day or greater reduced CRC risk by 91% compared to no treatment and was also supportive when taken at lower doses. They concluded that the benefit of regular consumption of 5-ASA was equal to frequent visits to a hospital physician.

References

1. Ekbom A, Helmick C, Zack M et al (1990) Increased risk of large bowel cancer in Crohn's disease with colonic involvement. Lancet 336:357–359
2. Langholz E, Munkholm P, Davidsen M et al (1992) Colorectal cancer risk and mortality in patients with ulcerative colitis. Gastroenterology 103:1444–1451
3. Choi PM, Zelig MP (1994) Similarity of colorectal cancer in CD and UC. Gut 35:950–954
4. Gyde S, Prior P, Dew MJ et al (1982) Mortality in ulcerative colitis. Gastroenterology 83:36–43
5. Munkholm P, Langholz E, Davidsen M, Binder V (1993) Intestinal cancer risk and mortality in patients with Crohn's disease. Gastroenterology 105:1716–1723
6. Jess T, Winther KV, Munkholm P et al (2002) Mortality and causes of death in Crohn's disease: follow-up of a population-based cohort in Copenhagen County, Denmark. Gastroenterology 122:1808–1814
7. Eaden JA, Abrams KR, Mayberry JF (2001) The risk of colorectal cancer in ulcerative colitis: a meta analysis. Gut 48:526–535
8. Ekbom A, Helmick C, Zack M, Ademi HO (1990) Ulcerative colitis and colorectal cancer. N Eng J Med 323:1228–1233
9. Rutter M, Saunders B, Wilkinson K et al (2004) Severity of inflammation is a risk factor for colorectal neoplasia in ulcerative colitis. Gastroenterology 126:451–459
10. Gyde SN, Prior P, Allan RN et al (1988) Colorectal cancer in ulcerative colitis: a cohort study of primary referrals from three centers. Gut 29:206
11. Lennard-Jones JE (1985) Cancer risk in ulcerative colitis: surveillance or surgery. Br J Surg 72(Suppl):84
12. Collins RH, Feldman M, Fordtran JS (1987) Colon cancer, dysplasia and surveillance in patients with ulcerative colitis: a critical review. N Engl J Med 316:1654
13. Levin B (1992) Inflammatory bowel disease and colon cancer. Cancer 70:1313
14. Marchesa P, Lashner BA, Lavery IC et al (1997) The risk of cancer and dysplasia among ulcerative colitis patients with primary sclerosing cholangitis. Am J Gastroenterol 92:1285
15. Pinczowski D, Ekbom A, Baron J, et al (1994) Risk factors for colorectal cancer in patients with ulcertive colitis: a case-control study. Gastroenterology 107:117–120
16. Lashner BA, Provencher KS, Seidner DL et al (1997) The effect of folic acid supplementation on the risk for cancer or dysplasia in ulcerative colitis. Gastroenterology 112:29–32
17. Lashner BA, Heindereich PA, Su GL et al (1989) Effect of folate supplementation on the incidence of dysplasia and cancer in chronic ulcerative colitis. Gastroenterology 97:255–259
18. Nuako KW, Ahlquist DA, Mahoney DW et al (1998) Familial predisposition for colorectal cancer in chronic ulcerative colitis: a case-control study. Gastroenterology 115:1079–1083
19. Askling J, Dickman PW, Karlen P et al (2001) Colorectal cancer rates among first-degree relatives of patients with inflammatory bowel disease: a population-based study. Lancet 357:262–266
20. Riegler G, Carratù R, Tartaglione MT et al (1988) Prevalence and relative risk of malignancy in relatives of inflammatory bowel disease patients an control subjects. J Clin Gastroenterol 27(3):211–214
21. Riegler G, Caserta L, Castiglione F et al (2006) Increased risk of breast cancer in first-degree relatives of Crohn's disease patients: an IG-IBD study. Dig Liv

Dis 38(1):18–23
22. Persson PG, Karlen P, Bernell O et al (1994) Crohn's disease and cancer: a population-based cohort study. Gastroenterology 107:1675–1679
23. Fireman Z, Grossman A, Lilos P et al (1989) Intestinal cancer in patients with Cron's disease: a population study in cental Israel. Scand J Gastroenterol 24:346–350
24. Jess T, Winther K, Munkholm P et al (2000) Is there an increased risk of intestinal and extra intestinal cancer in patients with Crohn's disease? A population based cohort followed from 1962 to 1997. Gastroenterology 118(Suppl 2):1472
25. Gillen CD, Walmsley RS, Prior R et al (1994) Ulcerative colitis and Crohn's disease: a comparison of the colorectal cancer risk in extensive colitis. Gut 35:651–5
26. Vogelstein B, Fearon ER, Hamilton SR et al (1988) Genetic alteration during colorectal tumour development. N Engl J Med 319:525
27. Itzkowitz SH, Greenwald B, Meltzer SJ (1995) Colon carcinogenesis in inflammatory bowel disease. Inflamm Bowel Dis 1:142
28. Burner GC, Rabinovitch PS, Haggit RC et al (1992) Neoplastic progression in ulcerative colitis: histology, DNA content, and loss of a p53 allele. Gastroenterology 103:1602
29. Riddell RH, Golman H, Ramsohoff DF et al (1983) Dysplasia in inflammatory bowel disease: standardized classification with provisional clinical application. Hum Pathol 14:931–968
30. Willenbucher RF (1996) Inflammatory bowel disease. Semin Gastrointest Dis 7:94–104
31. Lennard-Jones JE, Nelville DM, Morson BC et al (1990) Precancer and cancer in extensive ulcerative colitis: findings among 401 patients over 22 years. Gut 31:800–806
32. Goldman H (1996) Significance and detection of dysplasia in chronic colitis. Cancer 78:2261–2263
33. Blackstone MO, Riddell RH, Roger BHG et al (1982) Dysplasia-associated lesion or mass (DALM) detected by colonscopy in long-standing ulcerative colitis: an indication for colectomy. Gastroenterology 80:366–374
34. Torres C, Antonioli D, Odze RD et al (1998) Polypoid dysplasia and adenomas in inflammatory bowel disease. Am J Surg Pathol 22:275–284
35. Odze RD (1999) Adenomas and adenomas-like DALMs in chronic ulcerative colitis: a clinical, pathological and molecular review. Am J Gastroenterol 94:1746–1750
36. Suzuki K, Muto T, Shinozaki M et al (1998) Differential diagnoses of dysplasia associated lesion or mass and coincidental adenoma in ulcerative colitis. Dis Colon Rectum 41:322
37. Engelsgjerd M, Farraye FA, Odze RD (1999) Polypectomy may be adequate treatment for adenoma-like dysplastic lesions in chronic ulcerative colitis. Gastroenterology 117:1288
38. Rubin PH, Friedman S, Harpaz N et al (1999) Colonoscopy polypectomy in chronic colitis: conservative management after endoscopic resection of dysplastic polyps. Gastroenterology 117:1295
39. Morin PJ, Sparks AB, Korinek V et al (1997) Activation of B-catenin-Tcf signaling in colon cancer by mutations in B-catenin or APC. Science 275:1787
40. Munemitsu S, Albert I, Souza B et al (1995) Regulation of intracellular beta-catenin levels by adenomatous polyposis coli (APC) tumour suppressor protein. Proc Natl Acad Sci USA 92:3046
41. Vietri MT, Riegler G, Pappalardo D et al (2006) The Arg72Pro p53 polymorphism influences the clinical outcome of ulcerative colitis. Lab Invest (In press)
42. Ramsohoff DF, Riddell RH, Levin B (1985) Ulcerative colitis and colonic cancer: problems in assessing the diagnostic usefulness of mucosal dysplasia. Dis Colon Rectum 28:383
43. Taylor BA, Pemberton JH, Carpenter HA et al (1992) Dysplasia in chronic ulcerative colitis: implications for colonoscopic surveillance. Dis Colon Rectum 35:950
44. Warren R, Barwick KW (1983) Crohn's colitis with adenocarcinoma and dysplasia: report of a case and review of 100 small and large bowel resection for Crohn's disease to detect incidence of dysplasia. Am J Surg Pathol 7:151
45. Provenzale D, Wong JB, Onken JE, Lipscomb J (1998) Performing a cost effectiveness analysis: surveillance of patients with ulcerative colitis. Am J Gastroenterol 93:872
46. Fonkalsrud EW, Phillips JD (1990) Reconstruction of malfunctioning ileoanal pouch procedures as an alternative to permanent ileostomy. Am J Surg 160:245–251
47. Ruseler-Van Embden JGH, Schouten WR (1994) Pouchitis: result of microbial imbalance? Gut 35:658–664
48. Chaussade S, Denizot Y, Valleur P (1991) Presence of Paf-acether in stool of patients with pouch ileoanal anastomosis and pouchitis. Gastroenterology 100:1509–1514
49. Levin KE, Pemberton JH, Phillips SF (1992) Role of oxygen free radicals in the etiology of pouchitis. Dis Colon Rectum 35:452–456
50. Kroesen AJ, John M, Schofelder G (1997) Expression of inducible nitric oxide syntase (iNOS) in pouchitis after ileoanal pouch surgery for ulcerative colitis. Langenbecks Archiv fur Chirurgie 114:451–454
51. Clausen MR, Tvede M, Mortensen PB (1992) Short-chain fatty acids in pouch contents from patients with and without pouchitis after ileal pouch-anal anastomosis. Gastroenterology 103:1144–1153
52. Penna C, Dozois RR, Tremaine W (1996) Pouchitis after ileal pouch anal anastomosis for chronic ulcerative colitis occur with increased frequency in patients with associated primary sclerosing cholangitis. Gut 38:234–239
53. Teixeira WGJ, Silva JH, Texeira MG (1999) Pouchitis: extracolonic manifestation of ulcerative colitis? Rev Hosp Clin Fac Med S Paulo 54:155–158
54. Moody GA, Javanthi V, Probert CS et al (1996) Long-term therapy with sulphasalazine protects against colorectal cancer in ulcerative colitis: a retrospective study of colorectal cancer risk and compliance with treatment in Leicestershire. Eur J Gastroenterol Hepatol 8:1179–1183
55. Eaden J, Abrams K, Ekbom A et al (2000) Colorectal cancer prevention in ulcerative colitis: a case-control study. Aliment Pharmacol Ther 14:145–153

Colonic and Anorectal Motility in Inflammatory Bowel Disease

Beatrice Salvioli, Gabriele Bazzocchi

Introduction

Bowel disturbances in patients with inflammatory bowel disease (IBD) range from abdominal pain, tenesmus, diarrhea, rectal bleeding and passage of mucus. Intestinal pseudo-obstruction and toxic megacolon can occur as frightening complications of either ulcerative colitis (UC) or Crohn's disease (CD). Altered small and large intestinal motility patterns are a possible cause of the spectrum of symptoms of which patients complain [1]. Little is known about motility alterations in IBD and, most of all, how important they are in determining the patient's symptoms. Presumably, interactions between epithelial transport and abnormal motor activity are the key mechanisms. The disparity between severity of symptoms and degree of inflammation and small hard stools often passed with blood and mucus suggest a contribution of gut dysmotility to clinical features. Evidence of altered gut motility have been reported as being not only confined to the lower gut, but also to the small intestine, stomach and gallbladder [2, 3].

Patients with IBD generally experience periods of active disease followed by resolution of the mucosal injury and healing. This may be followed by a period of inactivity or quiescence that is interrupted by an acute relapse, the most frequent symptom of which is diarrhea. Impaired colonic absorption and/or increased secretion of fluids may partially explain liquid diarrhea [4].

Factors that might be involved in dysmotility include changes in the smooth muscle cell function, changes in innervation or variations in the sensory components. Herein, we try to give an overview of what has been discovered so far on motility modifications in patients with inflammatory bowel disease and in animal models.

Human In Vivo Studies

Colonic Motility

Studies on colonic motility in IBD patients date back decades and provide conflicting results. The discrepancies reflect differences of study design, pressure sensors and patients selection [5]. Diarrhea may partly be explained by changes in mucosal secretory and absorptive functions, but some authors also suggest that alterations in colonic motility may also contribute to increased urgency and frequency of defecation in patients with ulcerative colitis. The cause of diarrhea could be identified in an excessive propulsive activity [6, 7], or in rectosigmoid inflammation rather than by rapid transit [8]. The disease is often associated with right-sided constipation and left-sided diarrhea [9], reflecting proximal colonic stasis with rapid transit through the rectosigmoid region [8]. The paradoxical slowing of transit in the small intestine and proximal colon seem to be consequential to an increased sensitivity to normal colonic contents which delays transit [10]. Clinical studies suggest that active inflammation is accompanied by a reduction in contractile activity in the diseased area and it seems that a decrease in segmental contraction, which normally slows down movement of colonic contents, would exacerbate diarrhea by allowing rapid forward movement of the bowel content. Prolonged recordings of colonic motility show a circadian variation characterized by a marked reduction of contractile activity at night [11, 12] and increased non-propagating contractions after eating [13] in healthy subjects. Different studies in patients with UC reported either a reduced or an exaggerated postprandial colonic response [14]. A simultaneous study of postprandial colonic motility and transit measured by scintigraphy in patients with UC showed a decreased contractility and an increased low-amplitude propagating contractions in patients compared to healthy controls, while transit had a variable pattern [10]. A diminished colonic contractile response to meals has been recently confirmed by a study that examined the effect of ulcerative proctosigmoiditis on motor functions of an uninflamed segment of descending colon, whereas fasting motility was increased [15]. Colonic compliance was unaffected by these changes, suggesting that modifications occur in physiological responses, and not in intrinsic wall properties. Moreover, the same authors assessed the effect of nicotine on colonic motor functions, without drawing any conclusion on a beneficial role of nicotine on motility, since low doses did not have any effect on transit or motor function. To overcome the limits of short-time period studies, other authors evaluated colonic motor activity by means of 24-h manometry [16] in patients with active UC, diarrhea-predominant irritable bowel syndrome (IBS) patients and healthy controls. Patients with IBD and IBS had increased high and low-amplitude propagated activity, suggesting that an increased propulsive contractility is responsible for diarrheal states. Most of the studies published in literature have been performed in patients with UC, since studies in patients with CD are limited by the access in the small intestine. There is evidence of altered interdigestive motility in the small intestine in the majority of patients studied with inactive and uncomplicated disease [2]. This may result in changes in orocecal transit that could lead to the bacterial overgrowth [17] present in 23% of unselected patients with CD, which is associated with a prolongation of orocecal transit time (OCTT). Other authors describe a delayed OCTT in 75% of patients: both delayed OCTT and small-bowel bacterial overgrowth may be clinically relevant in CD, not only because of the contribution to symptoms but also because of the possible negative influence on the releasing of the drug in slow-release drug formulations. Small-intestinal transit time is significantly shorter in ileocecal-resected patients, which might influence small-intestinal pH and transit time. An ileocecal resection might, therefore, affect the delivery of active drugs from tablets with pH-dependent delivery [18].

Gallbladder motility has also been evaluated since patients with CD have an increased risk of developing gallstones. Fasting gallbladder volume is decreased in patients with large-bowel involvement or after ileocecal resection, whereas postprandial motility seems to be unaffected [19]. Impaired gastric emptying was found in a subgroup of CD patients who complained of mild upper gut symptoms such as bloating, early satiety and abdominal distention and in those with localization restricted to the colon [3]. The impact of psychological, physical, and immunological stressors on gastrointestinal secretion, motility, epithelial permeability, and inflammation is now thoroughly documented, and stress has a major influence on digestive diseases [20]. Psychological stress is one environmental factor which has long been reported as having a relationship with activity in IBD. Psychological (dichotomous listening tests, stressful interviews) and physical (cold hand immersion) stress modulates gut function by enhancing colonic motor activity [21]. Dichotomous listening tests and cold pain stress have also been shown to increase jejunal water and sodium and chloride ion secretion [22].

Data suggest that stress-induced alterations in gastrointestinal inflammation may be mediated through changes in the hypothalamic-pituitary-adrenal axis function and alterations in bacterial-mucosal interactions, and via mucosal mast cells and mediators such as corticotrophin releasing factor. A recent report indicates that the intestine produces the same stress peptides that are present in the central nervous system [23]. In particular, a bacterial toxin that is the principal cause of antibiotic-induced colitis and diarrhea, results in the local generation of stress peptides that regulate the transit of digested material through the intestine under normal conditions and mediate inflammation without involving the central nervous system. This intrinsic stress response mechanism may contribute to disorders such as IBD and IBS, for which stress exacerbates the symptoms. For a more comprehensive review, the reader is referred to a detailed paper review that explores the recent advances on the pathogenic role of psychological stress in IBD [24].

Anorectal Motility

Most of the studies on anorectal motility yielded different results, depending on the activity of disease, especially in the rectums of patients with ulcerative colitis. Reduction of anal sphincter pressures in active colitis may contribute to episodes of fecal incontinence in some patients; however, overall, resting and squeeze pressures are similar in patients, irrespective of disease activity [9]. Rectal inflammation seems to be responsible for the augmented sensitivity to air-filled balloon distention [7, 26] or to rectal saline infusion [5], as well as decreased rectal compliance and higher contractility, suggesting that symptoms of urgency of defecation and fecal incontinence may be due to a hypersensitive, hyperactive, and poorly compliant rectum [9]. The role of acute inflammation on rectal motility and sensory perception are corroborated by data showing that, despite decreased rectal compliance in active and quiescent disease [7], only patients with active UC are hypersensitive to distention compared to controls and patients during remission [9]. The increased rectal sensitivity in active colitis is associated with a marked decrease in rectal compliance, which is reduced in active disease, suggesting that reduced rectal size is due to loss of distensibility. Moreover, in patients, lower rectal volumes are required for initiating sustained anal relaxation than in controls and continence is threatened in the absence of a strong external anal sphincter contraction that counterbalances the prolonged sphincter relaxation. From these conflicting data, it is not clear whether rectal inflammation or decreased compliance are responsible for augmented sensation, or whether symptoms (e.g., abdominal pain) commonly present during flares depend on the inflammation grade of the mucosa. In order to shed light on this, some authors evaluated the rectosigmoid perception to balloon distention in patients with mild UC, patients with IBS and controls [27]. They found that despite mild rectal mucosa inflammation and similar mechanoelastic properties, patients with UC were hyposensitive to balloon distension compared to the other groups. Another interesting point was that repeated rectosigmoid stimulation induced hypoalgesia in more than 50% of the UC patients, as compared to the hyperalgesia detected in IBS patients [28]. The authors concluded that persistent peripheral irritation is associated with activation of counter-regulatory antinociceptive mechanisms which produce endogenous analgesia, and that acute symptoms during disease exacerbation are partially related to transient inflammatory mucosal events resulting in sensitization of visceral afferent pathways.

The different perceptual responses to rectosigmoid stimuli between mild chronic inflammatory and functional disease are confirmed by different regional activation (i.e., greater activation of limbic/paralimbic circuits in IBS and inhibition of these circuits by the right lateral frontal cortex in UC and controls) in cerebral PET studies [29].

Alterations of anorectal functions are not confined to UC, but are also recognizable in CD. A linear relationship between the degree of proctitis and the rectal maximal tolerated volume is observed in patients with CD involving the rectum [30]. Impairment of anorectal functions (i.e., lower anal resting and squeeze pressures, lower wave amplitude and frequency, altered perception and reduced compliance) is documented not only in simultaneous endoscopic and histologic lesions of the disease, but also in patients with sole microscopic lesion [31]. Moreover, in the absence of macroscopic anorectal disease, some alterations, specifically absence of rectoanal inhibitory reflex and hyposensitivity to rectal balloon distension, could be due to alterations in the enteric nervous system [32].

Another study evaluating visceral sensitivity in patients with ileal Crohn's disease presented evidence for reduced pain sensitivity, possibly related to descending bulbospinal inhibition of sacral dorsal horn neurons in response to chronic intestinal tissue irritation [33]. The presence of a hyposensitive rectum in CD was already observed by some authors years ago, where almost half of patients with a normal looking rectum could tolerate higher volumes of distension without reporting discomfort as opposed to healthy controls [30]. It is likely that a certain type of inflammation may reduce pain sensitivity by the production of endorphins at the seat of the injury [34]. In contrast to previously reported results, some data indicate that patients with CD limited to the ileum or colon, exhibit increased resting pressures in conjunction with rectal hypersensitivity, indicative of a potential role in the pathogenesis of fissures [35].

Human In Vitro Studies

The mechanisms underlying this colonic dysfunction are poorly understood, but may involve changes in smooth muscle contractility, enteric neurotransmission or afferent sensory input from the bowel wall. It is well recognized that inflammation is associated with alterations in mucosal and motor function in both the small intestine and the colon and that colonic motility varies with disease activity. As inflammation progresses, there are changes in the profile of the inflammatory/immune cells and associated mediators that may directly or indirectly affect smooth muscle contractility. Early clinical studies report both hypermotility and hypomotility in ulcerative colitis patients. Moreover, UC patients exhibit changes in the frequency of spontaneous contractions that vary with the duration of their disease. A number of studies have attempted to determine whether neurotransmission and neuromuscular function is altered in the colonic tissue of IBD-affected patients. The intrinsic properties of the circular muscle from patients with UC show few differences from those of healthy control subjects, but electrically or agonist-stimulated contraction are reduced [36, 37]. Altered motor function measured In Vitro may be evident through alterations in the cholinergic function or neurokinin (NK) receptor-mediated contraction in the smooth muscles in UC [38]. Extrinsic sensory neurons in the gut contain neurotransmitters such as calcitonin gene-related peptide (CGRP) and substance P (SP). Both have been implicated in the effects of colonic distension and capsaicin application to the colon and are considered to have an important role in normal digestive, secretory and motor functions in the gut [39, 40]. There is also strong evidence implicating sensory neuropeptides in the functional development of gastrointestinal inflammation, particularly in IBD [41]. Elevations of substance P (SP) peptide levels and immunoreactivity [42-43], and upregulation of receptors for SP and its mRNA [44, 45], influence inhibitory nerves including nerves containing vasoactive intestinal peptide (VIP). Reduction in excitatory transmit including SP [46] and altered NK-2 receptor-mediated contraction occur in IBD-affected colon [47].

Selective impairments in tachykinin and CGRP-mediated colonic motility are manifest in inflammatory bowel disease In Vitro [48]. Data show a reduction in motility in patients with active disease. In Vitro, there is evidence of impaired contractility of smooth muscle from UC patients, suggesting the physiological release of an inhibitory neurotransmitter [36]. There is a large neural inhibitory component to responses from inflamed tissue and these responses could be blocked through the inhibition of nitric oxide synthase (NOS), implicating nitric oxide (NO) as the mediator [49]. The role of NO in the pathophysiology of IBD is controversial. An immunoblot of biopsies revealed significant elevation of nitric oxide synthase isoform (iNOS) in active UC compared to uninflamed sites [50, 51], whereas in patients with CD, no significant changes were detected [52].

Recently, using a new investigative tool (chemiluminescence technique by means of a tonometric balloon), some authors detected higher rectal luminal levels of NO in IBD patients compared to IBS and healthy controls [53]. Nicotine appears to reduce circular muscle activity, predominantly through the release of NO that appears to be upregulated in active ulcerative colitis [54].

There is an increase in NO synthase activities in the nerve of the myenteric plexus as well as in smooth muscle cells in the colon in UC [55]. A report evaluating expression of the inducible isoform of nitric oxide synthase (iNOS) in UC suggested increased production of this inflammatory enzyme in the muscle layers of the colon and implicated the resultant nitric oxide as the mediator of the reduced contractility and consequent toxic megacolon [56].

One of the mechanisms responsible for the motility dysfunction observed in patients with UC could be due to increase level of cytokines (i.e., IL-1 beta) through production of hydrogen peroxide (H_2O_2) [57]. In UC, the mucosa releases IL-1beta, H_2O_2, and NO [58], and H_2O_2 is also produced in the muscle layer of UC [59], which may contribute to the impaired Ca2+ release and altered sigmoid muscle contractility. In both human and animal models of colitis there appears to be a relationship between altered colonic motility and abnormal local release of various inflammatory mediators of which prostaglandins such as PGE2 are of considerable importance [60, 61]. There is evidence of increased synthesis of prostaglandin (PGE2) in the rat myenteric plexus after appropriate cytokine stimulation [62] and also in the rectal mucosa of patients with active IBD [63].

Gastrin releasing peptide (GRP) receptor expression is decreased in the inflamed and non-inflamed colon of CD, while that is not the case in UC [64]. The cell types involved in the altered motor pattern include interstitial cells of Cajal [65], which are damaged and presumably contribute to altered motility. In tissues from Crohn's disease patients, the density of interstitial cells of Cajal is reduced throughout the tunica muscularis, suggesting that the disturbance of intestinal motility that occurs in patients with CD may be a consequence of the loss of or defects in specific populations of interstitial cells of Cajal within the tunica muscularis [66]. Hypersensitivity to cholinergic stimulation has been demonstrated in the colonic smooth muscle from patients with UC and it may result from increased calcium release from intracellular stores [67].

Animal in Vivo and in Vitro Studies

As already described, the mechanisms of altered motility in IBD are unclear but may reflect changes in the axon/smooth muscle cell relationship and data suggest that the enteric nervous system (ENS) has an important role in the motility defects [68]. A limitation in understanding the etiology of IBD is that few animals spontaneously develop colitis and several animal models, particularly the hapten 2,4,6-trinitrobenzenesulfonic acid (TNBS) in ethanol have been used to produce an acute inflammation that progresses over several weeks to a chronic stage that is morphologically similar to Crohn's disease. Data in animal models are controversial. Measurements of In Vivo motility patterns in dogs during acetic acid-induced ileitis showed that inflammation increased the frequency of giant migrating contractions and decreased the frequency of migrating motor complexes and tone [69, 70]. A study evaluating colonic motor response to a meal in acute colitis dogs showed an absence of motor response of the colon to a meal and increase in the postprandial frequency of giant migrating contractions associated with an increase in defecation frequency [71]. Data suggest that both the initial inflammation and recurrence of active disease induce a transient increase in contractile amplitude and duration and the effects of repeated episodes of acute inflammation (i.e., successive applications of TNBS in rats) have a different impact on spontaneous contractions of colonic circular muscle compared with a single TNBS application [72]. Acute inflammation of the colon significantly promotes the amplitude and duration of spontaneous contractions likely due to loss of NO control or to changes in excitatory neurotransmitters such as acetylcholine (Ach) [72]. Whereas, other data suggest that propulsive motility is reduced, since in rats with acute dextran sulfate sodium (DDS)-induced colitis, there was a reduced frequency of colonic giant migrating contractions in the proximal and middle colon [73] and reduced pellet propulsion In Vitro in isolated distal colon from TNBS-treated guinea pigs [74].

Many of the contractile abnormalities of muscle from animal models of colitis appear to be due to muscle specific defects, or alterations in signal transduction mechanisms rather than plasticity of the innervation of the muscle [75–77]. Indeed, morphological studies of canine colon suggest that NO is a crucial mediator in the communication between interstitial cells of Cajal, enteric inhibitory nerves, and smooth muscle in the generation of spontaneous contractions [78]. Impaired nitric oxide synthase (NOS) activity in nerves seems to be implicated in the reduced ability of smooth muscle to relax in colitis induced by dextran sulfate sodium in rats [79]. Modifications in excitatory reactions are illustrated by data showing an increased response to ACh and substance P during acute inflammation, an effect attributed to a loss of neural inhibition (i.e., NOS activity), rather than an increase in excitation, resulting in enhanced contractile amplitude [80].

The initial inflammation induces a long-lasting alteration in the frequency of spontaneous contractions, which suggests a remodeling of the interactions between smooth muscle and nerves. In TNBS colitis in the rat, it has been recently demonstrated that a loss of intrinsic axons is an early event in colitis and, although reversed by axonal proliferation, transient denervation may promote circular smooth muscle cell hyperplasia [81].

Specifically, chronic inflammation reduces smooth muscle contractility [80], and the thickening of the smooth muscle evident at 7 days post TNBS is consistent with reports of smooth muscle hyperplasia and hypertrophy in animal models [82] and in IBD patients [83].

In experiments with injections of indomethacin in rats, which induces inflammation, during the active phase there is a decrease of motor activity related to bacterial translocation [84]. The initial intestinal hypomotility seems associated to inhibitory effects of nitric oxide due to the increased levels of inducible NOS isoform, since after the administration of selective iNOS inhibitors, a reaction of hypermotility occurs. Nematode infection leads to direct effects of Th2 cytokines such as myocyte hypertrophy and hypercontractility similar to that seen because of exposure to IL-4 and IL-13 and is thought to be partly due to the signal transducer and activator of transcription factor STAT-6 in the affected myocytes, which is necessary for the effect of Th2 cytokines [85]. The impact of chronic inflammation on muscle contractility has been examined after 12 weeks of infection with *Schistosoma mansoni* in mice [86] and pigs [87]. The infection in the mice caused small intestinal hypercontractility on one side, that seemed to be due to increased postjunctional myocyte responsiveness to a released transmitter and a slow transit on the other side [86]. In the pigs, the severity of infection was inversely correlated with VIP immunoreactivity and directly correlated with SP and neuronal nitric oxide synthase (nNOS) levels [88].

In summary, as already stated, several factors contribute to alteration of muscle contractility. Some changes are due to prereceptor mechanisms, causing a reduced release of non-adrenergic, non-cholinergic inhibitory transmitters that diminish contractility and relaxation of the non-inflamed fundus in TNBS ileitis in rats. In fact, changes in muscle function are not limited to the region of the inflamed gut [89, 90]: noradrenaline and acetylcholine are reduced not only in the inflamed, but also in the unaffected segment in TNBS colitic rats. The reduced release of neurotransmitters during colitis can be explained by increased presynaptic inhibition of neurotransmitter release, either by augmented α2-adrenoceptor expression or by enhanced release of histamines from mast cells and elevated levels of cytokines such as IL-6 [91]. As well as in humans, stress has effects on the GI tract in animals. Gastrointestinal transit is differently affected by stress, varying from region to region: specifically the orocecal and colonic transit was accelerated, while gastric emptying was delayed [92].

Acute tissue irritation with chemical irritants such as turpentine, acetic acid, formalin, or zymosan induces visceral hyperalgesia in animal models of acute colitis, mediated by the activity of spinal N-methyl d-aspartate (NMDA) and non-NMDA receptors, as well as in rats treated with TNBS there is an enhanced visceromotor response to colorectal distension [93].

The reduced contractile activity in IBD [94] may be the result of altered serotonin (5-HT) availability (increase 5-HT availability and decrease 5-HT reuptake), likely due to desensitization of 5-HT receptors. These data suggest that abnormal 5-HT signaling at the afferent limb of intrinsic and extrinsic reflex pathways, due to increased 5-HT availability, could contribute to changes in gut function and sensitivity in the inflamed bowel [95].

Study in Ileal-Pouch Anal Anastomosis (IPAA)

Very few studies have described motor pattern in patients with IBD after surgery and with IPAA in particular. In a study of some years ago [96], our aim was to determine whether a meal induces specific motor patterns in longstanding IPAA. Nine patients (6M, 3F) aged 35–58 (median 49) years were studied 1–10 (median 6.8) years after ileostomy closure. Two had a W-pouch and seven had a J-pouch. None of the patients showed endoscopic findings of pouchitis; daily bowel movements were 2–6 (median 4.6). After at least 12 h of fasting, an 8-channel perfused catheter with an open central lumen was placed by means of a guide-wire inserted during a regular colonoscopy. Recording ports, 15 cm apart, were positioned such that four were in the proximal small bowel, three in the reservoir and one on the internal anal sphincter. After at least 1 h after colonoscopy, we recorded pressure signals for 120 min before the ingestion of a 1 000-Kcal meal with 40, 30 and 30% of lipids, proteins and carbohydrates respectively. Postprandial recording continued for a further 60 min. Small bowel and pouch contractile activity was characterized at rest by sequences of large, isolated contraction waves. Phase III of MMCs were recorded in 7 patients. However, they were not followed by quiescence phases (Phase I), entering the rhythmic contraction sequence. In two cases, MMCs propagated into the reservoir resulting in IAS relaxation (Fig. 1). A meal induced an immediate increase in amplitude and frequency of motor waves creating clusters of multiphasic contractions. The global motility index (area under the curve) in the ileoanal pouch increased from 397–794 (mean 590) and from 479–756 (mean 582) mm Hg-min/60 min in the two fasting periods to 621–1 710 (mean 863) postprandially ($p<0.04$; Wilcoxon test for matched pairs). We concluded that: (1) the fasting activity is not characterized by the typical sequences of the interdigestive motor activity in patients with longstanding ileoanal pouch; (2) the presence of altered MMC phases suggests that motor activity in the proximal small bowel is modified as a result of reservoir creation; (3) a meal induces significant changes in motor activity in the ileoanal reservoir, suggesting that "colonic" motility patterns arises in the most distal tract of the gut.

Conclusions

Evidence in the literature reports motility abnormalities in patients with inflammatory bowel disorders. Many of the symptoms reported by patients derive from alteration in gut physiology. The mechanisms of this dysmotility are uncertain but different factors, either direct or indirect, of muscles and nerves can produce alteration of gut functions through the involvement of endocrine and neural networks.

We can summarize that entry of new ingesta into the colon during the postprandial period stimulates enteric mechanisms to initiate an excessive number of both high and low-amplitude propagating contractions. The decreased contractile function of the smooth muscle further helps acceleration of propulsion by decreasing segmental contractions and allowing forward movement of the colonic contents with-

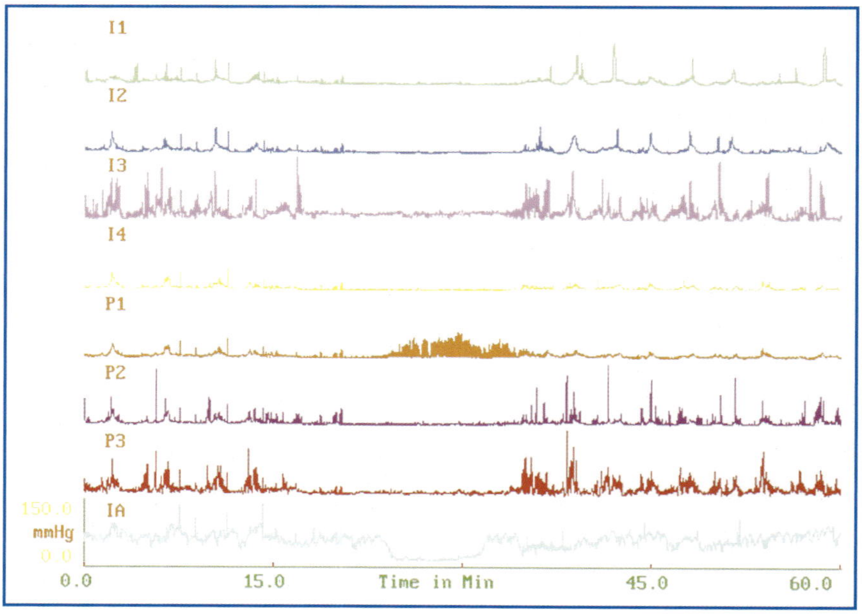

Fig. 1. One hour multilumen manometric recording in patients with ileal pouch-anal anastomosis during fasting. Four recording ports were placed in the afferent ileal tract (*I*), three recording ports were in the pouch (*P*) and one in the proximal anal canal (*IA*). Phase II motor pattern was abruptly interrupted simultaneously in all the recording sites: it was replaced by MMC phase 1-like motility for about 15 min. During this complete quiescent period, a phase III-like motor complex was recorded at the most proximal pouch level (*P1*): at the same time, relaxation of the internal anal sphincter occurs (*IA*). Phase II-like motility and basal anal tone resumed simultaneously in all the recording channels

out impediments. The anorectal region is characterized by increased sensitivity to distension and reduced compliance

References

1. Snape WJ Jr (1991) The role of a colonic motility disturbance in ulcerative colitis. Keio J Med 40:6–8
2. Annese V, Bassotti G, Napolitano G et al (1997) Gastrointestinal motility disorders in patients with inactive Crohn's disease. Scand J Gastroenterol 32:1107–1117
3. Annese V, Bassotti G, Napolitano G et al (1995) Gastric emptying of solids in patients with nonobstructive Crohn's disease is sometimes delayed. J Clin Gastroenterol 21:279–282
4. Greig E, Sandle GI (2000) Diarrhea in ulcerative colitis: the role of altered colonic sodium transport. Ann N Y Acad Sci 915:327–332
5. Rao SS, Read NW, Stobart JA et al (1988) Anorectal contractility under basal conditions and during rectal infusion of saline in ulcerative colitis. Gut 29:769–777
6. Bazzocchi G, Ellis J, Villanueva-Meyer J et al (1991) Effect of eating on colonic motility and transit in patients with functional diarrhea. Simultaneous scintigraphic and manometric evaluation. Gastroenterology 101:1298-1306
7. Loening-Baucke V, Metcalf AM, Shirazi S (1989) Rectosigmoid motility in patients with quiescent and active ulcerative colitis. Am J Gastroenterol 84:34–39
8. Rao SS, Read NW (1990) Gastrointestinal motility in patients with ulcerative colitis. Scand J Gastroenterol Suppl 172:22–28
9. Rao SS, Read NW, Davison PA, Thompson WG (1987) Anorectal sensitivity and responses to rectal distension in patients with ulcerative colitis. Gastroenterology 93:1270–1275
10. Reddy SN, Bazzocchi G, Chan S et al (1991) Colonic motility and transit in health and ulcerative colitis Gastroenterology 101:1289–1297
11. Rao SS, Sadeghi P, Beaty J et al (2001) Ambulatory 24-h colonic manometry in healthy humans. Am J Physiol 280:G629-G639
12. Bassotti G, Germani U, Morelli A (1995) Human colonic motility: physiological aspects. Int J Colorectal Dis 10:173–180
13. Moreno-Osset E, Bazzocchi G, Lo S et al (1989) Association between postprandial changes in colonic intraluminal pressure and transit. Grastroenterology 96:1265-1273
14. Snape WJ Jr, Matarazzo SA, Cohen S (1980) Abnormal gastrocolonic response in patients with ulcerative colitis. Gut 21:392–396
15. Coulie B, Camilleri M, Bharucha AE et al (2001) Colonic motility in chronic ulcerative proctosigmoiditis and the effects of nicotine on colonic motility in patients and healthy subjects. Aliment Pharmacol Ther 15:653-663
16. Bassotti G, de Roberto G, Chistolini F et al (2004) Twenty-four-hour manometric study of colonic propulsive activity in patients with diarrhea due to inflammatory (ulcerative colitis) and non-inflammatory (irritable bowel syndrome) conditions. Int J Colorectal Dis 19:493–497
17. Castiglione F, del Vecchio Blanco G, Rispo A et al (2000) Orocecal transit time and bacterial overgrowth in patients with Crohn's disease. J Clin Gastroenterol 31:63–66
18. Fallingborg J, Pedersen P, Jacobsen BA (1998) Small intestinal transit time and intraluminal pH in ileocecal resected patients with Crohn's disease. Dig Dis Sci 43:702–705
19. Vu MK, Gielkens HA, van Hogezand RA, et al (2000) Gallbladder motility in Crohn's disease: influence of disease localization and bowel resection. Scand J Gastroenterol 35:1157–1162
20. Tache Y, Martinez V, Wang L, Million M (2004) RF1 receptor signaling pathways are involved in stress-related alterations of colonic function and viscerosensitivity: implications for irritable bowel syndrome. Br J Pharmacol 141:1321–1330
21. Rao SS, Hatfield RA, Suls JM, Chamberlain MJ (1998) Psychological and physical stress induce differential effects on human colonic motility. Am J Gastroenterol 93:985–990
22. Barclay GR, Turnberg LA (1988) Effect of cold-induced pain on salt and water transport in the human jejunum. Gastroenterology 94:994–998
23. La Fleur SE, Wick EC, Idumalla PS et al (2005) Role of peripheral corticotrophin-releasing factor and urocortin II in intestinal inflammation and motility in terminal ileum. Proc Natl Acad Sci U S A 102:7647–7652
24. Mawdsley JE, Rampton DS (2005) Psychological stress in IBD: new insights into pathogenic and therapeutic implications. Gut 54:1481–1491
25. Loening-Baucke V, Metcalf AM, Shirazi S (1989) Anorectal manometry in active and quiescent ulcerative colitis. Am J Gastroenterol 84:892–897
26. Farthing MJG, Lennard-Jones JE (1978) Sensibility of the rectum to distention and the anorectal distention reflex in ulcerative colitis. Gut 19:64–69
27. Chang L, Munakataa J, Mayer EA et al (2000) Perceptual responses in patients with inflammatory and functional bowel disease. Gut 47:497–505
28. Munakata J, Naliboff B, Harraf F et al (1997) Repetitive sigmoid stimulation induces rectal hyperalgesia in patients with irritable bowel syndrome. Gastroenterology 112:55–63
29. Mayer EA, Berman S, Suyenobu B et al (2005) Differences in brain responses to visceral pain between patients with irritable bowel syndrome and ulcerative colitis. Pain 115:398–409
30. Buchmann P, Mogg GA, Alexander-Williams J et al (1980) Relationship of proctitis and rectal capacity in Crohn's disease. Gut 21:137–140
31. Chrysos E, Athanasakis E, Tsiaoussis J et al (2001) Rectoanal motility in Crohn's disease patients. Dis Colon Rectum 44:1509–1513
32. Mueller, M H, Kreis ME, Gross ML et al (2002) Anorectal functional disorders in the absence of anorectal inflammation in patients with Crohn's disease. Br J Surg 89:1027–1031
33. Bernstein CN, Niazi N, Robert M et al (1996) Rectal afferent function in patients with inflammatory and functional intestinal disorders. Pain 66:151–161
34. Porreca F, Lai J, Malan TP Jr (1998) Can inflammation

relieve pain? Nat Med 4:1359–1360
35. Andersson P, Olaison G, Hallbook O et al (2003) Increased anal resting pressure and rectal sensitivity in Crohn's disease. Dis Colon Rectum 46:1685–1689
36. Snape WJ, Williams R, Hyman PE (1991) Defect in colonic smooth muscle contraction in patients with ulcerative colitis. Am J Physiol 261:G987–G991
37. Green JT, Richardson C, Marshall RW et al (2000). Nitric oxide mediates a therapeutic effect of nicotine in ulcerative colitis. Aliment Pharmacol Ther 14:1429–1434
38. Cook TA, Brading AF, McMortensen NJ (2000) Abnormal contractile properties of rectal smooth muscle in chronic ulcerative colitis. Aliment Pharmacol Ther 14:1287–1294
39. Julia V, Morteau O, Bueno L (1994) Involvement of neurokinin 1 and 2 receptors in viscerosensitive response to rectal distension in rats. Gastroenterology 107:94–102
40. Plourde V, St-Pierre S, Quirion R (1997) Calcitonin gene-related peptide in viscerosensitive response to colorectal distension in rats. Am J Physiol 273:G191–G196
41. Holzer P (1998) Implications of tachykinins and calcitonin gene-related peptide in inflammatory bowel disease. Digestion 59:269–283
42. Goldin EF, Karmeli Z, Selinger Z, Rachmilewitz D (1989) Colonic substance P levels are increased in ulcerative colitis and decreased in chronic severe constipation. Dig Dis Sci 34:754–757
43. Mantyh CR, Vigna SR, Bollinger RR et al (1995) Differential expression of substance P receptors in patients with Crohn's disease and ulcerative colitis. Gastroenterology 109:850–860
44. Goode T, O'Connell J, Anton P et al (2000) Neurokinin-1 receptor expression in inflammatory bowel disease: molecular quantitation and localisation. Gut 47:387–396
45. Renzi D, Pellegrini B, Tonelli F et al (2000) Substance P (neurokinin-1) and neurokinin A (neurokinin-2) receptor gene and protein expression in the healthy and inflammed human intestine. Am J Pathol 157:1511–1522
46. Al-Saffar A, Hellstrom PM (2001) Contractile response to natural tachykinins and selective tachykinin analogs in normal and inflamed ileal and colonic muscle. Scand J Gastroenterol 36:485–493
47. Menzies JRW, McKee R, Corbett AD (2001) Differential alterations in tachykinin NK2 receptors in isolated colonic circular smooth muscle in inflammatory bowel disease and idiopathic chronic constipation. Regul Pept 99:151–156
48. Smith AS, Scott D SMID (2005) Impaired capsaicin and neurokinin-evoked colonic motility in inflammatory bowel disease. J Gastroenterol Hepatol 20(5):697-704
49. Tomita R, Fujisaki S, Tanjoh K, Fukuzawa M (2000) Role of nitric oxide in the left-sided colon of patients with diverticular disease. Hepatogastroenterology 47:692-696
50. Middleton SJ, Shorthouse M, Hunter JO (1993) Increased nitric oxide synthesis in ulcerative colitis. Lancet 341:465–466
51. Singer II, Kawka DW, Scott S et al (1996) Expression of inducible nitric oxide synthase and nitrotyrosine in colonic epithelium in inflammatory bowel disease. Gastroenterology 111:871–885
52. Palatka K, Serfozo Z, Vereb Z et al (2005) Changes in the expression and distribution of the inducible and endothelial nitric oxide synthase in mucosal biopsy specimens of inflammatory bowel disease. Scand J Gastroenterol 40:670–680
53. Reinders CI, Herulf M, Ljung T et al (2005) Rectal mucosal nitric oxide in differentiation of inflammatory bowel disease and irritable bowel syndrome. Clin Gastroenterol Hepatol 3:777–783
54. Green JT, Richardson C, Marshall RW et al (2000) Nitric oxide mediates a therapeutic effect of nicotine in ulcerative colitis. Aliment Pharmacol Therapeut 14:1429–1434
55. Boughton-Smith NK, Evans SM, Hawkey CJ et al (1993) Nitric oxide synthase activity in ulcerative colitis and Crohn's disease. Lancet 342:338–340
56. Mourelle M, Casellas F, Guiarner F et al (1995) 0Induction of nitric oxide synthase in colonic smooth muscle from patients with toxic megacolon. Gastroenterology 109:1497–1502
57. Vrees MD, Pricolo VE, Potenti FM, Cao W (2002) Abnormal motility in patients with ulcerative colitis: the role of inflammatory cytokines. Arch Surg 137:439–445
58. Cao W, Fiocchi C, Pricolo VE (2005) Production of IL-1beta, hydrogen peroxide, and nitric oxide by colonic mucosa decreases sigmoid smooth muscle contractility in ulcerative colitis. Am J Physiol Cell Physiol 289:C1408–C1416
59. Cao W, Vrees MD, Kirber MT et al (2004) Hydrogen peroxide contributes to motor dysfunction in ulcerative colitis. Am J Physiol 286:G833–G843
60. Caprilli R, Orion L (1992) Pathogenesis of gastrointestinal distension in severe ulcerative colitis: a hypothesis. Gastroenterol Int 5:268–272
61. Snape WJ, Kao HW (1988) Role of inflammatory mediators in colonic smooth muscle function in ulcerative colitis. Dig Dis Sci 33:655–705
62. Rühl A, Berezin I, Collins SM et al (1995) Involvement of eicosanoids and macrophage like cells in cytokine mediated changes in rat myenteric nerves. Gastroenterology 109:1852–1862
63. Hawkey CJ, Karmelli F, Rachmilewitz D et al (1983) Imbalance of prostacyclin and thromboxane synthesis in Crohn's disease. Gut 24:881-885
64. Beek WP, Muller ES, Van Hogezand RA et al (2004) Gastrin releasing peptide receptor expression is decreased in patients with Crohn's disease but not in ulcerative colitis. J Clin Pathol 57:1047–1051
65. Rumessen JJ (1996) Ultrastructure of interstitial cells of Cajal at the colonic submuscular border in patients with ulcerative colitis. Gastroenterology 111:1447–1455
66. Porcher C, Baldo M, Henry M et al (2002) Deficiency of interstitial cells of Cajal in the small intestine of patients with Crohn's disease. Am J Gastroenterol 97:118–125
67. Cook TA, Brading AF, Mortensen NJ MCC (2000) Abnormal contractile properties of rectal smooth muscle in chronic ulcerative colitis. Aliment Pharmacol Ther 14:1287–1294
68. Lomax AE, Fernandez E, Sharkey KA (2005) Plasticity

of the enteric nervous system during intestinal inflammation. Neurogastroenterol Mot 17:4–15
69. Jouet P, Sarna SK, Singaram C et al (1995) Immunocytes and abnormal gastrointestinal motor activity during ileitis in dogs. Am J Physiol 269:G913–G924
70. Sarna SK (2003) Neuronal locus and cellular signaling for stimulation of ileal giant migrating and phasic contractions. Am J Physiol Gastrointest 284:G789–G797
71. Sethi AK, Sarna SK (1991) Colonic motor activity in acute colitis in conscious dogs. Gastroenterology 100:954–963
72. Bossone C, Hosseini JM, Pineiro-Carrero V et al (2001) Alterations in spontaneous contractions in vitro after repeated inflammation of rat distal colon. Am J Physiol 280:G949–G957
73. Li M, Johnson CP, Adams MB, Sarna SK (2002) Cholinergic and nitrergic regulation of in vivo giant migrating contractions in rat colon. Am J Physiol 283:G544–G552
74. Linden DR, Chen JX, Gershon MD et al (2003) Serotonin availability is increased in mucosa of guinea pigs with TNBS-induced colitis. Am J Physiol 285:G207–G216
75. Lu G, Qian X, Berezin I et al (1997) Inflammation modulates in vitro colonic myoelectric and contractile activity and interstitial cells of Cajal. Am J Physiol 273:G1233–G1234
76. Grossi L, McHugh K, Collins SM (1993) On the specificity of altered muscle function in experimental colitis in rats. Gastroenterology 104:1049–1056
77. Lu G, Mazet B, Sun C et al (1999) Inflammatory modulation of calcium-activated potassium channels in canine colonic circular smooth muscle cells. Gastroenterology 116:884–892
78. Sanders KM (1996) A case for interstitial cells of Cajal as pacemakers and mediators of neurotransmission in the gastrointestinal tract. Gastroenterology 111:492–515
79. Borjesson L, Delbro DS (2003) Neurogenic and non-neurogenic mechanisms in response of rat distal colon muscle to dextran sulphate sodium treatment. Auton Neurosci 107:74–80
80. Hosseini JM, Goldhill JM, Bossone C et al (1999) Progressive alterations in circular smooth muscle contractility in TNBS-induced colitis in rats. Neurogastroenterol Motil 11:347–356
81. Lourenssen S, Wells RW, Blennerhassett MG (2005) Differential responses of intrinsic and extrinsic innervation of smooth muscle cells in rat colitis. Exp Neurol 195:497–507
82. Yamada T, Marshall S, Specian RD, Grisham MB (1992) A comparative analysis of two models of colitis in rats. Gastroenterology 102:1524–1534
83. Rowland R, Pounder DJ (1982) Crohn's colitis. Pathol Annu 17:267-290
84. Porras M, Martin MT, Soler M, Vergara P (2004) Intestinal motor disorders associated with cyclical bacterial overgrowth in a rat model of enteritis. Am J Physiol 287:G58–64
85. Zhao A, McDermott J, Urban JF Jr et al (2003) Dependence of IL-4, IL-13, and nematode-induced alterations in murine small intestinal smooth muscle contractility on Stat6 and enteric nerves. J Immunol 171:948–954
86. Moreels TG, De Man JG, Bogers JJ et al (2001) Effect of Schistosoma mansoni-induced granulomatous inflammation on murine gastrointestinal motility. Am J Physiol 280:G1030–G1042
87. Balemba OB, Mortensen K, Semuguruka WD et al (2002) Neuronal nitric oxide synthase activity is increased during granulomatous inflammation in the colon and caecum of pigs infected with Schistosoma japonicum. Auton Neurosci 99:1–12
88. Balemba OB, Semuguruka WD, Hay-Schmidt A et al (2001) Vasoactive intestinal peptide and substance P-like immunoreactivities in the enteric nervous system of the pig correlate with the severity of pathological changes induced by Schistosoma japonicum. Int J Parasitol 31:1503–1514
89. Moreels TG, De Man JG, De Winter BY et al (2001) Effect of 2,4,6-trinitrobenzenesulphonic acid (TNBS)-induced ileitis on the motor function of non-inflamed rat gastric fundus. Neurogastroenterol Motil 13:339–352
90. Jacobson K, McHugh K, Collins SM (1995) Experimental colitis alters myenteric nerve function at inflamed and noninflamed sites in the rat. Gastroenterology 109:718–722
91. Liu S, Xia Y, Hu H et al (2000) Histamine H3 receptor-mediated suppression of inhibitory synaptic transmission in the submucous plexus of guinea-pig small intestine. Eur J Pharmacol 397:49–54
92. Enck P, Merlin V, Erckenbrecht JF, Wienbeck M (1989) Stress effects on gastrointestinal transit in the rat. Gut 30:455-459
93. Julia V, Mezzasalma T, Bueno L (1995) Influence of bradykinin in gastrointestinal disorders and visceral pain induced by acute or chronic inflammation in rats. Dig Dis Sci 40:1913–1921
94. O'Brien MD, Phillips SF (1996) Colonic motility in health and disease. Gastroenterol Clin North Am 25:147–162
95. Linden DR, Foley KF, Mcquoid C et al (2005) Serotonin transporter function and expression are reduced in mice with TNBS-induced colitis. Neurogastroenterol Motil 17:565–574
96. Bazzocchi G, Gionchetti P, Diquattro C et al (1999) Small bowel and ileoanal pouch motility after feeding. Gastroenterology 116:A956

Extraintestinal Manifestations of Inflammatory Bowel Disease

Giacomo C. Sturniolo, Michela Barollo, Renata D'Incà

Introduction

Inflammatory bowel disease (IBD) mainly affects the gastrointestinal system but is associated with various chronic diseases of other organs that are jointly called extraintestinal manifestations (EIM). In some of these disorders, onset and clinical manifestations are associated with the course of the intestinal disease while in others they are independent of the intestinal disease. The former include peripheral arthritis, erythema nodosum or aphthous ulcers and episcleritis; the latter are pyoderma gangrenosum, uveitis, spondylarthropathy and primary sclerosing cholangitis (PSC). Other extradigestive-associated diseases are represented by gallstones and nephrolithiasis. Non-disease-specific complications such as amyloidosis, osteoporosis and thromboembolic complications are also common [1] (Table 1). EIM are more common when the colon is inflamed, i.e. in patients with Crohn's disease (CD) of the colon rather than small bowel involvement. EIM can involve many organs, such as the skin, joints, eyes, liver/biliary system and kidney. They significantly influence morbidity and mortality of bowel disease, so their treatment is of major importance in the course of the intestinal disease [2].

Pathogenesis

Just as the pathogenesis of IBD is the result of a genetic predisposition due to an altered mucosal barrier and disrupted immune system in response to environmental antigens, the development of EIM is

Table 1. Extraintestinal manifestations of inflammatory bowel disease (IBD)

Musculoskeletal
Arthritis: ankylosing spondylitis, isolated joint involvement
Hypertrophic osteoarthropathy: colitic type, clubbing, periosteitis, metastatic Crohn's disease
Miscellaneous: osteoporosis, aseptic necrosis, polymyositis

Skin and mouth
Reactive lesions: erythema nodosum, pyoderma gangrenosum, aphthous ulcers, vesiculopustular eruptions, necrotizing vasculitis
Specific lesions: fissures and fistulas, oral Crohn's disease, drug rashes
Nutritional deficiency: acrodermatitis enteropathica (Zn), purpura (vitamins C and K), glossitis (vitamin B), hair loss and brittle nails (protein)
Associated diseases: vitiligo, psoriasis, amyloidosis, epidermolysis bullosa acquisita

Hepatobiliary
Specific complications: primary sclerosing cholangitis and bile duct carcinoma
Associated inflammation: autoimmune chronic active hepatitis, pericholangitis, portal fibrosis and cirrhosis, granuloma in Crohn's disease
Metabolic: fatty liver, gallstones associated with ileal Crohn's disease

Ocular
Uveitis (iritis), episcleritis, scleromalacia, corneal ulcers, retinal vessel disease

Metabolic
Growth retardation in children and adolescents, delayed sexual maturation

also multifactorial (Fig. 1). Though pathogenesis of these manifestations has yet to be clearly understood, it seems to be immunologically mediated and probably involves an autoimmune process. Studies on families support a role for genes in the expression of EIM. The high prevalence of autoantibodies such as perinuclear antineutrophil cytoplasmic antibodies (p-ANCA) in PSC is suggestive of humoral immunity. Many studies have demonstrated that ulcerative colitis (UC) patients have other associated autoimmune diseases more often than normal individuals or CD patients, thus supporting the role of immunity [3]. In a large population study conducted in Sweden, 21% of patients with UC had EIM that were found correlated with the extent of colonic involvement. Genetic susceptibility was also supported by the higher prevalence of extracolonic manifestations in familial UC [4]. Moreover, the positive effect of immunosuppressants on many EIM substantiates the hypothesis that immunity has a major part to play.

Many humoral and cellular abnormalities have been found in patients with IBD [5]. The process leading to EIM is little known, but the inflamed colonic mucosa is probably the source of the immune responses in the other organs [6, 7]. Studies on rat models have pointed to the importance of mucosal barrier dysregulation and the crucial role of enteric bacteria in the onset of chronic inflammation of the colonic mucosa. In the transgenic model of rat expressing human leukocyte antigen (HLA)-B27, arthritis and psoriasis develop together with colitis, but in a germ-free environment, the animals develop no such colitis or other manifestations, suggesting a role for cross-reaction between colonic antigens and joints and the essential role of bacterial flora and genetic factors in disease induction [8, 9]. As for humoral immunity, autoantibodies cross-reactive to both colonic and biliary epithelium have been demonstrated in patients with PSC and UC. The factors capable of causing an autoimmune response include tissue damage, release of sequestered antigens, increased major histocompatibility complex (MCH) expression, ectopic expression of molecules and dysregulation of cytokines. Autoantibody production may also be triggered by molecular mimicry [10–12].

The importance of genetic factors in the onset of IBD with EIM has been demonstrated by familial studies showing high concordance for EIM in siblings with IBD [13]. In UC, HLA-DRB1*0103 has been associated with joint and eye complications. P-ANCA were reported in 59–84% of UC patients and 10–40% of CD patients; they were also frequent (80%) in cases of PSC and in 25% of family members of PSC patients, thus suggesting genetic susceptibility [14–16]. HLA-B27 is associated with the presence of spondylitis in UC. Colonic epithelium does not express class II MCH, but an aberrant expression has been reported in the inflamed colon of IBD patients, thus allowing presentation of autoantigens to T lymphocytes [17, 18].

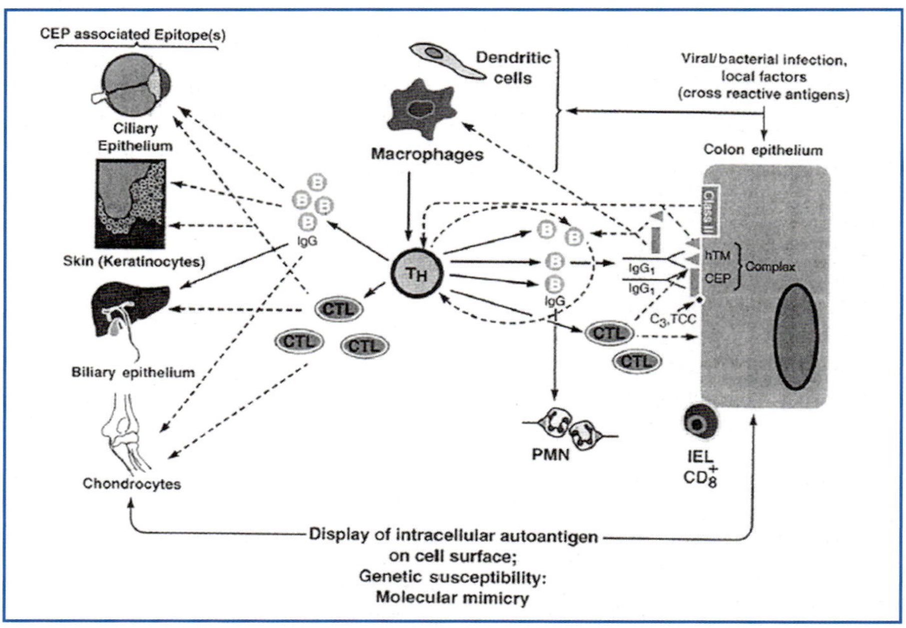

Fig. 1. A Proposed model for the pathogenesis of UC and extraintestinal manifestations based on the distribution of "shared autoantigens" (Modified from [1])

Joint Manifestations: Arthralgia, Arthritis and Ankylosing Spondylitis

Peripheral arthralgia and arthritis are the most common EIM in IBD patients and are mainly reactive. When the colon is inflamed, the prevalence of joint manifestations in both CD and UC varies between 26% and 39% whereas in Crohn's ileitis it is 8%. It has recently been demonstrated that lymphocytes from CD patients react with human synovia, thus confirming the importance of common antigens in the pathogenesis of these manifestations [19].

Arthritis in IBD is usually pauciarticular and asymmetrical, and it affects knees, ankles, wrists and elbows while joints such as the hands and shoulders are less involved. It has a migratory pattern and is transient and generally nondeforming although it may become chronic and erosive in 10% of patients [20]. The onset of arthralgia usually parallels intestinal disease activity whereas arthritis often develops independently, and joint manifestations may precede bowel disease by years [21].

Orchard distinguished between two types of arthritis: type 1 involves fewer than five joints, is self-limiting and associated with active bowel disease; type 2 involves more than five joints and symptoms persist for several months and independently from the activity of the underlying bowel disease [22]. There is no increased incidence of HLA-B27 in these two types. The presence of peripheral arthritis is frequently associated with other EIM, such as erythema nodosum and uveitis. Common blood markers of arthritis are difficult to interpret when such joint involvement is associated with IBD because there are two different inflammatory events involved. In our study, we evaluated human serum cartilage glycoprotein 39 (HC-gp39) in IBD patients with and without arthritis. HC-gp39 was higher in IBD patients with arthritis and correlated with the number of joints involved. HC-gp39 might be a marker of arthropathy in IBD and could also be proposed as a disease activity marker in arthritis associated with IBD [23].

Axial involvement includes sacroiliitis and spondylitis and affects a smaller proportion of IBD patients. Its onset is frequently insidious and its course independent of the bowel disease, making it indistinguishable from idiopathic ankylosing spondylitis. The prevalence of axial involvement is hard to estimate because a large number of patients with radiographically diagnosed sacroiliitis are asymptomatic, and it is hard to say how many will progress to symptomatic disease [24]. In a recent study, the prevalence of ankylosing spondylitis was 0.9% in UC and 1.2% in CD, but another study reported rates of 1.6–7% in UC and up to 8% in CD. Greenstein reported a prevalence of 3.8% in UC and 4% in CD, suggesting lack of predilection for either disease [19]. In our experience, we analysed 100 sacroiliac joints of 50 IBD patients with inflammatory back pain and found that 14% had no sacroiliac joint alterations, 38% had minimal alterations, 16% had monolateral sacroiliitis and 28% had ankylosing spondylitis. These data confirm the relevance of axial and peripheral joint symptoms in patients with IBD, who need to be carefully evaluated [25].

Symptomatic disease has a clinical pattern identical to that of idiopathic disease. Patients develop low back pain, especially during the night, followed by morning stiffness and buttock, chest or neck pain. The characteristic clinical signs are spine motility impairment and chest expansion. The main feature of axial involvement is that its onset and course are independent of the bowel disease. HLA-B27 has a high prevalence in ankylosing spondylitis (90%) while in patients with IBD and spondylitis, its prevalence varies from 50–75%. The simultaneous presence of HLA-B60 and HLA-B44 seems to increase the patient's susceptibility to axial involvement [26].

The approach to arthralgia and arthritis type 1 is to treat the bowel disease flare. Controlling disease activity with steroids leads to remission of joint manifestations. When arthralgia is independent of bowel disease activity, however, it should be treated with paracetamol because nonsteroidal anti-inflammatory drugs may activate and exacerbate the bowel disease [27]. Type 2 arthritis and ankylosing spondylitis (the course of which is independent of the bowel disease) should be treated preferably with sulphasalazine. Many studies have demonstrated the efficacy of this medication in patients with peripheral arthritis and, to a lesser degree, in spondylitis – especially in the long term. The use of methotrexate and 6-MP seems promising for controlling peripheral arthritis and spondylitis. In very severe and resistant cases, infliximab has been used successfully, but new randomised controlled trials are necessary [28].

Osteoporosis

Osteoporosis is a common skeletal health problem characterised by low bone mass and bone microstructural deterioration leading to bone fragility and susceptibility to fracture. Peak bone mass depends on many factors, such as nutritional, hormonal, genetic and environmental factors. Vitamin D and calcium absorption, and the consequent parathormone levels, determine the degree of bone loss. Low bone mass can derive from a diminished bone formation/resorption ratio and/or increased remodeling process. Bone mass is evaluated and diagnosed by measuring bone mass density [29]. Bone mass density is measured in many different ways, but the preferred method is dual energy X-ray absorptiometry (DEXA), which measures X-ray attenuation during its passage through bone. This method is highly sensitive and can evaluate bone mass in both cortical (radius) and trabecular (lumbar spine) bone.

Criteria for assessing bone loss are expressed by two densitometric parameters, called T and Z scores, which are standard deviation scores expressed in relation to reference values for young healthy subjects (T score) and for gender- and age-matched healthy controls (Z score). A review of studies using DEXA demonstrated that osteopenia occurs in 40–50% and osteoporosis in 30% of patients with IBD. Osteoporosis and osteopenia are also reportedly more frequent in CD than in UC [30]. A recent literature review showed that, in uncontrolled studies, patients with IBD had a prevalence of severe demineralisation ranging from 18% to 42%. On the other hand, larger studies including a healthy control group showed a prevalence of severe bone mass density reduction in only 2–16% of IBD cases [31, 32]. Bone disease is of relevance in IBD, but most data in studies on this issue are pooled from IBD clinics, so the problem may be overestimated. Longitudinal changes in bone mass in IBD patients were found much the same as in the general population.

Osteoporosis in IBD is probably caused by many factors, such as corticosteroid therapy, inflammatory cytokines and malnutrition/malabsorption. Dinca et al. evaluated the frequency and evolution of osteopenia in IBD patients and found that a low bone density is frequent in both CD and UC but apparently remains stable in CD. The evolution of bone mass density suggests that a low bone density is associated with the pathogenesis of CD whereas in UC, it seems to be correlated with the effects of corticosteroids [33].

Corticosteroids are an important cause of bone demineralisation in IBD patients. They suppress bone formation through a direct inhibitory effect on osteoblasts, inhibiting growth factors, increasing osteoblast apoptosis and accelerating bone resorption by reducing androgens and oestrogens and increasing secretion of parathyroid hormone. They also reduce intestinal calcium absorption and increase its renal excretion. Corticosteroids cause osteoporosis in 50% of treated patients, irrespective of the disease involved. The role of corticosteroids is hard to distinguish from the role of active inflammation. Bone loss occurs mostly during the first weeks of treatment and persists throughout the treatment. A study has demonstrated a 27% loss of bone mass density after 1 year of treatment with prednisone [34, 35]. Many studies have demonstrated a direct correlation between corticosteroid treatment and loss of bone mass density. A recent large population-based study showed that CD patients with fractures were significantly more likely to have used corticosteroids in the previous 2 years than those without fractures. Patients with CD and osteoporosis were also more likely to be on steroid treatment and at a higher cumulative dose than patients without osteoporosis. New bone formation is also reduced in IBD patients treated with steroids [36].

Other steroids, e.g. budesonide, are rapidly metabolised and poorly absorbed by comparison with standard steroids such as prednisone, but a recent study by Greenberg et al. demonstrated that budesonide offered no advantage over low-dose prednisone in terms of preserving bone mass density, possibly due to its more limited effect on inflammation [37]. Steroids are often prescribed for children with IBD, and a study on 119 children with IBD treated with corticosteroids at a dose of more than 7.5 mg/day for 12 months revealed a significant reduction in their bone mass density. A similar study reported that bone density of the lumbar spine was lower the higher the cumulative dose of prednisone. Other studies found no such bone loss correlating with concurrent or past corticosteroid intake, however, and osteoporosis has also been observed in IBD children who have never been exposed to corticosteroids.

Corticosteroids may be responsible for loss of bone mass, but their use may also be indicative of a more severe disease - which may be the real culprit [38]. Therapy with corticosteroids is only one of the many causes of bone loss in IBD. The inflammatory condition is characterised by an increase in circulating cytokines, which increases osteoclast activity. Tumour necrosis factor (TNF) alpha inhibits osteoblast differentiation and induces osteoclast differentiation, increasing osteoclast survival and decreasing osteoclast apoptosis. A recent study demonstrated that the TNF-receptor-based interaction between osteoblasts and osteoclasts is the common pathway of bone metabolism alteration [39]. Although inflammation itself is an important cause of bone metabolism alteration, malnutrition is common in IBD patients due to anorexia, malabsorption, greater loss of nutrients and increased metabolic demand. In some patients, calcium and vitamin D are low due to a poor dietary intake and malabsorption, and any reduction in these elements that are so important to bone metabolism may contribute to bone loss. Some studies on the weekly dietary records of inactive CD patients showed they had a lower vitamin D intake (1 μg/day) than the recommended daily amount of 5 μg/day. Similarly, IBD patients had a lower calcium intake than healthy people, and the active vitamin D levels were found significantly lower in CD and UC patients than in healthy controls. In CD patients with extensive ileal disease, bone loss was related not only to vitamin D deficiency but also with deficiency of vitamin-K-dependent proteins. Among these proteins is osteocalcin, the function of which is dependent on vitamin K; an altered gut microflora and fat malabsorption can cause vitamin K deficiency, which contributes to bone mass loss.

There are several pharmacological options for treating osteoporosis and, since its course varies in different patients and is not easily predictable, treatment of the bowel disease itself could be a kind of prophylaxis against bone disease, as inflammatory cytokines play an important role in altering bone metabolism [40]. Among treatment options for osteoporosis in IBD, hormone replacement therapy (HRT) has only been evaluated in an open study in postmenopausal women with CD. HRT has been shown to stop progression of bone loss in postmenopausal women and increase bone mass density in the long term although it does not seem to alter patients' fracture rate. HRT could be recommended in postmenopausal women with CD providing they have no contraindications, such as personal history or strong family history of breast cancer.

Dietary supplementation with calcium and vitamin D is one of the front-line therapies for preventing bone loss but is not enough in patients taking corticosteroids (such as IBD patients). A randomised controlled trial involving 103 patients comparing calcium (1,000 mg/qd) and calcitriol (0.6 mg/qd) showed that calcitriol prevented yearly bone loss from the lumbar spine more effectively than calcium alone [41]. Another study showed that long-term oral vitamin D substitution was able to prevent forearm bone loss in CD whereas in unsupplemented patients, bone mass density decreased significantly (7%). Combined calcium (800–1,000 mg) and vitamin D (800–1,000 IU) intake increased lumbar spine bone mineral density by 2.2–3.2% in the first year of treatment.

Calcitonin is a nonsteroidal hormone that directly inhibits osteoclast activity: its use seems to increase bone mass by 4–5% and it is now available in nasal sprays or rectal suppositories. It has not been approved for glucocorticoid-induced osteoporosis, however, and there are no published data available on its efficacy in this IBD patient population [42].

Sodium fluoride has been found to increase bone mass density in patients with CD, and its effect increases over 2 years of treatment whereas calcium and vitamin D supplementation is only beneficial in the first year of treatment.

Bisphosphonates are the only effective therapy for glucocorticoid-induced osteoporosis, and there are different types of medication that bind tightly to hydroxyapatite crystals in the bone and inhibit osteoclastic bone resorption. Recent meta-analyses demonstrated that etidronate, alendronate and risedronate increase bone mass density at the hip and spine in a dose-dependent manner, and their use is associated with a 30–50% reduction of vertebral fractures. Alendronate and risedronate also reduce rates of nonvertebral fractures both in women with osteoporosis and in adults with corticosteroid-induced osteoporosis. The efficacy of bisphosphonates beyond 1 year of treatment and on spinal fractures remains to be seen, however. Similarly, a recent review on etidronate demonstrated that it increased bone mass density in the lumbar spine and femoral neck, but the beneficial effect was only evident for vertebral fractures [43].

Adequate use of corticosteroids and agents that can facilitate their tapering are of fundamental importance in prevention of osteoporosis in IBD patients. The latter agents include: mesalamine, which has been effective in reducing the number of steroid-dependent CD patients, and azathioprine, 6-mercaptopurine and infliximab, which are also effective in reducing the number of steroid-dependent patients and treating refractory patients.

Many efforts have been made to reduce the use of conventional steroids, which should be used while maximising the use of other effective therapies to contain the risk of severe osteoporosis and fractures. Clinical evidence suggests that steroid dosage correlates with bone mass density but not with fracture risk and that ongoing steroid therapy only worsens bone mass density in cases of UC. There are scant data on the reversibility of these effects (only one small study on patients after colectomy), and topical steroids apparently offer no advantage because they may be less effective in controlling inflammation.

The most important measures in managing osteoporosis are treating intestinal inflammation, identifying patients with osteoporosis and promptly starting adequate therapy. Bone mass density measurements can be recommended at diagnosis and repeated every 2–3 years. In the event of osteopenia, or if corticosteroids are needed, then preventive therapy should be considered.

Skin Manifestations

Erythema nodosum (EN) and pyoderma gangrenosum (PG) are the most frequent cutaneous manifestations among skin lesions [44]. EN is the most frequent cause of inflammatory nodules in the lower extremities and is associated with IBD in 11% of cases. It occurs more often in UC than in CD, and it is three to six times more frequent in women than in men, with a peak incidence at the age of 20–30 years. There are several conditions associated with EN.

EN develops in parallel with the colitis whereas PG may be concomitant or subsequent, even developing years after colectomy [45]. EN is characterised by sudden onset of multiple, bilateral, symmetrical, painful, red and warm nodules arising mainly on the extensor surfaces of the arms and legs. These nodules are often associated with systemic symptoms, such as fever, malaise and joint pain. The typical course of the disease lasts 3–6 weeks, but the residual bruise-like lesions may last for months. As for the presence of different EIM in the same patient (i.e. EN, ankylosing spondylitis and uveitis), there are numerous hypotheses to explain overlapping syndromes, one of which is based on the assumption of a common antigen, an isoform of tropomyosin, in the eyes, skin and joints. The likely aetiology is a hypersensitive response due to deposition of immune complex in and around venules in the septa of connective tissue in subcutaneous fat. Treatment for EN usually focuses on the underlying disease since EN usually regresses when the bowel disease is brought under control and recurs when it flares up. Corticosteroids, 5-aminosalicylates (5-ASA), azathioprine, cyclosporine and other immunosuppressants are the main types of medication used. Topical hydrocortisone can also be used symptomatically. Supportive treatment includes leg elevation, support stockings and bed rest [46].

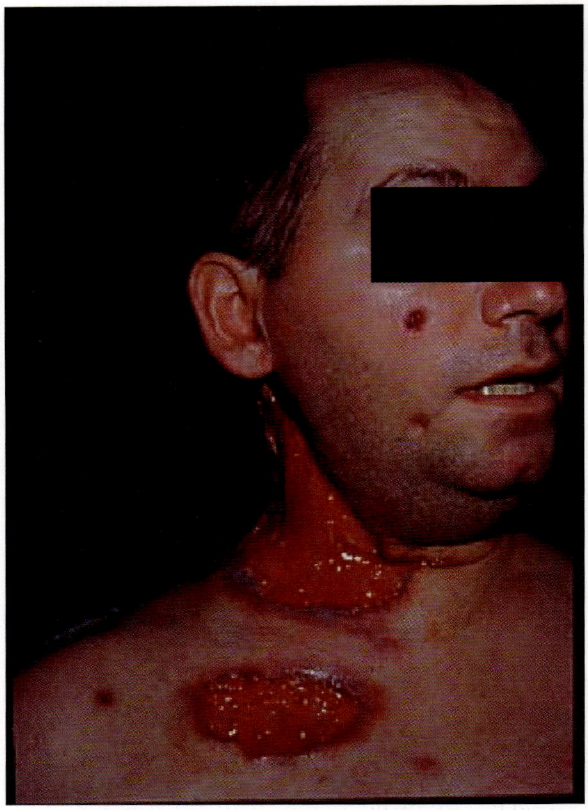

Fig. 2. A case of extended Pyoderma Gangrenosum (our experience)

PG is a rare, destructive skin lesion characterised by nodules and pustules, which can lead to formation of ulcers with necrotic bases (Fig. 2). PG is seen in 1–10% of UC patients and 0.5–20% of CD patients. It occurs equally in men and women, with a peak incidence between 25 and 54 years of age. From 50% to 78% of patients with PG have underlying disease, such as IBD, myeloproliferative or rheumatic disease. PG has been described in four variants: ulcerative, pustular, bullous and vegetative. Ulcerative and pustular PG are associated with IBD [47]. The pathogenesis of PG has not been clearly explained as yet but is probably due to a vasculitis caused by precipitation of immunocomplexes. PG is sometimes quite difficult to treat, depending on severity of the skin lesions and degree of bowel inflammation. In UC, appropriate treatment for the colonic inflammation is important, but neither medical nor surgical treatment can guarantee results in terms of healing the skin lesions [48]. It is now well established that topical treatment is usually insufficient, even in association with systemic treatment, so supportive treatment has to be combined with systemic therapy. Although measures to clean the lesions and prevent bacterial overgrowth are important, in-depth debridement is not encouraged because it can cause new lesions. Topical 5-ASA is not effective, and systemic 5-ASA has limited effect in treating the associated intestinal disease. Steroids are the most effective, first-line treatment for acute PG. High intravenous doses are used for refractory lesions. Initial doses range from 1 mg to 2 mg/kg per day. Among the immunosuppressants, cyclosporine and tacrolimus are effective in the treatment of PG. A retrospective study reported that 11 steroid-refractory cases of IBD with associated PG rapidly healed within 4–5 days of administering cyclosporine therapy, irrespective of intestinal disease activity; the authors suggested using 6-mercaptopurine and azathioprine as maintenance therapy and that long-term azathioprine is useful in PG for its steroid-sparing effect [49]. We reported on a case of PG refractory to cyclosporine that rapidly responded to oral therapy with tacrolimus (0.1 mg/kg per day), and the patient remained in remission with azathioprine therapy alone after discontinuing tacrolimus [50]. The effectiveness of infliximab has been reported in many studies. A recent randomised placebo-controlled study showed that it was superior to placebo in the treatment of PG. Patients randomised to receive infliximab were given a dose of 5 mg/kg weekly, and by the second week, 46% had improved as opposed to only 6% in the placebo group. There was no difference in outcome between PG patients with and without associated IBD. Other retrospective studies demonstrated the efficacy of infliximab in healing PG skin lesions but found that patients often require repeated courses of and had to be maintained on infliximab [51–53]. A recent case report described the efficacy of leukocyte apheresis (an extracorporeal leukocyte removal therapy) in a UC patient with PG who achieved a rapid and sustained remission of skin lesions [54].

Ocular Manifestations

Ocular manifestations include anterior uveitis, scleritis and episcleritis. They occur in about 5% of patients with UC; anterior uveitis is more frequent in UC whereas milder ocular manifestations are more frequent in CD. Rare ocular manifestations include scleromalacia, cataract and retinal vessel problems. Ocular complications are usually associated with active bowel disease.

Diagnosis of uveitis is made by slit-lamp examination and is found in both eyes in 50% of cases. Moreover, uveitis is more frequent in UC patients with other EIM, such as joint and skin lesions. Uveitis needs prompt treatment to avoid scarring complications. The treatment of choice is topical corticosteroids associated with systemic corticosteroids, azathioprine or cyclosporine. Colectomy has been shown to induce remission of ocular disease in half the cases. The effects of sulphasalazine are discouraging while the use of non-steroidal anti-inflammatory drugs is limited by the risk of inducing recurrent bowel disease [55, 56].

Hepatobiliary Complications

The incidence of hepatobiliary complications ranges from 5% to 15% in IBD patients. These complications include steatosis, cholelithiasis and PSC. An Italian study reported an overall prevalence of hepatobiliary alterations, e.g. steatosis and altered liver function test results, in 12% of IBD patients. A recent study by Bargiggia et al. reported gallstones, liver steatosis and liver enlargement in about 55% of 511 IBD patients undergoing abdominal ultrasound (Fig. 3).

Cholelithiasis is reportedly more frequent in patients with IBD, and the risk of gallstones was found increased in both CD and UC patients [odds ratio (OR) 3.6 for CD and 2.5 for UC]. The risk was also greater in patients with CD localised in the distal ileum (OR 4.5) and in UC patients with pancolitis (OR 3.3) [57]. In a study on 251 patients with CD, Hutchinson et al. found a 28% prevalence of gallstones and the only independent risk factor was prior surgery [58].

The most important and specific hepatobiliary complication in IBD is PSC, reported in up to 10% of patients, and 70–90% of PSC patients have associated UC. The clinically most severe consequence of this disease is increased risk of cholangiocarcinoma, the incidence of which is around 15% [59]. PSC is a chronic progressive disease of the biliary tree that

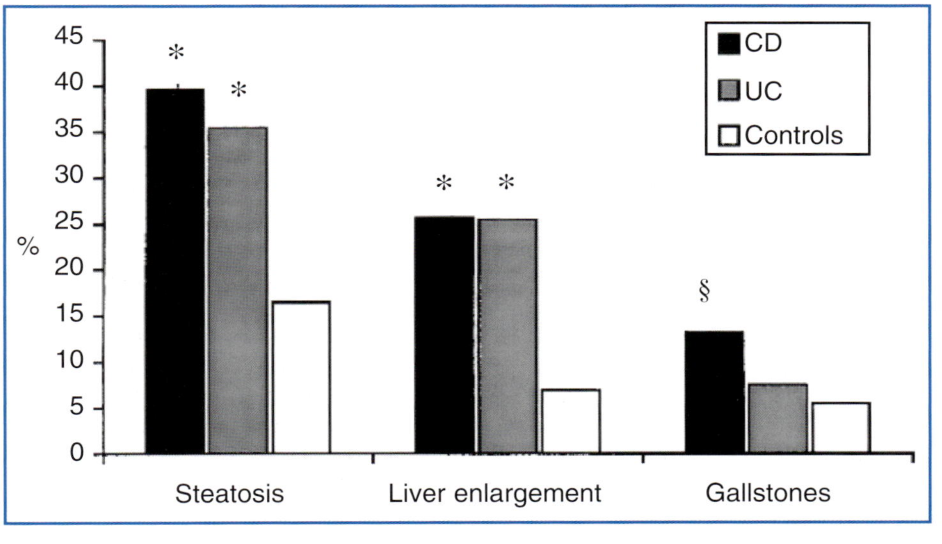

Fig. 3. Hepatobiliary abnormalities identified by ultrasonography in IBD patients.
* $p<0.001$ vs. controls
§ $p<0.016$ vs. controls
(Modified from [57])

can involve both the intra- and the extrahepatic bile ducts; it is characterised by duct strictures and dilations and concentric fibrosis of the intrahepatic bile ducts. Its clinical course does not parallel bowel disease activity, and it may progress in patients even years after proctocolectomy. The pathogenesis of PSC is still not clearly understood, but there is abundant evidence that immune dysregulation plays a crucial part in the development of this liver disease. Different studies have reported changes in tissue lymphocyte population, abnormal cytokine patterns and aberrant expression of HLA class II molecules on the bile duct epithelium. This provides indirect evidence that PSC is an immune-mediated disease, which causes immunological damage to the biliary tree. PSC also has some features of autoimmune disease, such as presence of autoantibodies, association with other autoimmune diseases and strong link with the haplotype B8-DRB1*0301-DQB1*0201. The mechanism by which immune tolerance is lost has yet to be fully understood, however [60]. Genetic susceptibility to PSC has been investigated, and a number of studies have reported that a pattern of genetic polymorphism is involved in generating the predisposition to develop this disease.

As a possible explanation for the correlation between intestinal and hepatic disease, some studies have suggested that the initial event could be passage of bacterial products through the inflamed mucosa into the portal circulation. These bacterial products could be cleared by hepatic macrophages, thus inducing an immune response that causes peribiliary duct fibrosis in a susceptible host. Another hypothesis, that is better able to justify the clinical course of the biliary disease, concerns the presence of enterohepatic circulation of lymphocytes between gut and liver: mucosal lymphocytes produced as a result of intestinal inflammation would remain as memory cells, causing hepatic inflammation under certain circumstances. This theory is supported by the finding that certain lymphocyte homing receptors are shared by the liver and gut [61]. Moreover, nitric oxide (NO) synthase overexpression has been found in biliary cell ducts in advanced PSC. Such synthase overexpression is not induced by different proinflammatory cytokines, and it produces a large amount of NO, resulting in production of reactive O species. These highly reactive substances damage many different cell functions and DNA repair enzymes and, in the long term, chronic inflammation may be responsible for the oncological complication of PSC [62].

Diagnosis of PSC is often incidental during follow-up of patients with IBD and, in most cases, patients are asymptomatic but have altered liver function test results. Symptoms of PSC include pruritus, fatigue, right upper quadrant pain, jaundice and often cholangitis. Only few patients present with symptoms of advanced liver disease or cholangiocarcinoma. Laboratory tests reveal cholestasis with increased alkaline phosphatase values whereas liver function test findings may be normal or fluctuate during the course of the disease, becoming worse in its advanced stages. Autoantibodies that have the strongest association with PSC are p-ANCA, found in 33–88% of cases. PSC is diagnosed by finding strictures and dilations of the intra- or extrahepatic bile ducts on magnetic resonance (MR) cholangiopancreatography (which has proved as sensitive as endoscopic retrograde cholangiopancreatography) (Fig. 4). Liver biopsy is also important to determine the stage of liver disease, rule out any biliary dysplasia and diagnose small-duct PSC. Small duct PSC affects a subgroup of patients with altered liver function test results and histological changes typical of PSC but with negative imaging tests. Recent studies have reported a better course of this disease, with only 12% of patients progressing to classical PSC and no cases of cholangiocarcinoma. A study conducted in Oslo reported that small-duct PSC is more frequent in CD than in UC.

Treatment for PSC is based on specific agents, such as immunosuppressants, antifibrogenic drugs and ursodeoxycholic acid. Cholestatic complications are treated with cholestyramine, ursodeoxycholic acid (UDCA) and antihistamines. End-stage liver disease requires orthotopic liver transplantation [63]. UDCA is a hydrophilic bile acid widely used in cholestatic liver disease. The positive effect of UDCA has yet to be fully explained, but it probably contrasts toxic effects of hydrophobic bile acids on hepatic cells. Therapeutic actions of UDCA are:

1. protecting cholangiocytes by displacing hydrophobic bile acid from the bile acid pool.
2. A choleretic effect that prevents retention of potentially toxic biliary products in the liver.
3. An antiapoptotic effect via activation of epidermal growth factor receptor and mitogen-activated protein kinases.
4. A potential immunomodulatory role on cytokine secretion by monocytes.

Many trials have been performed to understand the clinical efficacy of UDCA in the context of PSC, and almost all demonstrated improvement in liver function test findings while only the small trials by Stiehl et al. and Beuers et al. and the high-dose trial by Mitchel et al. have demonstrated improvement in liver histology. All trials using a standard dose of UDCA (13–15 mg/kg) failed to demonstrate any significant effect on disease progression despite the positive effect on liver function test findings [64–66]. As the biliary concentration of UDCA increases with

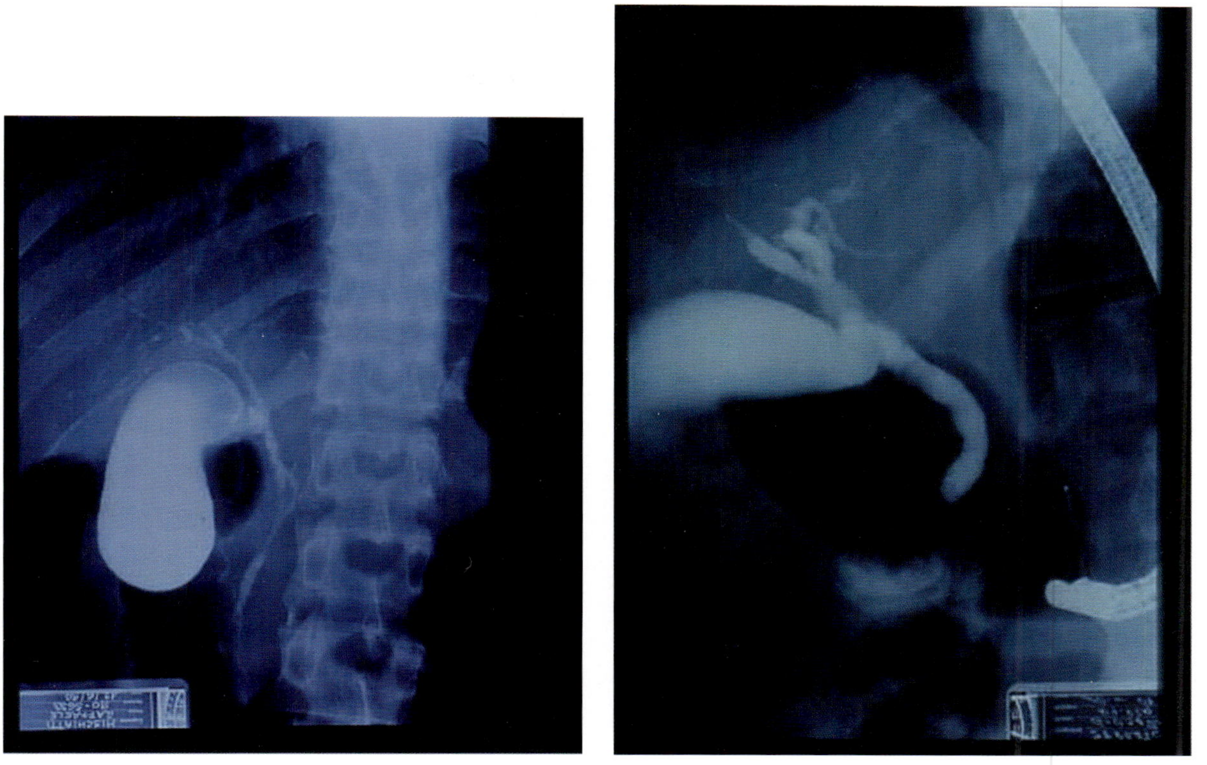

Fig. 4. Two ERCP images of primary sclerosing cholangitis (our experience)

increasing doses, reaching a plateau at a dose of 22–25 mg/kg, higher doses are likely to be more effective than lower doses. A small trial by the Oxford group using a high dose of UDCA demonstrated significant improvement in both the cholangiographic picture and degree of liver fibrosis but arrived at no conclusive results on how this treatment affects survival.

Steroids have been considered potentially useful for treatment of PSC because of their immunomodulatory effect, but no positive impact on the liver disease has been seen in patients administered cycles of steroids for their concomitant UC. Steroid therapy has been evaluated in a number of small, often uncontrolled, trials. Two such studies on PSC patients treated with steroids several years ago came to different conclusions, and another study combining prednisolone and colchicine therapy failed to demonstrate any positive effect on disease progression or survival [67, 68].

Various immunosuppressants have been studied for the treatment of PSC, most of them with disappointing results. Three trials failed to show any efficacy of methotrexate, alone or in combination with UDCA [69–71]. Cyclosporine has been found to prevent progression of histological changes in the liver in the 2-year follow-up of one randomised controlled trial involving 34 patients. In preliminary studies, tacrolimus proved capable of improving liver function test results, but further trials are needed [72]. The outcome of preliminary studies with pentoxifylline and etanercept revealed no clinical benefit [73, 74].

The course of colitis in patients with PSC is usually a mild pancolitis. A recent study comparing UC alone with UC associated with PSC reported a mild clinical course of colitis in the latter, characterised by fewer hospital stays and courses of steroid therapy [75].

The outcome of restorative proctocolectomy in UC complicated by PSC is not clear. A recent study compared outcome – in terms of risk of dysplasia/cancer, morbidity/mortality and long-term results – of IBD patients with and without PSC undergoing proctocolectomy. It revealed that IBD patients with PSC have higher risk of cancer in the resected colon after proctocolectomy and higher long-term mortality. Function and quality of life were similar in the two groups, but the presence of PSC was associated with worse survival [76].

The risk of colorectal cancer is reportedly higher (31%) in UC patients with PSC than in those with UC alone (5%) [77]. Since the original publication by Broomè et al. [78] in 1992, about 14 studies have appeared on the risk of colorectal cancer in patients with PSC. Some of these studies are difficult to interpret because all patients with colitis are cases of pancolitis, which is itself an independent risk factor for colorectal cancer in UC. There is nonetheless general consensus that patients with UC and associated PSC have higher risk of dysplasia and should undergo colonoscopy with multiple biopsies every year. A recent work has suggested that UDCA may have a role in preventing colorectal neoplasia because it can reduce the amount of toxic hydrophobic bile acids reaching the colon [79]. A small study on 59 PSC patients undergoing surveillance colonoscopy found a significantly lower prevalence of colonic dysplasia in patients taking UDCA. Another, larger study on 120 patients showed a small reduction in the amount of dysplasia in patients taking UDCA, but this failed to reach significance. A recent study by Wolf et al. compared 28 patients who were given UDCA for 6 months with 92 patients who were not, demonstrating that UDCA did not reduce the risk of developing cancer and dysplasia but did reduce the mortality rate [80]. Recent reports have suggested a worse course of colitis after liver transplantation despite immunosuppressant treatment, thus encouraging a more aggressive surgical approach to the management of colitis. Haagsma et al. studied 78 patients with end-stage PSC or autoimmune cirrhosis treated with liver transplantation and a median follow up of 7.2 years. They found that the cumulative risk for IBD was 3%, 12% and 20% at 1, 3 and 5 years, respectively, after liver transplantation. Moreover, IBD disease-free survival was higher in patients taking azathioprine. Pretransplantation IBD and the use of tacrolimus were independent predictors for IBD after liver transplantation. Prevalence of IBD after liver transplantation was found to be affected by the immunosuppresion used, and azathioprine seems to have a protective effect [81].

Dealing with PSC is a real challenge, especially when associated with UC, but more information is now emerging on the effects of PSC on clinical features of UC, and this is helpful in coping with the high risk of colorectal malignancies in these patients.

References

1. Das KM (1999) Relationship of extraintestinal involvements in inflammatory bowel disease. Dig Dis Sci 44(1):1–13
2. Bernstein CN, Blanchard JF, Rawsthorne P et al (2001) The prevalence of extraintestinal diseases in inflammatory bowel disease: a population-based study. Am J Gastroenterol 96(4):1116–1122
3. Snook JA, de Silva HJ, Jewell DP (1989) The association of autoimmune disorders with inflammatory bowel disease. Quart J Med 269:835–840
4. Brandtzaeg P, Halstensen TS, Kett K (1992) Immunopathology of inflammatory bowel disease. In: MacDermott RP, Stenson WF (eds) Inflammatory bowel disease, current topics in gastroenterology. Elsevier, London, pp 95–136
5. Padolsky DK (1991) Inflammatory bowel disease: Part 1. N Engl J Med 325:928–937
6. Sartor RB (1995) Microbial factors in the pathogenesis of Crohn's disease, ulcerative colitis and experimental intestinal inflammation. Inflammatory bowel disease. In: Kirsner JB, Shorter RJ (eds) Lea & Febiger, Philadelphia, pp 96–124
7. MacDermott RP, Elson CO (1991) Mucosal immunology I. Gastroenterol Clin North Am 20:397–627
8. Breban M, Hammer RE, Richardson JA et al (1993) Transfer of the inflammatory disease of HLA B27 transgenic rats by bone marrow engraftment. J Exp Med 178:1607–1616
9. Taurog JD, Richardson JA, Croft JT et al (1994) The germfree state prevents development of gut and joint inflammatory disease in HLA-B27 transgenic rats. J Exp Med 180:2359–2364
10. Mizoguchi A, Mizoguchi E, Chiba C et al (1996) Cytokine imbalance and autoantibody production in T cell receptor-a mutant mice with inflammatory bowel disease. J Exp Med 183:847–856
11. Chapman RW, Cottone M, Selby WS et al (1986) Serum autoantibodies in ulcerative colitis and primary sclerosing cholangitis. Gut 27:86–91
12. Tan EM (1991) Autoantibodies in pathology and cell biology. Cell 67:841–842
13. Satsagi J, Grootscholten C, Holt H et al (1996) Clinical pattern of familial inflammatory bowel disease. Gut 38:738–741
14. Rump JA, Scholmerich J, Gross V et al (1990) A new type of perinuclear anti-neutrophil cytoplasmatic antibody (p-ANCA) in ulcerative colitis but not in Crohn's disease. Immunobiology 181:406–413
15. Hoffenberg J, Fidanza S, Sauaia A (1999) Serologic testing for inflammatory bowel disease. J Pediatr 134:447–452
16. Lawrance IC, Murray K, Hall A et al (2004) A prospective comparative study of ASCA and pANCA in Chinese and Caucasian IBD patients. Am J Gastroenterol 99:2186–2194
17. Satsagi J, Grootscholten C, Holt H et al (1996) Clinical pattern of familial inflammatory bowel disease. Gut 38:738–741
18. Seibold F, Slametschka D, Gregor M et al (1992) Neutrophil autoantibodies: a genetic marker in primary sclerosing cholangitis and ulcerative colitis. Gastroenterology 107:532–536
19. Greenstein AJ, Janovitz HD, Sachar DB (1976) The extraintestinal complications of Crohn's disease and ulcerative colitis: a study of 700 patients. Medicine 5:401–412
20. Reinshagen M, Von Tirpitz C (2003) Osteoporosis and

other extraintestinal symptoms and complications of inflammatory bowel diseases. Dig Dis 21:138–145
21. Orchard TR (2001) Arthritis associated with inflammatory bowel disease. In: Bayless TM, Hanauer SB (eds) Advanced therapy of inflammatory bowel disease. Decker, Hamilton, London, pp 279–288
22. Orchard TR, Wordsworth BP, Jewell DP (1998) Peripheral arthropathies in inflammatory bowel disease: their articular distribution and natural history. Gut 42:387–391
23. Punzi L, Podswiadek M, D'Incà R et al (2003) Serum human cartilage glycoprotein 39 as a marker of arthritis associated with inflammatory bowel disease. Ann Rheum Dis 62(12):1224–1226
24. De Vos M, De Keyser F, Mielants H et al (1998) Review article: bone and joint disease in inflammatory bowel disease. Aliment Pharmacol Ther 12:397–404
25. Podswiadek M, Punzi L, Stramare R et al (2004) The prevalence of radiographic sacroiliitis in patients affected by inflammatory bowel disease with inflammatory low back pain. Reumatismo 56(2):110–113
26. De Vos M (2004) Review article: joint involvement in inflammatory bowel disease. Aliment Pharmacol Ther 20[Suppl 4]:36–42
27. Adler G, Reinshagen M (2003) Extraintestinale Manifestationen. Z Gastroenterol 41:54–61
28. Sieper J, Braun J (2001) New treatment options in ankylosing spondylitis: a role for anti-TNFa therapy. Ann Rheum Dis 60(Suppl 3):58–61
29. Compston JE (1995) Review article: osteoporosis, corticosteroids and inflammatory bowel disease. Aliment Pharmachol Ther 9:237–250
30. Bernstein CN, Leslie WD (2004) Review article: osteoporosis and inflammatory bowel disease. Aliment Pharmacol Ther 19:941–952
31. Schulte C, Dignass AU, Mann K et al (1998) Reduced bone mineral density and unbalanced bone metabolism in patients with inflammatory bowel disease. Inflamm Bowel Dis 4(4):268–275
32. Jahnsen J, Falch JA, Aadland E et al (1997) Bone mineral density is reduced in patients with Crohn's disease but not in patients with ulcerative colitis: a population based study. Gut 40:313–319
33. Dinca M, Fries W, Luisetto G et al (1999) Evolution of osteopenia in inflammatory bowel disease. Am J Gastroenterol 94(5):1292–1297
34. de Jong DJ, Corstens FH, Mannaerts L et al (2002) Corticosteroid-induced osteoporosis: does it occur in patients with Crohn's disease? Am J Gastroenterol 97(8):2011–2015
35. Dear KL, Compston JE, Hunter JO (2001) Treatments for Crohn's disease that minimise steroid doses are associated with a reduced risk of osteoporosis. Clin Nutr 20(6):541–546
36. Bernstein CN, Blanchard JF, Metge C (2003) The association between corticosteroid use and development of fractures among IBD patients in a population-based database. Am J Gastroenterol 98(8):1797–1801
37. Greenberg G, Feagan B, Martin F et al (1994) Oral budesonide for the treatment of active Crohn's disease. N Engl J Med 331:836–841
38. Manolagas SC, Jilka RL (1995) Bone marrow, cytokine and bone remodeling. Emerging insights into the pathophysiology of osteoporosis. N Engl J Med 332(5):305–311
39. Andreassen H, Rungby J, Dahlerup F et al (1997) Inflammatory bowel disease and osteoporosis. Scand J Gastroenterol 32:1247–1255
40. Lichtenstein GR (2003) Evaluation of bone mineral density in inflammatory bowel disease: current safety focus. Am J Gastroenterol 98(12):S24–S30
41. Sambrook P, Birmingham J, Kelly P et al (1993) Prevention of corticosteroids osteoporosis: a comparison of calcium, calcitriol and calcitonin. N Engl J Med 328:1747–1752
42. Bernstein CN, Seeger LL, Anton PA et al (1996) A randomized placebo-controlled trial of calcium supplementation for decreased bone density in corticosteroids-using patients with IBD: a pilot study. Aliment Pharmacol Ther 10:777–786
43. Cranney A, Welch V, Adachi JD et al (2001) Etidronate for treating and preventing postmenopausal osteoporosis. Cochrane Database Syst Rev (4):CD003376
44. Nousari HC, Provost TT, Anhalt GJ (2001) Cutaneous manifestations of inflammatory bowel disease. In: Bayless TM, Hanauer SB (eds) Advanced therapy of inflammatory bowel disease. B.C. Becker, Hamilton, pp 271–274
45. Tromm A, May D, Almus E et al (2001) Cutaneous manifestations in inflammatory bowel disease. Z Gastroenterol 39:137–144
46. Fleisher M, Rubin S, Levine A et al (2002) Infliximab in the treatment of refractory erythema nodosum of IBD. Gastroenterology 122(Suppl 1):A618
47. Bennet ML, Jackson JM, Jorizzo JL et al (2000) Pyoderma Gangrenosum. A comparison of typical and atypical forms with an emphasis on time to remission. Case review of 86 patients from 2 institutions. Medicine 79:37–46
48. Wollina V (2002) Clinical management of pyoderma gangrenosum. Am J Clinical Dermatol 3:14–58
49. Hohenleutner U, Mohr VD, Michel S et al (1997) Mycophenolate mofetil and cyclosporine treatment for recalcitrant pyoderma gangrenosum. Lancet 350:1748
50. D'Incà R, Fagiuoli S, Sturniolo GC (1998) Tacrolimus to treat pyoderma gangrenosum resistant to cyclosporine. Ann Intern Med 128:783–784
51. Regueiro M, Valentine J, Plevy S et al (2003) Infliximab for treatment of pyoderma gangrenosum associated with inflammatory bowel disease. Am J Gastroenterol 98:1824–1826
52. Brooklyn TN, Dunnill GS, Shetty A et al (2005) Infliximab for the treatment of pyoderma gangrenosum: a randomized, double-blind placebo controlled trial. Gut (Epub PMID:16188920)
53. Tavarela Veloso F (2004) Review article: skin complications associated with inflammatory bowel disease. Aliment Pharmacol Ther 20(Suppl 4):50–53
54. Fujimoto E, Fujimoto N, Kuroda K et al (2004) Leukocytapheresis treatment for pyoderma gangrenosum. Br J Dermatol 151:1090–1092
55. Soukiasian S, Foster CS, Raizman MB (1994) Treatment strategies for scleritis and uveitis associated with inflammatory bowel disease. Am J Ophthalmol 118:601–611

56. Lamers CBHW (1997) Treatment of extraintestinal complication of ulcerative colitis. Eur J Gastroenterol Hepatol 9:850–853
57. Bargiggia S, Maconi G, Elli M et al (2003) Sonographic prevalence of liver steatosis and biliary tract stones in patients with inflammatory bowel disease: study of 511 subjects at a single center. J Clinical Gastroenterol 36(5):417–420
58. Hutchinson R, Tyrrel PN, Kumar D et al (1994) Pathogenesis of gallstones in Crohn's disease: an alternative explanation. Gut 35(1):94–97
59. Wiesner RH (1994) Current concepts in primary sclerosing cholangitis. Mayo Clin Proc 69:969–982
60. Spurkland A, Saarinen S, Boberg KM et al (1999) HLA class II haplotypes in primary sclerosing cholangitis patients from five European populations. Tissue Antigens 53:459–69
61. Grant AJ, Lalor PF, Salmi M et al (2002) Homing of mucosal lymphocytes to the liver in the pathogenesis of hepatic complications of inflammatory bowel disease. Lancet 359:150–157
62. Spirli C, Fabris L, Duner E et al (2003) Cytokine-stimulated nitric oxide production inhibits adenyl cyclase and cAMP-dependent secretion in cholangiocytes. Gastroenterology 124:737–753
63. Cullen SN, Chapman RW (2005) Review article: current management of primary sclerosing cholangitis. Aliment Pharmacol Ther 21:933–948
64. Beuers U, Spengler U, Kruis W et al (1992) Ursodeoxycholic acid for treatment of primary sclerosing cholangitis: a placebo-controlled trial. Hepathology 16:707–714
65. Stiehl A, Walker S, Sthiel L et al (1994) Effect of ursodeoxycholic acid on liver and bile duct disease in primary sclerosing cholangitis. A 3-year pilot study with a placebo-controlled study period. J Hepatol 20:57–64
66. Mitchell SA, Bansi DS, Hunt N et al (2001) A preliminary trial of high dose ursodeoxycholic acid in primary sclerosing cholangitis. Gastroenterology 121:900–907
67. Buurgert SL, Brown BP, Kirkpatrick RB (1984) Positive corticosteroid response in early primary sclerosing cholangitis (abstract). Gastroenterology 86:1037(A)
68. Lindor KD, Wiesner RH, Colwell LJ et al (1991) The combination of prednisone and colchicine in patients with primary sclerosing cholangitis. Am J Gastroenterol 86:57–61
69. Knox TA, Kaplan MM (1991) Treatment of primary sclerosing cholangitis with oral methotrexate. Am J Gastroenterol 86:546–552
70. Knox TA, Kaplan MM (1994) A double-blind controlled trial of oral pulse methotrexate therapy in the treatment of primary sclerosing cholangitis. Gastroenterology 106:494–499
71. Lindor KD, Jorgensen RA, Anderson ML et al (1996) Ursodeoxycholic acid and methotrexate for primary sclerosing cholangitis: a pilot study. Am J Gastroenterol 91:511–515
72. Talwalkar JA, Lindor KD (2005) Primary sclerosing cholangitis. Inflamm Bowel Disease 11(1):62–72
73. Bharucha AE, Jorgensen R, Lichtman SN et al (2000) A pilot study of pentoxifylline for the treatment primary sclerosing cholangitis. Am J Gatroenterol 95:2338–2342
74. Epstein MP, Kaplan MM (2004) A pilot study of etanercept in the treatment primary sclerosing cholangitis. Dig Dis Sci 49:1–4
75. Moayyeri A, Daryani NE, Barhami H et al (2005) Clinical course of ulcerative colitis in patients with or without primary sclerosing cholangitis. J Hepatol Gastroenterol 20:366–370
76. Gorgun E, Remzi FH, Manilich E et al (2005) Surgical outcome in patients with primary sclerosing cholangitis undergoing ileal pouch-anal anastomosis: a case control study. Surgery 138(4):631–637
77. Chambers WM, Warren BF, Jewell DP et al (2005) Cancer surveillance in ulcerative colitis. Br J Surg 92(8):928–936
78. Broome U, Lindberg G, Lofberg R (1992) Primary sclerosing-cholangitis in ulcerative colitis: a risk factor for the development of dysplasia and DNA aneuploidy? Gastroenterology 102(6):1877-1880
79. Pardi DS, Loftus EV, Kremers WK et al (2003) Ursodeoxycholic acid acts as a chemopreventive agent in patients with ulcerative colitis and primary sclerosing cholangitis. Gastroenterology 124:889–893
80. Wolf JM, Rybicki LA, Lashner BA (2005) The impact of ursodeoxycholic acid on cancer, dysplasia and mortality in ulcerative colitis patients with primary sclerosing cholangitis. Aliment Pharmacol Ther 22:783–788
81. Haagsma EB, Van Den Berg AP, Kleinbeuker JH et al (2003) Inflammatory bowel disease after liver transplantation: the effect of different immunosuppressive regimens. Aliment Pharmacol Ther 18(1):33–44

Perianal Crohn's Disease: Assessment with Endoanal Ultrasonography

Giulio Aniello Santoro, Marianne Starck, Luca Campana, Bjørn Fortling

Introduction

Perianal disease is an important and distinguishing feature of Crohn's disease (CD). The incidence of perianal disease in patients with CD varies from 3.8% to 81% in different series [1, 2]. While perianal lesions occur more often in patients with colonic disease than in patients with small intestinal disease [2], 5% of patients with anorectal CD do not have proximal disease. Clinical features include hypertrophic skin tags, ulceration (Fig. 1), perianal abscesses and fistulae (Figs. 2 and 3), fissures, induration and anal stenosis [3]. A characteristic feature of perianal CD is that several abnormalities may coexist. Perianal abscesses occur in 23–62% of patients and are usually multiple and complex due to deep, cavitating ulcers that penetrate the anorectal wall [2]. Crohn's abscesses may also arise as a result of an infection of the intersphincteric anal glands. Anorectal fistulae in CD arise in 6–34% of patients [2]. According to their relationship with the sphincters [4], fistulae are classified in intersphincteric, transsphincteric, supralevator, extrasphincteric and submucosal. The American Gastroenterological Association recommended the division of fistulae into either simple or complex [5]. A simple fistula is a superficial, intersphincteric or low transsphincteric fistula, without secondary tracts, and it is not associated with an abscess. Com-

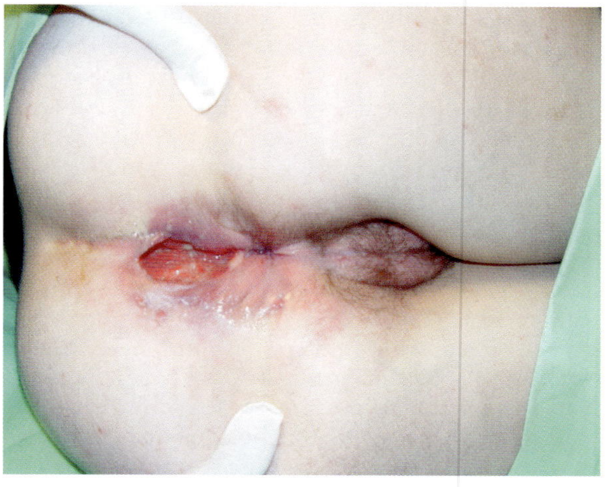

Fig. 1. Large cavitating ulcer in Crohn's disease

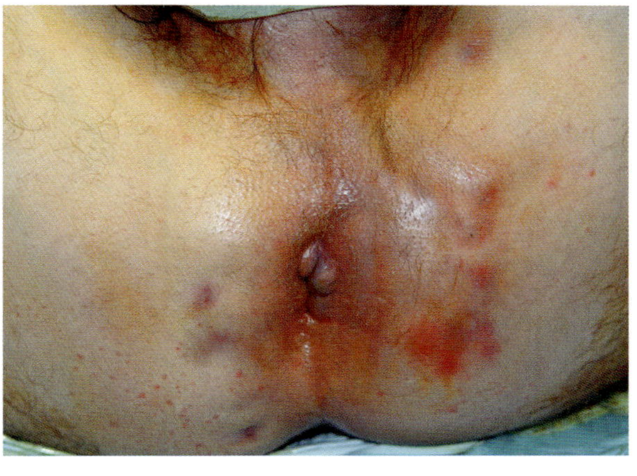

Fig. 2. Complex perianal sepsis in Crohn's disease with presence of multiple external fistulous openings

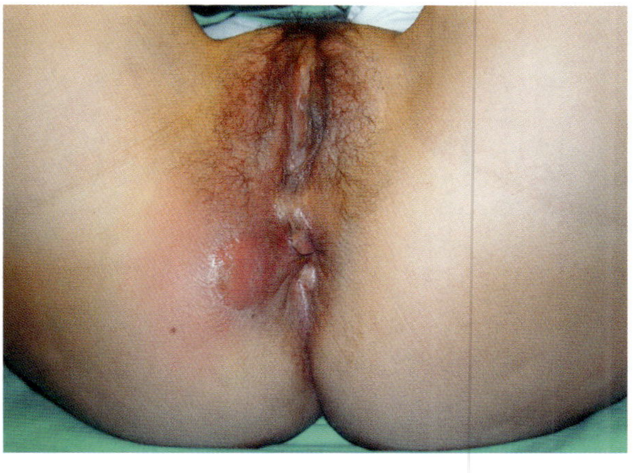

Fig. 3. Large perianal abscess in Crohn's disease extending to the anterior perineum

plex fistulae (high transsphincteric, suprasphincteric, or extrasphincteric fistulae, presence of multiple external openings, secondary tracts or large abscesses) may result from active rectal disease, which form deep, cavitating ulceration and fistulation. Rectovaginal fistula in CD occurs in 5.2–10% of patients [2]. In these fistulae, the internal opening may be present at the dentate line and the external opening at the fornix or low in the vagina (anovaginal), or the tract passes directly from the rectum to the vagina.

The diagnosis of perianal CD can be made when there is a persistent characteristic pathological lesion in association with the anal canal in a patient known to have at least two criteria for the diagnosis of the intestinal CD: clinical, radiological and histological. Perianal CD can be diagnosed in the absence of obvious clinical manifestations on intestinal CD, providing that there are typical perianal lesions showing histological evidence of granulomata in biopsies taken from ulcers or abscesses. Perianal CD is often difficult to treat, and different management modalities (surgery, medical therapy, diet) have been tried with variable results [6]. Disease activity appears to be associated with impaired wound healing, but wounds usually heal normally when the disease is inactive. Accurate evaluation is crucial for the treatment plan. Physical examination may reveal simple fistulae with a relatively superficial position; however, it is unable to identify ischiorectal, pelvirectal and horseshoeing tracts and most of the internal openings. When disease is active, the anal lesions have a characteristic swollen, translucent pink or bluish appearance with obvious ulceration. As disease activity resolves, oedema disappears, the tissue becomes opaque and ulcers heal with a fragile layer of epithelium. Inactive lesions may remain clinically significant because of the mechanical effects of the fistula or strictures.

Due to the limitations of conventional fistulography and pelvic computed tomography (CT) scanning [7], endoanal ultrasonography (EAUS) [8, 9] or pelvic magnetic resonance imaging (MRI) [10, 11] have been introduced as useful investigative modalities for perianal CD. In the following chapter, equipment, technique, endosonographic anatomy of the anal canal, accuracy and reliability of EAUS in the evaluation of perianal abscesses and fistulae in CD and comparison of EAUS with MRI is discussed.

Equipment

The most widely used EAUS system is the B-K Medical scanner (Pro-Focus 2202, B-K Medical A/S, Mileparken 34, DK-2730 Herlev, Denmark), with a hand-held rotating endoprobe type 1850, which gives a 360° axial view of the rectal wall (Fig. 4) [12]. The radial probe has a 24-cm metal shaft with a rotating transducer at its tip. This 8539 transducer has a frequency range from 5 MHz to 10 MHz with a focal length of 2–5 cm, and a 90° scanning plane and is rotated at four to six cycles per second to achieve a radial scan of the anus and surrounding structures. The end of the probe is covered with a cone made of sonolucent polymethyl pentene plastic and 1.7 cm in outer diameter, which is filled with degassed water to maintain acoustic coupling between the transducer and the tissue (Fig. 5). It is important to eliminate all bubbles within the hard anal cone, given that these may produce artifact and limit overall utility of the study. The outer walls of this cone are parallel so that

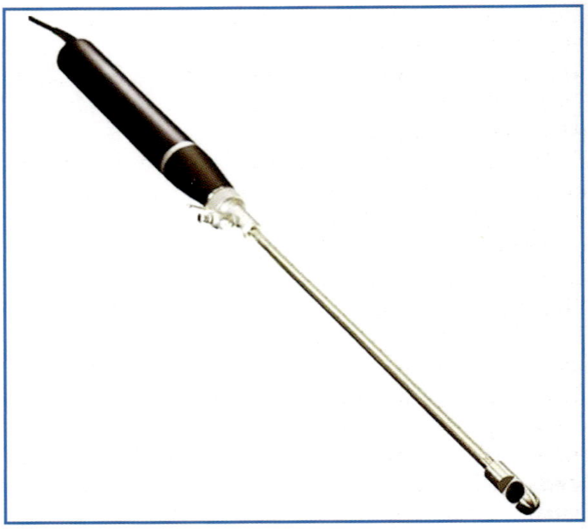

Fig. 4. B-K Medical anorectal probe type 1850

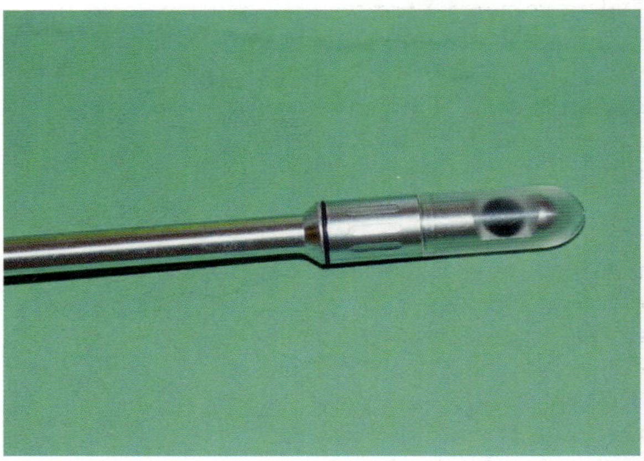

Fig. 5. The end of the probe is covered with a plastic cone

the probe may be moved within the anal canal without causing any anatomical distortion. In patients with a stenotic anus, a smaller endoprobe (7 MHz, type 6005, focal range: 0.5–3 cm) and cone (diameter 0.9 cm) can be used.

Technology progress allows the three-dimensional (3-D) reconstruction of two-dimensional (2-D) images [12]. It is not necessary to use new ultrasound probes but to connect the ultrasound apparatus to a computer equipped with a software (BK3Di). Three-dimensional reconstruction is based on a high number of parallel transaxial images acquired using a special colorectal pullback mover (UA0552) with the B-K Medical ultrasound probe type 1850. The colorectal pullback mover is a computer-controlled, motor-driven device that can be operated at different levels of resolution. For endoanal application, the usual setting is 0.2–0.3 mm between adjacent transaxial images. Scanning the anal canal with these settings over a pullback distance of 35 mm will typically yield 175 parallel images. Data from a series of closely spaced, 2-D images is combined to create a 3-D volume displayed as a cube. The 3-D image does not remain fixed; rather, it can be freely rotated, rendered, tilted and sliced to allow the operator to infinitely vary the different section parameters and visualise the lesion at different angles and to get the most information out of the data. After data is acquired, it is immediately possible to select coronal anterior–posterior or posterior–anterior as well as sagittal right–left views. The multiview function allows up to six different and specialised views at once with real-time reconstruction. If one wants to see the internal structure, a volume representation may be chosen. In this, one allows the ray to pass through the data, and contributions from different depths are added together in some way and used to construct the image pixel on the screen (volume rendering). "Volume render mode" is a special feature that successfully can be applied to high-resolution 3-D data volumes. Imaging processing includes maximum intensity, minimum intensity and summed voxel projections, combined with positional or intensity weighting. This technique changes the depth information of 3-D data volume so information inside the cube is reconstructed to some extent.

Extensive anorectal examinations, however, require moving the transducer head. Probe movement can cause artifacts and change anatomical presentation. The new B-K Medical 2050 anorectal transducer is designed so that no moving parts come into contact with human tissue (Fig. 6). The transducer's 360° rotating head, the proximal–distal actuation mechanism and the electronic mover are fully enclosed within the housing of the slim probe. Both 3-D data-set acquisition and high-precision positioning of the scan head over a longitudinal distance of 60 mm are accomplished at the touch of a button, allowing information gathering without having to move the probe's position. The 2050's double crystal covers a frequency range from 6 MHz to 16 MHz.

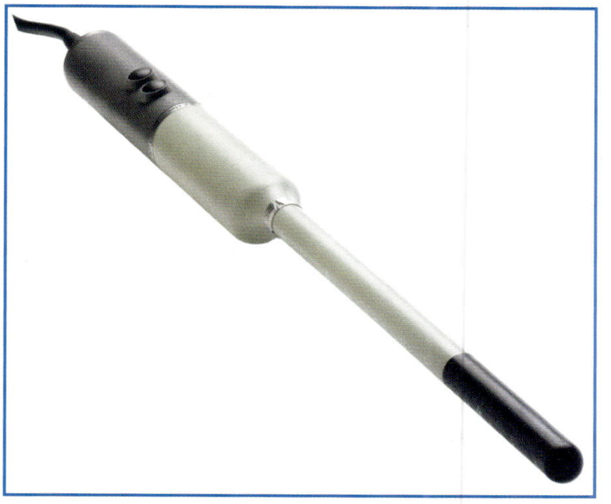

Fig. 6. B-K Medical anorectal probe type 2050

In females, transvaginal endosonography (TVS) can be performed in case of anal pain or stenosis or to obtain additional information using the same radial probes. Moreover, for sagittal and conventional transverse imaging of the pelvic floor, including color Doppler, a biplane, high-frequency transducer with a long linear and transverse array can be used (B-K Medical 8658 probe) (Fig. 7). Both arrays are placed at 90° to each other and at 90° to the longitudinal axis. The transducer can be placed resting on the posterior vaginal wall. With the patient lying on her back on a table or in a gynecological chair, the anterior vaginal wall will softly contact the surface of the ultrasound transducer without disturbing the functional anatomy.

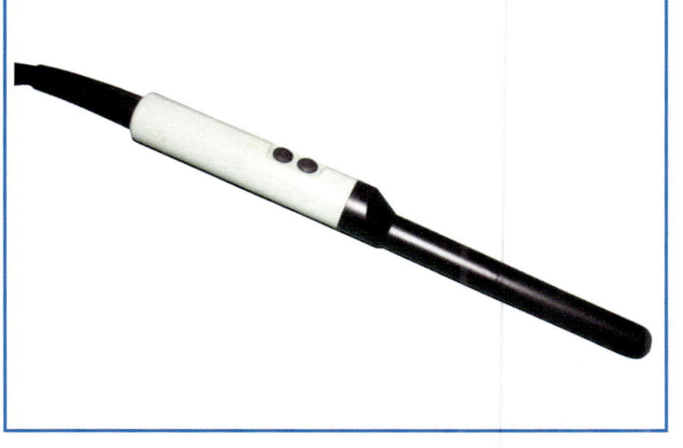

Fig. 7. B-K Medical linear probe type 8658

Transperineal ultrasound (TPUS) represents another method by which to detect perianal inflammatory disease, which can be performed using regular convex and linear high-resolution ultrasound probes [13]. A convex 3.5 -MHz probe provides a general overview over perianal anatomy, identifying bladder, rectum, prostate gland and urethra or vagina and uterus. Further investigation is performed with a 10-MHz linear probe for a much more detailed imaging of perianal inflammatory disease.

Technique

Endoluminal ultrasound is usually performed with the patient in the left lateral decubitus position. Before the probe is inserted into the anus, a digital rectal examination should be performed. If there is an anal stenosis, the finger can check to determine whether it will allow easy passage of the probe. A gel-containing condom is placed over the probe, and a thin layer of water-soluble lubricant is placed on the exterior of the condom. Any air interface will cause a major interference pattern. The probe is then ready for insertion through the anal canal. The patient should be instructed before the examination that no pain should be experienced. Under no circumstances should force be used to advance the probe.

When the spigot for introducing water into the plastic cone is pointing toward the ceiling, by convention, the anterior aspect of the rectum will be superior (12 o'clock) on the screen, right lateral will be left (9 o'clock) on the screen, left lateral will be right (3 o'clock) on the screen and posterior will be inferior (6 o'clock) on the screen (just as in the image on axial CT scan). Some adjustments may have to be made in the gain of the ultrasound unit to provide optimal imaging. It is always possible to perfectly depict all layers of the anal canal circumferentially. This is very important when assessing the canal at different levels. At the origin of the anal canal, the "U"- shaped sling of the puborectalis is the main landmark and should be used for final adjustment [12]. Once the entire canal down to the anal margin has been evaluated, the probe is removed. It is not uncommon to require several passes along the full length of the anus to gain all the information necessary. In some instances, two to six passes may be required to properly evaluate a complex perianal sepsis.

Endosonographic Anatomy of the Anal Canal

Knowledge of the anal canal and pelvic floor anatomy is required in order to better understand how

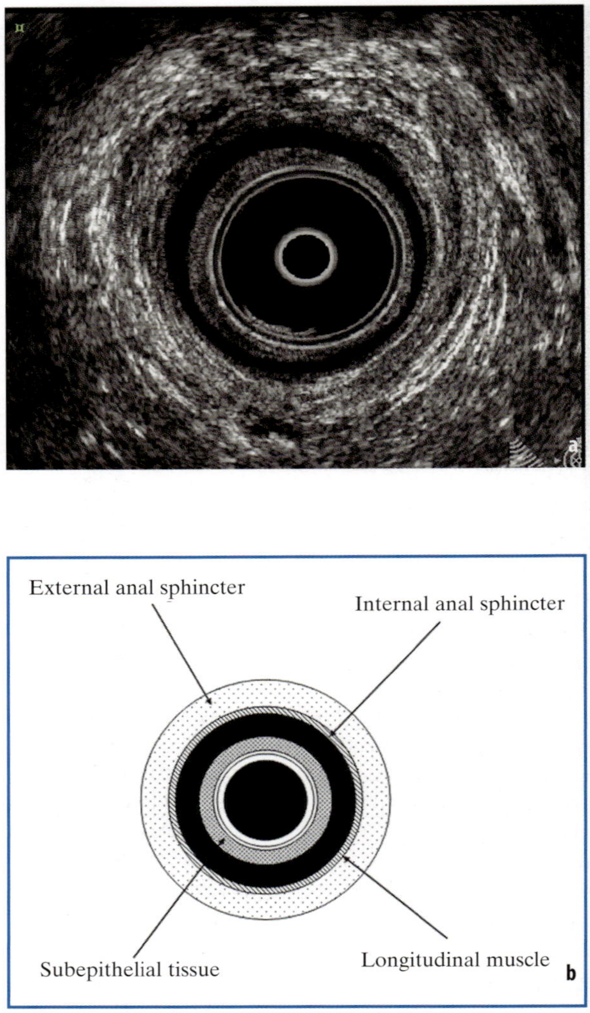

Fig. 8. Normal ultrasonographic six-layer structure of the mid anal canal in a male. Axial image (**a**), schematic representation (**b**)

perianal sepsis develops and to more accurately classify fistulae and abscesses. On ultrasound, six hypoechoic and hyperechoic layers can be seen in the normal anal canal [14]. The ultrasonographer must have a clear understanding of what each of these six lines represent anatomically. From inner to outer, the first hyperechoic layer corresponds to the interface of the plastic cone with the anal mucosal surface, the second hypoechoic layer to the mucosa, the third hyperechoic layer to the subepithelial tissues, the fourth hypoechoic layer to the internal anal sphincter (IAS), the fifth hyperechoic layer to the longitudinal muscle (LM) and the sixth mixed echogenic layer to the external anal sphincter (EAS) (Fig. 8). Three-dimensional endorectal ultrasound offers a valuable supplement to conventional ultrasound. The six layers of

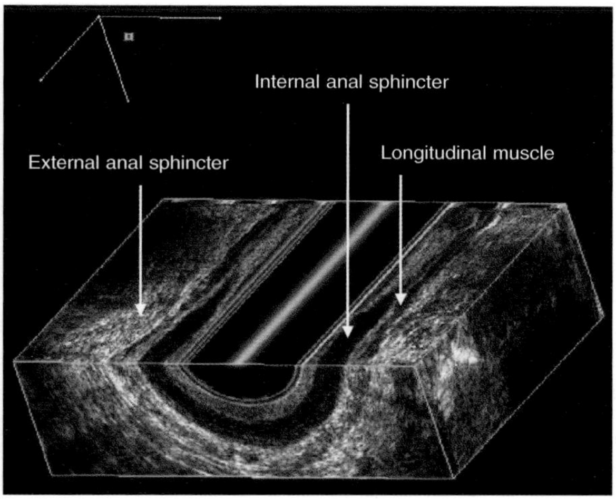

Fig. 9. Normal ultrasound anatomy of the sphincter complex in three-dimensional image

the anal canal are clearly illustrated in the coronal plane as well as in the transaxial and the longitudinal image planes (Fig. 9).

The hypoechoic layer that represents the IAS can be traced superiorly into the circular muscle of the rectum. Its thickness varies from 1.5 mm to 4 mm (mean 3.0±0.5 mm) and increases with age owing the presence of more fibrous tissue as the absolute amount of muscle decreases. The longitudinal muscle is 2.5±0.6 mm in males and 2.9±0.6 mm in females. This muscle is moderately echogenic, which is surprising, as it is mainly smooth muscle; however, an increased fibrous stroma may account for this. The average thickness of the EAS is 8.6±1.1 mm in males and 7.7±1.1 mm in females. Thickness of the IAS and EAS should be measured at the 3 o'clock and 6 o'clock positions in the midlevel of the anal canal.

Ultrasound imaging of the anus can be divided into three levels: deep, mid and superficial [14]. The level refers to the following anatomical structures: (1) deep: the sling of the puborectalis and the deep part of the EAS; (2) mid: the anococcygeal ligament, superficial part of the EAS, IAS and perineal body; and (3) superficial: the subcutaneous part of the EAS. The first ultrasound image recorded is normally at puborectalis level, where the perineal body is also seen in females. This image is normally documented and labeled HIGH (Fig. 10). In a normal patient, moving the probe a few millimetres in the distal direction will show an intact anterior EAS forming just below the superficial transverse perineal muscles. This image is a mid-canal projection where the IAS, conjoining longitudinal muscle and the superficial EAS all are identified. This image will be labeled MID (Fig. 11). When the probe is pulled further out, the image of the IAS will disappear and only the subepithelium and the subcutaneous segment of the LM + EAS will be seen. This last image will be labeled LOW (Fig. 12). The anterior part of the EAS differs between genders. In males, it is symmetrical at all levels; in females, it is shorter anteriorly and there is no evidence of anterior ring high in the canal (Fig. 13). In examining a female subject, the ultrasonographic differences between the natural gaps (hypoechoic areas with smooth, regular edges) and sphincter ruptures (mixed echogenicity, due to scarring, with irregular edges) occurring at the upper anterior part of the anal canal must be kept in mind [15].

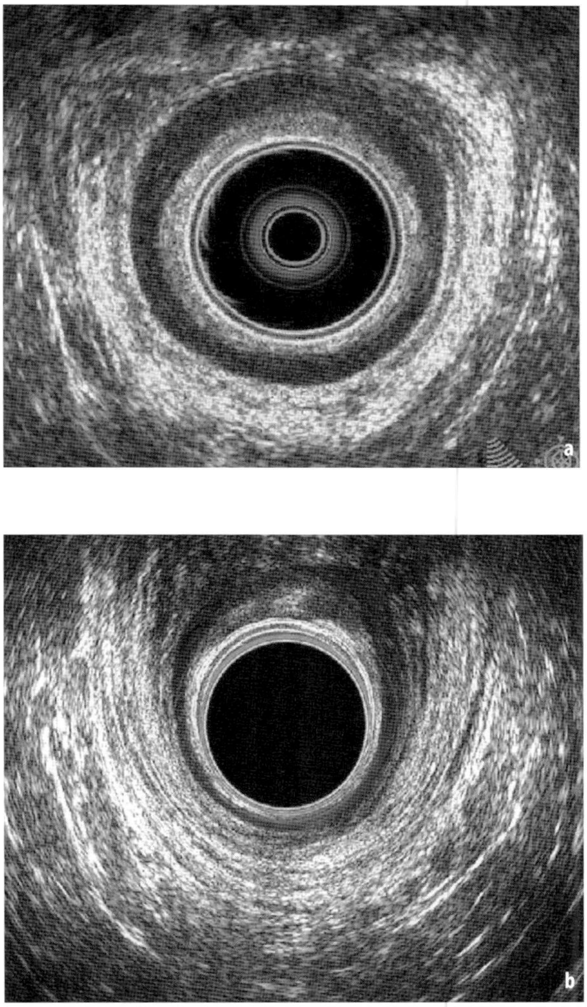

Fig. 10. Normal ultrasound anatomy of the deep level of the anal canal demonstrating the puborectalis. Anteriorly, a thin arc of muscle from the deeper part of the sphincter may be seen in males (**a**) whereas the deep part of the external sphincter is not recognisable in females (**b**)

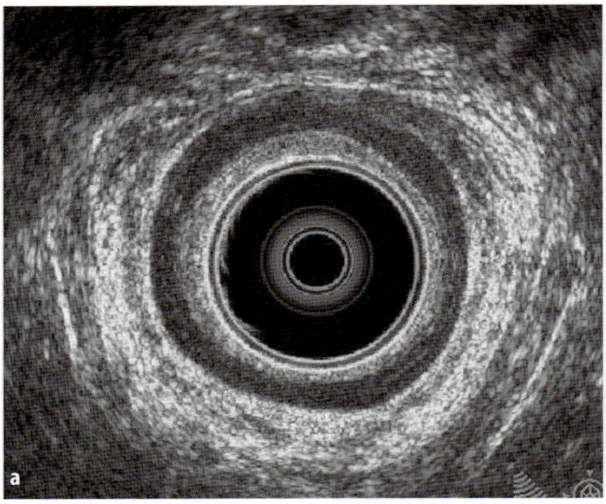

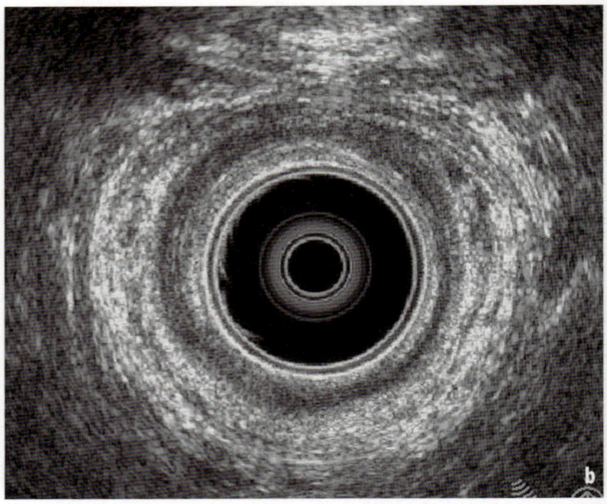

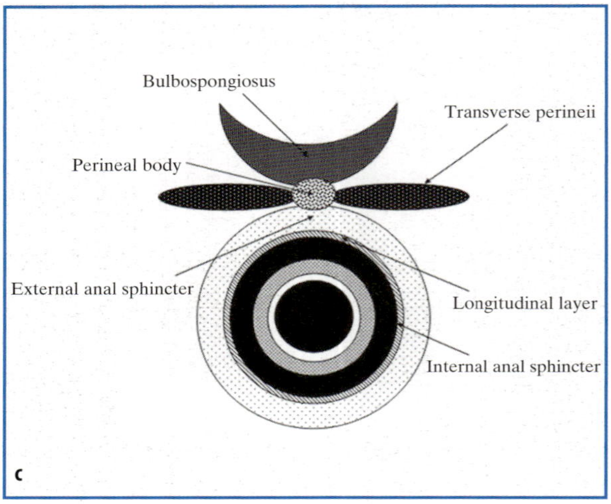

Fig. 11. Bulbospongiosus muscle, transverse perineal muscles and external anal sphincter meet in the perineal body. In males (**a**), a plane of fat persists between the transverse perinei and the external sphincter whereas in females (**b**), the transverse perinei fuse with the external sphincter. Schematic representation (**c**)

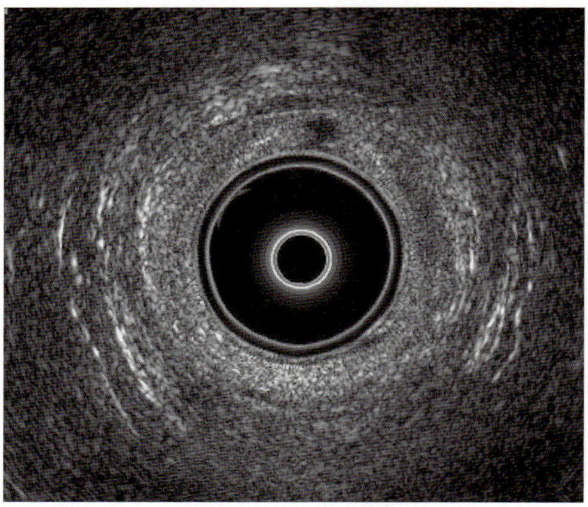

Fig. 12. Image at the superficial level demonstrating the subcutaneous external anal sphincter. The internal sphincter is absent at this level

Ultrasonographic Assessment of Perianal Crohn's Disease

Accurate identification of all loculate purulent areas and definition of the anatomy of the primary fistulous tract, secondary extensions and internal opening is crucial for the treatment plan. EAUS has been demonstrated to be a very helpful diagnostic tool in accurately assessing all fistula or abscess characteristics [8–11, 16, 17]. Ultrasound examination with the 2050 transducer is generally started using 13 MHz, changing to 12 MHz or 9 MHz to optimise visualisation of the deeper structures external to the anal sphincters. The puborectalis muscle and EAS, LM and IAS should always be identified and used as referents for the spatial orientation of the fistula or abscess.

An anal abscess appears as a hypoechoic, dishomogeneous area, sometimes with hyperechoic spots within it, possibly in connection with a fistulous tract directed through the anal canal lumen. Infection can spread in a number of directions, usually along the path of least resistance. Abscesses are classified as superficial, intersphincteric (Fig. 14), ischiorectal

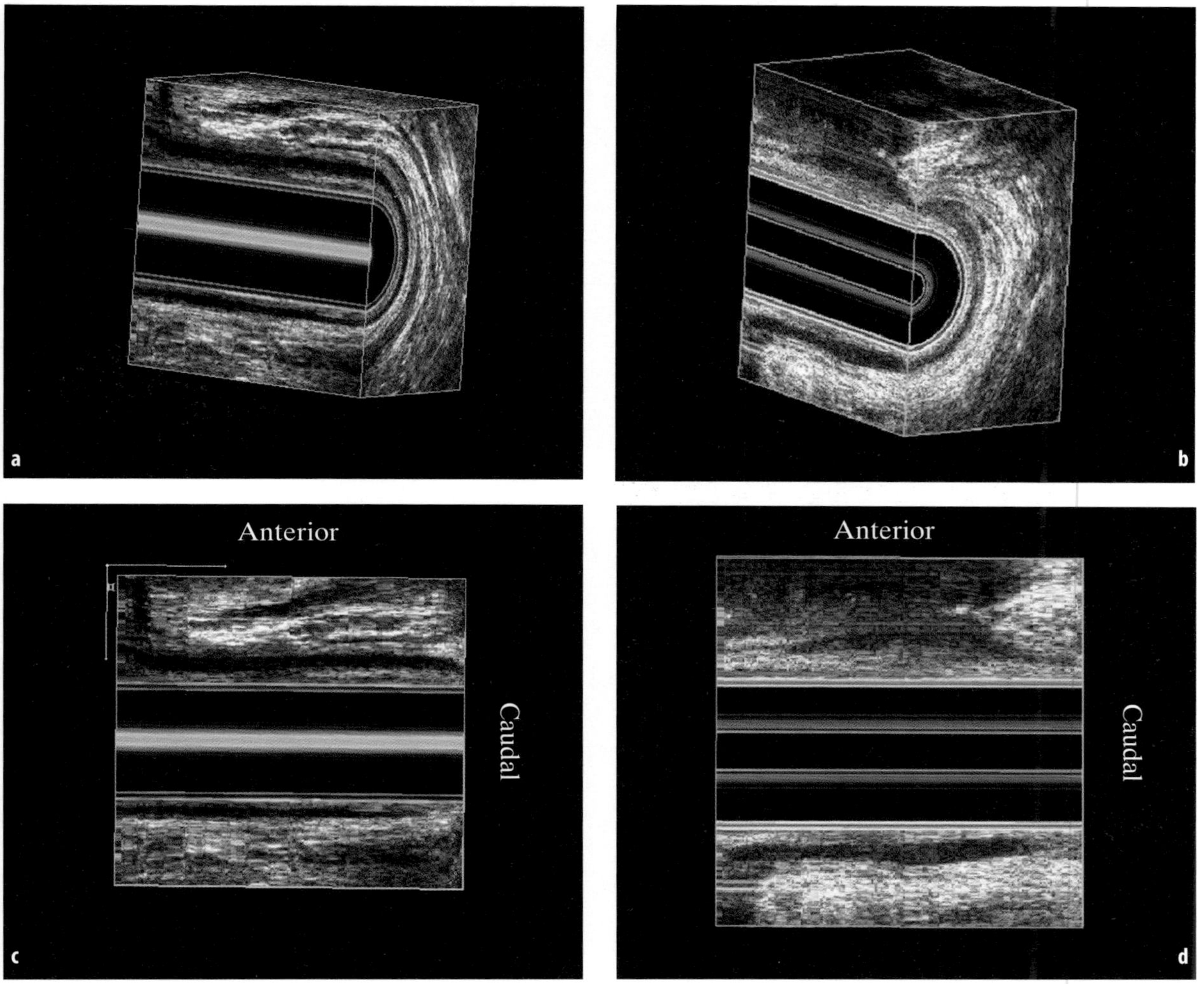

Fig. 13. Three-dimensional endosonographic reconstruction demonstrating that the anterior anal sphincter is shorter in the female: male (**a**), female (**b**). Sagittal images: male (**c**), female (**d**)

(Fig. 15), supralevator (Figs. 16, 17), pelvirectal and horseshoe (Fig. 18) [16]. An anal fistula appears as a hypoechoic tract, which is followed along its crossing of the subepithelium, internal or external sphincters and through the perianal spaces [16]. With regard to the anal sphincters, according to the classification by Parks et al. [4], the fistulous primary tract can be classified into four types:

1. Intersphincteric tract, which is presented as a band of poor reflectivity within the longitudinal layer, causing widening and distortion of an otherwise narrow intersphincteric plane (Fig. 19). The tract goes through the intersphincteric space without traversing the EAS fibres (Fig. 20).
2. Transsphincteric tract, in which the extension through the EAS is clearly shown by a poorly reflective tract running out through the EAS and disrupting its normal architecture (Figs. 21, 22). The point at which the main tract of the fistula traverses the sphincters defines the fistula level (high, medium or low). The low transsphincteric tract traverses only the distal third of the EAS at the lower portion of the medium anal canal. The medium transsphincteric tract traverses both sphincters, external and internal, in the middle part of the medium anal canal (Fig. 23). The high transsphincteric tract traverses both sphincters in the higher part of the medium anal canal in the space below the puborectalis (Fig. 24).
3. Suprasphincteric tract, which goes above or through the puborectalis level (Fig. 25).
4. Extrasphincteric tract, which may be seen close to but more laterally placed around the EAS (Fig. 26).

Rectovaginal fistula appears as a hypoechoic tract connecting the rectal wall and the vagina. It can be detected on endorectal ultrasonography with a stan-

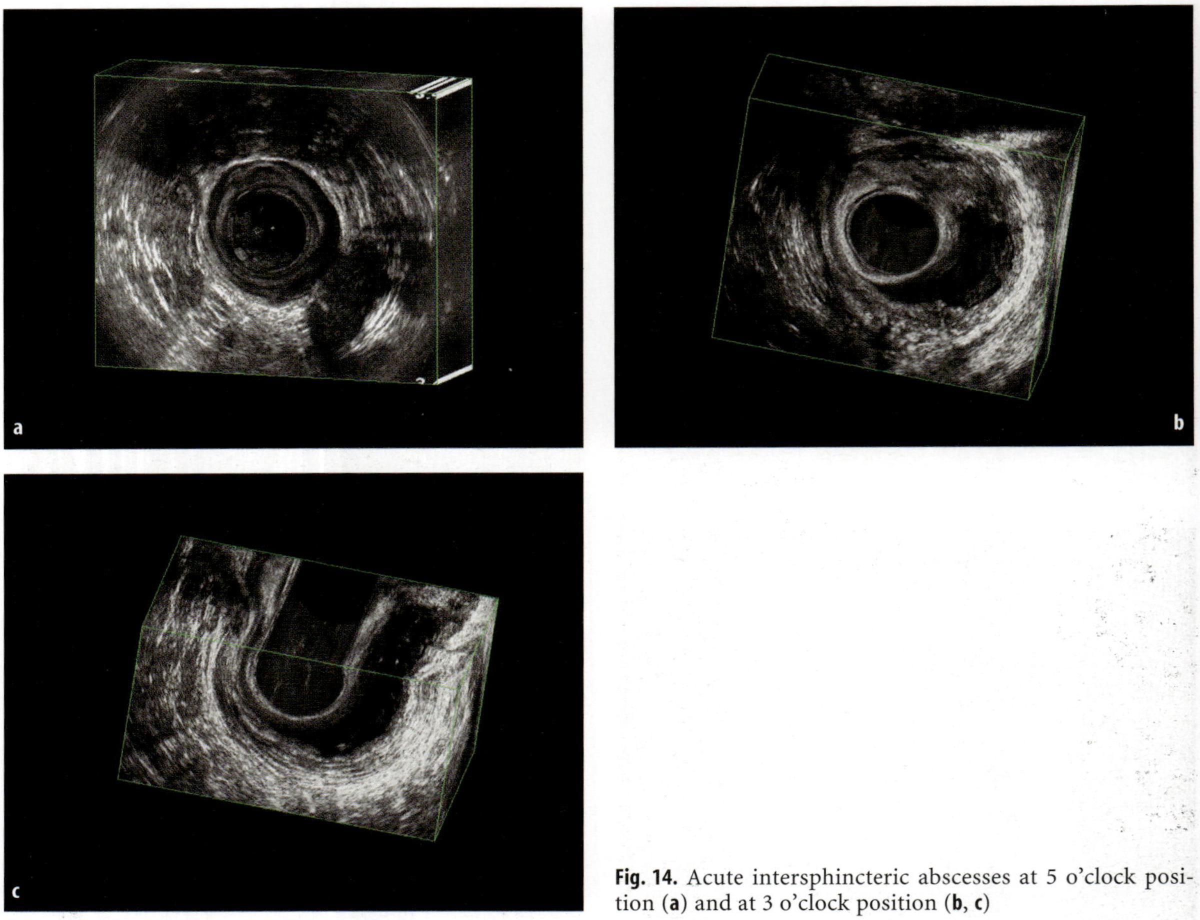

Fig. 14. Acute intersphincteric abscesses at 5 o'clock position (**a**) and at 3 o'clock position (**b**, **c**)

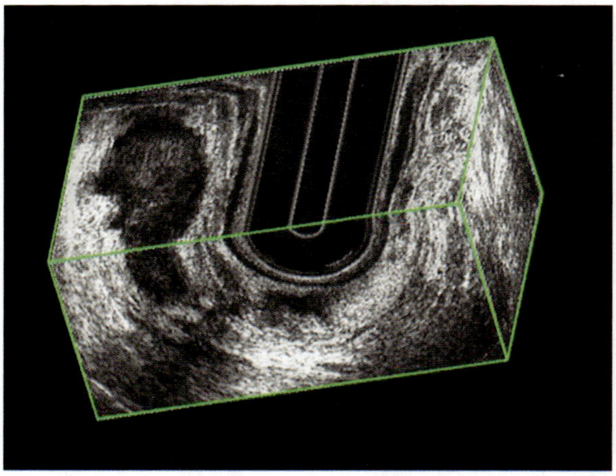

Fig. 15. Acute abscess in the right ischiorectal space

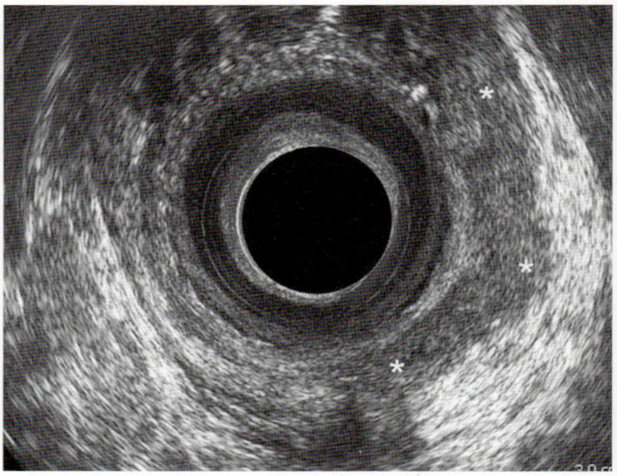

Fig. 16. Acute supralevator abscess presenting as an area of low reflectivity deep to the puborectalis muscle

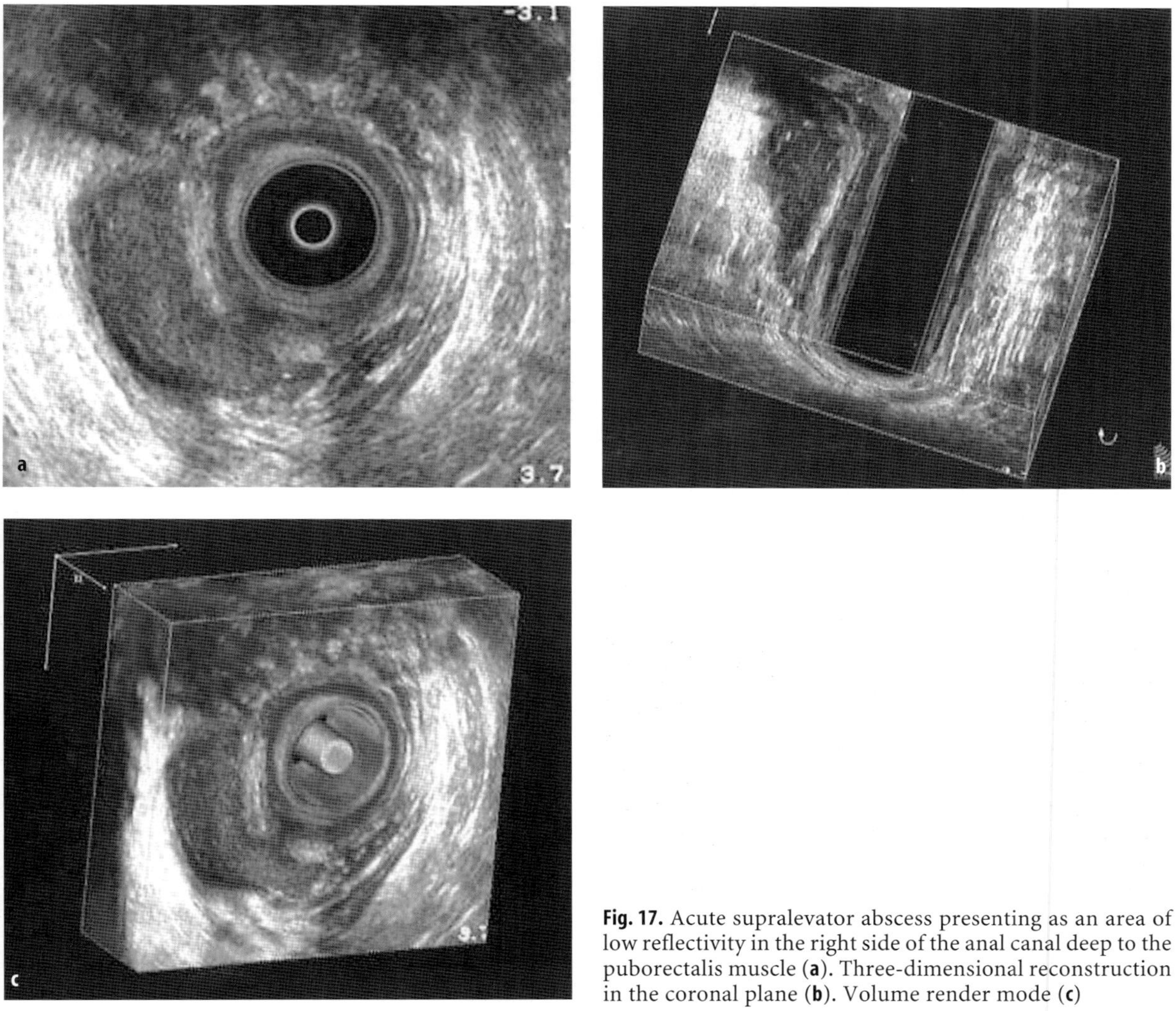

Fig. 17. Acute supralevator abscess presenting as an area of low reflectivity in the right side of the anal canal deep to the puborectalis muscle (**a**). Three-dimensional reconstruction in the coronal plane (**b**). Volume render mode (**c**)

dard water balloon, performed immediately after EAUS. Anovaginal fistulae are frequently small and collapsed, and their assessment may be problematic for both noncontrast and contrast-enhanced EAUS (Fig. 27). On the other hand, EAUS is very useful in the recognition of coexisting occult sphincter defects.

The major problems while investigating primary tracts with EAUS occur because of the structure alterations of the anal canal and perianal muscles and tissues, which can overstage the fistula, or poor definition of the tract when filled with inflammatory tissue, which can downstage the fistula. Differentiation between granulated tracts and scars is sometimes difficult. Straight tracts are easily identified, but smaller and oblique tracts are more difficult to image. Secondary tracts, when present, are related to the main one and are classified as intersphincteric, transsphincteric, suprasphincteric or extrasphincteric. Similarly, horseshoe tracts, when identified, are categorised as intersphincteric, suprasphincteric or extrasphincteric (Fig. 28-30). The use of 3-D EAUS, which enables reconstruction of transversal images of the anal canal in the coronal and sagittal planes, is very helpful in tracing the pathway of a tract.

The dentate line is not visible as an anatomical structure but is assumed to be just below the midpoint of the IAS. For this reason, the internal opening of an anal fistula is seldom clearly defined. Endosonographic criteria for the site of an internal opening, according to Cho [17], are the following: (1) an appearance of a root-like budding formed by the intersphincteric tract, which contacts the IAS; (2) an appearance of a root-like budding with an IAS defect; (3) a subepithelial breach connecting to the intersphincteric tract through an IAS defect. The site is categorised as being above, at or below the dentate

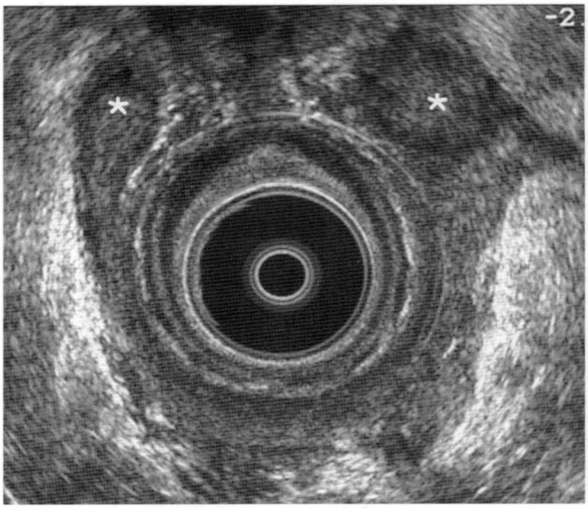

Fig. 18. Horseshoe collection in the intersphincteric space

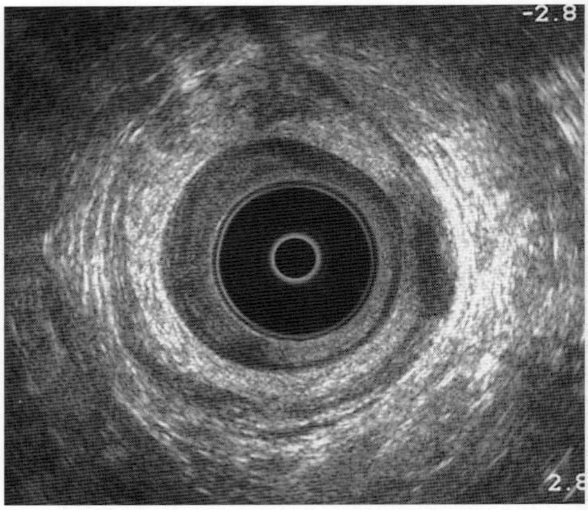

Fig. 19. Intersphincteric fistula at 3 o'clock position

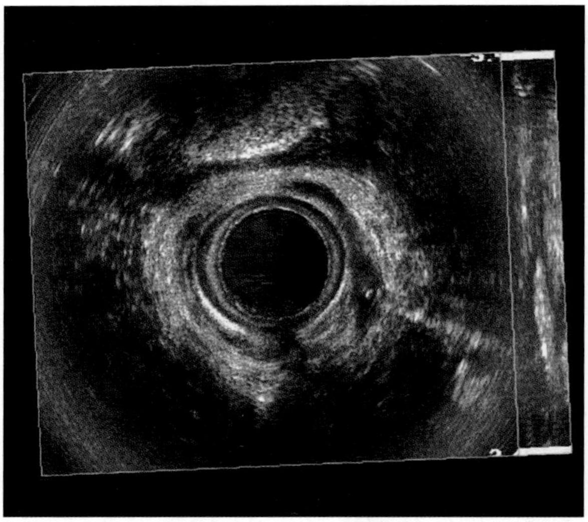

Fig. 20. Intersphincteric fistula with internal opening at 6 o'clock position and horseshoe extension in the left lateral intersphincteric space

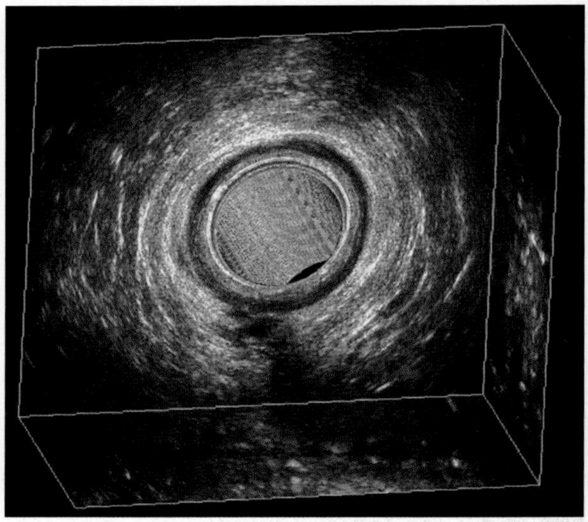

Fig. 21. Posterior transsphincteric tract extending through the external sphincter

line (in relation to the presumed location of the dentate line at the middle third of the anal canal) or in the rectal ampulla. In addition, the site of the internal opening can also be characterised by the clock position, being classified from 1 o'clock to 12 o'clock. The internal opening can be identified as hypoechoic (when acute inflammation is present) or hyperechoic (when chronically inflamed).

After standard EAUS examination, in patients in whom the external fistula opening is patent, 1.0–2.0 ml of 3% hydrogen peroxide (HP) can be injected very slowly using an 18-gauge plastic cannula via this opening while ultrasonic scanning of the anal canal is performed [16]. When no obvious external opening is present, a focal, elevated erythematous region immediately adjacent to the anal orifice is frequently identified. The soft catheter tip should be firmly pressed onto or probed into the center of this region, where the skin is easily broken, and the external opening located. Gas is a strong ultrasound

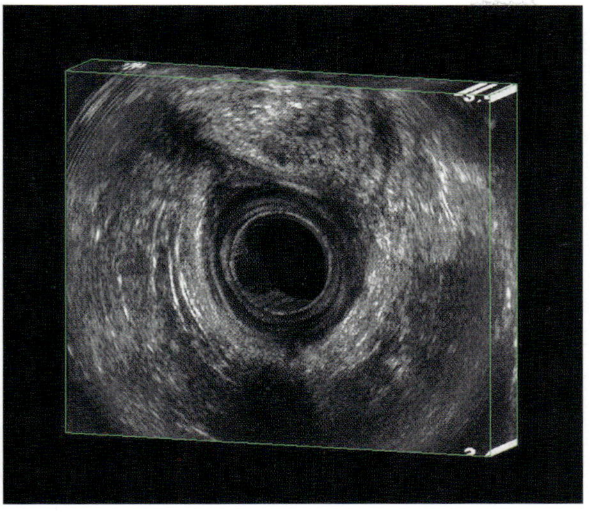

Fig. 22. Anterior transsphincteric tract at the level of transverse perineii

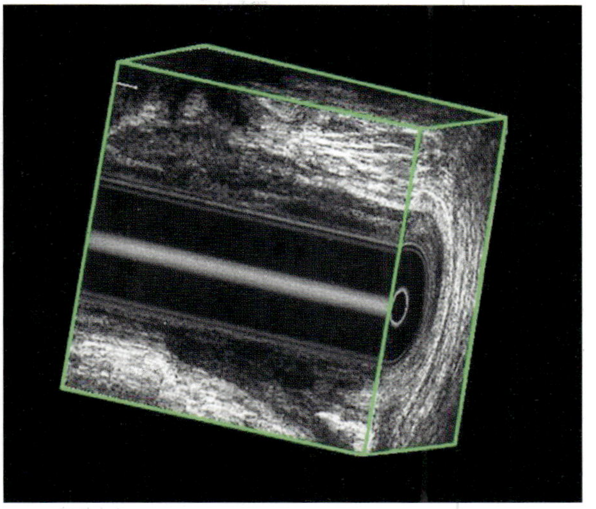

Fig. 23. Three-dimensional reconstruction in the sagittal plane showing a transsphincteric fistula that traverses the middle part of the external sphincter

reflector, and after injection, fistula tracks become hyperechoic, and the internal opening is identified as an echogenic breach at the submucosa (Figs. 31, 32). This method can be particularly useful when an active fistulous tract needs to be distinguished from postsurgical or posttraumatic scar tissue that can cause tissue alterations that are difficult to analyse. During this technique, however, the operator must be careful because the injected HP often results in bubbling into the anal canal, which then acts as a barrier to the ultrasound wave. Another disadvantage inherent to HP injection is the very strong reflection that occurs at a gas/tissue interface, which blanks out any detail deep into this interface. The bubbles produced by HP induce acoustic shadowing deep into the tract, so all information deep into the inner surface of the tract is lost. To reduce this potential pitfall of imaging, a volume-rendered 3-D data set can facilitate the following of a tortuous fistula tract due to the transparency and depth information (Fig. 33) [16].

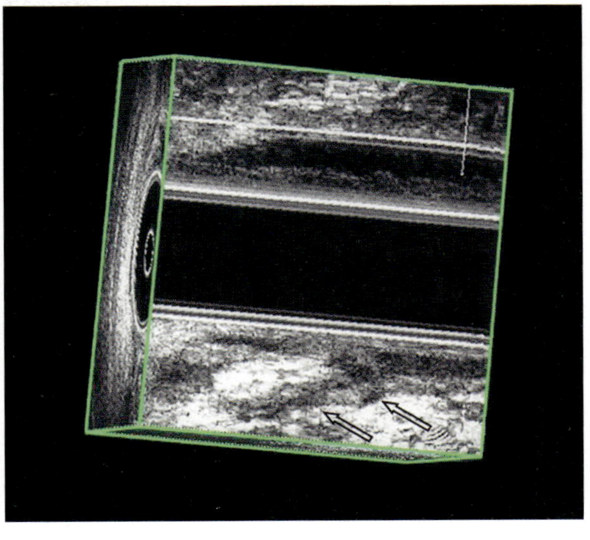

Fig. 24. Three-dimensional reconstruction in the sagittal plane showing a high transsphincteric tract traversing both sphincters in the higher part of the anal canal

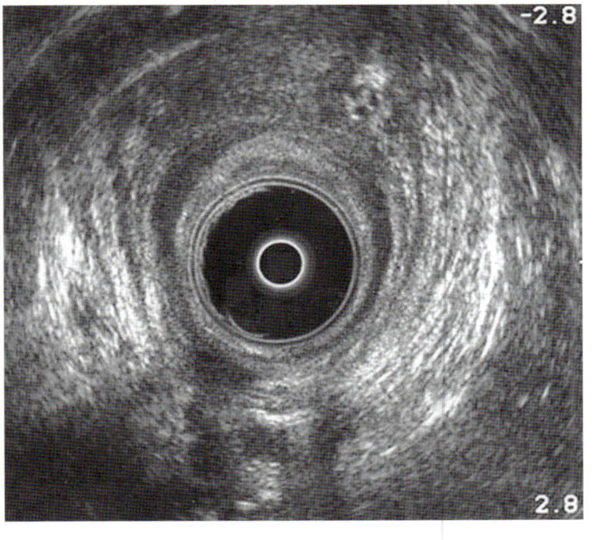

Fig. 25. Suprasphincteric tract extending through the puborectalis muscle

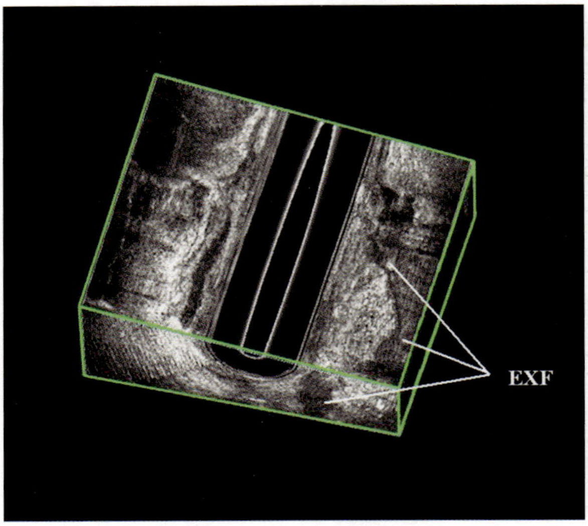

Fig. 26. Extrasphincteric fistula with direct communication between the perineum and rectum and no anal canal involvement

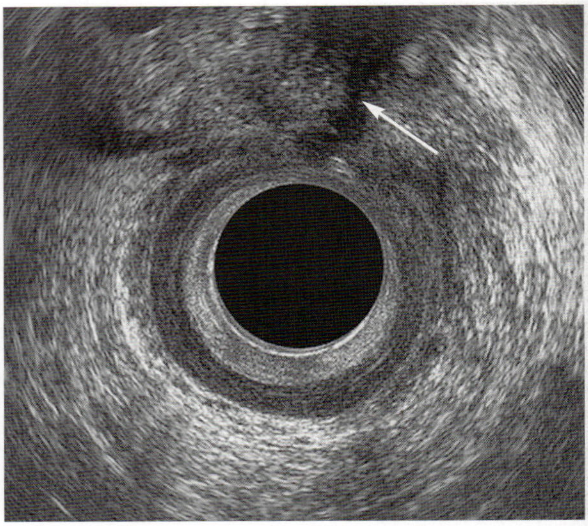

Fig. 27. Anovaginal fistula (*arrow*)

Accuracy

Imaging with EAUS has been shown to be a useful method (accuracy ranging from 63% to 100%) for evaluation of perianal abscesses and fistulae in CD [7–11, 13, 18]. Van Outryve et al. [8] reported that the routine proctological examination showed Crohn's lesions in 30% of patients and EAUS performed with a linear probe detected anorectal anomalies in 75% of patients. Moreover, EAUS was superior to CT scan in the study of pararectal and para-anal abscesses and fistulae. Schratter-Sehn et al. [19] demonstrated 46 fistulae, verified by surgery, in 36 patients with CD using EAUS performed with a 5-MHz sector (270°) scanner. Tio et al. [9] evaluated 36 patients with CD and suspected perianorectal disease. In the 17

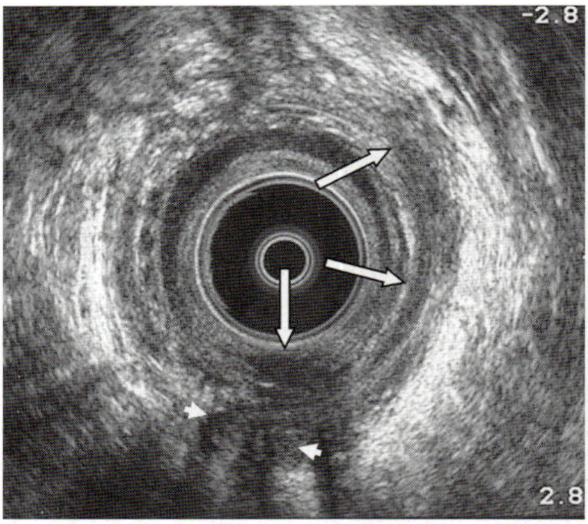

Fig. 28. Transsphincteric fistula (*small arrows*) with horseshoe secondary extension through the intersphincteric space (*large arrows*)

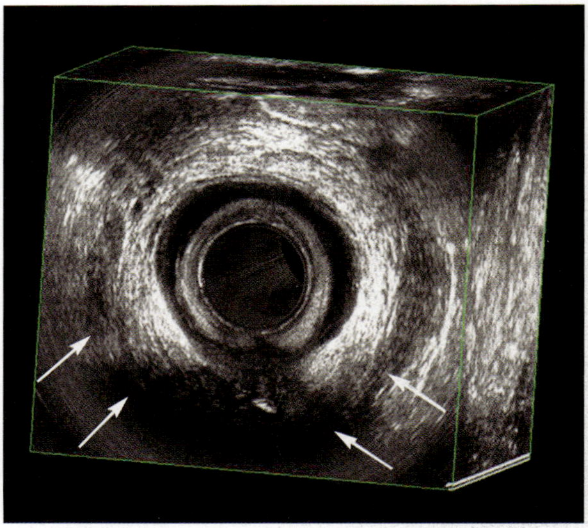

Fig. 29. Posterior transsphincteric fistula with horseshoe secondary extension in the ischioanal space (*arrows*)

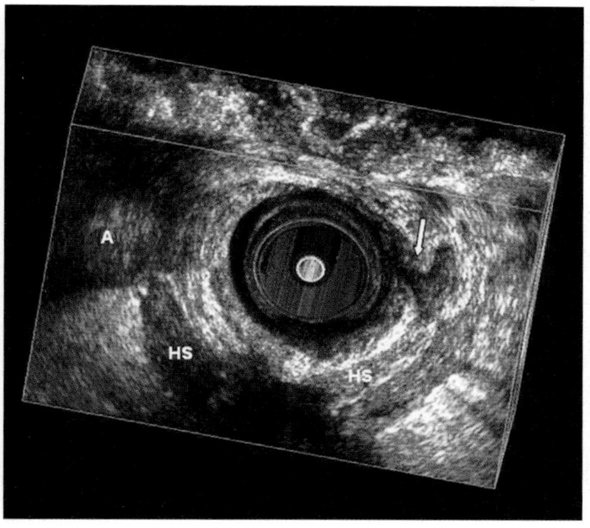

Fig. 30. Transsphincteric fistula at 3 o'clock position (*arrow*) with horseshoe secondary extension (*HS*) and forming an abscess into the right ischioanal space (*A*)

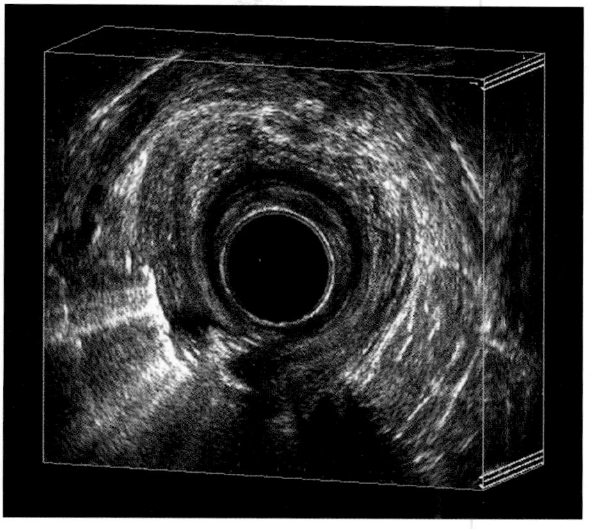

Fig. 31. Posterior transsphincteric fistula, after hydrogen peroxide injection, appearing as a hyperechoic tract extending through the external sphincter, with a secondary hyperechoic tract in the right ischioanal space

patients that had surgically confirmed fistulae, EAUS identified fistula in 14 (82.4%). Solomon [3] reported that patients with CD often have high and complex perianal fistulae. Using EAUS performed with a 7- to 10-MHz radial probe, they found that 40% of fistulae involved the upper half of the anal sphincter, 30% of patients had supralevator chronic abscess cavities and 29% of women had rectovaginal fistulae.

In the literature, several studies have reported on ultrasonographic findings after treatment. West et al. [20] evaluated the effect of combined ciprofloxacin and infliximab in perianal CD using HP-enhanced 3-D ultrasound (3-D HPUS). Only three of the 13 patients with a clinical response at week 18 also showed improvement on 3-D HPUS. This result is in agreement with van Bodegraven et al. [21], who reported that although clinical improvement was seen after short-term infliximab treatment, most fistulae still persisted on EAUS. These persistent lesions may lead to relapse of symptoms or abscess formation. In a long-term study, Rasul et al. [22] evaluated whether the clinical improvement after infliximab in 35 patients with Crohn's disease perianal fistulae was associated with endosonographic closure of fistula

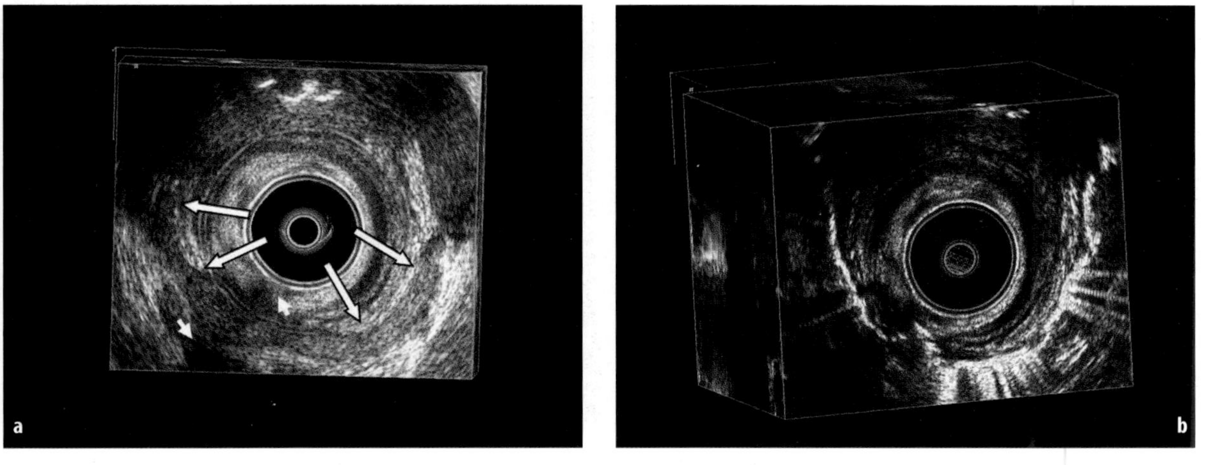

Fig. 32. Posterior transsphincteric fistula (*small arrows*) with horseshoe secondary intersphincteric extension (*large arrows*) before (**a**) and after (**b**) hydrogen peroxide injection

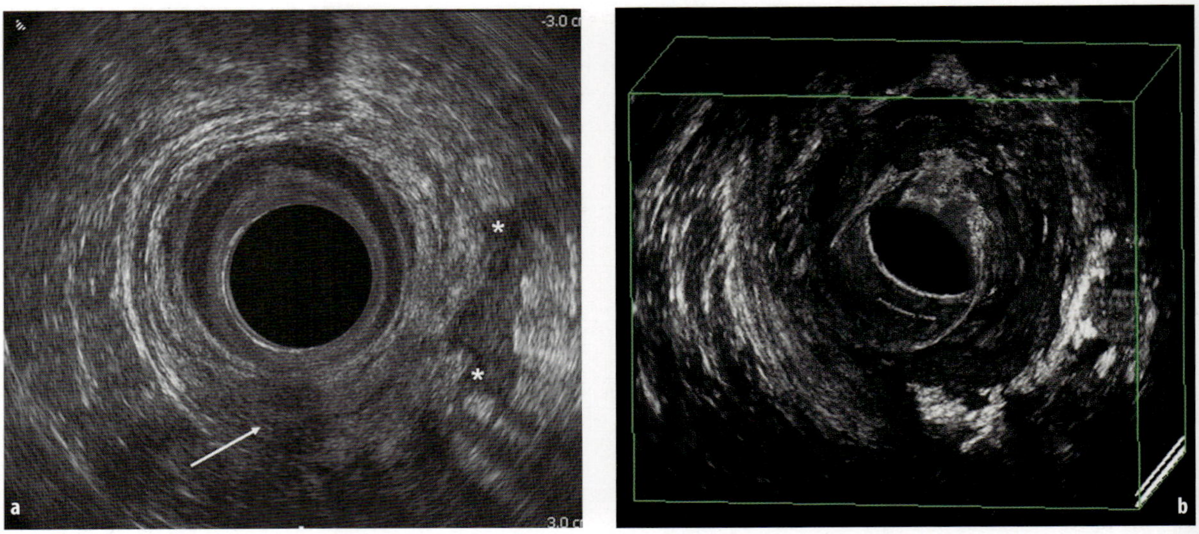

Fig. 33. Transsphincteric fistula (*arrow*) with an ischiorectal abscess (**a**). Three-dimensional reconstruction using "volume render mode" after hydrogen peroxide injection

tracts. TPUS identified more fistulae than appreciated clinically, as well as the presence of unsuspected fluid collections. Short-term clinical response was higher than radiographic response, and fistulous tracts on TPUS were still present in many clinical responders at week 8 (49% vs 14%, respectively). At week 56, complete clinical closure of fistulae remained in approximately one half of patients; however, ultrasonographic healing occurred in 46% of patients, and this correlated well with clinical healing. The main conclusion of this study is that even though fistulae clinically may have healed in the short term after initial treatment, further long-term therapy may be required if defects persist radiographically, even to a point that radiological improvement is seen so that symptom relapse and abscess formation can be prohibited.

A number of comparative studies have been performed to assess the efficacy of EAUS and MRI in evaluating perianal CD [8–11]. Some studies have shown superiority for MRI [23] whereas others have shown little difference [10, 11]. MRI scans can involve use of an endoanal coil or phased-array coil. Endoanal coil provides excellent spatial resolution but is unable to detect deeper fistula tracts and distant abscess collections, which are better assessed using phased-array coil [24]. MRI is useful for assessing the integrity of the IAS and EAS as well as identifying complex fistula tracts and abscesses [25]; however, pelvic MRI was shown to have a tendency to miss short or superficial fistula tracts. Orsoni et al. [11] conducted a prospective study comparing EAUS performed with a linear probe, pelvic MRI performed with body coil and examination under anaesthesia (EUA) in 22 patients and found EAUS to be the most sensitive modality. Agreement for fistulae with EAUS and MRI when compared with surgical findings was 82% and 50%, respectively. Schwartz et al. [10] compared the accuracy of MRI performed with phased-array coil, EAUS performed with both radial and linear probe and EUA in 34 patients with Crohn's perianal fistulae. All three methods demonstrated good agreement with the "consensus gold standard" (MRI, 87%; EAUS, 91%; EUA, 91%). In addition, when any two of the three methods were combined, accuracy was 100%. Maier et al. [23] showed that MRI was superior to EAUS performed with a radial probe in the assessment of fistulae in CD. Overall sensitivity of EAUS and MRI was 73% and 91% for primary fistulae and 69% and 88% for recurrent fistulae, respectively. Wedemeyer et al. [13] showed an excellent agreement (k >0.83) between MRI performed with a phased-array surface coil and TPUS in 25 patients with CD and clinical signs of perianal inflammatory disease. They recommended TPUS as a screening tool in acute perianal disorders in CD and to evaluate treatment outcomes.

Conclusion

EAUS evaluation of perianal complications of CD has been demonstrated to be superior to fistulography and CT and equal or superior to MRI. This imaging modality should be part of the diagnostic workup, helping guide therapy and preventing unnecessary surgery [26].

References

1. Frizelle FA, Santoro GA, Pemberton JH (1996) The management of perianal Crohn's disease. Int J Colorectal Dis 11:227–237
2. Singh B, Mortensen NJ, Jewell DP, George B (2004) Perianal Crohn's disease. Br J Surg 91:801–814
3. Solomon MJ (1996) Fistulae and abscess in symptomatic perianal Crohn's disease. Int J Colorectal Dis 11:222–226
4. Parks AG, Gordon PH, Hardcastle JD (1976) A classification of fistula-in-ano. Br J Surg 63:1–12
5. American Gastroenterological Association (2003) American Gastroenterological Association medical position statement: perianal Crohn's disease. Gastroenterology 125:1503–1507
6. Schwartz DA, Herdman CR (2004) Review article: the medical treatment of Crohn's perianal fistulas. Aliment Pharmacol Ther 19:953–967
7. Schratter-Sehn AU, Lochs H, Vogelsang H et al (1993) Endoscopic ultrasonography versus computed tomography in the differential diagnosis of perianorectal complications in Crohn's disease. Endoscopy 25:582–586
8. Van Outryve MJ, Pelckmans PA, Michielsen PP, Van Maercke YM (1991) Value of transrectal ultrasonography in Crohn's disease. Gastroenterology 101:1171–1177
9. Tio TL, Mulder CJ, Wijers OB et al (1990) Endosonography of perianal and pericolorectal fistula and/or abscess in Crohn's disease. Gastrointest Endosc 36:331–336
10. Schwartz DA, Wierse MJ, Dudiak KM et al (2001) A comparison of endoscopic ultrasound, magnetic resonance imaging, and examination under anesthesia for evaluation of Crohn's perianal fistulas. Gastroenterology 121:1064–1072
11. Orsoni P, Barthet M, Portier F, et al (1999) Prospective comparison of endosonography, magnetic resonance imaging and surgical findings in anorectal fistula and abscess complicating Crohn's disease. Br J Surg 86:360–364
12. Santoro GA, Di Falco G (2004) Endoanal and endorectal ultrasonographic techniques. In: Santoro GA, Di Falco G (eds) Atlas of endoanal and endorectal ultrasonography. Springer-Verlag. Milan, pp 11–21
13. Wedemeyer J, Kirchloff T, Sellge G et al (2004) Transcutaneous perianal sonography: a sensitive method for the detection of perianal inflammatory lesions in Crohn's disease. World J Gastroenterol 10:2859–2863
14. Santoro GA, Di Falco G (2004) Surgical and endosonographic anatomy of the rectum. In: Santoro GA, Di Falco G (eds) Atlas of endoanal and endorectal ultrasonography. Springer-Verlag, Milan, pp 37–41
15. Thakar R, Sultan A (2004) Anal endosonography and its role in assessing the incontinent patient. Best Pract Res Clinic Obstet Gynaec 18:157–173
16. Santoro GA, Ratto C (2006) Accuracy and reliability of endoanal ultrasonography in the evaluation of perianal abscesses and fistula-in-ano. In: Santoro GA, Di Falco G (eds) Benign anorectal diseases. Diagnosis with endoanal and endorectal ultrasound and new treatment options. Springer-Verlag, Milan, pp 142-157
17. Cho DY (1999) Endosonographic criteria for an internal opening of fistula-in-ano. Dis Colon Rectum 42:515–518
18. Tio TL, Kallimanis GE (1994) Endoscopic ultrasonography of perianorectal fistulas and abscesses. Endoscopy 26:813–815
19. Schratter-Sehn AU, Lochs H, Handl-Zeller L et al (1993) Endosonographic features of the lower pelvic region in Crohn's disease. Am J Gastroenterol 88:1054–1057
20. West RL, Van der Woude CJ, Hansen BE et al (2004) Clinical and endosonographic effect of ciprofloxacin on the treatment of perianal fistulae in Crohn's disease with infliximab: a double-blind placebo-controlled study. Aliment Pharmacol Ther 20:1329–1336
21. van Bodegraven AA, Sloots CE, Felt-Bersma RJ et al (2002) Endosonographic evidence of persistence of Crohn's disease-associated fistulas after infliximab treatment, irrespective of clinical response. Dis Colon Rectum 45:39–45
22. Rasul I, Wilson SR, MacRae H et al (2004) Clinical and radiological responses after infliximab treatment for perianal fistulizing Crohn's disease. Am J Gastroenterol 99:82–88
23. Maier AG, Funovics MA, Kreuzer SH et al (2001) Evaluation of perianal sepsis: comparison of anal endosonography and magnetic resonance imaging. J Magn Reson Imaging 14:254–260
24. deSouza NM, Gilderdale DJ, Coutts GA et al (1998) MRI of fistula-in-ano: a comparison of endoanal coil with external phased array coil techniques. J Comput Assist Tomogr 22:357–363
25. Borley NR, Mortensen NJ, Jewell DP (1999) MRI scanning in perianal Crohn's disease: an important diagnostic adjunct. Inflamm Bowel Dis 5:231–233
26. Lew RJ, Ginsberg GG (2002) The role of endoscopic ultrasound in inflammatory bowel disease. Gastrointest Endoscopy Clin N Am 12:561–571

Endoscopy in Crohn's Disease

Andrea Ederle, Paolo Inturri, Piero Brosolo, Alberto Fantin, Monica Preto

Endoscopic Diagnosis of Crohn's Disease

Endoscopy plays a major role in the diagnosis of Crohn's disease, especially with colonoscopy and ileoscopy; however, upper gastrointestinal endoscopy, enteroscopy, capsule endoscopy and endoscopic ultrasound (EUS) may help confirm and determine the extent of disease. Direct visualisation of mucosal lesions and the possibility of obtaining histologic specimens make endoscopic procedures the first-line tests in the evaluation of gastrointestinal diseases. However, radiology and magnetic resonance imaging (MRI) contribute to the diagnosis when visualising the small bowel [1].

Endoscopic Features of Crohn's Disease

Morphologic pictures observed during an endoscopic procedure are protean. The earliest endoscopic finding is the aphthous ulcer with a diameter of a few millimeters surrounded by a thin red halo of oedematous tissue [2], which is found in about 30–40% of patients with Crohn's colitis. Focal oedema and sporadic red spots are present in the "preaphthoid phase [3]. These lesions usually are multiple, becoming stellate or linear in shape, with normal intervening mucosa, and can be rounded or long and serpiginous. Cobblestone-like areas are formed when ulcers assume a longitudinal and transverse pattern forming a grid. This is due to submucosal oedema, including nonulcerated mucosa [4]. Sometimes, these lesions differ little from inflammatory polyps or pseudopolyps also often present in Crohn's colitis [5]. The presence of punched-out ulcers adjacent to inflamed mucosa gives rise after healing to mucosal bridges. Stenosis is often present in areas of severe inflammation, especially in the pyloric sphincter, ileocecal valve and rectosigmoid junction [6]. Length may vary from less than 3 cm to more than 10 cm and a width of less of 5 mm. Fistulae have been reported in more than 8% of patients affected by Crohn's colitis, often near stenoses [7]. Less common manifestations are diffuse mucosal irregularities with erythema, oedema, granularity.

Carrying out multiple biopsies in areas both involved and uninvolved by the disease increases diagnostic accuracy of endoscopy and pathology. The use of large biopsy forceps should be taken in consideration for obtaining a better specimen of the submucosa [8]. Finally, during colonoscopy, it is mandatory that intubation of the terminal ileum is performed in order to take biopsies that may increase the procedure's sensitivity and specificity [9].

Colonoscopy

Colonoscopy is an important aid in diagnosis and management of patients with inflammatory bowel disease (IBD). This procedure, with multiple biopsies, is indicated when adequate data are not available from clinical, sigmoidoscopic or radiologic studies and there is strong clinical suspicion of IBD. However, colonoscopy carries an increased risk of perforation when the bowel wall is inflamed and presents with ulcers and fistulae. Known or suspected severe inflammation is a relative contraindication to colonoscopy. Toxic megacolon is an absolute contraindication to endoscopy if performed only for diagnostic purpose because of the weakness of the colonic wall, which is paper thin [10]. Endoscopy monitoring to assess response to therapy has been evaluated by a randomised study in which patients were treated with steroids. In one group, steroid tapering was decided on following clinical remission; in the other group, the decision was based on endoscopic findings. The conclusion was that colonoscopy was not necessary to decide when to taper steroids, as the two groups did equally well [11].

Colonoscopy evaluation of the extent of disease is also part of preoperative assessment in order to decide the extent of resection and define the segments free from disease. The ileocecal area is the most frequent site of the disease, accounting for about 70% of cases. Of these, 20–30% involved the colon only, and 40–55% had ileocolic disease [12]. Although considered peculiar of Crohn's colitis, rectal sparing is found in less than half of patients. When the rectum is involved, the disease begins at the rectosigmoid junction or appears with anorectal inflammation. The entire rectum is affected by the disease from 5% to 10%. Lesion progression, from aphthous to serpiginous ulcers, has a discontinuous and asymmetric course, with the inflamed mucosa typically presenting normal "skip areas" [13]. Segmental localisation of the disease has a high predictive value [14].

Other endoscopic features found during a colonoscopy include pseudopolyps, erosions and stenosis. A prospective study evaluated the incidence of different lesions found during a colonoscopy. All the patients were affected by Crohn's disease and underwent the procedure before beginning therapy. Endoscopy showed the following findings: 93% superficial erosions, 74% deep erosions, 48% mucosal oedema, 44% erythema, 41% pseudopolyps, 10% aphthous ulcers, 8% ulcerated stenosis and 2% nonulcerated stenosis [15].

Pseudopolyps represent regenerative epithelium and may include granulation tissue without premalignant potential. They are often multiple and bright, with a fragile surface that bleeds very easily when biopsies are taken. Endoscopic differential diagnosis with adenomas can be difficult, and only biopsy will provide definitive diagnosis [16]. They need to be resected if bleeding or causing obstruction, and polypectomy is performed in the same way as in the general population [17].

Colonoscopy allows direct investigation of strictures. Biopsies are mandatory to rule out stenoses caused by carcinoma. Malignant lesions are usually eccentric, rigid and may present nodules within the stricture or at its margins [18]. The colonoscope should go beyond the stenosis in order to carry out a thorough inspection, using a pediatric instrument if needed, avoiding the standard colonoscope to act as a dilator [19]. Endoscopic features may also have prognostic value, as reported by Allez and collaborators [20]. They found that patients with deep and extensive ulcerations of the colon are at higher risk of penetrating complications and undergoing surgery. Distribution of severe endoscopic lesions was the following: rectum 13%, sigmoid colon 77%, left colon 62%, transverse colon 51%, right colon 28%.

When disease involves the colon only, the main differential diagnosis is between Crohn's disease and ulcerative colitis (UC) (Table 1). Usually, the two entities can be differentiated endoscopically, and inflammation distribution can aid diagnosis. Crohn's colitis is more likely in the presence of skip areas or when the rectum is spared. In UC, the rectum may be spared by local treatment or when the proximal colon is more involved than the rectum during an acute severe attack [21]. Moreover, peculiar to Crohn's disease is the presence of deep linear ulcerations separated by areas of normal mucosa as well as terminal ileum involvement. Inflamed mucosa extends for more than a few centimeters, and ulcerations are present in this portion of the small intestine. Although the small bowel is not involved by UC, a few centimeters of inflamed mucosa without ulceration may be present in the terminal ileum (backwash ileitis) in 15–20 % of patients with pancolitis.

When extensive inflammation of the colon is present, differential diagnosis between Crohn's disease and UC may be very difficult. Patients presenting features of both diseases are considered to have indeter-

Table 1. Crohn's disease and ulcerative colitis: endoscopic differential diagnosis

Crohn's disease	Features	Ulcerative colitis
Any portion of gastrointestinal tract	Distribution	Contiguous involvement of the colon starting from rectum
Often stenotic or ulcerated	Ileocecal valve	Without ulcerations
Frequent	Lesions to terminal ileum	Backwash ileitis (15–20%)
Sometimes	Lesions proximally to terminal ileum	Not present
25–50%	Rectal involvement	95–100%
Rare	Continuous colitis	Yes
Asymmetric inflammation	Mucosal involvement	Circumferential inflammation
Yes	Segmental inflammation	No
Yes	Skip areas	No
Frequent	Cobblestones-like areas	Rare
Aphthoid/deep	Ulcerations	Shallow
Frequent	Fistulas	Rare
Frequent	Stenosis	Rare

minate colitis, and at least 10% of patients who present with an IBD is regarded as having indeterminate colitis [22]. Usually, they are treated and monitored as are patients with UC unless signs of Crohn's disease develop. Other diseases that may resemble Crohn's disease are functional disorders (e.g. irritable bowel syndrome), immunomediated (e.g. connective tissue diseases), drug induced [(e.g. nonsteroidal anti-inflammatory drugs (NSAID)], vascular (e.g. intestinal ischaemia), neoplastic (e.g. carcinoma, lymphoma), infective or diverticular disease.

Upper- and Small-Bowel Endoscopy

Esophagus, stomach and duodenum may be involved by Crohn's disease [23]. Even in the upper gastrointestinal tract, aphthous ulcer is the most common lesion, but mucosal nodularity and stenosis may be seen [24]. The presence of inflamed mucosa in this portion of the digestive tract is important for differential diagnosis between Crohn's disease and UC. Radiologic procedures with barium as small-bowel follow-through or enteroclysis are important for diagnosis of Crohn's disease localised in the small bowel and for demonstration of strictures and fistulae [25]. However, a study comparing small-bowel barium examination with enteroclysis and ileoscopy showed that the radiology missed 27% of severe inflammatory changes and 50% of mild inflammatory changes [26]. Push enteroscopy allows evaluation of the proximal small bowel whereas intraoperative enteroscopy is used to explore the distal small intestine [27]. The former procedure is useful especially in patients without known Crohn's disease but who are suspected to have small-bowel involvement. However, a recent study reported that in patients with known Crohn's disease, capsule endoscopy has a higher yield in detecting mucosal involvement of the small bowel than does push enteroscopy and enteroclysis [28]. Intraoperative enteroscopy compared with preoperative radiography is able to find more intestinal lesions, especially small ulcers and inflammatory polyps [29].

A new method of carrying out enteroscopy consists of using a double-balloon technique in which a first balloon is placed on the tip of the enteroscope and the second balloon on the tip of the overtube. This technique allows far better insertability and maneuverability compared with conventional methods. Preliminary experience reported the performance of this procedure on eight patients with abdominal symptoms, three of whom were diagnosed with Crohn's disease [30]. Enteroscopy with the double-balloon technique was carried out using the oral approach in all patients and additionally with the anal approach in four patients. In two patients, it was possible to examine the whole small bowel, with a visualised total length of between 180 cm and 500 cm. Recently, Yamamoto reviewed the publications on double-balloon endoscopy, concluding that this method has the potential to be the standard of enteroscopy by replacing conventional push and intraoperative enteroscopy for diagnosis by means of bioptic specimens and therapeutic endoscopy of the small bowel [31].

Endoscopic Retrograde Cholangiopancreatography

Primary sclerosing cholangitis is a complication of IBD, present especially in patients affected by UC with an incidence between 1% and 4% and with lower frequency in Crohn's disease [32]. Patients with IBD and abnormal liver function test need to be evaluated for hepatobiliary complications. Depending on local availability, MR cholangiography or endoscopic retrograde cholangiopancreatography should be performed as the initial diagnostic test in the suspicion of sclerosing cholangitis. The latter procedure is indicated as the procedure of choice when biliary stenosis is suspected or evident.

Endoscopic Ultrasound

EUS is a procedure for imaging the intestinal wall at high resolution. The use of EUS shows findings that distinguish normal colon from IBD as increased wall thickness, lymphadenopathy or enlarged perirectal vessels [33]. In particular, vessel enlargement is more likely associated with patients with acute Crohn's disease whereas adenopathy is associated with acute UC. Therefore, this procedure could be helpful in differentiating the two diseases. An alternative to EUS is the high-frequency ultrasound catheter probe. In one study, a 20-MHz radial catheter was used to evaluate the colorectal wall in patients with IBD [34]. Crohn's disease was associated with thickening of the fourth hypoechoic layer (muscularis propria) or loss of layer structure, and mucosal and submucosal thickening was more likely in ulcerative disease.

Moreover, EUS plays a major role in diagnosis and assessment of Crohn's anorectal and perineal complications, such as abscesses or fistulae. Barium fistulography and computed tomography (CT) of the pelvis have been less sensitive for perianal disease [35] than EUS of the rectum [36]. One study demonstrated that rectal EUS had a diagnostic accuracy of at least 85%, as with examination under anesthesia and pelvic MRI, when evaluating the anatomy of perianal fistulae [37]. When any two tests were combined, the accuracy was 100%.

Finally, endoscopic-ultrasound-guided fine-needle aspiration may help confirm the diagnosis for suspected abscesses and provide therapeutic procedures [38].

Intestinal Strictures are a Commonly Encountered Problem in Patients with Crohn's Disease

Management of Strictures

Intestinal strictures are a commonly encountered problem in patients with Crohn's disease, resulting in bowel obstruction and eventually in repeated bowel resection and short bowel disease. Over one third of patients with Crohn's disease have a clear stenosing disease phenotype, often in the absence of luminal inflammatory symptoms [39]. At the foundation, as in other organs and tissues, there is transformation and activation of fibroblasts and smooth muscle cells that underlie fibrogenesis in the gut. Endoscopic balloon dilation is the preferred initial therapeutic modality in anastomotic strictures. In fact, endoscopic management with hydrostatic balloon dilation is an effective alternative to surgery in patients with endoscopically accessible lesions shorter than 7–8 cm [40], but careful patient selection is of great importance to ensure favourable long-term results. The presence of inflammation near the stricture should not be considered a contraindication to dilation, and intralesional steroid injection should be considered in these patients.

Among the three clinical patterns of Crohn's disease (inflammatory, penetrating/fistulising and obstructive/fibrostenotic), the latter is a frequent cause of symptoms and is an indication for surgery in over half of operations for Crohn's disease. Small-intestinal strictures are found in 21% of patients, duodenale strictures in 5% [41], colonic strictures range from 4% to 9% [42, 43] and anorectal strictures in 7.5% [44]. Strictures may also arise from surgical treatment for Crohn's disease, with reported rates of 17–81%.

To avoid surgery in patients with symptomatic Crohn's strictures, various endoscopic techniques have been successfully utilised: balloon dilation with or without corticosteroid injection, Savary dilation, endoscopic needle knife incisions and self-expandable metal stents, but no randomised clinical trials compare these methods for dilation. However, clinical situations in which to consider endoscopic management of Crohn's strictures are: endoscopic accessibility, multiple previous intestinal resections and short strictures (<8 cm). It is important to consider intralesional steroid injection if significant inflammation is present.

Intestinal balloon dilation is attractive due to the ability to directly apply the radial force achieved during balloon insufflation, in contrast to the shearing force applied during bougienage [45]. Balloon dilation is the most widely reported method for nonsurgically dilating intestinal strictures in Crohn's disease [46, 47] resistant to medical therapy, with endoscopic incisions of the stricture or electroincision with or without intralesional steroid injection [48]. The balloon, with a diameter from 18 mm to 25 mm, was inflated for 1–4 min and repeated two to four times per session [49]. Successful dilation was generally defined as allowing the passage of a standard adult colonoscope. One author [50] made four radial incisions into the stricture with a standard papillotome if the colonoscope could not pass the stricture. In this way, dilation sufficient to allow passage of the adult colonoscope was achieved in every patient, with 3% of complications (minor bleeding and perforation) in a total of 137 dilations, with complete symptom relief achieved in 66% of patients over a mean follow-up of 19 months. It was suggested that the nonresponse group had more aggressive disease. Other authors performed hydrostatic balloon dilation with inflation diameters from 12 mm to 18 mm [51]. Immediate symptomatic relief was noted in 77% of patients, with persistent long-term relief in 44% after a mean follow-up of 25 months. Longer strictures and active inflammation were characteristics that portended poor response. The same authors, in a follow-up study of a larger number of patients undergoing hydrostatic balloon dilation for symptomatic ileocolonic stricture in Crohn's disease resistant to medical treatment and followed up over a 5-year period, suggested that dilation can be successful in the setting of inflammation [52]. Technical success was achieved in 90% of procedures, with best results in ileocolic anastomoses. Overall relief of symptoms was achieved in 62% of patients after mean follow-up of 33.6 months, with 8% of complications and no deaths for a total of 76 dilations. Lack of success was noted in strictures with tight angulation and longer lenght.

Based on the success of using intralesional corticosteroids in caustic lesions, dilation followed by intralesional steroid injection was performed in Crohn's strictures [53]. Following hydrostatic dilation, approximately 5 mg betamethasone dipropionate diluted into 5–10 ml of normal saline as 0.5- to 1-ml aliquots was injected into the most narrowed area using a standard sclerotherapy needle. Immediate symptom relief was always achieved without complications, and 84% of patients achieved a prolonged symptom-free period during a follow-up of 6 years after combination dilation/injection without need for surgery. Use and control of a precut papillotome for luminal incision, followed by injection of triamcinolone, is more difficult than hydrostatic balloon dilation and limited to short strictures although success rate is high [54]. Another study evaluated efficacy and safety of endoscopic balloon dilation with or without intralesional steroid injection for symptomatic upper and lower gastrointestinal Crohn's disease strictures [55]. Using a mean follow-up of 18.8 months, technical success was achieved in 96.5% of 17 patients. Recurrence rate in the steroid group was 10% and that in the nonsteroid group 31%. Overall, long-term success was achieved in 76.5% of patients, with a complication rate of 10% with no mortality.

Experience with self-expanding metal stents in Crohn's disease has been very limited [56], with complete relief of obstructive symptoms after placement despite stent migration some months after insertion. Similarly, minimal data exist on endoscopic treatment of gastroduodenal strictures in Crohn's disease. In one study, a 20-mm balloon was utilised, and symptomatic relief was achieved in every patient, with all responding to repeat dilation [57].

Fistulae Management

Currently, there are no data supporting the role of endoscopy as primary treatment of fistulising Crohn's disease. Nevertheless, aside from guiding medical and surgical therapy of a fistula, endoscopy may indirectly and directly impact the treatment of fistulising Crohn's disease [58]. Indirectly, endoscopy may allow for dilation of obstructing strictures that prevent the closure of the fistula. Directly, may treat the fistula via an injection of fibrin-based sealants or anticytokine therapy. A fistula located proximal to an obstructive stricture does not heal due to an increase in luminal pressure. Endoscopic balloon dilation of the stricture would reduce intraluminal pressure and the amount of bowel contents passing through the fistula, and allow for a better chance of closure. For endoscopic dilation to be successful, the stricture must be accessible, short (<8 cm) and not significantly inflamed, conditions that are often not the present in fistulising Crohn's disease. Nevertheless, in a patient with a symptomatic fistula that is proximal to a short, noninflammatory stricture, endoscopic balloon dilation offers an alternative to surgery.

There are case reports of injecting fibrin tissue sealant into a perineal fistula of patients with IBD [59]. Results of an external fistula closure with fibrin sealants are disappointing. Recently, there have been several reports on the endoscopic treatment of a gastrointestinal fistula with various tissue sealants as fibrin-based, collagen or amino-acid solutions [60, 61]. However, these reports were not related to IBD but to fistulas secondary to other diseases, and endoscopically administered tissue sealants are unlikely to play a role in the treatment of Crohn's disease fistulas [62]. To date there are no studies that have evaluated the role of endoscopically administered biologic therapy for treatment of Crohn's fistula, and there is only one published abstract that has evaluated local injection of infliximab into a perianal fistula. As new therapies becomes available, there will be a greater need for therapy administered directly to the mucosa, and therapeutic endoscopy may play a role in the treatment of fistulising Crohn's disease. One study was performed using EUS to assess and guide combination medical and surgical therapy for patients with Crohn's perianal fistulas [63]. The presence of fistula healing on EUS was used to guide seton removal and discontinuation of infliximab or antibiotics, demonstrating that EUS may identify a subset of patients who can discontinue infliximab without recurrence of fistula drainage.

Although there are no reports of stricture dilation in Crohn's disease patients with ileal or colonic stomas, the same principles as with ileocolonic or colonic strictures apply [51]. Endoscopic management of these strictures may be more desirable in many of these patients who have already undergone multiple bowel resections. Radiologic contrast imaging and endoscopy will provide information on whether the stricture is amenable to hydrostatic balloon dilation. The procedure may be repeated with progressively larger-diameter balloons until a satisfactory result is obtained, such as being able to pass a standard colonoscope through the stricture. Contraindications to dilation include coagulopathy and strictures associated with large and deep ulcerations.

Capsule Endoscopy in Crohn's Disease

Video capsule endoscopy (VCE) is a new, noninvasive imaging technique for the complete small bowel. The video capsule is a small device with a diameter of 11 mm and a length of 26 mm, which can be swallowed. It contains six light-emitting diodes, a lens, a colour camera chip and two batteries. The video capsule obtains two images per second. Video images are transmitted by means of radiotelemetry to the sensor array attached to the body with a belt. Images from a period of time as long as 8 h are stored in a portable recorder.

There are no standard preparations before the examination: certain operators prescribe only a liquid diet after lunch on the day preceding the capsule endoscopy and a fast for 8 h before the procedure.

Others recommend more complex preparation with various combinations of laxatives [sennoside, polyethylene glycol (PEG) solution]. After swallowing the capsule endoscope with 100–200 ml of water containing 100 mg of simethicone, the patient could drink 2 h later and eat 4 h later. In patients who have undergone gastric surgery or those with gastroparesis, the video capsule could be inserted endoscopically in the small intestine. Stomach passage takes an average of 34 min, and passes through the small intestine in about 4 h. Complete visualisation of the small bowel up to the caecum is achieved in 80% of patients. Most operators recommend a plain abdominal X-ray be performed 7–14 days after the examination if the capsule examination does not show images of the colon and the patient does not see the capsule passage in the stool. The capsule is designed to be used once, and after it is passed with the stool, it is not reusable [64]. On completion of the examination, the recorded images are downloaded and converted into a movie by connecting the recorder to a workstation. Data are reviewed by an operator in about 1 h with dedicated software.

The main contraindication is the presence of small-bowel stenosis that may lead to capsule retention and obstruction (see below). Other contraindications are a patient with difficulty swallowing, pregnancy or the presence of implanted medical devices such pacemakers. Capsule endoscopy is very useful in the management of patients with suspected small-bowel disease.

The diagnosis of Crohn's disease is difficult. Current radiologic and endoscopic studies are limited in the diagnosis of early small-bowel mucosal disease in patients with this disease. VCE detects early lesions in the small bowel of patients with Crohn's disease and is effective in diagnosing patients with suspected Crohn's disease undetected by small-bowel series and enteroclysis [65, 66] and in some cases of Crohn's disease with intestinal strictures missed by enteroclysis. Enteroclysis in patients with Crohn's disease has a diagnostic yield of 37% while capsule endoscopy has a yield of 70%. This is not surprising since enteroclysis will not easily detect flat or mucosal abnormalities [67]. VCE is also superior to CT enteroclysis [5] in patients with known or suspected Crohn's disease, especially in the detection of significantly more inflammatory lesions in the proximal and middle part of the small bowel. VCE probably is less effective than radiology at detecting fistulae, and this might be a reason for sometimes choosing radiological investigations in preference to VCE [68].

There is concern that a capsule might become stuck or impacted against a stricture. In fact, capsule impaction does occur approximately in the 2–5 % of cases. Most capsule impactions are asymptomatic and rarely produce obstructive symptoms. A "patency" capsule has been developed to detect possible strictures noninvasively and more accurately than enteroclysis. This device has the same dimensions as the VCE but has a dissolving body. Use of the patency capsule may be of value to rule out the possibility of intestinal strictures in patients with Crohn's disease and suspected small-bowel obstruction although the patency capsule can also cause transient obstruction.

The major difficulty of VCE is the definition of a gold standard for diagnosis. Crohn's disease produces mucosal inflammation and ulceration of various intensities in different bowel areas. The earliest lesion in Crohn's disease displays tiny mucosal foci of chronic inflammation and, more recently, a focal loss of villi [69]. Another early lesion is aphthoid ulceration. The finding of one or two aphthous ulcers or erosion in patients during capsule endoscopy is common, and it is likely that many of these do not have Crohn's disease [70].

It must be remembered that all ulceration is not indicative of Crohn's disease. Clinically relevant points to keep in mind are the difficulty in differentiating ulcers of Crohn's disease from those of NSAID use and the high prevalence of NSAID-induced ulcers in 71% of NSAID users [71]. Hence, it is critical to evaluate the history of NSAID use in every patient undergoing VCE. In the absence of NSAID use, diagnosis of Crohn's disease was purposed by certain authors on the presence of multiple aphthous or erosive lesions (>10) that were either continuous or segmentally distributed [72]. Infections must be excluded by duodenal biopsy, stool microbiology or serology.

It is known from older studies that the small bowel is affected in Crohn's disease in about one third of cases [73, 74]. Newer studies based on VCE show that the small bowel could be involved in approximately 60% of patients with Crohn's disease. This might be kept in mind in case of lack of response in patients treated with drugs released into the terminal ileum or colon [66, 68].

Diagnostic costs for Crohn's disease can be very high. This is probably due to the low diagnostic yield of certain diagnostic procedures. VCE has a higher average diagnostic yield than comparative procedures due to imaging clarity and the ability to visualise the entire small bowel [75–77]. Literature review found the average diagnostic yield of small-bowel follow-through (SBFT) and colonoscopy of Crohn's disease to be 53% whereas VCE had a diagnostic yield of 69%. Recent economic analysis comparing VCE with traditional diagnostic procedures demonstrates that employing VCE as a first-line diagnostic procedure appears to be less costly than current common procedures for diagnosing suspected Crohn's disease in the small bowel [77].

Risk of Cancer and Endoscopic Surveillance

The first description of a cancer of the colon complicating "regional enteritis" was described in 1948 [79]. After this, published works abounded with reports of colorectal cancer in series of patients with Crohn's disease [80]. In a recent population-based study [81], Bernstein et al. determined the incidence of cancer by linking records from the IBD and non-IBD cohort with the Comprehensive Cancer Care Manitoba Registry. IBD patients were matched 1:10 to randomly selected members of the population without IBD based on year, age gender and postal area of residence. There was an increased risk of colon carcinoma for both Crohn's disease patients [2.64: 95% confidence interval (95% CI), 1.69–4.12) and UC patients (2.75; 95% CI, 1.91–3.97]. There was an increased IRR of rectal carcinoma only among patients with UC (1.90; 95% CI, 1.05–3.43) and an increased IRR of carcinoma of the small intestine only in Crohn's disease patients (17.4; 95% CI, 4.16–72.9). An increased IRR of extraintestinal tumours was observed only for the liver and biliary tract in both Crohn's disease patients (5.22; 95% CI, 1.05–14.9) and UC patients (3,96; 95% CI, 1.05–14.9). Gillen et al. [82] concluded that when cases of ulcerative and Crohn's colitis of similar anatomic extent are followed for similar durations, the two diseases may ultimately prove to have similar increases in risk for colorectal cancer [83]. In fact, they compared the cancer risk in two hospital-referred but identically selected cohorts of patients with extensive UC and equally extensive Crohn's disease of the colon. As in the classic 1973 paper by Weedon et al. [84], the overall risk of colorectal cancer was increased nearly 20-fold over the general population. Moreover, both relative risks and absolute 20-year cumulative incidences of cancer were virtually identical in the ulcerative and Crohn's colitis cohorts. This study, therefore, conclusively establishes the previously reported [85–87] but still underappreciated similarity between cancer risks in these two diseases.

Friedman et al. [88] in 2001 concluded that colonoscopy surveillance should be strongly considered in chronic extensive Crohn's colitis. In fact, they reported on 259 patients with chronic Crohn's colitis who underwent screening and subsequent surveillance colonoscopy and biopsy since 1980. Biopsies were performed at 10-cm intervals and from strictures and polypoid masses. A total of 663 examinations were performed on 259 patients. Median interval between examinations was 24 months. The screening and surveillance programme detected dysplasia or cancer in 16%. A finding of definite dysplasia or cancer was associated with age >45 years and increased symptoms. By life table analysis, the probability of detecting dysplasia or cancer after a negative screening colonoscopy was 22% by the fourth surveillance examination. It is interesting from a clinical point of view that the pediatric colonoscope helped increase the yield of neoplasia by 19%. Despite this report, Mpofu et al. [89] concluded a review indicating that there is no clear evidence that surveillance colonoscopy prolongs survival in patients with IBD with extensive colitis.

There is evidence that cancers tend to be detected at an earlier stage in patients who are undergoing surveillance, and these patients have a correspondingly better prognosis but lead-time bias could contribute substantially to this apparent benefit. There is indirect evidence that surveillance is likely to be effective at reducing the risk of death from IBD-associated colorectal cancer and indirect evidence that it is acceptably cost effective. Therefore, the follow-up of colonic Crohn's disease must be similar to the follow-up of ulcerative colitis. Itzkowitz et al. suggested [90], awaiting more data about Crohn's and colorectal cancer, that it seems prudent to follow a UC-based surveillance strategy for patients with at least 8 years of Crohn's colitis involving at least one third of the colon. The suggested surveillance strategy is reported in Fig. 1 with the performance reported in Table 2 indicated by these authors. Information on family history of colorectal cancer may be a simple way to identify individuals with extensive colonic Crohn's disease at more and more elevated risk of developing colorectal cancer [91], especially with a first-degree diagnosed with colorectal cancer before 50 years of age.

Cases of colorectal cancer in Crohn's disease are in reality few, less than in UC, because many patients with extensive Crohn's colitis have early surgical resection, eliminating the risk of cancer [82]. An increased number of small intestinal carcinoma in patients affected by Crohn's disease has been reported although the strength of this association (age, length of disease, characteristics and distribution) still has to be elucidated. Relative risk is estimated between six and 50 times by different authors, but small intestinal cancer is very rare, and this relative risk does not justify endoscopic surveillance. Longstanding disease, previous intestinal exclusion surgery and enterocutaneous or other types of fistulae should probably be considered for the development of cancer [92] for eventual clinical suspicion but not for scheduled endoscopic surveillance. Small intestinal cancer in Crohn's disease usually arises in distal ileum [93], and therefore it seems reasonable to attempt to extend surveillance colonoscopy to this

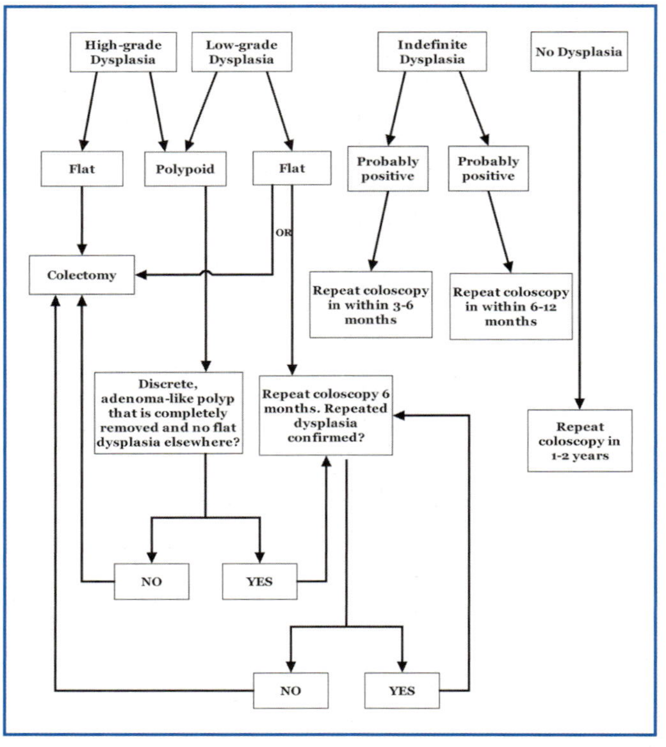

Fig. 1. Suggested surveillance strategy. See "Recommended Surveillance Strategy" section in text for explanation

Table 2. Suggested performance of surveillance colonoscopy

- Obtain four biopsy specimens of flat mucosa every 10 cm (consider sampling every 5 cm in the rectosigmoid)
- Place each quadruplicate set in a separate specimen jar (as opposed to pooling biopsy specimens from several colonic segments)
- Sample suspicious lesions or polyps
- Make sure to biopsy flat mucosa around the base of any suspicious polyp and submit specimen in a separate container
- Consider suppressing symptoms of active inflammation with medical therapy prior to surveillance colonoscopy
- In Crohn's colitis, strictures may require using a thinner calibre colonoscope
- Consider brush cytology or barium enema to evaluate impassible strictures

bowel tract, dilating and biopsying stenosis, if possible.

References

1. Scholmerich J (2003) Inflammatory bowel disease. Endoscopy 35:164–170
2. Morson BC (1972) The early histological lesion of Crohn's disease. Proc R Soc Med 65:71– 72
3. Watier A, Devroede G, Perey B et al (1980) Small erythematous mucosal plaques: an endoscopic sign of Crohn's disease. Gut 21:835–839
4. Meuwissen SGM, Pape KSSB, Agenant D (1976) Crohn's disease of the colon: analysis of the diagnostic value of radiology, endoscopy and hystology. Am J Dig Dis 21:81–88
5. Waye JD (1977) The role of colonoscopy in the differential diagnosis of inflammatory bowel disease. Gastrointest Endosc 23:150–154
6. Blackstone MO (1984) Inflammatory bowel disease. In: Blackstone MO (ed) Endoscopic Interpretation. Raven Press, pp 464–494
7. Mekhjian HS, Switz DM, Melnyk CS et al (1979) Clinical features and natural history of Crohn's disease. Gastroenterology 77:898–906
8. Sands BE (2002) Crohn's disease. In: Feldman, M, Friedman LS, Sleisenger, MH (eds) Sleisenger and Fordtran's gastrointestinal and liver disease. Saunders, Los Angeles, pp 2011–2044
9. Marshall JK, Hewak J, Farrow R et al (1988) Terminal ileal imaging with ileoscopy versus small-bowel meal with pneumocolon. J Clin Gastroenterol 27:217–222
10. Waye JD (1990) Endoscopy in inflammatory bowel disease: indications and differential diagnosis. Med Clin North Am 74:51–65
11. Landi B, Anh TN, Cortot A et al (1992) Endoscopic

monitoring of Crohn's disease treatment: a prospective, randomized clinical trial. Gastroenterology 102:1647–1653

12. Farmer RG, Hawk WA, Turnbull RB (1975) Clinical patterns in Crohn's disease: a statistical study of 615 cases. Gastroenterology 68:627–635
13. Hogan WJ, Hensley GT, Geenen JE (1980) Endoscopic evaluation of inflammatory bowel disease. Med Clin North Am 64:1083–1102
14. Pera A, Bellando P, Caldera D et al (1987) Colonoscopy in inflammatory bowel disease. Diagnostic accuracy and proposal of an endoscopic score. Gastroenterology 92:181–185
15. Modigliani R, Mary J, Simon J et al (1990) Clinical, biological, and endoscopic picture of attacks of Crohn's disease: evolution on prednisone. Gastroenterology 98:811–818
16. Waye J (1978) Colitis, cancer and colonoscopy. Med Clin North Am 62:211–224
17. Forde K, Gold RP, Holck S et al (1978) Giant pseudopolyposis with colonic intussusception. Gastroenterology 75:1142
18. Hunt R, Teague R, Swarbrick E et al (1975) Colonoscopy in the management of colonic strictures. BMJ 2:360
19. D'Haens G, Rutgeerts P (1996) Endoscopic evaluation. In: Prantera C, Korelitz BI (eds) Crohn's disease. Marcel Dekker, New York, pp 117–127
20. Allez M, Lemann M, Bonnet J et al (2002) Am J Gastroenterol 97:947–953
21. Whitehead R (1989) Ulcerative colitis. In: Whitehead R (ed) Gastrointestinal and oesophageal pathology. Churchill Livingstone, Edinburgh, p 522
22. Riegler G, Arimoli A, Esposito P et al (1997) Clinical evolution in an outpatients series with indeterminate colitis. Dis Colon Rectum 40:437–439
23. Yardley JH, Hendrix TR (1997) Gastroduodenal Crohn's disease: the focus is on focality. Gastroenterology 112:1031–1033
24. Levine MS (1987) Crohn's disease of the upper gastrointestinal tract. Radiol Clin North Am 25:79–91
25. Dijkstra J, Reeders JWAJ, Tytgat GNJ (1995) Idiopathic inflammatory bowel disease: endoscopic-radiologic correlation. Radiology 197:369–375
26. Tribl B, Turetschek K, Mostbeck et al (1998) Conflicting results of ileoscopy and small bowel double-contrast barium examination in patients with Crohn's disease. Endoscopy 30:339–344
27. Keuchel M, Hagenmuller F (2005) Small bowel endoscopy. Endoscopy 37:122–132
28. Chong AK, Taylor A, Miller A et al (2005) Capsule endoscopy vs. push enteroscopy and enteroclysis in suspected small-bowel Crohn's disease. Gastrointest Endosc 61:262–263
29. Esaki M, Matsumoto T, Hizawa K et al (2001) Intraoperative enteroscopy detects more lesions but is not predictive of postoperative recurrence in Crohn's disease. Surg Endosc 15:455–459
30. May A, Nachbar L, Wardak A et al (2003) Double-balloon enteroscopy: preliminary experience in patients with obscure gastrointestinal bleeding or chronic abdominal pain. Endoscopy 35:985–991
31. Yamamoto H, Kita H (2005) Double-balloon endoscopy. Curr Opin Gastroenterol 21:573–557
32. Mihas AA, Murad TM, Hirshowitz BI (1978) Sclerosing cholangitis associated with ulcerative colitis. Am J Gastroenterol 70:614–619
33. Gast P, Belaiche J (1999) Rectal endosonography in inflammatory bowel disease: differential diagnosis and prediction of remission. Endoscopy 31:158–167
34. Sowed AM, Chak JA, Katz JA, Sivak MV (1999) Catheter probe-assisted endoluminal US in inflammatory bowel disease. Gastrointest Endosc 50:41–46
35. Schratter-Sehn AU, Lochs H, Vogelsang H et al (1993) Endoscopic ultrasonography versus computed tomography in the differential diagnosis of perianorectal complications in Crohn's disease. Endoscopy 25:582–586
36. Tio TL, Mulder CJ, Wijers OB et al (1990) Endosonography of peri-anal and peri-colorectal fistula and/or abscess in Crohn's disease. Gastrointest Endosc 36:331–336
37. Schwartz DA, Wiersema MJ, Dudiak KM et al (2001) A comparison of endoscopic ultrasound, magnetic resonance imaging, and exam under anesthesia for evaluation of Crohn's perianal fistulas. Gastroenterology 121:1064–1072
38. Chang K, Chaurasia O, Albers C et al (1994) Endoscopic ultrasound guided fine needle aspiration in the evaluation of extrinsic lesions adjacent to the lower gastrointestinal tract. Gastrointest Endosc 40:61
39. Van Asshe G, Geboes K, Rutgeerts P (2004) Medical therapy for Crohn's disease strictures. Inflamm Bowel Dis 10:55–60
40. Legnani PE, Kornbluth A (2002) Therapeutic options in the management of strictures in Crohn's disease. Gastrointest Endoscopy Clin N Am 12:589–603
41. Goldberg HI, Caruthers SB, Nelson JA (1979) Radiographic findings of the National Cooperative Crohn's Disease Study. Gastroenterology 77:925–937
42. Farmer RG, Hawke WA, Turnbull RB (1976) Indication for surgery in Crohn's disease. Analysis of 500 cases. Gastroenterology 71:245–250
43. Waye JD (1980) Endoscopy in inflammatory bowel disease. Clin Gastroenterol 9:279–296
44. Greestein AJ, Sachar DB, Kark AE (1994) Strictures of the anorectum in Crohn's disease: resection or stricturoplasty. Semin Colon Rectal Surg 5:193–198
45. Morini S, Hassan C, Cerro P et al (2001) Management of an ileocolic anastomotic stricture using polyvinyl over-the-guidewire dilators in Crohn's disease. Gastrointest Endosc 53:584–586
46. Brower RA (1986) Hydrostatic balloon dilation of a terminal ileal stricture secondary to Crohn's disease. Gastrointest Endosc 32:38–40
47. Williams AJK, Palmer KL (1991) Endoscopic balloon dilation as a therapeutic option in the management of intestinal strictures resulting from Crohn's disease. Br J Surg 78:453–454
48. Dieruf L, Prakash C. (2001) Endoscopic incision of a postoperative colonic stricture. Gastrointest Endosc 54:522–524
49. Blomberg B, Rolny P, Jarnerot G (1991) Endoscopic treatment of Anastomotic strictures in Crohn's disease. Endoscopy 23:195–198
50. Blomberg B (1991) Endoscopic treatment of anastomotic strictures in Crohn's disease. Endoscopy 23(4):195-198

51. Breysem Y, Yanssens JF, Coremans G et al (1992) Endoscopic balloon dilation of colonic and ileo-colonic Crohn's strictures: long-term results. Gastrointest Endosc 38:142–147
52. Couckuyt H, Gevers AM, Coremans G et al (1995) Efficacy and safety of hydrostatic balloon dilation of ileo-colonic Crohn's strictures: a prospective long-term analysis. Gut 36:577–580
53. Ramboer C, Verhamme M, Dhondt E et al (1995) Endoscopic treatment of stenosis in recurrent Crohn's disease with balloon dilation combined with local corticosteroids injection. Gastrointest Endosc 2:252–255
54. Lavy A. (1997) Triamcinolone improves outcome in Crohn's disease strictures. Dis Colon Rectum 40:184–186
55. Singh VV, Draganov P, Valentie J. (2005) Efficacy and safety of endoscopic balloon dilatino of symptomatic upper and lower gastrointestinal Crohn's disease strictures. J Clin Gastroenterol 39:284–290
56. Matsuhashi N, Nakajima A, Suzuki A et al (2000) Long term outcome of non surgical stricturoplasty for intestinal strictures in Crohn's disease. Gastrointest Endosc 51:343–345
57. Matsui T, Hatakemaya S, Ikeda K et al (1997) Long-term outcome of endoscopic balloon dilation in obstructive gastroduodenal Crohn's disease. Endoscopy 29:640–645
58. Blomberg B (1992) Endoscopic treatment modalities in inflammatory bowel disease. Endoscopy 24:578–581
59. Ambrose NS, Alexander-Williams J (1988) Appraisal of a tissue glue in the treatment of persistent perineal sinus. Br J Surg 75:484–485
60. Jung M, Raute M, Menegold BC (1986) Endoscopic therapy of fistulae with fibrin sealant. Fb Seal Op Med 173–178
61. Lange V, Meyer C, Wenk F, Schildberg FW (1989) Fistuloscopy – a further approach to the sealing of gastrointestinal fistulae. In: Waclawizek HW (ed) Progress in fibrin sealing. Springer Verlag, Berlin, Heidelberg, New York pp 453–464
62. – (2002) Fistulas. Gastrointest Endoscopy Clin N Am, P 12
63. Schwartz DA, White CM, Wise PE, Herline AJ (2005) Use of endoscopic ultrasound to guide combination medical and surgical therapy for patients with Crohn's perianal fistulas. Inflamm Bowel Dis 11(8):727–732
64. Van Tuyl SAC, Kuipers EJ, Timmer R, Stolk MFJ (2004) Video capsule endoscopy: procedure, indications and diagnostic yield. Neth J Med 62:225–228
65. Liangpunsakul S, Chadalawada V, Rex DK et al (2003) Wireless capsule endoscopy detects small bowel ulcers in patients with normal results from state of the art enteroclysis. Am J Gastroenterol 98:1295–1298
66. Chong AK, Taylor A, Miller A et al (2005) Capsule endoscopy vs. push enteroscopy and enteroclysis in suspected small-bowel Crohn's disease. Gastrointest Endosc 61:255–261
67. Costamagna G, Shah SK, Riccioni ME et al (2002) A prospective trial comparing small bowel radiographs and video capsule endoscopy for suspected small bowel disease. Gastroenterology 123:999–1005
68. Voderholzer WA, Beinhoelzl J, Rogalla P et al (2005) Small bowel involvement in Crohn's disease: a prospective comparison of wireless capsule endoscopy and computed tomography enteroclysis. Gut 54:369–373
69. Swain P. (2005) Wireless capsule endoscopy and Crohn's disease. Gut 54:323–326
70. Mitty R, Cave DR (2002) Focal villous denudation: a precursor to aphthoid ulcers in Crohn's disease as detected by video capsule endoscopy. Gastroenterology 122:A217
71. Dubcenco E, Jeejeebhoy KN, Petroniene R et al (2005) Capsule endoscopy findings in patients with established and suspected small-bowel Crohn's disease: correlation with radiologic, endoscopic, and histologic findings. Gastrointest Endosc 62:538–544
72. Graham DY, Opekun AR, Willingham FF (2005) Visible small-intestinal mucosal injury in chronic NSAID users. Clin Gastroenterol Hepatol 3:55–59
73. Mekhjian HS, Switz DM, Melnyk CS et al (1979) Clinical features and natural history of Crohn's disease. Gastroenterology 77:898–906
74. Steinhardt HJ, Loeschke K, Kasper H et al (1985) European Cooperative Crohn's Disease Study (ECCDS): clinical features and natural history. Digestion 31:97–108
75. Kornbluth A, Colombel JF, Leighton JA, Loftu E and ICCE (2005) Consensus for Inflammatory Bowel Disease. Endoscopy 37:1051–1054
76. Raju GS, Samir Kumar (2005) Nath Capsule Endoscopy. Curr Gastroenterol Rep 7:358–364
77. Cave D (2005) Capsule Endoscopy and Crohn's disease. Gastrointest Endosc 61(2):262–263
78. Goldfarb NI, Pizzi LT, Fuhr JP Jr et al (2004) Diagnosing Crohn's disease: an economic analysis comparing wireless capsule endoscopy with traditional diagnostic procedures. Dis Manag 7(4):292–304
79. Warren S, Sommers SC (1948) Cicatrizing enteritis (regional enteritis) as a pathologic entity: analysis of one hundred and twenty cases. Am F Pathol 24:475–501
80. Gyde SN, Prior P et al (1980) Malignancy in Crohn's, Macartneyt JC disease. Gut 21:1024–1029
81. Bernstein CN, Blanchard JF, Kliewer E, Wajda A (2001) Cancer risk in patients with inflammatory bowel disease: a population-based study. Cancer 91:854-862
82. Gillen CD, Prior P, Andrews HA, Allan RN (1994) Ulcerative colitis and Crohn's disease: a comparison of the colorectal cancer risk in extensive colitis. Gut 35:1590–1592
83. Sachar DB (1983) New concepts of cancer. Mt Sinai F Med 50:133–7
84. Weedon DD, Shorter RG, Ilstrup DM et al (1973) Crohn's disease and cancer. N Engl J Med 289:1099–1102
85. Greestein AJ, Sachar DB, Smith H et al (1981) A comparison of cancer risk in Crohn's disease and ulcerative colitis. Cancer 48:2742–2745
86. Softley A, Clamp SE, Watkinson G et al (1988) The natural history of inflammatory bowel disease: has there been a change in the last 20 years? Scand F Gastroenterol 23(Suppl 144):20–24
87. Ekbom A, Helmick C, Zack M, Adami H-O (1990) Increased risk of large-bowel cancer in Crohn's disease with colonic involvement. Lancet 336:357–359
88. Friedman S, Rubin PH, Bodian C et al (2001) Screening and surveillance colono scopy in chronic Crohn's colitis. Gastroenterology 120(4):820-826
89. Mpofu C, Watson AJ, Rhoders JM (2004) Strategies for

detecting colon cancer and/or dysplasia in patients with inflammatory bowel disease. Cochrane Database Syst Rev (2):CD000279
90. Itzkowitz SH, Harpaz N (2004) Diagnosis and management of dysplasia in patients with inflammatory bowel diseases. Gastroenterology 126:1634- 1648
91. Askling J, Dickman PW, Kaklen P et al (2001) Family history as a risk factor for colorectal cancer in inflammatory bowel disease. Gastroenterology 120:1356–1362
92. Prati M, Quadri F, Botti F et al (2002) Intestinal carcinoma in Crohn's disease. Report of four cases and review of the literature. Minerva Chir 57(1):29–33
93. Senay E, David B, Sachar B et al (1989) Small bowel carcinoma in Crohn's disease. Cancer 63:360–363

Role of Endoscopy in Ulcerative Colitis

Giampaolo Angelini, Laura Bernardoni

Introduction

The need to formulate a correct diagnosis of ulcerative colitis (UC), based also on histopathological findings, for differential diagnosis from Crohn's disease (CD) and to establish site and extension of the disease are indications for colonoscopy in UC patients. In patients with certain diagnosis, colonoscopy is the gold standard to identify preneoplastic lesions (dysplasia) during surveillance for colorectal cancer (CRC), which is more common in patients with UC than in the general population (Table 1).

Table 1. Colonoscopy role in management of ulcerative colitis (UC)

Diagnostic validation
Extension of UC
Conventional medical therapy failure
Complication onset (stenosis, dysplasia, cancer)

Diagnosis

A colonoscopy with visualisation of the entire colon and terminal ileum allows a correct differential diagnosis from CD in 85–90% of patients, but in 10–15% of patients, only a diagnosis of indeterminate colitis can be established [1]. In severe disease, endoscopic examination must be limited (proctosigmoidoscopy), with careful insufflation, due to high risk of perforation and toxic megacolon.

Active Disease

Endoscopic lesions change with inflammation degree. In mild disease, the mucosa is hyperaemic, with abnormal vascular pattern; in moderate disease, vascular pattern vanishes and the mucosa is friable, easily bleeding at instrument touch, with superficial ulcerations. Severe disease is characterised by spontaneously bleeding deep ulcerations, with mucopurulent exudate. Characteristically in UC, the rectum is involved at all times and, differently from CD, lesions are extended continuously from rectum to proximal colon. Therefore, inflammation can involve the sigma and rectum (proctosigmoiditis), extend to the splenic curve (left-side colitis) or affect the entire colon (extensive colitis). Before colonoscopy the patient's pharmacological history should be obtained because the use of medical enemas can normalise the rectal mucosae and induce erroneous CD diagnosis.

Ileal lesions are characteristic of CD and represent major macroscopic criteria to differentiate UC from CD. In 17% of patients with pancolitis, severe inflammation can induce incompetence of the ileocecal valve and consequent faecal reflux, causing inflammation (backwash ileitis). Generally, extension and severity of colitis are correlated to severity of ileum inflammation, even if 2% of backwash ileitis is associated to severe left-side colitis or mild extensive colitis. It seems that other pathogenetic factors are implicated to backwash ileitis (infections, bacterial overgrowth, reaction to drugs, etc.). Backwash ileitis does not seem to correlate with increased CRC development risk nor to higher incidence of complication after proctocolectomy with an ileal pouch [2].

In course of the first colonoscopy biopsies for histopathological definition of colitis type are necessary; in any cases, only biopsies can distinguish idiopathic colitis from infectious colitis. Biopsies must be taken from inflamed mucosae, healthy mucosae and ileum since real UC extension and existence of microscopic inflammation must be evaluated because therapy and prognosis can change accordingly. A new approach to microscopic inflammation is confocal endoscopy (see below), which allows targeted biopsies.

Silent Disease

During silent disease (remission phase), haustrae are reduced and the colon is tube like; characteristic lesions are pale and sometimes granulose mucosae (atrophy) is apparent and there is a loss of vascular pattern and presence of pseudopolyps. The so-called inflammatory polyps are present in acute and quiescent disease and are composed of regenerating mucosae and inflammatory cells without dysplastic epithelium. Therefore, they do not degenerate to CRC. The use of A video capsule is very limited in UC. It can play a marginal role in indeterminate colitis, showing unknown lesions in the small intestine that can contribute to a diagnosis of CD [3].

Disease Activity

In clinical practice, Truelove-Witts index is used to establish disease activity, but many endoscopic scores are used to measure UC activity [for example, St. Mark's index, UC disease activity index (UCDAI), Mayo score), but endoscopy gives little additional information to clinical indexes of disease activity in UC. In clinical practice, it seems appropriate to treat these patients on the basis of symptoms [4, 5].

Follow-Up of US

After correct diagnosis and obtaining remission maintained by correct medical therapy, a second colonoscopy within 8 years from the beginning of the symptoms, is indicated only in case of relapse not responsive to therapy [6–9]. Refractory disease can be caused by viral infection (most commonly by cytomegalovirus), primarily in patients on immunosuppressant maintenance therapy. In this case, the endoscopist has a front-line role taking biopsies from the bottom of the ulcers, where CMV implant, during proctosigmoidoscopy.

After 8 Years from the Beginning

The main role of colonoscopy during follow-up of UC is screening and surveillance for CRC. The lifetime prevalence of CRC in patients with UC is estimated to be 3.7% and 5.4% among those with total colitis. Rates are higher in patients with longstanding disease, and the cumulative probabilities at 10, 20 and 30 years increase to 2%, 8% and 18%, respectively. Compared with age-matched members of the general population, the relative risk of cancer is 20% for extensive colitis and 4% for left-side colitis [10]. The main risk factors for CRC in patients with UC are reported in Table 2.

Table 2. Risk factors for colorectal cancer (CRC) in ulcerative colitis (UC) patients [11].

Disease standing
Anatomic extension
Positive family history for CRC
Age at onset of UC
Severe or chronic inflammation
Primary sclerosing cholangitis

Before 8 Years from the Beginning

Disease Standing

Disease standing is an independent risk factor for CRC development in patients suffering from UC. There is no standard definition for the duration of UC. Although some studies define duration based on the date of radiological, endoscopic or histological diagnosis, a preferred approach is to define it in relationship to the onset of UC-like symptoms. Since the risk of CRC becomes greater than in general population after 8–10 years from disease onset [12], the Crohn's and Colitis Foundation of America (workshop: "Colon cancer in IBD: science and surveillance", Palm Harbor, Florida, March 2000recommends that a screening colonoscopy be performed 8–10 years after onset of symptoms attributable to UC to redefine extension and cutoff dysplasia. Then, a regular surveillance program should be carried out.

Anatomic Extension

As disease standing it is an independent risk factor for CRC, extension should be defined by both endoscopic and histological evaluation, whichever reveals more extensive involvement, not with radiological images since cancer and dysplasia can arise in areas of the colon that show histological evidence of disease even without macroscopic abnormalities [13].

Primary Sclerosing Cholangitis

All patients with primary sclerosing cholangitis (PSC) without prior diagnoses of irritable bowel disease (IBD) should undergo a colonoscopy to determine their status. This procedure should include biopsies from normal-appearing mucosae because microscopic evidence of colitis may not be visually apparent. For patients suffering from IBD, screening and subsequent yearly surveillance should begin at the time of PSC onset.

Age of Onset

Although there is some evidence to support a higher relative risk for CRC among UC patients diagnosed at a young age [12], there is insufficient evidence to support starting screening and surveillance before 8 years of disease onset.

Positive Family History of CRC

This is an additional risk factor for development of CRC in patient with UC [14], but there is insufficient evidence to warrant a closer follow-up.

In a recent study, Rutter et al. [15] demonstrated that some endoscopic lesions were correlated to higher risk of CRC development and, on the contrary, that normal endoscopy testified a low risk of neoplasia. Mainly, pseudopolyps were correlated to higher risk of CRC development not because of direct degeneration but because they are an expression of severe and constant inflammation. Some drugs may modify risk of development of CRC; aminosalicylate use, perhaps folic acid intake and ursodeoxycholic acid in the subset of colitis patients with PSC have been suggested to be cancer chemopreventive agents [16, 17]. A screening colonoscopy must be done to rule out dysplasia or cancer after 8–10 years from the onset of the disease. The accuracy of intestinal washout is very important because, in these patients, minimal lesions can be in situ carcinoma.

The cornerstone of endoscopic surveillance in UC is dysplasia, which is defined as unequivocal neoplastic alteration of the colonic epithelium. Dysplasia represents the histological manifestation of widespread chromosomal instability caused by the effects of persistent inflammation. Most cancers in colitis are preceded by dysplasia, and approximately 75% of cases have coexisting dysplastic change elsewhere in the colon. The detection of dysplasia in colitis is used as a clinical marker of imminent or established carcinoma. During examination, multiple biopsies must be taken, even on normal mucosae, to assess extension increase of UC [18].

After screening, patients with UC must begin a regular surveillance program (Fig. 1). Patients with extensive colitis or left-side colitis who have a negative screening colonoscopy should begin surveillance within 1–2 years. After 2 negative examinations, the next surveillance colonoscopy can be performed every 3 years until UC has been present for 20 years. At that time, consideration should be given to shorten the surveillance times to 1–2 years since CRC risk increases with longer duration of colitis. Patients with PSC should undergo yearly surveillance. Patients with proctosigmoiditis, who have little or no increased risk of CRC compared with the general population, should be managed according to standard CRC prevention measures as defined in guidelines [11].

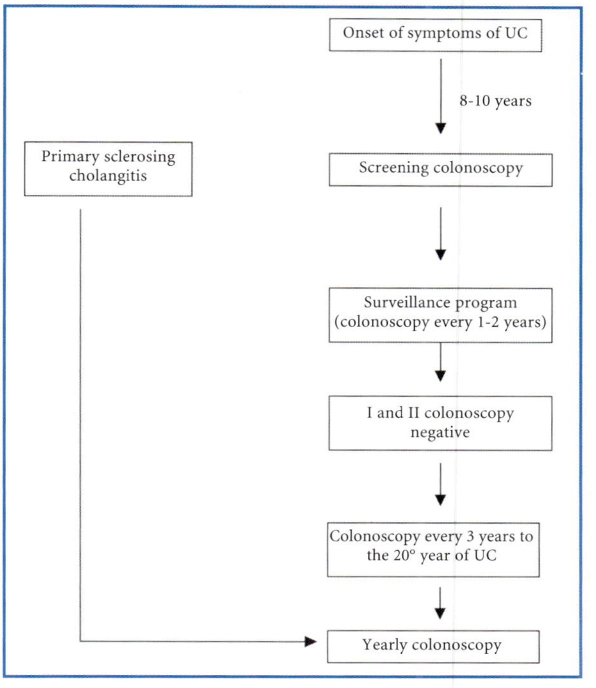

Fig. 1. Follow-up in UC

Screening colonoscopy must be performed during quiescent UC because the presence of severe inflammation can cause an erroneous histological differential diagnosis from dysplasia. Standard examination must include the entire colon and the collection of 4 random biopsies every 10 cm of mucosae since it has been estimated that 33 biopsies are required to provide a 90% chance of finding the highest degree of present dysplasia [19]. In UC, dysplasia on flat mucosae is distinguished by dysplasia associated to lesions or mass (DALM) because there is a significant major risk that these harbour cancer, even if a recent study showed that in 90% of patients a scrupulous colonoscopy can detect dysplastic lesions even on flat mucosae [20].

New Endoscopic Techniques

New endoscopic techniques are being introduced to improve early identification of even minimal lesions and to take targeted biopsies in suspicious areas. These techniques do not replace colonoscopy but are second-level examinations [21].

Chromoendoscopy

Endoscopic dye-spraying can improve dysplasia detection [7, 19]. This procedure involves the application of a mucosal stain or pigment, usually by injection through an endoscopic spray catheter. Chromoendoscopy improves the detection of minimal colonic lesions, raising the sensitivity of the endoscopic examination and, once a lesion is detected, can allow lesion characterisation, increasing the specificity of the examination [21–24]. There are 3 general classes of stain:

- Contrast dyes (for example, indigo carmine 0.1%): These coat the colonic mucosal surface and neither react with nor are absorbed by it. When dye is sprayed on the surface, groove patterns becomes evident and so mucosal lesions are highlighted.
- Absorptive dyes: These are absorbed by different cells to different degrees. Methylene blue 0.1% after few minutes avidly stains noninflamed mucosae but is poorly taken up by areas of active inflammation and dysplasia.
- Reactive dyes: These react with epithelium or mucosal secretion, producing detectable colour change.

  Colour use seems to be safe. The indigo carmine is poorly absorbed from the gastrointestinal tract. There is a theoretical risk of allergic reaction, but this has not been reported with intraluminal use. A recent study suggests that methylene blue can cause DNA damage after chromoendoscopy in patients with Barrett's oesophagus.

Description of Procedure

On insertion, all faecal fluid should be aspirated and adherent stool washed off to ensure optimal mucosal views. Any abnormalities seen on insertion should be biopsied or removed, as they may not be easily identified on extubation. When the cecal pole has been reached, intravenous drugs (scopolamine 20 mg or glucagon 1 mg) should be given to reduce spasm and haustral-fold prominence. Adequate air insufflation is necessary. A dye-spray catheter is inserted down the instrumentation channel and the tip protruded 2–3 cm, and an assistant can spray the stain with a syringe. Spraying should be done in segments of 5–15 cm. Once a segment has been sprayed, excess dye must be suctioned and mucosal examination begins; it is necessary to wait few seconds for indigo carmine to settle into the mucosal contours; methylene blue takes about 60 s to be absorbed. Once this segment has been examined, the next segment is sprayed and so on until the anal margin. On average, 60–100 ml of solution is required to spray the entire colorectal mucosa. Suspicious areas should be photographed, biopsied and the site endoscopically resected or tattooed if necessary. Patients with multiple postinflammatory polyps present a dilemma because the mucosa is not smooth, making dysplasia detection difficult. The colonoscopist must remain alert for any polypoid lesion that does not have a smooth surface and should take biopsies.

Magnifying Colonoscopy

New-generation colonoscopes with lens system on the tip enlarge the imagine up to 140 times [25–27]. Magnifying colonoscopes can show anatomic details to discriminate inflammatory from neoplastic lesions and to establish inflammation extension [27, 28], which previously was detectable only by histopathological examination. It has been reported that microscopic disease activity can predict relapse in patients with UC and so influence the treatment plan.

By matching chromoendoscopy and magnifying colonoscopy, it is possible to obtain a very detailed mucosal examination, and even to distinguish polyp types (pseudopolyp, hyperplastic and adenomatous). Kudo et al. [29] confirmed the feasibility of applying the "pit patterns" of the colonic polyp to distinguish them via magnifying colonoscopy and indigo carmine dye contrast (Table 3) [28, 30].

Confocal Endoscopy

Today it is possible to obtain in vivo microscopic imagines by introducing a catheter into the operative

Table 3. Kudo et al classification for "pit pattern" [29]

	Non neoplastic polyp	Neoplastic polyp
Type I	Normal round pit	
Type II	Small or large asteroid pit	
Type III s		Smaller than normal tubular or round pit
Type III l		Larger than normal tubular or round pit
Type IV		Dendritic or gyrous-like pit
Type V		Nonstructural pit

endoscopic channel [31, 32]. A fluorescent contrast agent is used to achieve high-contrast images. Fluorescein used systemically is preferred to acriflavine, tetracycline or cresyl violet used topically, since these agents have mutagenic potential cell's structure in a dedicated monitor. This new technology should allow histological diagnosis during conventional colonoscopy, but at the moment, accuracy is no better than 60%.

Management of Abnormal Findings

A finding of histologic lesions "indefinite for dysplasia", confirmed by 2 expert pathologists, warrants strict surveillance with repeat endoscopy within 3 months [33]. A finding of high-grade dysplasia indicates total colectomy because of the high risk of synchronous or metachronous CRC [34, 35]. Management of low-grade dysplasia is uncertain because it can progress to high-grade dysplasia or cancer in approximately 35–50% of patients within 5 years. Hence, 20% of patients with low-grade dysplasia have a CRC diagnosed at prophylactic total colectomy. Therefore, different therapeutic options should be considered. Prophylactic colectomy should be recommended if the number of specimens is poor or in multifocal dysplastic areas. If the patient declines prophylactic colectomy, careful surveillance should be carried out by a colonoscopy with adequate biopsies every 3–6 months. Negative sequential colonoscopy should not encourage patient or physician, and surveillance must continue every 6 months [33].

In the case of polyps in UC mucosae [adenoma-like mass (ALM)], polypectomy is indicated and, moreover, biopsies should be taken in the surrounding area (for separate examination). If those are negative for dysplasia, surveillance should be carried out every 6 months; however, if dysplasia is present on the mass or in the adjacent area, colectomy is indicated because of the high risk of synchronous CRC [11, 19, 36–38]. If the polyp is on either macroscopically or microscopically healing areas, follow-up is similar to those of sporadic adenoma.

Stenosis

Restorative proctocolectomy with ileal pouch-anal anastomosis is the surgical treatment of choice for patients with medically refractory UC or UC with dysplasia. A well-known complication of surgery is the stricture of the pouch outlet (pouch-anal anastomosis) or pouch inlet (the junction of neoterminal ileum and pouch). Both can benefit from endoscopic balloon dilatation associated with topical injection of long-acting steroids. This procedure appears safe and effective in treating pouch outlet and inlet anastomosis and can avoid or delay surgery [39].

References

1. Guindi M, Riddell RH (2004) Indeterminate colitis. J Clin Pathol 57:1233–1244
2. Haskell H, Andrews CW Jr, Reddy SI et al (2005) Pathologic features and clinical significance of "backwash" ileitis in ulcerative colitis. Am J Surg Pathol 29(11):1472–1481
3. Kornbluth A, Legnani P, Lewis SB (2004) Video capsule endoscopy in inflammatory bowel disease. Past, present and future. Inflamm Bowel Dis 10:278–285
4. Higgins P, Schwartz M, Mapili J, Zimmermann EM (2005) Is endoscopy necessary for the measurement of disease activity in ulcerative colitis? Am J Gastroenterol 100:355–361
5. Maunder RG, Greenberg GR (2004) Comparison of a disease activity index patients'self-reported symptom severity in ulcerative colitis. Inflamm Bowel Dis 10:632–636
6. Fefferman DS, Farrell RJ (2005) Endoscopy in inflammatory bowel disease: indications, surveillance, and use in clinical practice. Clin Gastroenterol Hepatol 3(1):11–24
7. Gearry RB, Barclay ML, Burt MJ et al (2004) Surveillance for dysplasia in patients with inflammatory bowel disease: a national survey of colonoscopic practice in New Zealand. Dis Colon Rectum 47(3):314–322
8. Inadomi JM (2003) Cost-effectiveness of colorectal cancer surveillance in ulcerative colitis. Scand J Gastroenterol Suppl (237):17–21
9. Hata K, Watanabe T, Kazamas S et al (2003) Earlier surveillance colonoscopy programme improves survival in patients with ulcerative colitis associated colorectal cancer: results of a 23-year surveillance programme in the Japanese population. Br J Cancer 89(7):1232–1236
10. Bernstein CN (2004) A balancing view: Dysplasia surveillance in ulcerative colitis–sorting the pro from the con. Am J Gastroenterol 99(9):1636–1637
11. Itzkowitz S, Present DH (2005) Consensus conference: colorectal cancer screening and surveillance in inflammatory bowel disease. Inflamm Bowel Dis 11:314–321
12. Eaden JA, Abrams KR, Mayberry JF (2001) The risk of colorectal cancer in ulcerative colitis: a meta-analysis. Gut 48:526–535
13. Mathy C, Schneider K, Chen Y (2003) Gross versus microscopic pancolitis and occurence of neoplasia in ulcerative colitis. Inflamm Bowel Dis 9:351–355
14. Askling J, Dickman PW, Karlen P (2001) Family history as a risk factor for colorectal cancer in inflammatory bowel disease. Gastroenterology 120:1356–1362
15. Rutter MD, Saunders BP, Wilkinson KH et al (2004) Cancer surveillance in longstading ulcerative colitis: endoscopic appearances help predict cancer risk. Gut 53:1813–1816
16. Itzkowitz SH, Harpaz N (2004) Diagnosis and manage-

ment of dysplasia in patients with inflammatory bowel diseases. Gastroenterology 126(6):1634–1648
17. Tung BY, Emond MJ, Haggitt RC et al (2001) Ursodiol use is associated with lower prevalence of colonic neoplasia in patients with ulcerative colitis and primary sclerosing cholangitis. Ann Intern Med 134(2):89–95
18. Taylor BA (1992) Dysplasia in chronic ulcerative colitis: implications for colonoscopic surveillance. Dis Colon Rectum 35(10):950–956
19. Rutter M, Bernstein C, Matsumoto T et al (2004) Endoscopic appearance of dysplasia in ulcerative colitis and the role of staining. Endoscopy 36(12):1109–1114
20. Rutter MD, Saunders BP, Wilkinson KH et al (2004) Most dysplasia in ulcerative colitis is visible at colonoscopy. Gastrointest Endosc 60(3):334–339
21. Mpofu C, Watson AJ, Rhodes JM (2004) Strategies for detecting colon cancer and/or dysplasia in patients with inflammatory bowel disease. Cochrane Database Syst Rev 2:CD000279
22. Sada M, Igarashi M, Yoshizawa S et al (2004) Dye spraying and magnifying endoscopy for dysplasia and cancer surveillance in ulcerative colitis. Dis Colon Rectum 47(11):1816–1823
23. Bernstein CN (2003) The color of dysplasia in ulcerative colitis. Gastroenterology 124(4):1135–1138
24. Matsumoto T, Nakamura S, Jo Y et al (2003) Chromoscopy might improve diagnostic accuracy in cancer surveillance for ulcerative colitis. Am J Gastroenterol 98(8):1827–1833
25. Hurlstone DP, Shorthouse AJ, Cross SS et al (2004) High-magnification chromoscopic pouchoscopy: a novel in vivo technique for surveillance of the anal transition zone and columnar cuff following ileal pouch-anal anastomosis. Tech Coloproctol 8(3):173–178
26. Hata K, Watanabe T, Motoi T et al (2004) Pitfalls of pit pattern diagnosis in ulcerative colitis-associated dysplasia. Gastroenterology 126(1):374–376
27. Kunihiro M, Tanaka M (2004) Magnifying colonoscopic features of ulcerative colitis reflect histologic inflammation. Inflamm Bowel Dis 10:737–744
28. Su M-Y, Ho Y-P (2004) Magnifying endoscopy with Indigo carmine contrast for differential diagnosis of neoplastic and nonneoplastic colonic polyps. Dig Dis Sci 49:1123–1127
29. Kudo S, Hirota S, Nakajiama T (1994) Colorectal tumors and pit pattern. J Clin Pathol 47:880–885
30. Kudo S, Rubio CA, Teixeira CA et al (2001) Pit pattern in colorectal neoplasia: Endoscopic magnifying view. Endoscopy 33(4):367–373
31. Evans JA, Nishioka NS (2005) Endoscopic confocal microscopy. Curr Opin Gastroenterol 21(5):78–84
32. Kiesslich R, Neurath M (2005) Endoscopic confocal imaging. Clin Gastroenterol Hepatol 3:S58–S60
33. Bernstein CN (2004) Ulcerative colitis with low-grade dysplasia. Gastroenterology 127(3):950–956
34. Connell WR, Lennard-Jones JE, Williams CB et al (1994) Factors affecting the outcome of endoscopic surveillance for cancer in ulcerative colitis. Gastroenterology 107(4):934–944
35. Bernstein CN, Shanahan F, Weinstein WM (1994) Are we telling patients the truth about surveillance colonoscopy in ulcerative colitis? Lancet 343:71–74
36. Sinicrope FA, Wang K (2004) Treating polyps in ulcerative colitis: adenoma-like lesions and dysplasia-associated mass lesions. Clin Gastroenterol Hepatol 2(7):531–533
37. Chawla A, Judge TA, Lichtenstein GR (2002) Evaluation of polypoid lesions in inflammatory bowel disease. Gastrointest Endosc Clin N Am 12(3):525–534
38. Rubin PH, Friedman S, Harpaz N et al (1999) Colonoscopic polypectomy in chronic colitis: conservative management after endoscopic resection of dysplastic polyps. Gastroenterology 117(6):1295–1300
39. Shen, B, Fazio VW (2004) Endoscopic balloon dilatation of ileal pouch strictures. Am J Gastroenterol 99:2340–2347

Nutrition and Malnutrition in Inflammatory Bowel Disease

Italo Vantini, Fosca De Iorio, Naika Tacchella, Luigi Benini

Introduction

Nutrition and nutritional status can be affected by IBD. If one looks at patients with IBD referred to an outpatient clinic or admitted to a ward, patients with ulcerative colitis usually do not have an overt impairment in nutritional status, but in acute and severe attacks it is possible that they only need nutritional support. Patients affected by Crohn's disease more frequently suffer from overt or subtle nutritional problems, both in childhood and as in the adult life. Despite the fact that most patients' survival expectancy is not impaired and most cases remain productive [1], Crohn's disease can be associated with impairment in QoL scores, disability, and failure to thrive, which is also frequently associated with nutritional problems. It has been estimated that 25–75% of patients suffer from varying degrees of malnutrition; however, the first figure appears more realistic. Impairment in nutritional status more frequently occurs in patients with unremitting and/or complicated disease, but others factors can contribute to malnutrition, particularly in children. Concomitant factors can be shared by the same patient: (1) anorexia and reduced calorie intake; (2) reduced ingestion of foods because of abdominal pain; (3) diarrhoea, malabsorption and protein-loosing enteropathy, especially if the disease is extensive and involves the jejunum; (4) bacterial overgrowth; (5) increased intestinal permeability and chronic inflammation contributing to a chronic hypermetabolic state, which is frequently found in malnourished patients with active disease; (6) GI fistulas, intestine narrowing and infections; (7) subtle deficiency of vitamins and oligoelements that complicate and/or are capable of favouring malnutrition; (9) aftermath of extensive surgical resection with chronic intestinal failure (short-bowel syndrome). Energy requirements and expenditure may increase in the presence of persisting inflammation, and protein synthesis and catabolism appear to correlate with disease activity, even doubling it in the moderate to severe activity phase [2]. An energy requirement of up to 40 KCal/kg/day with a protein requirement of 1.8 g/kg/day has been estimated [3]. However, in adult patients with Crohn's disease without fever and infections, the resting energy expenditure (REE) measured by indirect calorimetry appeared to correlate well with, and to be practically identical to, the expenditure estimated by the Harris-Benedict formula. This suggests, that in about 90% of patients, it is equal to 25±4 KCal/kg/day and that it exceeds 30 KCal/kg/day in only 10% of patients. Therefore, energy and protein requirements depend on the disease activity, the presence of complications, and in most patients, nutritional requirements are not significantly greater than might be theoretically expected.

Some topics deserve a lot of attention because of their frequency, impact on quality of life, therapeutic implications such as : (1) problems of malnutrition in children with IBD and the role of an early nutritional approach in improving growth not just as calorie administration, but as a real therapy; (2) indications and role of artificial nutrition in IBD and of enteral nutrition as primary care; (3) the effect of enteral formulas on some inflammation and mucosal mechanisms in IBD; (4) bone changes in IBD, prevention and treatment.

Clinical Studies on Artificial Nutrition in Crohn's Disease

Artificial nutrition (enteral and parenteral) represents a widespread approach to many gastrointestinal disorders such as intestinal failure and chronic intestinal pseudo-obstruction, inflammatory bowel disease (IBD), severe exocrine pancreatic insufficiency due to cystic fibrosis, enteric and pancreatic fistulas, swallowing disorders, and other conditions secondary to other severe gastrointestinal disease or major digestive surgery leading to malnutrition. The availability of different enteral nutritional formulas, improvements in assessing nutritional status and its relationships with the digestive tract, as well as the progress in the management of artificial nutrition procedures have enhanced its safety, efficacy and scale of use.

Crohn's disease can be an indication for artificial nutrition, improving patient management and also providing some insights into the nature of the disease, for example with regard to the role of dietary antigens, intestinal permeability and the intestinal inflammatory and immunological response in the pathogenesis and clinical course of the disease. At this point, there is no medical or surgical treatment capable of curing the disease, and the only realistic therapeutic objectives consist of achieving remission of the active phases, treatment of complications, and an attempt to maintain remission with immunosuppressive agents and more recently with long-term infliximab treatment. Though the obvious aim of artificial nutrition is to improve or restore adequate nutritional status in the presence of malnutrition by artificially administering nitrogen together with an energy source, in Crohn's disease, an increasingly investigated aspect is the assessment of whether or not enteral nutrition (EN) may have the role of primary care.

Nutritional Care in Children with Crohn's Disease

Between 15 to 40% of children with Crohn's disease suffer from malnutrition and growth failure, puberty retardation and development of secondary sexual characteristics retardation [4]. The slowing down of height velocity has been also observed [4, 5]. What is clinically relevant is that malnutrition may affect as many as 25% of children even before the apparent onset of the disease [5]. Some factors are involved such as the catabolic state during the acute and/or persistent active phase, anorexia leading to insufficient calorie intake to cater to the subject's needs during the critical growth phase, malabsorption and protein dispersion, and deficiencies of zinc, calcium, magnesium and phosphorus. Moreover, steroid treatment plays its most detrimental role in children. A number of hormone deficiencies have been considered such as GH, thyroid hormones and cortisol. A significant correlation between height and bodyweight deficits and low circulatory levels of IGF-I has been found [6], which increases with the improvement in the nutritional status induced by adequate feeding (as can be achieved artificially) [6].

Nutritional support and rehabilitation, by administering defined oral, enteral formulas or parenteral infusion of nutrients plays a major role in childhood. Several studies have shown a positive role of parenteral nutrition in increasing weight and height, and in inducing puberty in children with Crohn's disease [7–12], with better results being obtained if the nutritional approach begins in the prepubertal period and the disease has been in remission for some time [13, 14]. Though the growth phase covers a limited period, the earliest possible nutritional therapy is distinctly indicated in order to exploit the child's growth potential to the full. Parenteral nutrition is able to favour clinical remission of the acute phase in children [7, 8], and to trigger body growth after surgical treatment [12]. In some cases, long-term parenteral nutrition has been used [15].

A substantial number of controlled and uncontrolled trials have provided suggestions on the usefulness of both orally and enterally administered defined formulas (continuously or intermittently), depending on the indication, facilities, and patient's compliance, in inducing an increase in height or body weight and in accelerating the onset of puberty.

Elemental, semi-elemental and polymeric enteral formulas have been tested with no substantially different degrees of efficacy [16–23] and they have proved capable of facilitating remission of the acute phase [21, 24], and of having efficacy comparable (though less quickly) to prednisolone [25]. In a meta-analysis of randomised studies, EN was as effective as steroids in achieving clinical remission [26]. Though long-term nocturnal enteral protocol was able to contribute towards keeping the disease in remission [23], its long-term efficacy is not yet proven.

Re-feeding allows an improvement in the nutritional status, growth rate and height, remission of the acute phase and, in certain circumstances, reduction in relapses. The main goal in children affected by Crohn's disease is taking the patient off steroids, thereby avoiding their detrimental influence in this phase of life and hastening the onset of puberty with the development of secondary sexual characteristics. This is more conveniently achieved with EN, which plays its greatest role in children with Crohn's disease, bringing about a major change for the better in the patient's quality of life, in the sense of actual treatment and nutritional rescue and rehabilitation.

Artificial Nutrition in Crohn's Disease

Usually, TPN is indicated when the digestive tract cannot be used for nutrition. Its aim is to promote bowel rest, to avoid any contact between bowel and dietary antigens and to improve the nutritional status. Despite some detrimental effects which the absence of nutrients may have on the gut, the role of TPN has been investigated in both retrospective and controlled clinical studies [25]. In the retrospective studies, TPN was used alone or in combination with steroids, and hospital remission of Crohn's disease was obtained within a wide 28–100% range of patients [27]. If we do not consider the extreme figures and trials enrolling less than 20 patients, the overall hospital remission quoted about 50%; however, it rose to 77% in the largest study in which 100 patients were enrolled [28]. Long-term remission over 3–49 months ranged from 0 to 69%, and 1-year remission was registered in about 40% of patients.

Some prospective trials have assessed the efficacy of TPN with a fairly homogeneous overall hospital remission rate of about 80%, but with a wide long-term [20–48 months) remission rate ranging from 18 to 69% [29–32]. The remission rate for TPN, as compared to steroids, does not appear significantly different, though it is consistently numerically lower [32, 33]. In some studies, numerically (though not statistically) higher remission rates were reported with TPN when combined with steroids [34].

A number of studies have reported some positive effects of TPN in the conservative treatment of fistulas in Crohn's disease, with closure rates of 43% [34], 59% [35], 44% [36] and 62% [27], and some superiority of TPN over EN has been described [38]. However, other studies did not confirm any advantage of TPN [29, 39–41]. Short-term fistula closure is probably to be expected in approximately 40% of cases treated with TPN, with a relapse rate varying from 10 to 60% [28, 37]. The use of EN for fistula closure has yielded contradictory results: while a promising effect [42] or results comparable to those achieved with TPN were reported [43], in other trials, EN has failed to be effective [44]. Moreover, TPN has been tried preoperatively to reduce disease activity and to limit the length of resected bowel. Reduction of approximately 20 cm of small bowel and 11 cm of the ileum and caecum has been measured in patients treated preoperatively with TPN [45]. Moreover, in a single study, TPN has been tried as an alternative to surgery in Crohn's disease of the colon, but not in patients with small-bowel disease where it failed to obviate the need for surgery [46].

The role of TPN has been also assessed in patients resistant to steroids (remission observed in 40–80% of cases) [28, 47–49], and in steroid-dependent patients (remission observed in 100% of cases) [50, 51]. Steroid treatment does not improve the response to TPN [50].

Although available data are not homogeneous and the quality of studies is not always high, there is sufficient evidence that, in adults, TPN improves nutritional status, can be used preoperatively, may offer an alternative to surgery in selected patients with Crohn's disease of the colon, is helpful in patients with GI tract fistulas, and can favour remission of the acute phase of the disease.

Nevertheless, elemental diets has proved as effective as TPN in inducing remission of the active phase at rates of 87.5% *vs.* 85% [52], 62% *vs.* 75% [53] and 70% *vs.* 80% respectively [54]. It has also been found to be just as effective as both TPN and partial parenteral nutrition (EN: 58%; TPN: 71%; partial parenteral nutrition: 60% remission observed, respectively) [55]. Moreover, long-term remission rate following TPN does not seem to be different from that observed after an elemental diet (27% *vs.* 32% long-term remission, respectively) [53, 55], but contradictory features have been reported for TPN *vs.* steroids (17 and 3%) [33] and 33% *vs.* 28.6% remission rates respectively [56]. Some studies have compared long-term remission after TPN and after EN: no substantial differences were found by comparing long-term remission rates, active disease persisted in 60% *vs.* 41% and in 50% *vs.* 37% respectively [54, 55]. Therefore, bowel rest would not appear necessary for inducing remission of the acute phase and, because of its cost and side effects, TPN should be restricted to selected patients only.

In Crohn's disease, an altered immunological and inflammatory response to endoluminal antigens is present, and an increased intestinal permeability has been reported [57]. On the basis of some candidate interactions between the luminal contents and the intestinal mucosa, EN and oral elemental or semi-elemental formulas have been investigated as a primary care for Crohn's disease. Elemental formulas (40–50% of whose nitrogen are amino acids), possess low antigenicity, are easily proximally absorbed, and are generally endowed with a low lipid content often in the form of MCT. In Crohn's disease, some intolerance to intraluminal food antigens has been postulated, but in rechallenge and double-blind rechallenge studies, less than half of the patients in whom remission was achieved with an elemental diet, and who presented apparent sensitivity to a number of foodstuffs, proved to have benefited from food exclusion diets [58]. On the other hand, despite the fact that oral liquid formulas were associated with a clinical remission rate comparable to that achieved with first-line drugs, a minority of patients complained about the oral liquid formula so much that its use was curtailed [59]. Despite this drawback, elemental formulas are capable of improving intestinal permeability, and of reducing mucosal inflammation in Crohn's disease [60].

Clinical studies have shown that EN used with elemental formulas is associated with remission rates comparable to those obtained with steroids at a figure approximately as high as 75% [21, 25, 28, 61–64], and in a single trial it was superior to prednisolone [62]. However, the relapse rate or remission length after an elemental diet is quite variable. In one study, following a good 83% remission rate, the amount of patients remaining in remission at 6 and 12 months were less than 50%, which was lower than in the group that had achieved remission with prednisolone [64]. In a large retrospective study, the frequency of lasting remission rates at 6, 12, 24, 36, 48 and 60 months after remission achieved with elemental EN did not significantly differ (37–45% at 3 years) from those observed following steroids (24% at 3 years) [65]. Thus, elemental EN nutrition appears as effective as steroid therapy and TPN in favouring remission, but it is questionable whether the relapse rate is greater, equal to, or even lower than that after steroid-induced remission.

Semi-elemental and elemental formulas have yielded identical results in inducing remission of active Crohn's disease [24, 66, 67]. In one study, a semi-elemental formula gave results comparable to those of prednisolone (remission rates: semi-elemental 89%, prednisolone 87%) [24], but this was not confirmed in two controlled trials [59, 68] in which prednisolone was superior to EN.

In clinical studies with polymeric EN, with one exception [69], remission was observed in at least 60% of patients, with an average rate of about 70%, but up to 80% in three trials [70–72]. With the exception of the above-mentioned study [69] in which better results were observed with an elemental diet, comparison between elemental and polymeric formulas confirmed that they were equally effective in inducing remission [71, 73, 74]. One study showed that a polymeric formula (remission rate: 94%) and prednisolone (remission rate: 88%) were equally effective in inducing remission of Crohn's disease and in reducing the van Hees index. Additionally, a greater number of patients who had achieved remission with EN were still in remission 12 months later [72]. Thus, polymeric enteral diets are also associated with similar remission rates as elemental diets and steroids, but there is no sufficient evidence that they promote longer clinical remission.

The increasing evidence that intestinal environment and microflora, genetic factors and altered immune mucosal response can account for the mechanisms triggering and perpetuating the inflammatory process, may give new insights for understanding why EN may have a role of primary care in Crohn's disease. Though mechanisms of elemental diets (and generally of EN) in IBD are incompletely understood, there is evidence of an anti-inflammatory action. A 4-week elemental diet impacts with cytokines, decreasing mucosal IL-1b, IL-1ra, IL-6, IL-8 TNF-alfa to healthy control levels in patients with active Crohn's disease. The IL-1ra/IL-1beta ratio, which was lowered before EN, increased to control values after EN. Clinical remission can be achieved in 71%, endoscopic healing in 44% (ileum) and 39% (colon), and histological healing in about 20% of the treated cases [74]. Moreover, endoscopic and histological healing was associated with a decline in cytokine concentration and with an improvement in pro-inflammatory/anti-inflammatory cytokine imbalance [74]. In Vitro incubation in an elemental diet-like environment of colonic or ileal biopsies of patients with IBD (but not of control patients), increased the interleukin-1 receptor antagonist/inteleukin-1 beta ratio [75]. Though in vitro/in vivo pathways can be different and the former features should be considered with caution, these data suggest that an elemental diet "environment" increases the anti-inflammatory/pro-inflammatory cytokine ratio.

Exclusive polymeric EN in children was associated with an early increase in IGF-1 and decrease in pro-inflammatory cytokine IL-6, C-reactive protein, ESR and the Crohn's disease activity index [76]. An increased resistance of T-cells to apoptosis is induced by IL-6, but also it has been shown to interfere with bone metabolism leading to osteopenia [77, 78]. IL-6 is over-expressed in Crohn's disease, and its blockade experimentally leads to partially reverse growth failure [79]. A relationship between increased IL-6 levels and decreased IGF-1 levels was found in children [79]. Increase in IGF-1 levels was obtained by both steroids and elemental diet, but body growth was promoted solely by the latter [80]. However, environmental (dietary and even more bacteria) factors directly influenced by EN and cellular mechanisms by which inflammatory and immune response can be modulated, have not been elucidated so far. Because of comparable results given by semi-elemental and polymeric diets, it is clear that dietary antigen exclusion alone, as inferred by earlier studies with elemental diets, or the so-called bowel rest, are not the mechanisms involved. Effects on intestinal permeability, cytokine expression, intraluminal products of nutrient substrates by the microflora, and perhaps some components of defined EN formulas (such as anti-inflammatory cytokines and/or lipids) remain the main candidates in support of using the nutritional approach as primary care in Crohn's disease.

Though some contradictory results of clinical trials could be partly explained by different composition and selection of patient samples and by concomitant treatments, some data suggest that the composition of EN formulas may influence their effects in Crohn's disease. Different peptide lengths, and varying fat content and quality as substrates for the arachidonic and eicosanoid acid cascade, with down-regulation of pro-inflammatory compounds, could account for the actions of EN in Crohn's disease. On the other hand, supplements with dietary n-3 PUFA have been successfully employed both in an animal model of inflammation [83] and in rheumatoid arthritis [84].

An excellent analysis of clinical trials suggested that lipid composition may play a major role in the effect of EN as primary care in Crohn's disease [82]. High-lipid formulas, particularly linoleic acid formulas, were associated with worse results, whereas low-lipid formulas and those with large amounts of MUFA have yielded better results. Linoleic acid is the precursor of arachidonic acid, which constitutes the substrate for the synthesis of factors with a substantial pro-inflammatory action (IL-6, LTB-4, PGE_2, thromboxane A_2), the content of which is increased in the active phases of Crohn's disease. EN formulas rich in n-6 PUFA such as linoleic acid, which is capable of inducing marked synthesis of arachidonic acid and of pro-inflammatory factors, would be, therefore, less indicated than diets with a low content of PUFA or containing PUFA of the n-3 series which induces the synthesis of factors with a less pronounced pro-inflammatory activity (LTB-5, PGE_3 and PGI_2)—the synthesis of which competes with that of the factors with stronger pro-inflammatory action. Furthermore, this would also reduce the synthesis of cytokines—tumour necrosis factor (TNF-alfa) and platelet activating factor (PAF)—involved in tissue-damaging mechanisms. Dietary n-3 PUFA promoted an anti-inflammatory effect in experimental colitis, by affecting the immune cell function, by reducing myeloid cell recruitment and activation of myofibroblasts, pro-inflammatory cytokines, by enhancing epithelial barrier function and by acting on the tight junction and up-regulation of occludines. The ratio n-6/n-3, more than their absolute levels, with competition for COX and 5-LOX, seems to determine the final eicosanoid balance [85]. However, increased biosynthesis, consumption of PUFA and high circulating levels of n-3 PUFA in active Crohn's have been described [86], raising some doubts on the need for high n-3 content enteral formulas.

Bone Disease in IBD

Reduced bone mineral density (BMD) is frequently associated with Crohn's disease (CD). Early studies have described a high prevalence of osteopenia (a T-score of −1 or lower) and osteoporosis (a T-score of −2.5 or lower) in inflammatory bowel disease (IBD). Uncontrolled studies gave a prevalence of severe demineralisation determined by dual-energy absorptiometry (Z-score of lower than −2 or T-score of lower than −2.5) that ranged from 18 to 42%, while larger studies with a healthy control group showed prevalence rates of only 2–16% [87]. It is important to notice that these studies are prone to selection bias as they are conducted in specialised IBD centres. In fact, in prospective longitudinal studies, changes in BMD in patients with IBD were similar to those of the general population [88]. The most relevant clinical question is to determine whether alterations in BMD can affect the fracture risk. There have been four large population-based studies describing fracture risk in patients with IBD. A survey was mailed to members of the Danish Crohn's/Colitis Association regarding fractures [89]. The authors concluded that patients with UC had similar overall fracture rates compared with control subjects. Crohn's disease patients had a relative risk of 1.7 for all fractures (RR for female patients 2.5, 2.9 among premenopausal females, 1.8 among postmenopausal women and 0.6 among men) compared to the control group. A family fracture history (RR 2.4) especially paternal (RR 3.6) increased the risk of fracture among patients with CD. Among UC patients, maternal fracture history (RR 2.4) and smoking (RR 3.8) were additional risk factors. There was no correlation between fracture risk and steroid use in both CD and UC. It is important to notice that the control subjects were not matched to patients by age and gender and were more likely to be older and male, and less likely to be current smokers or on hormone replacement therapy than patients with Crohn's disease. Furthermore, there may have been a bias in the nature of patients who returned the questionnaire, as those who were at higher risk may have been more likely to respond. In population-based studies, the same authors observed that the relative risk of sustaining a fracture requiring hospitalisation in CD was 1.9, whereas at 1.08 in UC it had not significantly increased [90].

There have been two North American population-based studies of fracture risk in IBD [91, 92]. The first study, published by Bernstein et al., identified hospital and out-patient fractures by collecting the data via administrative databases for the Canadian province of Manitoba. The overall fracture rate for patients with IBD was found to be approximately 1 per 100 patient-years and this increased to a relative risk of 1.41 compared with an age-gender- and geographical residence-matched control group. There was an increased fracture risk of the hip and of the spine, which was evidenced in patients over 60 years of age. No differences were observed between men and women and between CD and UC patients. However, there was a significantly increased fracture risk for UC male patients compared with females. The other North American study used the Olmsted County population-based database of 243 CD patients. Compared with controls, the overall risk ratio for any fracture was 0.9, whereas the relative risk for an osteoporotic fracture was 1.4. The risk ratio for thoracolumbar vertebral fracture was 2.2. Thus, the risk of fracture was not greater than in the general population, except in the elderly. The last study was a primary care-based nested-case control study which used a General Practice Research Database in the UK that included 683 patients [93]. The overall odds ratio for IBD patients compared with a matched control group was 1.21 without differences between males and females. After accounting for a measure of disease severity, there were no significant differences in the fracture risk between patients with CD and UC; the risk of fracture correlated with the number of symptoms and with age.

The collective messages of these studies are the following: (1) patients with IBD may have increased fracture rates but the magnitude of the excess risk is small and most evident in the elderly; (2) fracture risk is generally similar in CD and UC; (3) osteoporosis is gender neutral among patients with IBD.

Risk Factor for Osteoporosis in IBD

The mechanisms underlying bone loss in IBD are still unclear. Several factors that also contribute to osteoporosis in the general population are implicated: physical inactivity, hypogonadism, underweight, calcium and vitamin D deficiency, malnutrition, smoking (most commonly in CD), treatment with steroids and the effects of inflammatory cytokines related to the disease activity. As noted before, among patients with IBD, fracture risk, which is similar in CD and UC, is gender neutral and most evident in adults. In the following, we will briefly discuss the other main risk factors.

Onset of inflammatory bowel disease. A recent analysis of premenopausal adult women with early onset IBD did not provide evidence that an early onset of disease is a major risk factor for early onset osteoporosis [94].

Steroid use. Systemic steroid therapy is associated with rapid bone loss, particularly in the trabecular bone of the lumbar spine. Steroid use is a major factor in IBD-associated bone loss. Nevertheless, it is difficult to separate the effects of corticosteroid use from those of disease activity. Bernestein et al. observed that corticosteroid use in the 2-year period preceding fracture was more frequently in patients experiencing fracture compared with those not experiencing fractures [94]. Few studies have examined BMD in newly diagnosed patients. Gosh et al. observed reduced BMD in patients with CD, but not with UC [95]. This could be explained by the relative lower age and hence higher BMD of the UC patients and by the high preponderance of proctitis with less deleterious systemic consequences. BMD was unaffected by the subsequent use of steroids over a 1-year period. Schoon et al. [96] found BMD to be normal at diagnosis. It has been suggested that the high prevalence of oral contraceptives used in this study (92% of the women) may have provided protection against bone loss. Lamb et al. [97] observed a reduced BMD at diagnosis, prior to corticosteroid treatment in 34 IBD patients.

Calcium intake, vitamin D deficiency, malabsorption, intestinal resection, body mass index. Adequate calcium-intake has been suggested as being an important determinant of optimal bone mass. Bernstein et al. observed, in a cohort of premenopausal women prior to 20 years of age, that the average BMD was not different than in controls and only 3% had BMD in the osteoporotic range [94]. Therefore, IBD children achieve normal BMD as adults and it is possible that during remission periods or steroid-free periods there is a sufficient opportunity to achieve normal bone mineralisation. In this same study, oral calcium and vitamin D intake were measured by a 4-day food record and no correlation was observed between the intake of these nutrients and BMD [98]; this is similar to a previous report in 168 CD patients [99]. Hence, a 4-day record can be beneficial in determining the quantity of calcium supplementation required. One variable often cited as being important in CD is the relationship between osteomalacia, the skeletal hallmark of vitamin D deficiency, and reduced vitamin D intake and/or absorption. Factors contributing to vitamin D deficiency in CD include malabsorption of dietary vitamin D and 25-hydroxy vitamin D undergoing enterohepatic circulation, lack of adequate sun exposure, a low dietary vitamin D intake and the ingestion of drugs interacting with the intestinal absorption of vitamin D. The majority of the studies suggest that low dietary intake of vitamin D is not an important determinant of BMD in IBD patients [100]. Cholestyramine is often used to control postresectional diarrhoea due to bile acid malabsorption. Both resection of the terminal ileum and cholestyramine therapy lead to the depletion of bile acids, which are essential for vitamin D absorption; ensuring adequate intake of vitamin D is highly recommended especially in patients with small-bowel resection. Most of the studies on the importance of vitamin D deficiency come from literature in the early 1980s that specifically addressed BMD in a selected group of CD patients with decreased serum 25-OHD. A recent study showed that vitamin D absorption in CD patients is normal [101]. Some studies have shown no relationship between BMD and measured serum 25-OHD [102–104]. Two studies have found that serum 25-OHD levels are actually lower in UC than in CD [105, 106]. Relative malnutrition and low body weight are important risk factors. In the general population, body mass index is strongly correlated with BMD [107] and meta-analysis has concluded that a low body weight is a significant and consistent risk factor for fracture in the general population, although the 51 studies used were dominated by older women [108]. The same appears true for CD patients. In a population-based study of 60 CD patients, 60 UC patients and 60 healthy controls, those with CD had both a lower BMD as well as lower lean mass [109]. This effect was only seen in those with current or past systemic steroid use, which is consistent with the known adverse drug effects on both bone and muscle tissue. Among 168 CD patients, the BMI was significantly correlated with BMD ($p<0.0001$) [110].

Inflammation-mediated bone loss. The link between inflammation and bone loss may be of particular interest in IBD-associated osteopenia. The recently discovered receptor activator of nuclear factor κB (RANK) ligand (RANKL) osteoprotegerin (OPG), may be the important link between systemic inflammation and osteoporosis. The OPG molecule binds to the receptor activator of nuclear factor κB (RANK). The effect of this ligation is to regulate T cell–dendritic cell communications, dendritic cell survival and lymph node organogenesis. The interaction of RANK on the surface of the osteoclasts with its ligand RANKL induces osteoclastogenesis. Osteoprotegerin (OPG) can be secreted by osteoblasts and serves as a decoy receptor that prevents the ligation of RANKL, which can interfere with osteoclastogenesis. The balance between RANKL and OPG is of major importance for the regulation of osteoclastogenesis. The way in which compounds stimulate RANK ligand or OPG will affect whether they inhibit or induce osteoclastogenesis. Certain pro-inflammatory cytokines such as IL-1 and TNF alfa, induce RANKL and displace the balance of bone formation and bone reabsorption in favour of bone reabsorption causing bone loss. Corticosteroids partially exert their toxic effects on bone by the same mechanism and they also inhibit OPG production.

Genetic risk factors of rapid bone loss. An interesting report linked potential fracture risk as a measure of bone mineral density by DXA with the presence or absence of specific alleles for certain proinflammatory cytokines [111]. Eighty-three patients with IBD were enrolled and went through a follow-up with BMD measurements over 1.6±0.3 years: 17% had a T-score below –2.5 at the spine and 11% had a T-score below –2.5 at the hip. They observed that the extent of bone loss was not correlated to clinical severity of disease or administration of steroids. Non-carriage of the 240-base pair allele of the IL-1ra gene and carriage of the 130-base pair allele of IL-6 were independently associated with increased bone loss, and their combined presence was significantly associated with increased bone loss. Todhunter et al. [112] investigated the influence of IL-6, collagen type 1a1 (COL1A1) and vitamin D receptor gene (VDR) single nucleotide polymorphisms (SNP) on BMD in a cohort of 245 patient's with CD. They observed that lumbar spine and total hip BMD was higher in patients with CC genotype compared to GG ($p=0.041$ and $p=0.014$ respectively). In patients genotyped for COL1A1, (hip, but not lumbar spine), BMD was higher in the homozygous wild type GG than in the heterozygous GT. No differences were observed either between BMD VDR Taq 1 and Fok 1 genotypes or between BMD and CARD 15 genotypes. The authors observed that in CD, a condition characterised by increased levels of IL-6, the genotype CC is protective against IL-6 mediated bone reabsorption. Furthermore, COL1A1 gene polymorphisms at the Sp1 binding sites are thought to influence the properties of bone by altering the level of transcription and production of collagen. It has been observed that bone strength is reduced in heterozygous compared to wild type subjects [113].

Clinical Trials on Prevention and Therapy of IBD-Associated Bone Disease

Therapeutic intervention studies focussing on IBD are sparse and no clinical trials with the aim of fracture prevention are available. Extrapolating results from fracture prevention trials in osteoporotic and steroid-induced osteoporosis may be tricky for several reasons: (1) orally administered agents, especially biphosphonates whose absorption is only 1–5% even in healthy subjects, may not be adequately absorbed in those with intestinal disease (in patients with active disease, especially of the upper gastrointestinal tract, parenteral administration of biphosphonates may be appropriate); (2) IBD is under-represented in the larger intervention trials on steroid-induced osteoporosis, making the conclusions arguable; (3) younger men and premenopausal women—patients of special interest with regard to IBD-associated bone disease—have not been subjected to therapeutic intervention trials outside the context of steroid-induced osteoporosis. Taking all these drawbacks as a whole, review articles on the therapy of IBD-associated bone disease should be considered with caution. Experts emphasise lifestyle modifications (physical exercise, no smoking and alcohol excess), vitamin D (400–800 IE daily) and calcium (1 000–1 500 mg/day) supplementation and hormone replacement therapy (oestrogens or selective oestrogens receptor modulators in women; testosterone in hypogonadal men). However, these recommendations are far from fully evaluated. The factors that are known at the present are discussed in the following.

Firstly, vitamin D supplementation is relatively inexpensive and does not necessitate control of calcium levels at regular intervals. It should be considered for all older patients (>60 years) because of the known high prevalence of vitamin D deficiency. In contrast, active vitamin D metabolites are expensive, necessitate control of calcium serum levels and have not been shown to be effective for fracture reduction. Secondly, calcium supplementation does not appear to be essential in patients who are being supplemented with genuine vitamin D. In addition, calcium is not well tolerated. Thirdly, early menopause or male hypogonadism should be corrected with hormone replacement therapy and fourthly, the dose of corticosteroids should be kept to a minimum and non-systemic or controlled-release formulations should be advised [114].

Previous short-term studies have indicated that biphosphonates and slow release sodium fluoride can improve BMD. No effects were seen after 1 year in a randomised study of corticosteroid-using patients with IBD with the administration of calcium and vitamin D alone [115]. One small, randomised placebo-controlled study of 32 CD patients addressed the changes in BMD after a year-long therapy with the oral bisphosphonate alendronate 10 mg/day [116]. After one year, the bone mineral density had increased significantly at the spine in the alendronate-treated group compared with the control group and showed a trend for recovery at the femoral neck. However, several issues have to be considered when interpreting the data of this study. First of all, the patients were selected for disease quiescence, and patients with active disease, whose bone microenvironment may be more exposed to bone-resorbing cytokines or whose ability to absorb oral biphosphonates may be compromised, were excluded. Additionally, although the study was randomised, the alendronate-treated group had significantly higher levels of biochemical markers of bone reabsorption at baseline, which may have improved the response to anti-reabsorptive therapy. There are, however, some encouraging aspects: the favourable response of CD patients to oral and the good tolerability of the drug in these patients. In a more recent randomised controlled study, Von Tirpitz et al. randomised 84 CD patients with reduced BMD to receive calcium citrate (800 mg/day plus vitamin D 1 000 IU/day) alone (n=13) or with either slow release sodium fluoride (25 mg twice daily; n=36) or ibandronate (1 mg intravenously every 3 months; n=35) [117]. The randomisation was unbalanced as patients with osteoporosis were assigned either to the fluoride group or to the ibandronate group. Other problems were the shorter average disease duration in the fluoride group and incomplete follow-up. At 27 months, lumbar bone density increased by 2.6% (p=0.066) for the group given only calcium and vitamin D, 5.7% (p=0.003) for those given fluoride and 5.4% (p=0.003) for those given ibandronate; this effect was particularly evident during the first year. Femoral BMD did not change in any group and no participant suffered a new vertebral fracture. Thirty-five patients who received steroids at least once during the study showed a mean increase in BMD similar to that observed in those who did not receive steroids. A significant correlation was observed between BMI and the BMD during the observational period and improved nutrition may alone contribute to the improvement of BMD (p<0.001), emphasising that treatment of underlying bowel disease and associated improvement of body weight may be important factors in the management of osteoporosis. Bernstein et al. [118] measured the BMD in 46 CD patients treated with infliximab for 1 year. At baseline, reduced BMD occurred in 43% of patients at the lumbar spine and 46% at the left femur; after 1 year of therapy, BMD was significantly increased. BMD gain between the groups with and without osteopenia was not different. Changes in BMD were not correlated to concurrent steroid therapy, calcium supplementation or changes in C-reactive proteins.

Conclusions

Malnutrition is rather frequent in Crohn's disease, particularly in children and in adults with unremitting and/or complicated disease. Several factors can contribute to malnutrition and some of them can be shared by the same patient. Early and/or subtle nutritional changes should be considered in the comprehensive evaluation of patients affected by IBD. Bone changes and increased fracture risk have been described in both Crohn's disease and ulcerative colitis. Though chronic use of steroids has been considered a determinant in BMD impairment, the relationship between steroid administration and fracture risk has recently been questioned. Increasing attention has been focused on the role of the underlying chronic inflammatory process as a major factor of bone disease. In any case, the use of vitamin D and calcium supplementation is highly recommended, especially in those that have been steroid treated and elderly patients. Bisphosphonate can be useful in preventing and treating bone changes, but indications and selection of patients still remains unclear. Further studies on genetic determinants of bone changes in IBD could probably improve our ability in selecting patients for appropriate treatment. On the other hand, it has been shown that maintenance therapy with infliximab can improve BMD, which underscores the role of inflammation in IBD-related bone disease.

A nutritional approach in IBD, namely in Crohn's disease, is not just calorie supplementation [119]. It is mainly recommended in children with active Crohn's disease, where it constitutes a major therapeutic tool, not only in improving nutritional status, but also in favouring clinical remission, in sparing or avoiding steroids, in allowing and accelerating growth, in hastening the onset of puberty (especially if the treatment is started early and in the prepubertal period) and in improving school performance and social activities. In Crohn's disease, EN should be preferred to parenteral treatment due to its lower cost and side effects. Moreover, EN may have the role of primary care in this disorder. Improvement in intestinal permeability and modulation of the inflammatory response are candidates for mechanisms that have a positive effect in active Crohn's disease. An imbalance between Th1 and Th2 (and related cytokines) is considered to be associated with pathological response, and recognition of commensal bacteria contributes to the Th1-Th2 cytokine balance, underscoring that gut bacteria are necessary for maintaining the immune homeostasis. This balance is altered in Crohn's disease, leading to chronic inflammation. However, no information is currently available on the effect of defined EN formulas in modifying or modulating microflora and related action on gut mucosa and inflammatory response.

Comparable clinical results have been shared by different EN formulas, and special formulas have not shown any superiority over "regular" ones. Since the basic composition of polymeric EN does not substantially differ from foods and, although there is evidence of actions on some inflammation-related mechanisms, one might speculate whether the effect is related to specific components, to some balance or imbalance between them or whether it is aspecific and related to the presence of nutrients in an inflamed intestine.

In adult EN, although it offers some alternative to drug therapy for inducing remission, in clinical practice it is actually restricted to patients suffering from severe and persisting anorexia and from malnutrition due to unremitting disease and/or complications. It has not proven to be effective in poor or nonresponders to first-line drug therapy, and few data support its use in patients with suspected or effective food intolerance, not amenable by means of food exclusion diets.

Therapeutic improvement via infliximab in inducing remission and in long-term management of Crohn's disease, in treating fistulas, and its role in promoting better quality of life scores could restrict indications for the nutritional approach as primary care in Crohn's disease. Nutritional care will probably maintain its role in children in complicated cases in which drug therapy (namely steroids) can be associated with a higher rate of long-term side effects on growth, bone and endocrine system. Mechanisms whereby EN formulas have a real therapeutic effect on the immune and inflammatory response represent an intriguing research field for improving our understanding of the pathophysiology of IBD. In a practical setting, oral nutrition should always be preferred and promoted via nutrient and energy dense foods with good calcium content, according to local nutritional habits and individual preferences.

References

1. Sonnenberg A (1992) Disability and need for rehabilitation among patients with inflammatory bowel disease. Digestion 51:168–178
2. Powell-Tuck J, Garlick PJ, Lennard-Jones JE, Waterlow JC (1984) Rates and whole body protein synthesis and breakdown increase with the severity in inflammatory bowel disease. Gut 25:460–464
3. Smith RC, Burkinshaw L, Hill GL (1982) Optimal energy and nitrogen intake for gastroenterological patients requiring intravenous nutrition. Gastroenterology 82:445–452
4. Kirschner BS (1990) Growth and development in chronic inflammatory bowel disease. Acta Pediatr Scand 366:98–104
5. Kanof ME, Alan AL, Bayless TM (1988) Decreased height velocity in children and adolescents before the diagnosis of Crohn's disease. Gastroenterology 95:1523–1527
6. Kirshner BS, Sutton MM (1986) Somatomedin-C levels in growth-impaired children and adolescents with chronic inflammatory bowel disease. Gastroenterology 91:830–836
7. Whittington PF, Barnes HV, Bayless TM (1977) Medical management of Crohn's disease in adolescence. Gastroenterology 72:1338–1344
8. Layden T, Rosenberg J, Nemchausky B et al (1976) Reversal growth arrest in adolescent with Crohn's disease after parenteral alimentation. Gastroenterology 70:1017–1021
9. Grand RJD, Homer DR (1975) Approaches to inflammatory bowel disease in childhood and adolescence. Pediat Clin North Am 22:835–838
10. Kelts DG, Grand RJ, Shen G et al (1979) Nutritional basis of growth failure in children and adolescents with Cohrn's disease. Gastroenterology 76:720–727
11. Strobel CT, Byrne WJ, Ament ME (1979) Home parenteral nutrition in children with Crohn's disease: an effective management alternative. Gastroenterology 77:272–279
12. Mock DM (1986) Growth retardation in chronic inflammatory bowel disease. Gastroenterology 91:1019–1023
13. Homer DR, Grand RJ, Colodny AH (1977) Growth,

course, and prognosis after surgery for Crohn's disease in children and adolescents. Pediatrics 59:717–725
14. Amarnath RP, Fleming CR, Perrault J (1987) Home parenteral nutrition in chronic intestinal diseases: its effect on growth and development. J Pediatr Gastroenterol Nutr 6:89–95
15. Fleming CR, McGill DB, Berkner S (1977) Home parenteral nutrition as primary therapy in patients with extensive Crohn's disease of the small bowel and malnutrition. Gastroenterology 73:1077–1081
16. Siedman EG, Roy CC, Weber AM (1987) Nutritional therapy of Crohn's disease in childhood. Dig Dis Sci 32:82–88
17. Morin CL, Roulet M, Roy CC, Weber A (1980) Continuous elemental enteral alimentation in children with Crohn's disease and growth failure. Gastroenterology 79:1205–1210
18. Kirschner BS, Klich JR, Kalman SS (1981) Reversal of growth retardation in Crohn's disease with therapy emphasizing oral nutrition restitution. Gastroenterology 80:10–15
19. Navarro J, Vargas J, Cezard JP et al (1982) Prolonged constant rate elemental enteral nutrition in Crohn's disease. J Pediatr Gastroenterol Nutr 1:541–546
20. Motil KJ, Grand RJ, Maletskoses CJ, Young VR (1982) The effect of disease, drug and diet on whole body protein metabolism in adolescents with Crohn's disease and growth failure. Pediatrics 101:345–351
21. O'Morain CA, Segal A, Levi AJ (1984) Elemental diet as primary treatment of acute Crohn's disease: a controlled trial. BMJ 288:1859–1862
22. Saverymuttu S, Hodgson HJF, Chadwick VS (1985) Controlled trial comparing prednisolone with an elemental diet plus non-absorbable antibiotics in active Crohn's disease. Gut 26:994–998
23. Belli DC, Seidman E, Bouthillier L et al (1988) Chronic intermittent elemental diet improves growth failure in children with Crohn's disease. Gastroenterology 94:603–610
24. Sanderson IR, Boulton P, Menzies JA, Walker-Smith JA (1987) Improvement of abnormal lactulose/rhamnose permeability in active Crohn's disease of the small bowel by an elemental diet. Gut 28:1073–1076
25. Afonso JJ, Rambeau JL (1990) Nutritional care for patients with Crohn's disease. Hepatogastroenterology 37:32–41
26. Heuschkel RD, Monache CC, Megerian JT, Baird AE (2000) Enteral nutrition and corticosteroids in the treatment of acute Crohn's disease in children. J Pediatr Gastroenterol Nutr 31:8–15
27. Hansen JDL, Freeseman C, Moodie AD, van der Spuy HI (1971) What does nutritional growth retardation imply? Pediatrics 47:299–313
28. Ostro MJ, Greenberg GR, Jeejeebhoy KN (1985) Total parenteral nutrition and complete bowel rest in the management of Crohn's disease. JPEN 9:280–287
29. Greenberg GL, Haber GB, Jeejeebhoy KN (1976) Total parenteral nutrition (TPN) and bowel rest in the management of Crohn's disease. Gut 12:828
30. Elson CO, Layden TJ, Nemchausky BA et al (1980) An evaluation of total parenteral nutrition in the management of inflammatory bowel disease. Dig Dis Sci 25:42–48
31. Muller JM, Keller HW, Erasmi H, Pichlmaier H (1983) Total parenteral nutrition as the sole therapy in Crohn's disease: a prospective study. Br J Surg 70:40–43
32. Lerebours EB, Messing B, Chevalier B et al (1986) An evaluation of total parenteral nutrition in the management of steroid-dependent and steroid-resistant patients with Crohn's disease. JPEN 10:274–278
33. Dickinson RJ, Ashton MG, Axon ATR et al (1980) Controlled trial of intravenous hyperalimentation and total bowel rest as an adjunct to the routine therapy of acute colitis. Gastroeneterology 79:1199–1204
34. McIntyre PB, Powell-Tuck J, Wood SR et al (1986) Controlled trial of bowel rest in the treatment of severe acute colitis. Gut 27:481–485
35. Driscoll RH Jr, Rosenberg IH (1978) Total parenteral nutrition in inflammatory bowel disease. Med Clin North Am 62:185–201
36. Gouma DJ, Meyenfeldt MF, Rouflart M, Soeters PB (1988) Preoperative total parenteral nutrition (TPN) in severe Crohn's disease. Surgery 103:648–652
37. Mullen JL, Hargrove C, Dudrick SJ et al (1978) Ten years experience with intravenous hyperalimentation and inflammatory bowel disease. Ann Surg 187:523–529
38. Dudrick SJ, Latifi R, Schrager R (1991): Nutritional management of inflammatory bowel disease. Surg Clin North Am 71:609–623
39. Shiloni E, Coronado E, Freund HR (1989) Role of total parenteral nutrition in the treatment of Crohn's disease. Am J Surg 157:180–185
40. Bos LP, Weterman I (1980) Total parenteral nutrition in Crohn's disease. World J Surg 4:163–166
41. Eisenberg HW, Turnbull RB, Weakley FL (1974) Hyperalimentation as preparation for surgery in transmural colitis (Crohn's disease). Dis Colon Rectum 17:469–475
42. Rombeau JL, Rondanelli R (1987) Enteral and parenteral nutrition in patients with enteric fistulas and short bowel syndrome. Surg Clin North Am 67:551–571
43. Klein S (1993) Nutritional therapy for patients with gastrointestinal diseases. In: Sleisenger MH, Fordtran JS (eds) Gastrointestinal disease. Saunders, Philadelphia
44. Voitk AJ, Echave V, Feller JH et al (1974) Experience with elemental diet in the treatment of inflammatory bowel disease. Arch Surg 107:329–333
45. Lashner BA, Evans AA, Hanauer SB (1989) Preoperative total parenteral nutrition for bowel resection in Crohn's disease. Dig Dis Sci 34:741–746
46. Shiloni E, Freund HR (1983) Total parenteral nutrition in Crohn's disease: Is it a primary or supportive mode of therapy? Dis Colon Rectum 26:275–278
47. Vogel CM, Corwin TR, Baue AE (1974) Intravenous hyperalimentation in the treatment of inflammatory diseases of the bowel. Arch Surg 108:460–467
48. Dean RE, Campos MM, Barret B (1976) Hyperalimentation in the management of chronic inflammatory bowel disease. Dis Colon Rectum 19:601–604
49. Sanderson IR, Udeen S, Davies PSW et al (1987) Remission induced by an elemental diet in small bowel Crohn's disease. Arch Dis Chil 61:123–127
50. Babb RR (1978) The role of parenteral nutrition in the treatment of inflammatory bowel disease. Am J Gastroenterol 70:506–509

51. Matuchanski C (1986) Parenteral nutrition in inflammatory bowel disease. Gut 27:81–84
52. Alun Jones V (1987) Comparison of total parenteral nutrition and elemental diet in induction remission of Crohn's disease: long-term maintenance of remission by personalized food exclusion diets. Dig Dis Sci 32:S100–S107
53. Wright RA, Adler EC (1990) Peripheral parenteral nutrition is no better than enteral nutrition in acute exacerbation of Crohn's disease. J Clin Gastroenterol 12:396
54. Lochs H, Meryn S, Marosi L (1983) Has total bowel rest a beneficial effect in the treatment of Crohn's disease? Clin Nutr 2:61
55. Greenberg GR, Fleming CR, Jeejeebhoy KN et al (1988) Controlled trial of bowel rest and nutritional support in the management of Crohn's disease. Gut 29:1309–1315
56. McIntyre PB, Powell-Tuck J, Wood SR et al (1986) Controlled trial of bowel rest in the treatment of severe acute colitis. Gut 27:481–485
57. Hollander D, Vadheim C, Brettholz E et al (1986) Increased intestinal permeability in patients with Crohn's disease and their relatives. Ann Intern Med 105:883–885
58. Lochs H, Steinhardt HJ, Klaus-Wentz B et al (1991) Comparison of enteral nutrition and drug treatment in active Crohn's disease: results of the European Cooperative Crohn's Disease Study IV. Gastroenterology 101:861–888
59. Malchow H, Steinhardt HJ, Lorenz-Meyer H et al (1990) Feasibility and effectiveness of a defined-formula diet regimen in treating active Crohn's disease: European Cooperative Crohn's Disease Study III. Scand J Gastroenterol 25:235–244
60. Teahaon K, Smethurst P, Pearson M et al (1991) The effect of elemental diet on intestinal permeability and inflammation in Crohn's disease. Gastroenterology 101:84–89
61. Seidman EG, Boutillier L, Weber AM et al (1986) Elemental diet versus prednisone as primary treatment of Crohn's disease. Gastroenterology 90:A1625
62. Okada M, Yao T, Yamamoto T et al (1990) Controlled trial comparing elemental diet with prednisolone in the treatment of active Crohn's disease. Hepato-Gastroenterol 37:72–80
63. Gorard DA, Hunt JB, Payne-James JJ et al (1993) Initial response and subsequent course of Crohn's disease treated with elemental diet or prednisolone. Gut 34:1198–1202
64. Gorard DA, Hunt JB, Payne-James JJ et al (1991) Early response and subsequent course of Crohn's disease treated with elemental diet or prednisolone: a controlled trial. Gut 100:A213
65. Tehaon K, Bjarnason I, Pearson M, Levi AJ (1990) Ten years' experience with an elemental diet in the management of Crohn's disease. Gut 31:1133–1137
66. Middleton SJ, Riordan AM, Hunter JO (1991) Comparison of elemental and peptide-based diets in the treatment of acute Crohn's disease. Ital J Gastroenterol 23:609
67. Royall D, Kahan I, Baker JP et al (1992) Clinical and nutritional outcome of an elemental versus semi-elemental diet in active Crohn's disease. Gastroenterology 10:A576
68. Lochs H, Steinhardt HJ, Kiaus-Wentz B et al (1991) Comparison of enteral nutrition and drug treatment in active Crohn's disease: results of the European Cooperative Crohn's Disease Study IV. Gastroenterology 101:861–888
69. Giaffer MH, North G, Holdsworth CD (1990) Controlled trial of polymeric versus elemental diet in treatment of active Crohn's disease. Lancet 335:816–819
70. Bodemar G, Nillson L, Smedh K, Larsonn J (1991) Nasogastric feeding with polymeric, whole protein low fat diet in Crohn's disease. J Clin Nutr Gastroenterol 6:75–83
71. Park RHR, Galloway A, Danesh BJZ, Russell RI (1991) Double-blind controlled trial of elemental diet and polymeric diets as primary treatment in active Crohn's disease. Eur J Gastroenterol Hepatol 3:483–490
72. Gonzales-Huix F, de Leon R, Fernandez-Benares F et al (1993) Polymeric enteral diets as primary treatment of active Crohn's disease: a prospective steroid controlled trial. Gut 34:778–782
73. Raouf AH, Hildrey V, Walker RJ et al (1991) Enteral feeding as sole treatment for Crohn's disease: controlled trial of whole protein v. amino acid based feed and a case study of dietary challenge. Gut 32:702–707
74. Yamamoto T, Nakahigashi M, Umegae S et al (2005) Impact of elemental diet on mucosal inflammation in patients with active Crohn's disease: cytokine production and endoscopic and histological findings. Inflamm Bowel Dis 6:580–588
75. Meister D, Bode J, Shand A, Ghosh S (2002) Anti-inflammatory effects of enteral diet components on Crohn's disease-affected tissues in vitro. Dig Liver Dis 34:430–438
76. Bannerjee K, Comacho-Hubner C, Babinska K et al (2004) Anti-inflammatory and growth-stimulating effects precede nutritional restitution during enteral feeding in Crohn's disease. J Pediatr Gastroenterol Nutr 38:270–275
77. Atreya R, Mudter J, Finotto S et al (2000) Blockade of interleukin 6 trans signaling suppresses T-cell resistance against apoptosis in chronic intestinal inflammation: evidence in Crohn's disease and experimental colitis in vivo. Nat Med 6:583–588
78. Sylverster FA, Wizga N, Hyams JD, Gronowicz GA (2002) Effect of Crohn's disease on bone metabolism in vitro: a role for interleukin-6. J Bone Miner Res 17:695–702
79. De Benedetti F, Alonzi T, Moretta A et al (1997): Interleukin 6 causes growth impairment in transgenic mice through a decrease in insulin-like growth factor-I: a model of stunted growth in children with chronic inflammation. J Clin Invest 99:643–650
80. Thomas AG, Holly JM, Taylor F, Miller V (1993) Insulin like growth factor-I, insulin like growth factor binding protein-1, and insulin in childhood Crohn's disease. Gut 34:944–947
81. Rigaud D, Cosnes J, Le Quintrec Y et al (1991) Controlled trial comparing two types of enteral nutrition in treatment of active Crohn's disease: elemental vs. polymeric diet. Gut 32:1492–1497
82. Fernandez-Banares F, Cabrè E, Gonzalez-Huix F, Gassull MA (1994) Enteral nutrition as primary therapy in

Crohn's disease. Gut 1:S55–S59
83. Vilaseca J, Salas A, Guarner F, Rodriguez R et al (1990) Dietary fish oil reduces progression of chronic inflammatory lesions in a rat model of granulomatous colitis. Gut 31:539–544
84. Kremer JM, Jubiz W, Michalek A et al (1987) Fish-oil fatty acid supplementation in active rheumatoid arthritis. Ann Intern Med 106:497–503
85. Whiting CV, Bland PW, Tarlton JF (2005) Dietary n-3 polyunsaturated fatty acids reduces disease and colonic proinflammatory cytokines in a mouse model of colitis. Inflamm Bowel Dis 11:340–349
86. Esteve-Comas M, Ramirez M, Fernandez-Benares F et al (1992) Plasma polyunsaturated fatty acid pattern in inflammatory bowel disease. Gut 33:1365–1369
87. Bernstein CN, Leslie WD (2004) Review article: osteoporosis and inflammatory bowel disease. Aliment Pharmacol Ther 19:941–952
88. Bernstein CN, Leslie WD LeBoff MS (2003) AGA technical review on osteoporosis in gastrointestinal diseases. Gastroenterology 124:795–841
89. Vestergaard P, Krogh K , Rejnmark L et al (2000) Fracture risk is increased in Crohn's disease but not in ulcerative colitis. Gut 46:176–181
90. Vestergaard P, Mosekilde L (2002) Fracture risk among patients with celiac disease, Crohn's disease and ulcerative colitis: a nationwide follow-up study of 16,416 patients in Denmark. Am J Epidemiol 156:1–10
91. Bernstein CN Blanchard JF, leslie W et al (2000) The incidence of fractures among patients with inflammatory bowel disease: a population based cohort study Ann Intern Med 133:795–799
92. Loftus EV Jr, Crowson CS, Sandborn WJ et al (2002) Long-term fracture risk in patients with Crohn's disease: a population based-study in Olmsted County, Minnesota. Gastroenterology 123:468–475
93. Van Staa TP, Cooper C, Brusse LS et al (2003) Inflammatory bowel disease and the risk of fracture. Gastroenterology 125:1591–1597
94. Bernstein CN, Leslie WD, Tabacck SP (2003) Bone density in a population-based cohort of premenopausal adult women with early onset inflammatory disease Am J Gastroenterology 98:1094–1100
95. Gosh S, Cowen S, Hannah WJ, Ferguson A (1994) Low bone mineral density in Crohn's disease, but not in ulcerative colitis, at diagnosis. Gastroenterology 107:1031–1039
96. Schoon EJ, Block BM, Geerling BJ et al (2000) Bone mineral density in patients with recently diagnosed inflammatory bowel disease. Gastroenterology 19:1203–1208
97. Lamb EJ, Wong T, Smith DJ (2002) Metabolic bone disease is present at diagnosis in patients with inflammatory bowel disease. Aliment Pharmacol Ther 16:1895–1902
98. Bernstein CN, Bector S, Leslie WD (2003) Lack of relationship of calcium and vitamin D intake to bone mineral density in premenopausal women with inflammatory bowel disease. Am J Gastroenterol 98:2468–2473
99. Habtezion A, Silverberg MS, Parkes R et al (2002) Risk factors for low bone density in Crohn's disease. Inflamm Bowel Dis 8:87–92
100. Andreassen H, Rix M, Brot C, Eskildsen P (1998) Regulators of calcium homeostasis and bone mineral density in patient's with Crohn's disease. Scand J Gastroenterol 33:1087–1093
101. Vogelsang H, Schofl R (1997) 25-hydroxy-vitamin D absorption in patients with Crohn's disease and with pancreatic insufficiency. Wien Klin Wochesnschr 109:678–682
102. Compston JE, Judd D (1987) Osteoporosis in patients with inflammatory bowel disease. Gut 28:410–415
103. Andreassen H, Rungby J, Dahlerup JF, Mosekilde L (1997) Inflammatory bowel disease and osteoporosis. Scand J Gastroenterol 32:1247–1255
104. Silovennd Bnoinen J (1996) Relationship between vitamin D, parathyroid hormone and bone mineral density in inflammatory bowel disease. J Intern Med 239:131–137
105. Abitbol V, Roux C, Chaussade S et al (1995) Metabolic bone assessment in patients with inflammatory bowel disease. Gastroenterology 108:417–422
106. Bernstein CN, Seeger LL, Sayre JW et al (1995) Decreased bone density in inflammatory bowel disease is related to corticosteroid use and not disease diagnosis. J Bone Miner Res 10:250–256
107. Reid IR (2002) Relationships among body mass index, its components, and bone. Bone 31:547–555
108. Espallargues M, Sampietro-Colom L, Estrada MD (2001) Identifying bone-mass related risk factors for fracture to guide bone densitometry: a systematic review of the literature. Osteoporos Int 12:811–822
109. Jahnsen J, Falch JA, Mowinckel P, Aadland E (2003) Body composition in patients with inflammatory bowel disease: a population-based study. Am J Gastroenterol 98:1556–1562
110. Habtezion A, Silverberg MS, Parkes R et al (2002) Risk factors for low bone density in Crohn's disease. Inflamm Bowel Dis 8:87–92
111. Schulte CM, Dignass AU, Goebell H et al (2000) Genetic factors determines the extent of bone loss in inflammatory bowel disease. Gastroenterology 119:909–920
112. Schulte CM (2004) Review article: bone disease in inflammatory bowel disease. Aliment Pharmacol Ther 20(Suppl 4):43–49
112. Todhunter CE, Sutherland-Craggs A, Bartram SA et al (2005) Influence of IL6, COL1A, and VDR gene polymorphisms on bone mineral density in Crohn's disease. Gut (54):1579–1584
113. Mann V, Hobson E, Li B et al (2001) A COL1A1 Sp1 binding site polymorphism predisposes to osteoporotic fracture by affecting bone density and quality. J Clin Invest 107:899–907
114. Scott EM, Gaywood I, Scott BB (2000) Guidelines for osteoporosis in coeliac disease and inflammatory bowel disease. Gut 46(Suppl 1):i1–i8
115. Bernstein CN, Seeger LL, Anton PA et al (1996) A randomized placebo controlled-trial of calcium suplemetation for decreased bone density in corticosteroid-using patients with inflammatory bowel disease: a pilot study. Aliment Pharmacol Ther 10:777–786
116. Haderslev KV, Tjellesen L, Sorensen HA, Staun M (2000) Alendronate increases lumbar spine bone mineral density in patient's with Crohn's disease. Gastroenterology 119:639–46
117. Von Tirpitz C, Klaus J, Steinkamp M et al (2003) Ther-

apy of osteoporosis in patients with Crohn's disease: a randomized study comparing sodium fluoride and ibandronate. Aliment Phamacol Ther 17:807–816

118. Bernstein M, Irwin S, Greenberg GR (2005) Maintenance infliximab treatment is associated with improved bone mineral density in Crohn's disease. Am J Gastroenterol 100:2031–2035

119. Heuschekel R (2004) Enteral nutrition in Crohn's disease: more than just calories. J Pediatr Gastroenterol Nutr 38:239–241

Probiotics in Inflammatory Bowel Diseases

Paolo Gionchetti, Fernando Rizzello, Claudia Morselli, Rosy Tambasco, Massimo Campieri

Introduction

The rationale for using probiotics in inflammatory bowel disease (IBD) is based on convincing evidence implicating intestinal bacteria in their pathogenesis. The distal ileum and the colon are the areas with the highest bacterial concentrations and represent the sites of inflammation in IBD; similarly pouchitis, the non-specific inflammation of the ileal reservoir after ileo-anal anastomosis, appears to be associated with bacterial overgrowth and dysbiosis. Enteric bacteria or their products have been found within the inflamed mucosa of patients with Crohn's disease (CD) [1].

There is evidence of a loss of immunologic tolerance to commensal bacteria in patients with IBD [2, 3]. Patients with CD respond consistently to diversion of the faecal stream, with immediate recurrence of inflammation after restoration of intestinal continuity [4] or infusion of luminal content into the bypassed ileum [5], and pouchitis does not occur before the ileostomy closure.

Patients with IBD have altered composition of enteric flora with increase of aggressive bacteria such as *Bacterioides*, adherent/invasive *Escherichia coli*, *Enterococci*, and decrease of protective *Lactobacillus* and *Bifidobacterium* species [6]. However, the most compelling evidence is derived from animal models; despite great diversity in genetic defects and immunopathology, a consistent feature of many transgenic and knockout mutant murine models of colitis is dependency on the presence of normal enteric flora for full expression of inflammation [7]. All these observations have suggested the possibility of preventing or treating IBD by manipulating intestinal microflora and increasing evidence supports the potential therapeutic role of probiotics in IBD [8].

Probiotics

The first to propose the use of probiotics for the purpose of health maintenance and disease prevention was Elie Metchnikoff, the Russian Nobel Prize winner, who at the turn of the last century suggested that high concentration of *Lactobacilli* in the intestinal flora was important for health and longevity in humans [9]. Probiotics are defined as "living organisms, which upon ingestion in certain numbers, exert health benefits beyond inherent basic nutrition" [10].

Table 1. Organisms associated with probiotic activity

Lactobacilli
Bifidobacteria
Streptococci
Others bacterial strains
Enterococci, non-pathogenic *E. coli*
Non bacterial organisms
Yeasts (*Saccharomyces boulardii*)

Bacteria associated with probiotic activity are most commonly *Lactobacilli*, *Bifidobacteria* and *Streptococci* but other non-pathogenic bacteria such as some strains of Escherichia coli and non-bacterial organisms such as the yeast *Saccharomyces boulardii* have been used (Table 1). For clinical application probiotic strains must possess certain characteristics. They need to be resistant to acid and bile, and must have the ability to be metabolically active within the luminal flora, where, ideally, they should survive, but not persist in the long term. They should be antagonistic against pathogenic bacteria and, obviously, they must be safe for human use and should maintain their viability and beneficial properties during manufacturing processes [11].

Mechanisms of Action

Several mechanisms have been proposed to account for probiotic action including the antagonistic activity against pathogenic bacteria either by inhibition of adherence and translocation or by production of anti-bacterial substances such as anti-microbial pep-

Table 2. Mechanisms of action of probiotics

Inhibits pathogenic enteric bacteria
Decreases luminal pH
Secretes bacteriocidal proteins
Colonisation resistance
Blocks epithelial binding
Improves epithelial and mucosal barrier function
Produces SCFA
Enhances mucus production
Increases barrier integrity
Alters immunoregulation
Increases IL-10 and TGFβ and decreases TNF
Increases IgA production

tides (bacteriocins) and hydrogen peroxide. Probiotics also stimulate mucosal defence both at the level of immune and epithelial function with an increase in sIgA production, blockade of pro-inflammatory cytokines, enhancement of anti-inflammatory cytokines levels, stimulation of intestinal mucin expression and improvement of gut permeability. Finally they are able to produce nutrients of special importance to the intestine such as short-chain fatty acids and vitamins (Table 2).

Animal Models Studies

Encouraging results have been obtained with probiotic therapy in experimental colitis. Administration of *Lactobacillus reuteri* was shown to significantly reduce inflammation in acetic acid- and methotrexate-induced colitis in rats [12, 13]. More recently *Lactobacillus sp.* was shown to be able to prevent the development of spontaneous colitis in interleukin-10 (IL-10) deficient mice [14], and continuous feeding with *Lactobacillus plantarum* could attenuate an established colitis in the same knockout model [15]. A strain of *Lactobacillus salivarius* (subsp. *Saliva rius*) reduced the rate of progression from inflammation through dysplasia and colonic cancer in IL-10 deficient mice [16], and a strain of *Bifidobacterium, infantis* and of *Lactobacillus salivarius* were able to attenuate inflammation with a reduced ability to produce Th1-type cytokines in the IL-10 knockout model [17]. Using a cocktail of probiotic bacteria (VSL#3), Shibolet and colleagues have shown a significant attenuation of inflammation with a decrease of MPO (myeloperoxidase) and NOS (nitric oxide synthase) activity in iodoacetamide-induced colitis in rats [18], while Madsen and colleagues have reported a significant improvement of inflammation together with a reduction in mucosal levels of pro-inflammatory cytokines and a normalization of colonic barrier integrity in IL-10 KO mice [19].

Ulcerative Colitis

The efficacy of a non-pathogenic strain of *Escherichia coli* Nissle 1917 in the treatment of IBD has been tested in three recent trials. In the other three controlled studies, *E. coli* Nissle 1917 has been found to exhibit efficacy similar to that of mesalazine in maintenance treatment of ulcerative colitis (UC) [20–22].

We have explored another strategy, using a probiotic preparation (VSL#3) characterised by very high bacterial concentration (each packet containing 450 billion viable bacteria) and the presence of a cocktail of eight different bacterial species. This product contains viable lyophilised bacteria of four strains of *Lactobacilli* (*L. casei*, *L. plantarum*, *L. acidophilus*, *L. delbrueckii* subsp. *Bulgaricus*), three strains of *Bifidobacteria* (*B. longum*, *B. breve*, *B. infantis*) and one strain of *Streptococcus salivarius* subsp. *Thermophilus*.

We carried-out a pilot study using VSL#3 as maintenance treatment in patients with UC in remission, who are allergic or intolerant to sulphasalazine and mesalazine, to verify the impact on the faecal flora of this preparation. Twenty patients received 6 g per day of VSL#3 (1 800 billion bacteria) for 12 months and were assessed clinically and endoscopically at baseline and at 6 and 12 months or in case of relapse. Stool culture and determination of faecal pH were also performed at different intervals.

Microbiological determination showed a significant increase in concentration of *Lactobacilli*, *Bifidobacteria* and *Streptococcus thermophilus*, which was already evident after 20 days and persisted through the treatment period with return to basal levels within 15 days after stopping the treatment without modification of the faecal concentration of *Bacteroides*, *Enterococci*, *Coliforms*, *Clostridia* and the total anaerobes and aerobes. Faecal pH was significantly reduced by the treatment and 15 of the 20 patients (75%) remained in remission [23].

In an uncontrolled pilot study VSL#3, at a very high dose (3 600 billion), was able to induce remission in 63%, with a positive response in another 23% of patients with active mild-to-moderate disease [24]. Similarly, in an open, uncontrolled 4-week study, the yeast *Saccharomyces boulardii* induced remission in 71% of patients with mild to moderate ulcerative colitis [25].

Pouchitis

In a double-blind study, we have compared the efficacy of VSL#3 with placebo in the maintenance treatment of chronic pouchitis. Forty patients who obtained clinical and endoscopic remission after 1 month of combined antibiotic treatment (rifaximin 2 g/day plus ciprofloxacin 1 g/day) were randomised to receive VSL#3 6 g daily (1 800 billion bacteria/day) or an identical appearing placebo for 9 months. Clinical assessment was done every month; endoscopic and histological assessment were performed at entry and every 2 months thereafter. Stool culture was done before and after antibiotic treatment and subsequently every month during maintenance treatment. Relapse was defined as an increase of at least 2 points in the clinical portion of pouchitis activity index that should be confirmed endoscopically and histologically. All the 20 patients treated with placebo had a relapse in the follow-up period; in contrast 17 of the 20 (85%) patients treated with VSL#3 were still in remission after 9 months. Interestingly, all these 17 patients had a relapse within 4 months after suspension of the active treatment. Faecal concentration of *Lactobacilli*, *Bifidobacteria* and *Streptococcus salivarius subsp.* Thermophilus were significantly increased within 1 month after starting VSL#3 treatment and remained stable throughout the study. However, this increase did not affect concentration of the other bacterial groups, suggesting that the effect was not mediated by suppression of endogenous luminal bacteria [26]. These results have been recently replicated by a study evaluating the efficacy of VSL#3 in maintaining antibiotic-induced remission (obtained after a 1-month treatment with metronidazole 800 mg/day plus ciprofloxacin 1 g/day) for 1 year in patients with refractory or recurrent pouchitis: 20 patients received VSL#3 1 800 billion bacteria once a day for one year and 16 patients received a placebo during the same period. Clinical, endoscopic and histological evaluations were made before, 2 and 12 months after the randomisation. A parallel assessment of the quality of life (QoL) was obtained with IBDQ. This study has substantially confirmed the observations made previously, with maintenance remission rate at 1 year for 85% in the VSL#3 group and 6% in the placebo group. A high QoL score was obtained by the group treated with VSL#3 [27].

As regards the mechanisms of action, in these patients we found that continuous administration of VSL#3 determined a significant increase of IL-10 tissue levels together with a significant decrease of tissue levels of the pro-inflammatory cytokines TNF alfa, IL-1 and IFN gamma, and a decrease of matrix metalloproteinase activity [28]. On the other hand, *Lactobacillus GG* was ineffective in preventing relapses in patients with chronic pouchitis in a placebo-controlled trial [29].

We have also carried-out a double-blind placebo controlled trial to evaluate the efficacy of VSL#3 in the prevention of pouchitis onset in patients operated for ileal pouch-anal anastomosis (IPAA) for UC. Within 1 week after ileostomy closure, 40 patients, were randomised to receive VSL#3 3 g per day (900 billion bacteria/day) or an identical placebo for 12 months; patients were assessed clinically endoscopically and histologically at 1, 3, 6, 9, 12 months according to PDAI.

Patients treated with VSL#3 had a significantly lower incidence of acute pouchitis compared to those treated with placebo during the first year after ileostomy closure (10 *vs.* 40%; $p<0.05$). Moreover, IBDQ was significantly improved only in the group treated with VSL#3, and median stool frequency in patients who did not develop pouchitis, was significantly less in the VSL#3 group compared to the placebo group [30].

Crohn's Disease

Results with probiotics in Crohn's disease are conflicting. In a small pilot study, treatment with capsules containing *E. coli* Nissle 1917 was compared to the administration of placebo in maintenance of steroid-induced remission of colonic CD. Twelve patients were treated with *E. coli* Nissle 1917 and 11 with placebo; at the end of the treatment period (12 weeks) relapse rates were 33% in the *E. coli* group and 63% in the placebo group, but unfortunately, because of the very small number of patients treated this difference did not reach statistical significance [31].

In a small comparative open study, the association of *Saccharomyces boulardii* 1 g/day plus mesalamine 2 g/day was significantly superior to mesalamine 3 g/day in maintenance of remission in a 6-month trial [32]. Prantera et al. have reported no benefit for *Lactobacillus GG* in preventing post-operative recurrence [33] in 1-year double-blind placebo-controlled trial. Additionally, more recently the same strain was shown not to be superior to placebo as an adjunct to standard treatment in the maintenance of medically induced remission in children [34].

We carried-out a single-blind study to compare a sequential antibiotic-probiotic treatment with mesalazine in the prevention of the post-operative recurrence of CD; 40 patients within 1 week after curative surgery were randomised to receive a high dose of rifaximin, a non-absorbable wide spectrum antibiotic, for 3 months followed by VSL#3 6 g per day for 9 months or mesalazine 4 g per day for 12 months. Patients were assessed clinically and endoscopically at 3 and 12 months; the combined antibiotic-probiotic treatment determined a significant lower incidence of severe endoscopic recurrence both at 3 and 12 months (10% and 20% *vs.* 40% and 40%, respectively; $p<0.01$) [35].

Conclusions

Many clinical and experimental observations do suggest an involvement of the intestinal microflora in the pathogenesis and in the perpetuation of IBD. Probiotics may provide a simple and attractive way to prevent or treat IBD, and patients find the probiotic concept appealing because it is safe, non-toxic and natural. A highly concentrated cocktail of probiotics (VSL#3) is effective in the prevention of pouchitis onset and relapses. Results in ulcerative colitis are promising both in prevention of relapses and treatment of mild to moderate attacks. Results in Crohn's disease are not yet clear because of conflicting data and the limited number of well-performed studies.

It is important to select a well-characterised probiotic preparation; in fact viability and survival of bacteria in many available preparations are unproven. It should be remembered that the beneficial effect of one probiotic preparation does not imply the efficacy of other preparations containing different bacterial strains, because each individual probiotic strain has unique biological properties. There is the need to improve our knowledge on the composition of enteric flora or "the neglected organ" and of the intestinal physiology and its relationship with the luminal ecosystem.

References

1. Guarner F, Casellas F, Borruel N et al (2002) Role of microecology in chronic inflammatory bowel diseases. Eur J Clin Nutr 56(Suppl 4):S34–S38
2. Duchmann R, Kaiser I, Hermann E et al (1995) Tolerance exists towards resident intestinal flora but is broken in active inflammatory bowel disease (IBD). Clin Exp Immunol 102:104–108
3. MacPherson A, Khoo UY, Forgacs I et al (1996) Mucosal antibodies in inflammatory bowel disease are directed against intestinal bacteria. Gut 38:365–375
4. Janowitz HD, Croen EC, Sachar DB (1998) The role of the faecal stream in Crohn's disease: an historical and analytic perspective. Inflamm Bowel Dis 4:29–39
5. D'Haens GR, Geboes K, Peeters M et al (1998) Early lesions of recurrent Crohn's disease caused by infusion of intestinal contents in excluded ileum. Gastroenterology 114:771–774
6. Neut C, Bulois P, Desreumaux P et al (2002) Changes in the bacterial flora of the neoterminal ileum after ileocolonic resection for Crohn's disease. Am J Gastroenterol 97:939–946
7. Sartor RB (1995) Insights into the pathogenesis of inflammatory bowel disease provided by new rodent models of spontaneous colitis. Inflam Bowel Dis 1:64–75
8. Campieri M, Gionchetti P(1999) Probiotics in inflammatory bowel disease: new insight to pathogenesis or a possible therapeutic alternative? Gastroenterology 116:1246–1249
9. Metchnikoff E (1907) The prolongation of life: optimistic studies. Heinemann, London, pp 161-183
10. Schaafsma G (1996) State of the art concerning probiotic strains in milk products. IDF Nutr News l5:23–42
11. Lee YK, Salminen S (1995) The coming age of probiotics. Trends Food Sci Technol 6:241–245
12. Fabia R, Ar'rajab A, Johansson M-L et al (1993) The effect of exogenous administration of *Lactobacillus reuterii* R2LC and oat fiber on acetic acid-induced colitis in the rat. Scand J Gastroenterol 28:155–162
13. Mao Y, Nobaek S, Kasravi B et al (1996) The effects of *Lactobacillus* strains and oat fibre on methotrexate-induced enterocolitis in rats. Gastroenterology 111:334–344
14. Madsen KL, Tavernini MM, Doyle JSG, Fedorak RN (1999) *Lactobacillus* sp prevents development of enterocolitis in interleukin-10 gene-deficient mice. Gastroenterology 116:1107–1114
15. Schultz M, Veltkamp C, Dieleman LA et al (2002) *Lactobacillus plantarum* 299V in the treatment and prevention of spontaneous colitis in interleukin-10 deficient mice. Inflamm Bowel Dis 8:71–80
16. O'Mahony L, Feenex M, O'Halloran S et al (2001) Probiotic impact on microbial flora, inflammation and tumour development in IL-10 knockout mice. Aliment Pharmacol Ther 15:1219–1225
17. McCarthy J, O'Mahony L, O'Callaghan L et al (2003) Double-blind, placebo-controlled trial of two probiotic strains in interleukin 10 knockout mice and mechanistic link with cytokine balance. Gut 52:975–980
18. Shibolet O, Karmeli F, Eliakim R et al (2002) Variable response to probiotics in two models of experimental colitis in rats. Inflamm Bowel Dis 8:399–408
19. Madsen K, Cornish A, Soper P et al (2001) Probiotic bacteria enhance murine and human intestinal epithelial barrier function. Gastroenterology 121:580–591
20. Kruis W, Schuts E, Fric P (1997) Double-blind comparison of an oral Escherichia coli preparation and mesalazine in maintaining remission of ulcerative colitis. Aliment Pharmacol Ther 11:853–858
21. Rembacken BJ, Snelling AM, Hawkey P (1999) Non pathogenic Escherichia coli vs mesalazine for the treatment of ulcerative colitis: a randomised trial. Lancet 354:635-639
22. Kruis W, Fric P, Potrotnieks J et al (2004)Maintaining remission of ulcerative colitis with *Escherichia Coli* Nissle 1917 is as effective as with standard mesalazine. Gut 53:1673–1623
23. Venturi A, Gionchetti P, Rizzello F et al (1999) Impact on the faecal flora composition of a new probiotic preparation. Preliminary data on maintenance treatment of patients with ulcerative colitis (UC) intolerant or allergic to 5-aminosalicylic acid (5 ASA). Aliment Pharmacol Ther 13:1103–1108
24. Bibiloni R, Federak RN, Tannock GW et al (2005) VSL#3 probiotic-mixture induces remission in patients with active ulcerative colitis. AM J Gastroenterol 100(7):1539–1546

25. Guslandi M, Giollo P, Testoni PA (2003) A pilot trial of *Saccharomyces boulardii* in ulcerative colitis. Eur J Gastroenterol Hepatol 15:697–698
26. Gionchetti P, Rizzello F, Venturi A et al (2000) Oral bacteriotherapy as maintenance treatment in patients with chronic pouchitis: a double-blind, placebo-controlled trial. Gastroenterology 119:305–309
27. Mimura t, Rizzello F, Helwig U et al (2004) Once daily high dose probiotic therapy for maintaining remission in recurrent or refractory pouchitis. Gut 53:108–114
28. Ulisse S, Gionchetti P, D'Alò S et al (2001) Increased expression of cytokines, inducible nitric oxide synthase and matrix metalloproteinases in pouchitis: effects of probiotic treatment (VSL#3). Gastroenterology 120(Suppl):A281
29. Kuisma J, Mentula S, Kahri A et al (2003) Effect of *Lactobacillus rhamnosus GG* on ileal pouch inflammation and microbial flora. Aliment Pharmacol Ther 17:509–515
30. Gionchetti P, Rizzello F, Venturi A et al (2000) Prophylaxis of pouchitis onset with probiotic therapy: a double blind, placebo controlled trial. Gastroenterology 118:A190
31. Malchow HA (1997) Crohn's disease and *Escherichia coli.* a new approach in therapy to maintain remission of colonic Crohn's disease? J Clin Gastroenterol 25:653–658
32. Guslandi M, Mezzi G, Sorghi M et al (2000) *Saccharomyces boulardii* in maintenance treatment of Crohn's disease. Dig Dis Sci 45:1462–1464
33. Prantera C, Scribano ML, Falasco G et al (2002) Ineffectiveness of probiotics in preventing recurrence after curative resection for Crohn's disease: a randomised controlled trial with *Lactobacillus GG.* Gut 51:405–409
34. Bousvaros A, Guandalini S, Baldassano RN et al (2005)A randomised, double-blind trial of *Lactobacillus GG* versus placebo in addition to standard maintenance therapy for children with Crohn's disease. Inflamm Bowel Dis 11:833–839
35. Campieri M, Rizzello F, Venturi A et al (2000) Combination of antibiotic and probiotic treatment is efficacious in prophylaxis of post-operative recurrence of Crohn's disease: a randomised controlled study vs. mesalazine. Gastroenterology 118:A781

Quality of Life in Patients Undergoing Colorectal Surgery

Mike Keighley

Introduction

The issues that most concern patients requiring colorectal surgery are as follows:

1. The fear of cancer.
2. The fear of having a permanent intestinal stoma.
3. The fear of bowel incontinence.

The problem in evaluating quality of life issues in colorectal surgery are largely based on the methodology used for assessing quality of life. Most assessments of quality of life are based on questionnaires. Sometimes these questionnaires are difficult to interpret and difficult to understand. Face-to-face interviews often provide more in depth information but the results of interviews are difficult to quantify. In essence, quality of life assessment attempts to numerically assess abstract issues.

Spectrum of Inflammatory Bowel Disease

The spectrum of inflammatory bowel disease results in major differences with respect to quality of life among patients with ulcerative colitis compared to those with Crohn's disease. In ulcerative colitis, only the colon and rectum is involved, the sphincters are spared and there is no small-bowel involvement. Although many of these patients present with acute fulminating colitis requiring an emergency colectomy, a high proportion of these patients can today be reassured that the stoma might be temporary and that there is an 80–95% chance of full continence, albeit with some diarrhoea after colorectal excision and pouch construction. There is of course a risk of malignancy and there is the risk that conventional surgery may be associated with complications resulting in a permanent stoma.

At the other end of the spectrum is Crohn's disease, which may affect any part of the gastrointestinal tract. The anal sphincters are commonly affected. There is a high risk of incontinence and repeated operations for recurrence. There is particularly a high risk of unavoidable complications: abscess, obstruction and fistula. Surgical treatment rarely cures Crohn's disease and there is constant worry about relapse requiring medication with potential serious side effects.

Between these two extremes is indeterminate colitis. Most cases of indeterminate colitis present as acute colitis and eventually turn out to behave more like ulcerative colitis than Crohn's disease. However, some cases of indeterminate colitis will, over time, develop the manifestations of Crohn's disease associated with all the co-morbidity of Crohn's disease and its negative impact on the quality of life.

Issues that Impact on Quality of Life in Inflammatory Bowel Disease

1. Body image is a major issue which influences quality of life in patients with inflammatory bowel disease. There is the fear of unsightly scars, impaired continence, stomas and psychosexual issues which result in isolation and have a major impact on social well being.
2. There is the fear of operations and the complications thereof, particularly of recurrence and of malignant disease which influences the patient's well being.
3. There is the issue of general health, particularly anaemia, malnutrition and lack of energy, which has a profound influence on quality of life.
4. Bowel function has a profound impact on quality of life, especially pertaining to uncontrollable incontinence.
5. Quite apart from the above issues, there are the psychosexual issues related to inflammatory disease as well as mental health, pain and the complications of medication.
6. The severity of bowel incontinence is closely associated with the gastrointestinal quality of life index score.

Ulcerative Colitis: Pouch Surgery

Measurement of quality of life, especially in pouch patients is fraught by methodological problems [1]. Quality of life varies on a daily basis and depends on mood, expectations and anal function. The instruments of measurements are usually based on questionnaires which attempt to quantify abstract issues [2].

Even though pouch surgery is generally successful, there is always a fear of incontinence, which would require a permanent stoma. High bowel frequency, which is not uncommon following pouch surgery, is less demoralizing than urgency. The most debilitating symptom, however, is passive incontinence [3].

Quality of life is said to be normal in well-motivated individuals who are treated by proctocolectomy and permanent ileostomy; although it is accepted that patients make considerable adjustments to their life [4]. Consequently pouch surgery has to ensure that imperfections of continence, bowel frequency and sexual dysfunction do not compromise the generally better image and social ease of patients who no longer require a permanent stoma [5, 6]. Pouch surgery for dysplasia or malignancy often is performed in a rather older population with quiescent colitis and the functional results may not be as good as pouch surgery for patients with chronic relapsing colitis where medical treatment has failed. Nevertheless, even minor imperfections of incontinence do not appear to have a major impact on quality of life after pouch surgery [6–9].

Data from three large North American series has indicated that all of those patients who held a job prior to the pouch operation returned to their original place of employment afterwards [10]. However, it has been reported [11] that 13% had to change their employment, a finding almost mirrored in a study from Vancouver [12]. Another study reported that 75% of those in military service were able to return to the armed services after pouch surgery [13]. Normal sporting activities could be pursued by all patients after pouch surgery. Furthermore, children and adolescents were able to complete their education without any detriment to their academic achievement [14].

Pezim and Nicholls [15] conducted a questionnaire survey among patients with a pouch to assess their preferences compared to their life when they had a protecting ileostomy. This is not an entirely fair comparison as loop stomas are usually more troublesome than an end ileostomy. Furthermore, patients were self selected, having undergone a major operation to avoid a stoma. Nevertheless, 87% said that they were more confident, 89% felt that they were cleaner and 87% said that their sex image was better than it had been with a stoma. Similarly, 87% said that they were more at ease socially and 87% that they were more able to pursue normal sporting interests. In our own series, the functional outcome and quality of life was as follows: 73% said that they had unquestionably improved, 89% stated that having a pouch operation was definitely worth the effort, none regretted the pouch but 16% were uncertain whether this was the best operation for them. Despite this, 73% would definitely recommend the operation to a friend. When this cohort of patients was interviewed by an independent assessor, 38% stated that they were concerned about going out, 32% said that they were often worried about taking holidays, 26% had minor concerns about normal sexual activity and 7% had severe sexual morbidity.

The impact of having a permanent intestinal stoma must be acknowledged. Quite apart from the cost of the ileostomy appliance and the surgical complications that often occur, the impact of a stoma on social well being, sexual fulfilment and religious acceptability is often not fully recognised [16]. A study of attitudes amongst Asian migrants and the endogenous public in the United Kingdom has highlighted the anxieties expressed in both groups in relation to having an abdominal stoma [17]. This morbidity is largely eliminated by a modern pouch-anal reconstruction, provided that patients are appropriately counselled and properly selected. Naturally, quality of life is seriously impaired if there are major complications following pouch surgery. Any assessment of the impact of pouch surgery on quality of life must include a thorough pre-operative assessment as well as a thorough pre-operative counselling process [18].

Sagar et al. [19] compared the quality of life of patients in Leeds treated by restorative proctocolectomy with a matched group of quiescent colitics in remission. Bowel frequency was lower in those with quiescent colitis, but even in the absence of severe active disease, urgency was a serious problem in 72% of those with colitis, compared with only 12% after pouch construction. There was more anxiety and depression in the colitics compared with the pouch patients, but there was no difference between the groups in terms of leakage, use of pads, perianal irritation or time spent in the lavatory.

Perhaps some of the most interesting data on quality of life in pouch patients emanate from longitudinal studies [20]. Berndtsson and Oresland [21] from Göteborg, used a modified Olbrisch adjustment scale and found that the initial subtotal colectomy and ileostomy provided little improvement for patients within the group when medically treated for colitis. Only after pouch construction was there a significant improvement in quality of life. Sexual satisfaction improved, there was much greater freedom to move about and travel without urgency, there was greater confidence and self respect, patients enjoyed a normal social life and there was improved work performance. Perhaps this was somewhat surprising given that 51% reported perianal soreness, 40% nocturnal evacuation and 58% consumed regular antidiarrhoea medication. The Cork Group [22] showed that parous patients and those with repeated pouchitis had a compromised quality of life after pouch surgery. They showed that despite a favourable quality of life, some form of dietary restriction was reported by 93%, especially the avoidance of eating late in the day. Elderly patients studied at the Cleveland Clinic had a higher incidence of impaired continence compared with the younger pouch patients [23]. Quality of life parameters when compared between indeterminate colitis and ulcerative colitis at the Cleveland Clinic were indistinguishable [24]. However, the impact of a diagnosis of Crohn's disease, especially if complicated by sepsis, fistula and failure, has a devastating impact on quality of life after pouch surgery [25]. Impaired fertility may also tarnish the image of the apparently successful pouch. Weinryb et al. [26] followed 40 patients for seven years and showed that quality of life improved with time and that there was remarkably little individual variation from day to day. The Amsterdam group reported a better global quality of life when laparoscopic pouch surgery was compared with conventional pouch construction [27]. We believe that this is a particularly important issue in asymptomatic individuals having prophylactic pouch surgery for familial adenomatous polyposis [28].

If a patient is dissatisfied with the functional outcome of restorative proctocolectomy or is dissatisfied because of repeated episodes of pouchitis, then the question of pouch excision and conversion to a conventional ileostomy or a reservoir ileostomy must be addressed. Patients must be counselled carefully and be warned that, although it is sometimes possible to salvage some ileum from the pouch, generally the whole pouch must be sacrificed, resulting in a rather liquid ileostomy and the loss of 40–50 cm of ileum. Nevertheless, for well-counselled patients who have had a poor functional outcome following pouch surgery, quality of life may be greatly improved by conversion to a conventional ileostomy and excision of the anorectum. However, there is a risk of pelvic nerve damage with potential impotence or retrograde ejaculation in men and urinary dysfunction as well after pouch excision. A quality of life survey was undertaken in patients who had had a pouch excision for ulcerative colitis compared with the responses of those of age and sex-matched patients having conventional proctocolectomy over the same time span. The results of the survey showed that the quality of life was broadly comparable, the only exception was the increased ileostomy losses from the stoma in the pouch-excision patients compared with conventional proctocolectomy [29]. Despite this optimistic report, the Helsinki group reported that pouch failures have a compromised quality of life with impaired general health and emotional well being, reduced energy, increased pain and disordered sexual function [30].

Generally pouch surgery results in improved quality of life, provided there is minimal soiling and a bowel frequency of less than seven or eight stools per day. If there are serious complications or if the underlying diagnosis proves to be Crohn's disease, then the quality of life is generally much worse with pouch surgery and the majority of these individuals would be better served by a conventional ileostomy.

Crohn's Disease

There are very few studies on quality of life issues in Crohn's disease. The issues that impact principally on quality of life are as follows:

1. The fear of recurrent Crohn's disease.
2. The fear of ill health and compromised work prospects.
3. Perianal disease often with psychosexual complications.
4. Impact of bodily image from multiple scars and anorectal sepsis and stomas.
5. Sexual morbidity and infertility.
6. A permanent stoma.
7. Incontinence.

In Crohn's disease there are often long periods of quiescence between successful surgical treatments. Nevertheless, Crohn's disease is associated with potential life-long disability. Factors which influence recurrence in ileal Crohn's disease are:

1. Early onset of disease.
2. Cigarette smoking.
3. Diffuse small-bowel disease.
4. Possibly a narrow ileocolonic anastomosis.

Diffuse small bowel disease has a high recurrence rate and a high reoperation rate [31], which is associated with a high incidence of interpersonal morbidity, loss of time from work, fear of repeated operations and the use of medical treatment associated with unpleasant side effects [32]. Diffuse small-bowel disease also has a major impact on social activities, fertility and normal home family life.

Crohn's disease is associated with a higher risk of losing one's job, early retirement or modification of employment. Patients with Crohn's disease have fewer children, than age and sex-matched normal subjects. Quality of life in Crohn's disease is generally associated with relapse, which compromises work, leisure and social activities [33, 34]. Quality of life is often compromised by growth retardation especially in diffuse disease.

The issues we found as having a major impact on quality of life in Crohn's disease were as follows:

1. Bowel frequency
2. Appetite and diet
3. Sleep
4. Dependence on others
5. Mental health
6. Psychosexual morbidity.

We found that during remission, quality of life in Crohn's disease did not differ from controls. In comparison, patients with active disease had a compromised quality of life. In Crohn's disease the impact of the underlying disease process on quality of life is largely influenced by individual's personality and motivation. Males seem to be more seriously affected than women. Generally minimally invasive surgery in Crohn's disease is associated with less of an impact on quality of life, particularly strictureplasty and segmental colonic resection [35].

The main message in managing Crohn's disease is the need for close collaboration between the gastroenterologists, surgeons, healthcare professionals and the patient and their families. Patients with Crohn's disease do better if they are provided with regular professional nutritional advice, appropriate medical therapy and the support of clinical nurse specialists. It is essential for surgeons involved in the management of Crohn's disease to spend time in the counselling process. There are fundamental surgical issues which also affect quality of life. In high-risk individuals, a proximal defunctioning stoma is always advised. Anastomoses should be avoided in the presence of severe sepsis because of the risk of breakdown. It is paramount that the surgeon preserves as much of the small bowel as possible and avoids major complications. Appropriate attention to these issues will have a considerable impact on the overall quality of life of patients with intestinal Crohn's disease.

References

1. Hauser W, Karl-Heinz J, Stallmach A (2005) Mental disorder and psychologic distress in patients with ulcerative colitis after ileal pouch-anal anastomosis. Dis Colon Rectum 48:952–962
2. Berndtsson IEK, Lindholm E, Oresland T, Hulten L (2004) Health-Related quality of life and pouch function in continent ileostomy patients: a 30-year perspective. Dis Colon Rectum 47:2131–2137
3. Rothbarth J, Bemelman WA, Meijerink WJH et al (2001) What is the impact of fecal incontinence on quality of life? Dis Colon Rectum 44:67–71
4. Camilleri-Brennan J, Steele RJC (2001) Objective assessment of quality of life following panproctocolectomy and ileostomy for ulcerative colitis. Ann R Coll Surg Engl 83:321–324
5. Richards DM, Hughes SA, Irving MH, Scott NA (2001) Patient quality of life after successful restorative proctocolectomy is normal. Colorectal Dis 3:223–226
6. Wheeler JMD, Banerjee A, Ahuja N et al (2005) Long-term function after restorative proctocolectomy. Dis Colon Rectum 48:946–951
7. Holubar S, Hyman N (2003) Continence alterations after ileal pouch-anal anastomosis do not diminish quality of life. Dis Colon Rectum 46:1489–1491
8. Scarpa M, Angriman I, Ruffulo C et al (2004) Health-related quality of life after restorative proctocolectomy for ulcerative colitis: long-term results. World J Surg 28:124–129
9. Swenson BR, Hollenbeak CS, Poritz LS, Koltun WA (2005) Modified two-stage ileal pouch-anal anastomosis: equivalent outcomes with less resource utilization. Dis Colon Rectum 48:256–261
10. Cohen Z (1986) Symposium: restorative proctocolectomy with ileal reservoir. Int J Colorectal Dis 1:2–19
11. Wexner SD, Jensen L, Rothenberger DA et al (1989) Long-term functional analysis of the ileoanal reservoir. Dis Colon Rectum 32:275–281
12. Skarskard ED, Atkinson KG, Bell GA et al (1989) Function and quality of life results after ileal pouch surgery for chronic ulcerative colitis and familial polyposis. Am J Surg 157:467–471
13. Bamberger PK, Otchy DP (1997) Ileoanal pouch in the active duty population. Dis Colon Rectum 40:60–66
14. Fonkalsrud EW (1984) Endorectal ileoanal anastomosis with isoperistaltic ileal reservoir after colectomy and mucosal proctectomy. Ann Surg 119:151–157
15. Pezim ME, Nicholls RJ (1985) Quality of life after restorative proctocolectomy with pelvic ileal reservoir. Br J Surg 72:91–93
16. McLeod RS, Baxter NN (1998) Quality of life of patients with inflammatory bowel disease after surgery. World J Surg 22:375–381
17. Bahkta P, Probert CSJ, Javanthi V, Mayberry JF (1992) Stoma anxieties: a comparison of the attitudes of Asian migrants and the indigenous population in the United Kingdom towards abdominal surgery and the role of intestinal stomas. Int J Colorectal Dis 7:1–3
18. Jimmo B, Hyman NH (1998) Is ileal pouch-anal anastomosis really the procedure of choice for patients with ulcerative colitis? Dis Colon Rectum 41:43–45
19. Sagar PM, Lewis W, Holdsworth et al (1993) Quality of life after restorative proctocolectomy with a pelvic ileal reservoir compares favourably with that of patients with medically treated colitis. Dis Colon Rectum 36:584–592
20. Tiainen J, Matikainen M (1999) Health related quality of life after ileal J-pouch-anal anastomosis for ulcerative colitis: long-term results. Scand J Gastroenterol 34:601–605
21. Berndtsson L, Oresland T (2003) Quality of life before and after proctocolectomy and IPAA in patients with

ulcerative proctocolitis: a prospective study. Colorectal Dis 5:173–179

22. Coffey JC, Winter DC, Neary P et al (2002) Quality of life after ileal pouch anal anastomoses: an evaluation of diet and other factors using the Cleveland global quality of life instrument. Dis Colon Rectum 45:30–38
23. Delaney CP, Dadvand B, Remzi FH et al (2002) Functional outcome, quality of life, and complications after ileal pouch-anal anastomosis in selected septuagenarians. Dis Colon Rectum 45:890–894
24. Delaney CP, Fazio VW, Remzi FH et al (2003) Prospective, age-related analysis of surgical results, functional outcome, and quality of life after ileal pouch-anal anastomosis. Ann Surg 238:221–228
25. Brown CJ, MacLean AR, Cohen Z, MacRae HM (2005) Crohn's disease and indeterminate colitis and the ileal pouch-anal anastomosis: outcomes and patterns of failure. Dis Colon Rectum 48:1542–1549
26. Weinryb RM, Liljeqvist L, Poppen B, Gustavsson P (2004) A longitudinal study of long-term quality of life after ileal pouch-anal anastomosis. Am J Surg 185:333–338
27. Dunker MS, Bemelman WA, Slors JF et al (2001) Functional outcome, quality of life, body image, and cosmesis in patients after laparoscopic-assisted and conventional restorative proctocolectomy: a comparative study. Dis Colon Rectum 44:1800–1807
28. Ky AJ, Sonoda T, Milsom JW (2002) One-Stage laparoscopic restorative proctocolectomy. Dis Colon Rectum 45:207–211
29. Tan HT, Connolly AB, Morton D, Keighley MRB (1997) Results of restorative proctocolectomy in the elderly. Colorectal Dis 12:319–322
30. Lepisto A, Luukkonen P, Jarvinen HK (2002) Cumulative failure rate of ileal pouch-anal anastomosis and quality of life after failure. Dis Colon Rectum 45:1289–1204
31. Tan WC, Allan RN (1993) Diffuse jejunoileitis of Crohn's disease. Gut 34:1374–1378
32. Gazzard BG, Price HL, Libby GW, Dawson AM (1978) The social toll of Crohn's disease. BMJ 2:1117–1119
33. Moody GA, Mayberry JF (1992) Quality of life: its assessment in gastroenterology. Eur J Gastroenterol Hepatol 4:1025–1030
34. Gazzard BG (1987) The quality of life in Crohn's disease. Gut 28:378–381
35. Ressiman P, Salky BA, Pfeifer J et al (1996) Laparoscopic surgery in the management of inflammatory bowel disease. Am J Surg 171:47–51

IBD and Pregnancy

Gianluca Colucci, Gian Gaetano Delaini, Filippo Nifosì

Introduction

Intestinal inflammatory diseases [irritable bowel disease (IBD)], including ulcerous rectocolitis [ulcerative colitis (UC)] and Crohn's Disease (CD), are pathologies primarily affecting young adults during the reproductive age, often causing a decrease of the patients' quality of life [1] because of the psychosocial impact caused by the chronic nature of the disease and consequently the therapy and clinical problems connected with complex and sometimes disabling symptomatological patterns, which can negatively affect both social and emotional living [2].

Patients of both genders suffering from such diseases must frequently face problems concerning sex life, fertility and, for woman, pregnancy [3]. Patients of child-bearing age often express doubts about their ability to have children because of psychological consequences of their disease in relation to interpersonal relationships and qualms about harmful effects to the foetus caused by relapse of disease activity stages and the drugs they have to take to prevent and/or treat them during pregnancy [4].

Fertility and IBD

One frequently asked question by young patients suffering from IBD concerns its possible impact on fertility [5, 6]. Generally, the infertility rate is similar to that in the healthy population, which is more or less 8–10%. However, epidemiologic studies show that these patients deliver fewer children than the general population. This fact might be ascribable to reduced fertility due to physical damage caused by the disease and by a decision not to have children because of difficulty developing interpersonal relationships due to poor self-image of their body and their sexuality and fears regarding pregnancy.

Prospective studies revealed that in patients suffering from UC, fertility is not affected except in cases in which the patient has undergone surgery [7]. This topic will be discussed later in the chapter. For women suffering from CD, fertility is reduced exclusively during the stages of the disease activity, probably due to inflammation and accretions involving tubes and ovaries. Control of disease recrudescences usually restores reproductive ability.

As for male patients, there is no certain evidence [8] that CD may cause infertility even if malnutrition and stages of disease activity are negative influences. As for the influence of the drugs prescribed for patients with IBD, there is considerable proof of the negative but temporary impact caused by the pharmacologic therapy [9], by sulfasalazine, in particular, which causes dose-related anomalies of seminal fluid and fertility in about 60% of men. The effect may be potentially reversible 2 months following interruption of therapy [10]. When sulfasalazine is replaced with another drug belonging to the 5-aminosalicylates group, fertility improves.

In both men and women, psychological attitude towards the disease is important as, even more so than the physical condition, it affects the sex life and, consequently, the ability to conceive.

Sexuality and IBD

Regarding the effect of IBD on interpersonal relationships and sexuality, it must be emphasised that, especially at a young age, patients are considerably affected psychologically, not only because their disease is chronic but because of some peculiar aspects of the disease. Direct and indirect effects of IBD, such as asthenia, diarrhoea, faecal incontinence, consequences of surgery and drug side effects generally cause a psychophysical condition of discomfort, making interpersonal relationships difficult both publicly and privately. In the light of these remarks, recent research pointed out the importance of not only clinical but also psychosocial patient evaluation, creating the basis for a multidisciplinary management of the disease that could considerably improve the patient's quality of life.

Young women suffering from IBD in particular

must be carefully examined in regard to physical problems, difficulties relating to their sex life and the possibility of pregnancy [11]. Women with UC usually do not present a higher incidence of gynaecological diseases, except those who have undergone ileal pouch anal anastomosis (IPAA) and presenting a higher incidence of dyspareunia. In women with CD, approximately 25% develop organic and functional gynaecological complications such as menstrual irregularity, amenorrhoea, inflammatory pelvic masses, abscesses and fistulae that, in the case of failure of medical therapy, require surgery, which is psychologically invalidating and greatly affect their quality of life and sexuality, especially if associated with laparotomies and creation of stomas.

Heredity

Another problem that often affects the reproductive and affective environment of patients with IBD is the fear that their children may inherit the same disease [12]. There is a 10.5% risk that the children of a parent with IBD may develop the disease, and 10% of patients have a first-degree relative with the disease, attesting to the role of heredity and genetic susceptibility to these morbid conditions in which multifactorial pathogenesis requires triggering factors of an environmental origin.

The modality of transmission of the genes that may cause the development of IBD is complex and cannot be explained with a mere Mendelian pattern. Studies on twins revealed that, in the case of MC, consistency is 44–50% in monozygotic twins and 0–3% in zygotic twins whereas in the case of UC, consistency is lower, at 6–14% in monozygotic twins and 0-5% in heterozygotic twins [12]. Some studies revealed that there is a stronger familial tendency in CD, attesting to the importance of the genetic arrangement in determining the tendency to develop the disease [12]. Recent researches [13] began to detect the chromosome regions that are probably involved in order to determine susceptibility to the disease. Some of these regions seem to be specific in CD and UC whereas others have a lower specificity. These discoveries are relevant in light of the possibility, from studying the genotype of a certain patient, of anticipating phenotypical features of the disease, distinguishing – for example, in the case of CD – types with a higher risk of fistulisation from those with a predominant tendency to form stenosis. Knowledge of a patient's genetic arrangement could help in the evaluation of risk of extraintestinal manifestations and the probability of response to medical and surgical therapy. For example, a gene was detected, called CARD 15, situated on chromosome 16, which codifies for a protein involved in the primary immune response to infections through the activation of the NF-kB. In patients with MC, mutations of this gene seem to be associated with a tendency to ileal localisation, an earlier age of onset and a higher tendency to stenosis. In the light of these considerations, it is reasonable to think that, in a more or less remote future, physicians may be able to anticipate features of the evolutive course of the disease in each patient by targeted genetic studies, optimising management by individualising medical-surgical therapy [13].

Effect of IBD on Pregnancy

As for the progress of pregnancy during IBD, many studies show that pregnant patients may have an ordinary gestational course during the stages of disease quiescence even if there still is, for reasons not yet explained, a risk that is about twice as high compared with healthy women to have complications such as delay of foetal intrauterine growth, prematurity and low birth weight. Therefore, strict obstetrical follow-up, particularly during the third trimester, is necessary [14, 15].

There is much evidence that any relapse of the disease, especially CD, increases considerably the risk of adverse events such as foetal malformations, premature delivery and miscarriage, emphasising the importance of planning for conception during the quiescence stage and the use of all diagnostic and therapeutical tools available to prevent or intensively treat any relapse of the activity stage during the entire course of pregnancy [16].

As for UC, any activity stage during pregnancy often determines a state of weakness for the expectant mother that frequently affects foetal growth negatively, causing low birth weight and premature delivery. This fact emphasises the importance of thorough and early nutritional therapy and intensive support of the overall conditions of the expectant mother. A recent study revealed the likely association between UC relapse during pregnancy and an increased tendency of foetal malformations [17]. The percentage of miscarriage–premature delivery associated with CU in the active non-fulminating stage is 18–40%, with values up to 60% in the case of fulminating relapses.

Effect of Pregnancy on IBD Course

Many studies have been conducted on the effect of pregnancy on the course of intestinal inflammatory diseases [18–20]. From available meta-analytical data, we found that the probability of relapse of disease activity stages did not increase considerably during pregnancy or during puerperium. A study of over 500 pregnancies in patients suffering from UC in a quiescent stage revealed that the percentage of patient at risk for relapse of the active stage is 34%, similar to the rate of recrudescence of patients suffering from UC who are not pregnant [20]. Most relapses take place during the first trimester, partly because of the high frequency of therapy interruption during the pregnancy period.

In the abcence of therapy, UC in the active stage at the moment of conception shows a further worsening during pregnancy in 45% of patients; in 26%, it remains unchanged. In a small percentage of women, pregnancy causes improvement or remission during the disease activity stage, mostly during the first trimester. If conception occurs during the active stage, it is likely that the latter does not change during the entire course of pregnancy in about two thirds of patients. It may happen that the first acute onset of UC coincides with the beginning of pregnancy; in this case, its disease course tends to be particularly aggressive. Moreover, in some patients, the disease stays subclinical in the extra-pregnancy periods and becomes symptomatic only during pregnancy.

The course of CD during pregnancy is similar to UC. The patient with quiescent disease at the time of conception usually does not present a higher risk of a relapse during pregnancy whereas the patient conceiving during the activity stage presents a further worsening in one third of cases, and in one third they show no change at all [21]. There are no definitive data regarding desirable optimal duration of remission prior conception in order to assure a high probability of a favourable pregnancy course for both the expectant mother and the foetus; however, the longer the quiescence stage, the better the outcome.

In addition to disease activity state at the time of conception, according to two recent studies [22], a previous pregnancy might affect the overall course of IBD. In particular, in patients with UC, it seems that the more the parity increases, the lower the need for surgery. Moreover, patients with a history of multiple pregnancies would present, in comparison with nonparous patients, a need for a lower number of intestinal resections and a higher interval among the various surgeries besides a reduction of the rate of disease. These remarks should partly be explained by the effect of pregnancy on the immune system [22].

Diagnostic Tools Usable During Pregnancy in Patients Suffering from IBD

Laboratory

Regarding possible diagnostic means to monitor the disease and for early recognition of recrudescences, the role of laboratory parameters is limited, as they are undermined by poor reliability of values during pregnancy. Constant physiological modification, connected with hemodilution, is necessary for some parameters that do not present suitable specificity to monitor pregnant women with IBD. These physiological changes include reduction of haemoglobin of about 1 g/dl, reduction of blood iron level, a two- to three-fold increase in erythrocyte sedimentation rate (ESR), reduction of about 1 g/dl of blood albumin and an increase of alkaline phosphatase of about 1.5% . As these parameters may be analogously modified even during the early stages of IBD relapse, they should not be used as diagnostic tools during pregnancy to avoid false positivities, or at least they should always be set in a wider clinical evaluation. For example, if a pregnant patient with CD shows good health conditions but her hematocrit decreased and her ESR increased, she probably is in a quiescent stage of the disease and does not need further examination. On the contrary, a pregnant patient showing ingravescent diarrhoea, abdominal pain and highly altered laboratory parameters does require further diagnostic examination, possibly including an endoscopic evaluation.

Radiology

During pregnancy, it would be best to avoid whenever possible the use of ionising radiation and all examinations emitting them, such as abdominal-X-ray, barium meal, barium follow-through or computed tomography, given their likely teratogenic, genotoxic and carcinogenic effect [19], particularly during the first trimester. According to the American Radiology Society, exposition to a radiation dose lower than 5 rads does not considerably increase the risk of foetal damage. For this reason, if a certain radiologic procedure is highly suggested, it should be performed after a careful discussion with the patient regarding cost/benefit ratios and after exclusion of any additional diagnostic procedures that are safer but equally effective.

Gastrointestinal Endoscopy

Many studies have found that flexible colonoscopy frequently necessary to examine pregnant patients with IBD is relative safe, with no considerable risk of complications for the expectant mother or the foetus [19]. The main indications for endoscopy during pregnancy and IBD are the need to confirm clinical suspicion of disease relapse and for management of complications such as gastrointestinal bleeding and biliary obstructions. Indications for flexible colonoscopy include haematochezia, chronic diarrhoea and abdominal and rectal pain. Moreover, this procedure is necessary in patients in the active disease stage who do not respond to medical therapy. Also, it may help those with atypical symptoms. As to colonoscopy during pregnancy, few data are available because of the limited casuistics although generally it should be reserved exclusively for patients where the diagnostic benefit is higher than the risk. Endoscopic examination of the superior intestinal tract is usually used less frequently than other procedures even although many studies emphasise good tolerability both for the expectant mother and the foetus as well as its high diagnostic value in the case of gastrointestinal bleeding.

Pharmacological Therapeutical Management of IBDs During Pregnancy

As for therapeutic management of IBD during pregnancy, recent studies have shown that pregnant patients should continue pharmacological therapy for the duration of the pregnancy, with the primary aim being to prevent disease relapse given the high risk of negative effects on the foetus. It is necessary that the physician perform a careful preliminary evaluation of the risk/benefit ratio associated with therapy during pregnancy, comparing any harmful effect on the foetus and the expectant mother caused by drugs on one hand and by disease relapse in the absence of pharmacological treatment on the other hand. The results of many studies [23] suggest that it would be best to continue therapy during the disease quiescent stage, treating intensively any recrudescences given the higher danger of the latter in comparison with most available drugs [24].

For patients with IBD, the 5-aminosalicylate (5-ASA) group (mesalamine, sulfasalazine, balsalazide), which have become the mainstay of pharmacological therapy of intestinal inflammatory diseases, may be used on pregnant patients to induce and maintain remission, as there is significant evidence regarding their safety during pregnancy. Many patients may be treated with aminosalicylates only [25–27].

However, for nonresponsive patients or for those allergic to 5-ASA and/or suffering from a more extended disease, corticosteroids are frequently prescribed [28]. Corticosteroids are particularly indicated during the stages of moderate–serious activity analogous to cases of the disease outside the pregnancy period. Many study attest to sufficient tolerability of these drugs and their poor effect on the risk of foetal malformations; despite their ability to cross the placental barrier, they are rapidly transformed by placental 11-hydroxigenasis in less active metabolites with a consequent reduction of their levels in placental blood, especially in the case of some types of steroids, such as prednisone. For this reason, suppression of the hypothalamus-hypophysis-suprarenal axis of the foetus is rare. Among the latest steroidal compounds, Budesonide – a synthetic glucocorticoid selectively released in the small bowel and therefore particularly indicated in the case of ileal localisation of CD – falls into classification category C of drugs that may be used during pregnancy, as a teratogenic effect was found in animals but not in humans.

Another likely therapeutic option in non-responsive patients or in patients allergic to first-choice drugs is represented by immunosuppressant drugs [30]. Rationale for their use is based on the recognised immunomediated pathogenesis of IBDs, including azathioprine, 6-mercaptopurine, cyclosporine, methotrexate and infliximab. Azathioprine and 6-mercaptopurine [29], taken in the usual doses, showed no negative effect on gametogenesis or evidence of a likely teratogen effect. However, given the poor number of studies investigating their use in pregnant patients with IBD, it would be best not to begin therapy with these agents during pregnancy.

Cyclosporine is not associated with an increased risk of teratogenesis [29], but given the high incidence of hepatic and kidney toxicity in the expectant mother, it must be exclusively used in pregnant women suffering from fulminating colitis who are non-responsive to steroids in order to avoid an urgent proctocolectomy, which is associated with a high risk of losing the foetus.

Methotrexate [31] is an antimetabolite drug and antagonist of folic acid. It is a teratogen and mutagen and therefore is contraindicated during pregnancy in those planning a pregnancy. Guinea pigs in utero exposed to methotrexate develop craniofacial and cardiovascular malformations and flaws of the neural tube caused by this drug's antagonism of folic acid. For these reasons, patients with IBD beginning therapy with methotrexate should use effective contraceptive methodologies. If conception takes place and interruption of pregnancy is not considered, high doses of folic acid should be administered during the entire course of pregnancy.

Recently, monoclonal antibodies (infliximab) against tumour necrosis factor (TNF) [32] were introduced as therapy for CD. In guinea pigs, these molecules, belonging to the class of biologic drugs, were not associated with a high risk of toxicity, embryotoxicity or teratogenic effect, and from data presently available, there is no definite evidence on the outcome of a woman's pregnancy. As rare cases of foetal death secondary to cerebral and/or pulmonary haemorrhage were found, as well as cardiac malformations such as Fallot's tetralogy and premature delivery, and given the small amount of studies regarding the effect of these drugs during pregnancy, their use is contraindicated in pregnant patients with CD and those planning to become pregnant.

In patients with IBD, some antibiotics, such as metronidazole and the fluoroquinolones, are sometimes used [33] not only to treat intervening infections but as primary therapy to treat CD. However, little data exists regarding the safety of antibiotics during pregnancy. In particular, metronidazole is the teratogen, foetotoxin and carcinogen in the mouse but these effects were not found in humans. For this reason short cycles of therapy with metronidazole may be used relatively safely to treat vaginal candidosis during pregnancy.

Regarding fluoroquinolones such as ciprofloxacin, there is no evidence of possible harmful effect on the foetus although available data are still limited.

In addition to the above-mentioned drugs, many studies show that the quality of life of pregnant patients may be incredibly improved by aspecific symptomatic drugs active on more frequently reported symptoms, such as abdominal pain, nausea and diarrhoea [34]. Among these drugs, metoclopramide (Plasil) may be used as an antiemetic without risk of foetal damage. On the contrary, given the small quantity of available data, loperamide, an antihemorrhoidal drug frequently used by patients with IBD, must be taken cautiously and exclusively by patients where probable benefits are higher than the risks. An alternative to loperamide, kaolin with pectin or cholestyramine may be used, the latter being suggested especially in ileal localisation of CD or in patients with gravidic cholestasis.

Musculoskeletal and some other forms of abdominal pain may be treated safely with acetaminophen whereas non-steroidal anti-inflammatory drugs (NSAIDs), such as aspirin, are contraindicated because of the risk of premature delivery, extended labour and extended postpartum haemorrhage [35].

How to Approach Delivery in Patients with IBD

On the basis of data given in the literature, patients with RCU may expect ordinary labour and a transvaginal delivery unless there are contraindications connected with concomitant morbid conditions. This consideration is generally valid also for patients who underwent IPAA, as transvaginal delivery does not seem to considerably compromise the integrity of anastomosis [36]. However, as will be discussed later, there is still no consensus regarding this subject.

Differently from pregnant women with UC, most patients with CD, especially those with active perineal involvement, should have a caesarean deliver. If transvaginal delivery cannot be avoided, episiotomy should be avoided [37]. If unavoidable, a mediolateral episiotomy is preferable in order to avoid anal sphincter damage. According to recent studies, development of new perineal complications after transvaginal delivery, usually associated with episiotomy, in patients without previous perineal disease is 17.9%. Moreover, while planning how to perform the delivery, the obstetrician should take into account the specific features of each patient.

Restorative Proctocolectomy with Ileal Pouch Anal Anastomosis and Women's Health

The restorative proctocolectomy with IPAA (RP-IPAA) is now a standard operation proposed for the treatment of UC. It is a complex operation requiring an expert surgical team. Despite the fact that it is generally performed in third-level centres only, complication rate is extremely high, varying in the studies reported in the literature between 13% and 64% [37–39]. Indications for this procedure are different in emergency or elective surgery: toxic megacolon, perforation or massive bleeding (in emergency surgery] or failure of medical therapy and rectal dysphasia/cancer (in elective surgery]. The operation greatly modifies the anatomy of the pelvic space because, after resection of the entire colon and rectum, an ileal reservoir (pouch] is engaged in the top of the anal canal. Since 1978, the year of the first formal description of the operation, many women of child-bearing age have undergone this operation. In the last 20 years, many studies have been published attempting to analyse two aspects: how this operation may influence female reproductive health and whether pregnancy affects functionality of the ileal pouch.

RP-IPAA and Menses

In the literature, four major works analyse this aspect [40–43]. These studies found that most patients noted no change in menses or that initial cycle irregularity eventually disappeared.

IPAA and Pelvic Anatomy

As we will soon see, most studies show a reduction in fertility after RP-IPAA. One hypothesis to explain this phenomenon is the presence of postoperative adhesions. Oresland [41] observed that, even if 20/21 women who underwent RP-IPAA had a normal physical examination, a hysterosalpingography showed some anomalies in 67% of subjects (14/21). Finding such as tubes adhered to the pelvis (48%) or bilateral tubal occlusion (10%) may certainly explain the decreased fertility, as recently emphasised by Diamond [44]. An important bias in this work, however, is the lack of performance of an examination before surgery, making the comparison between the pre- and postoperative situation impossible. Also, a study by Sjogren [45] showed an altered endopelvic status with reduced uterine mobility in 47% of women after RP-IPAA or the presence of adnexal tenderness in 13%.

Female Sexual Function After RP-IPAA

Many studies examined sexual function after RP-IPAA and particularly sexual satisfaction, desire, ability to experience orgasm and coital frequency [40, 43, 45, 46]. Results were satisfactory, as most of these aspects are influenced very little by surgery. However, a percentage of patients, ranging from 3% to 18%, were afraid of having stool leaks during intercourse. In contrast, especially in those with postoperatively unchanged or increased coital frequency from 82% to 100%, the appearance of dyspareunia was a rather frequent complication. Incidence varied considerably, from 0% to 38% [41, 42], stabilising in most works at 25%. Moreover, Farouk found that the incidence of this complication after surgery seems to increase over time [47].

RP-IPAA and Fertility

The desire to have a child is one of the primary instincts of the woman. This may explain why many women, despite the sequelae of such a serious surgery, decide to have a child. As already seen, UC in itself does not seem to influence fertility [6]. Almost all studies present in the literature agree on ascribing the serious negative effect of RP-IPAA on fertility [40, 41, 43, 45]. However, these works contained important methodologic bias or included a small number of participants. Three recent publications stand out, being points of reference on this topic.

Johnson et al. [48] compared 153 patients who underwent RP-IPAA with 60 patients with UC but treated with medical therapy. In this study, we come to two essential conclusions:

1. Women who underwent surgery had an infertility rate significantly higher in comparison with women who did not undergo surgery (28.1% vs 13.3%).
2. Surgery is the key element to explaining this difference. If the infertility rate in women before surgery matched that of patients treated with medical therapy only (odds ratio 0.68, P=0.23), reduction of the fertility rate in the same study group of women evaluated before and after surgery is very high (odd ratio 0.021, P<0,0001).

Moreover, through univariate data analysis, the authors attempted to identify which variables might influence the reduction in fertility. Surprisingly, only the increase of age seemed to have a statistically higher influence on fertility while the history of small-intestinal obstruction, the number of abdominal operations and postoperative pelvic sepsis (three events predisposing the development of adhesions) did not seem to have any influence.

The other two important studies come from the same Scandinavian group. In the first, the fertility rate of a cohort of patients who underwent RP-IPAA was compared with the expected number of births in the general population [49]. Also in this study, the fertility of patients with UC seemed to be slightly reduced in the preoperative stage but is halved after surgery. This reduction reaches the 35% if operated patients who underwent in vitro fertilisation are not included. In the second study, the fecundity rate of 290 women with UC who underwent surgery was compared with 661 healthy women, showing in this case also a reduction of fertility of 80%.

The implications of these studies are very important for preoperative counselling, which must explore the desire for maternity of women waiting to undergo RP-IPAA and, if the clinical situation allows, advise postponement of surgery until after pregnancy.

Ileal Pouch Function, Pregnancy and Delivery

There are at least two theoretical premises regarding a negative effect of pregnancy on pouch function. The first concerns the volumetric increase of the uterus, with a consequent increase of endoabdominal pressure (besides a direct compression effect on the reservoir). The second concerns the worsening of sphincterial function (it may already have been compromised after surgery) after vaginal delivery [50]. Surprisingly, most authors emphasise that pregnancy influences pouch functionality in a small way [47, 51–53], limited to a few cases of slight worsening and temporary incontinence, which generally disappears after delivery.

Even though this topic has been discussed for a long time, vaginal delivery is considered safe by most authors. Two large, retrospective, controlled series compare pouch function after vaginal delivery with pouch function in nulliparous [47] or after caesarean delivery [52], showing no differences. All authors emphasise, moreover, that episiotomy, especially medial episiotomy, must be avoided. We should conclude, therefore, considering the risks connected with caesarean delivery, it must be reserved for cases in which there is obstetrical indication.

In 2005, the authoritative group of Fazio [54] published a work that seems to refute what has been so far written. Recognising that the effects of delivery on sphincterial function in the short term are reduced, it emphasises a high incidence of sphincter injuries that can be detected with endorectal ultrasonography. Using the words from the title of this work, "a word of caution" is essential because, in the long run, functional response to this sphincter damage will need to be assessed. The authors suggested the opposite of what thus far appears in the literature, as they advise a planned caesarean delivery. In light of this work, it is necessary to carefully evaluate each patient in an attempt to assess the risk/benefit ratio between the two delivery modalities.

Conclusion

UC and CD are inflammatory diseases of the intestine, with a multifactor pathogenesis and the tendency to especially afflict young women of reproductive age, affecting their quality of life as well as their interpersonal relationships. In reference to this aspect, it is important to emphasise the psychological effect of the disease on patients' sexual life, which can undermine the opportunity of having children despite the fact that IBD itself does not considerably affect fertility. Moreover, even if pregnant women suffering from IBD require strict monitoring, particularly concerning the nutritional aspect and the need for aggressive treatment of any disease relapses, risk to the foetus or the expectant mother are moderate in suitably controlled disease, and many concerns about pregnancy and its possible consequences are not justified.

Risks increase in insufficiently treated disease, as in this case, relapses are frequent and invariably influence foetal growth negatively, resulting in low birth weight, premature delivery and miscarriage. For this reason, it is necessary when treating young women with IBD to apply a multidisciplinary approach involving careful evaluation of patients' psychosocial status and including discussion about medical, psychological and sexual problems, informing and educating them about the peculiar aspects of pregnancy and its management during IBD.

On the basis of the present trend, a patient with IBD that is kept in a quiescent stage thanks to increasingly effective medical therapies, most of which are well tolerated during pregnancy, may expect pregnancy course and outcome not too different from those expected in young healthy women.

Acknowledgment

The authors thank Dr. Isabella Pichiri for her precious help and assistance.

References

1. Irvine EJ, Feagan B, Rochon J et al (1994) Quality of life: a valid and reliable measure of therapeutic efficacy in the treatment of inflammatory bowel disease. Gastroenterology 106:287–296
2. Alstead EM, Nelson-Piercy C (2003) Inflammatory bowel disease in pregnancy. Gut 52:159–161
3. Moody G, Probert G, Srivasta E et al (1993) Sexual dysfunction amongst patients with Crohn's disease, a hidden problem. Digestion 52:179–183
4. Moody G, Mayberry J (1993) Perceived sexual dysfunction amongst patients with inflammatory bowel disease. Digestion 52:256–260
5. Mayberry JF, Weterman IT (1986) European survey of fertility and pregnancy in women with Crohn's disease: a case control study by European collaborative group. Gut 27:821–825
6. Hudson M, Flett G, Sinclair TS, et al (1997) Fertility and pregnancy in inflammatory bowel disease. Int J Gynaecol Obstet 58:229–237
7. Ravid A, Richard C, O'Connor BI et al (2001) Fertility after ileal pouch-anal anastomosis in women with ulcerative colitis. Gastroenterology 120:2417
8. Narendranathan M, Sandler RS, Suchindran M et al (1989) Male fertility in inflammatory bowel disease. J Clin Gastroenterol 11:403–406
9. O'Morain C, Smethurst P, Dore CJ et al (1984) Reversible male infertility due to sulphasalazine: studies in man and rat. Gut 25:1078–1084
10. Moody GA, Probert C, Jayanthi V et al (1997) The effect of chronic ill health and treatment with sulphasalazine on fertility amongst men and women with inflammatory bowel disease in Leicester. Int J Colorectal Dis 12:220–224
11. Trachter AB, Rogers AI, Leiblum SR (2002) Inflammatory bowel disease in women: impact on relationship and sexual health. Inflamm Bowel Dis 8(6):413–421
12. Peeters M, Nevans H, Baert F et al (1996) Familial aggregation in Crohn's disease. Increased age, adjusted risk and concordance in clinical characteristics. Gastroenterology 111:597–603
13. Sartor RB (2003) Clinical applications of advances in the genetics of IBD. Rev Gastroenterol Disord 3(Suppl1)S9–S17
14. Fonager K, Sorensen HT, Olsen J et al (1998) Pregnancy outcomes in women with Crohn's disease: a follow up study based on linkage between national registries. Am J Gastroenterol 93:2426–2430
15. Norgard B, Fonager K, Sorensen HT et al (2000) Birth outcomes in women with ulcerative colitis: a nation-

wide Danish cohort study. Am J Gastroenterol 95:3165–3170

16. Dominitz JA, Young JC, Boyko EJ (2002) Outcomes of infants born to mothers with inflammatory bowel disease: a population based cohort study. Am J Gastroenterol 97:641–648
17. Baird DD, Narendranathan M, Sandler RS (1990) Increased risk of pre-term birth for women with inflammatory bowel disease. Gastroenterology 99:987–994
18. Fedorkow DM, Persaud D, Nimrod CA (1989) Inflammatory bowel disease: a controlled study of late pregnancy outcome. Am J Obstet Gynaecol 160:998–1001
19. Cappell MS (1998) The safety and efficacy of gastrointestinal endoscopy during pregnancy. Gastroenterol Clin NA 27:37–71
20. Mogadam M, Korelitz BI, Ahmed SW et al (1981) The course of inflammatory bowel disease during pregnancy and postpartum. Am J Gastroenterol 18:735–742
21. Christian Mottet, Pascal Juillerat et al (2005) Pregnancy and Crohn's disease. Digestion 71:54-61
22. Castiglione F, Pignata S, Morace F et al (1996) Effect on pregnancy on the clinical course of a cohort of women with inflammatory bowel disease. Ital J Gastroenterol 28:199–204
23. Connel W, Miller A (1999) Treating inflammatory bowel disease during pregnancy: risk and safety of therapy. Drug Saf 21:311–323
24. Moskovitz DN, Carol Bodian et al (2004) The effect on the fetus of medications used to treat pregnant inflammatory bowel disease patients. Am J Gastroenterol 100(8)1897–1898
25. Habal FM, Hui G, Greenberg Gr (1993) Oral 5 aminosalicylic acid for inflammatory bowel disease in pregnancy: safety and clinical course. Gastroenterology 105:1057–60
26. Trallori G, d'Albasio G, Bardazzai G, et al (1994) 5-aminosalicylic acid in pregnancy: clinical report. Ital J Gastroenterol 26:75–78
27. Newman NM, Correy JF (1983) Possible teratogenicity of Sulphasalazine. Med J Aust 1(11):528–529
28. Reinisch SM, Simon NG, Karwo WG et al (1978) Prenatal exposure to prednisone in Humans and animals retards intrauterine growth. Science 202:436–438
29. Scott JR (1977) Fetal growth retardation associated with maternal administration of immunosuppressive drugs. Am J Obstet Gynecol 128(6):668–676
30. Marion JF, Present DH (1996) 6-MP maintains cyclosporine induced response in patients with severe ulcerative colitis with inflammatory bowel disease. Am J Gastroenterol 91:A1975
31. Weinstein GD (1977) Methotrexate. Ann Intern Med 86:199–204
32. Srinivasan R (2001) Infliximab treatment and pregnancy outcome in active Crohn's disease. Am J Gastroenterol 96:2274–2275
33. Burtin P, Taddio A, Ariburnu O et al (1995) Safety of metronidazole in pregnancy: a meta-analysis. Am J Obstet Gynecol 172:525–529
34. Lewis JH, Weingold AB (1985) The use of the gastrointestinal drugs during pregnancy and lactation. Am J Gastroenterol 80:912–923
35. Modigliani R (1997) Drug therapy for ulcerative colitis in pregnancy. Eur J Gastroenterol Hepatol 9:854–857
36. Scott HJ, McLeod RS, Blair J et al (1996) Ileal pouch-anal anastomosis: pregnancy, delivery and pouch function. Int J Colorectal Dis 11:84–87
37. Fazio VW, Ziv Y, Church JM et al (1995) Ileal pouch-anal anastomoses complications and function in 1005 patients. Ann Surg 222:120–127
38. Dayton MT, Larsen KP (1997) Outcome of pouch-related complications after ileal pouch-anal anastomosis. Am J Surg 174:728–731
39. Meagher AP, Farouk R, Dozois RR et al (1998). Ileal pouch-anal anastomosis for chronic ulcerative colitis: complication and long-term outcome in 1310 patients. Br J Surg 85:800–803
40. Metcalf AM, Dozois RR, Kelly KA (1986) Sexual function in women after proctocolectomy. Ann Surg 204:624–627
41. Oresland T, Palmblad S, Ellstrom M et al (1994) Gynaecological and sexual function in women after proctocolectomy. Int J Colorectal Dis 9:77–81
42. Damgaard B, Wettergren A, Kirkegaard P (1995) Social and sexual function following ileal pouch-anal anastomosis. Dis Colon Rectum 38:286–289
43. Tainen J, Matikainen M, Hiltunen KM et al (1999) Ileal J pouch anal anastomosis, sexual dysfunction and fertility. Scand J Gastroenterol 34:185–188
44. Diamond MP, Freeman ML (2001) Clinical implication of post-surgical adhesion. Hum Reprod Update 7:567–576
45. Sjogren B, Poppen B (1995) Sexual life in women after colectomy-proctomusectomy with S-pouch. Acta Obstet Gynecol Scand 74:51–55
46. Bambrick M, Fazio VW, Hull T et al (1996). Sexual function following restorative proctocolectomy in women. Dis Colon Rectum 39:610–614
47. Farouk R, Pemberton JH, Wolff BG et al (2000) Functional outcomes after ileal pouch-anal anastomosis for chronic ulcerative colitis. Ann Surg 231:919–926
48. Johnson P, Richard C, Ravid A et al (2004) Female infertility after ileal pouch-anal anastomosis for ulcerative colitis. Dis Colon Rectum 47:1119–1126
49. Olsen KO, Joelsson M, Lauberg S et al (1999) Fertility after ileal pouch anal anastomosis in women with ulcerative colitis. Br J Surg 86:493–495
50. Donnelly V, Fynes M, Campbell D et al (1998) Obstetric events leading to anal sphincter damage. Obstet Gynecol 92:955–961
51. Pezim ME (1984) Successful childbirth after restorative proctocolectomy with pelvic ileal reservoir. Br J Surg 71:292
52. Juhasz ES, Fozard B, Dozois RR et al (1995) Ileal pouch-anal anastomosis function following childbirth. An extended evaluation. Dis Colon Rectum 38:159–165
53. Scott HJ, McLeod RS, Blair J et al (1996) Ileal pouch-anal anastomosis: pregnancy, delivery and pouch function. Int J Colorectal Dis 11:84–87
54. Remzi FH, Gorgun E, Bast J et al (2005) Vaginal delivery after ileal pouch-anal anastomosis: a word of caution. Dis Colon Rectum 48:1691–1699

Urinary and Sexual Involvement in IBD

Luigi Zorcolo, Giuseppe Casula

Introduction

Urogenital involvement is not rare in patients with inflammatory bowel disease (IBD), but its real incidence has not been defined yet, as demonstrated by the wide range (4–27%) of percentages reported in literature [1–6]. In 1943, Hyams et al. [7] described a ureteral obstruction secondary to chronic enteritis. According to them, that was the first case of urinary disorder of the earliest 1 000 patients suffering from Crohn's disease (CD). In contrast, 40 years later, Kyle stated that as many as 27% of patients with CD will experience urinary disturbances during their life [2]. This apparent discrepancy simply reflects the fact that urinary diseases in IBD patients were (and still are!) often missed or misunderstood. This happens mainly because symptoms are frequently absent or modest and easily obscured by the more severe intestinal problems. However, since minor urinary involvement can result in serious illness (i.e. chronic renal failure), it is important for surgeons and physicians who deal with IBD patients, to be aware of these frequent complications in order to know how to prevent them, to be able to identify high-risk patients, and to chose the most appropriate treatment when these problems occur.

People with inflammatory bowel disease can also experience sexual difficulties. The exact incidence of this phenomenon is not known, as patients may feel embarrassed in discussing it with the doctor. However, it seems to be a common finding which is directly related to the duration and extent of the disease [8]. This is obviously an important problem, especially considering that IBD often affect young adults for a long period of their life.

In 1992, a prospective case-control study among 50 women with CD which had been not surgically treated, showed that although 45 of them had a stable relationship, 24% had no intercourse, compared to 4% of the control group, and the reason for this was mainly the frequent presence of abdominal pain and diarrhoea or the fear of faecal incontinence [9].

As shown in Table 1, some of the urologic and sex-

Table 1. Classification of urinary and sexual manifestations and complications

Urinary involvement

- Related to the disease
  - Indirectly related (secondary to metabolic derangements):
    - Urinary tract calculi
    - Cystitis
    - Amyloidosis
    - Nephritis (glomerulonephritis, interstitial nephritis)
  - Directly related (secondary to the inflammatory process):
    - Perirenal or perivesical abscesses
    - Entero-urinary fistulas
    - Ureteral obstruction
- Related to medical treatment
  - Nephrotoxicity from medical treatment
    - Related to surgical treatment
      - Urinary tract calculi
      - Urinary retention
      - Ureteral injury

Sexual involvement

- Related to the disease
  - Psychological aspects
  - Loss of libido
  - Generalised debility
  - Presence of cutaneous/perianal disease
  - Dyspareunia secondary to pelvic/perineal inflammation
- Related to medical treatment
  - Loss of libido
  - Impotence
  - Infertility
  - Vaginal dryness and atrophy
- Related to surgical treatment
  - Neurological damage (impotence, retrograde ejaculation)
  - Vaginal dislocation (dyspareunia)
  - Presence of stoma

ual manifestations are the consequence of the metabolic derangement associated with IBD, while others result from a direct involvement of the urinary tract due to the intestinal inflammatory process. In addition, some of them can be caused or favoured by medical or surgical treatment.

Urinary Manifestations Related to the Disease

Urinary Tract Calculi

The risk of developing urinary tract calculi is 10–100 times greater in patients with IBD than in the general population (Fig. 1) [3]. The reported incidence ranges from 1 to 25% [1–3, 6, 10–12]. The metabolic derangement leading to this complication can be either related to the disease itself or a consequence of its treatment. Patients with CD are much more affected than those with ulcerative colitis (UC) [10, 13], and the risk is increased after surgery.

Calculi are primarily composed of calcium oxalate or uric acid. In general, calcium oxalate stones are more frequent in patients who have extensive ileal disease or an ileal resection but who also have a functioning colon [14, 15], while uric acid calculi are typical of patients with chronic diarrhoea due to extensive colitis or ileostomy diversion. Because of their different pathogeneses they will be discussed separately.

Uric Acid Stones

Generally, uric acid renal stones are likely to form in the following circumstances: (1) increased excretion of uric acid in the urine, (2) persistently concentrated urine, (3) persistently low urinary pH. The last two conditions are often present in IBD patients; in fact, chronic diarrhoea secondary to UC or to an ileostomy generates a loss of water, sodium and bicarbonate salt, which are able to concentrate the urine and lower its pH.

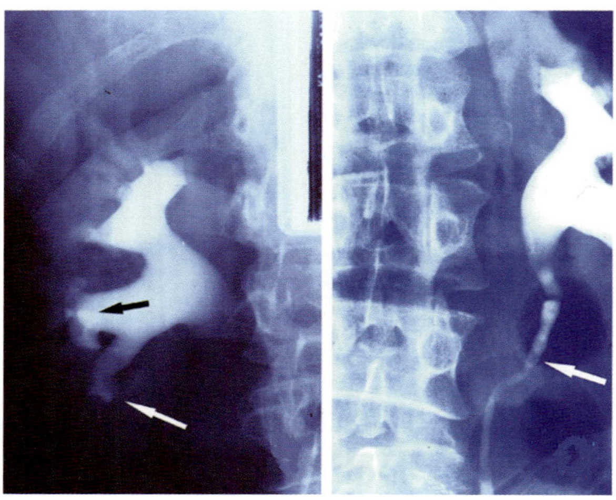

Fig. 1. Bilaterally dilated renal calices, renal and ureteral calculi (*white arrows*) and calcifications (*black arrow*) in a patient with longstanding CD

Clarke et al. [16] noticed that people with ileostomy produced about 300 ml less urine in a day than the control population; moreover the mean urinary pH was 5.05. At these levels, the solubility of uric acid (which has a pKa of 5.7) is almost 12 times lower [10], and this predisposes to crystallization and formation of uric stones, even in the absence of hyperuricemia and hyperuricosuria [17]. Other circumstances like urinary tract infection, chronic ureteral obstruction, high urinary calcium and oxalate concentration, steroid use (because they increase intestinal calcium absorption), prolonged bed rest (which favours calcium mobilisation from the bones), all increase the chance of stone formation.

Calcium Oxalate Stones

Calcium oxalate is the most common type of kidney calculi not only in IBD patients but also in the general population. However, in the latter, urinary oxalate concentration is often normal and the formation of stones is mainly secondary to the abnormalities in its solubility.

In contrast, the pathogenesis in IBD patients appears to be related to hyperoxaluria combined with fluid depletion. It has been shown that hyperoxaluria is present in two thirds of patients with ileal disease, or those that have had extensive ileal resection [18], and this condition renders these patients more prone to develop calculi. Hyperoxaluria, as demonstrated by Chadwick et al. [15] via the use of C14-labelled oxalate, is the consequence of an increased enteric absorption of dietary oxalate, which is 5 times greater in people with ileal disease compared to control population (30% *vs.* 6%). Since excessive oxalate is mainly absorbed by colonic mucosa, colectomy or ileostomy patients do not manifest this phenomenon [15, 19, 20]. Enteric hyperoxaluria mainly depends on two mechanisms, both of which are related to bile salt and the consequent fat malabsorption.

The first mechanism regards oxalate solubility. Under normal conditions, oxalate binds with dietary calcium to form insoluble calcium-oxalate, which is eliminated with the faeces. However, the affinity of calcium is higher for fatty acids than for oxalate. Thus, in the presence of malabsorption, calcium is mainly bound by non-absorbed fatty acids and this leads to an indirect augmentation of the soluble oxalate which can be easily absorbed by the colonic mucosa [19, 21]. It has been estimated that hyperoxaluria occurs if steatorrhea exceeds 12–15 g/day [15].

The second mechanism is an increase in permeability of colonic mucosa which is irritated by non-absorbed fatty acid and bile salts [20, 22]. A third described effect of bile salt malabsorption is the inhibition of a bacterium (*Oxalobacter formigenes*) which normally degrades oxalate in the colon [23–25]. Other factors such as excessive fluid loss, hypomagnesuria and hypocitruria due to hypokalemia [26], metabolic acidosis, steroid use and prolonged bed rest, predispose to stone formation.

Treatment

Treatment of urinary stones in IBD patients does not differ from treatment in the general population: extra-corporeal shock wave lithotripsy (ESWL) is the gold standard. When it fails, endoscopic procedures are an option, while open surgery is rarely required [27]. In case of complete persistent obstruction, especially if associated with infection, an immediate decompression with either a ureteral stent or nephrostomy may be necessary.

Prevention

Whatever the nature of calculi, the mainstay of prevention is maintaining a good hydration and minimising diarrhoea or ostomy output in order to have a urine volume of 1 500–2 000 ml/day. Patients at risk should regularly have urinary measurements of uric acid, oxalate, calcium, citrate, phosphate and pH, to keep them in the proper range.

In the presence of low pH, potassium/sodium citrate (30–60 mEq/day) can be used to alkalinise the urine [28]. Sodium bicarbonate (650 mg x 3/day) is an alternative but this can increase the risk of forming calcium stones [29]. If hyperuricosuria persists despite fluid intake and correction of urinary pH, the patient can start allopurinol (300 mg/day). However, it should be kept in mind that this drug may interact with azathioprine/6MP [30].

Table 2. Food with high concentration of oxalate

Spinach
Beets
Nuts
Wheat bran
Wild fruits
Chocolate
Tea
Cola

Prevention of hyperoxaluria is mainly obtained with diet: avoiding food high in oxalate (see Table 2) may be sufficient, but generally it is more effective to assume a low-fat diet and to substitute fats with medium-chain triglycerides in order to reduce fat malabsorption.

Different cations may be added to bind excessive oxalatum resistant to dietetic measures, but all of them have side effects. In fact, extra calcium (1–2 g/day), which is often necessary in patients with malabsorption, may lead to formation of calcium-phosphate calculi [31]; aluminium may interfere with phosphate absorption, while magnesium can exacerbate diarrhoea, thus minimising its potential benefit. A good oxalate binder is cholestyramine (4–10 g/day) [14]. Still, it may also increase bile salt losses and worsen steatorrhea. To date there is not a single accepted strategy for enteric hyperoxaluria and treatment needs to be personalised on the basis of haematological and urinary parameters (see algorithm in Table 3).

Table 3. Treatment of enteric hyperoxaluria as adapted from Pardi et al. [30]

Phase I	Warning
Increase fluid intake for urine output of 3 L/day	
Low-oxalate diet	
Low-fat (50 g/day) diet	
Calcium supplementation (1–2 g/day)	Needs monitoring of urinary Ca; potential high risk of Ca-phosphate stones
Cholestyramine (4 g × 4 day)	May exacerbate steatorrhea
Phase II (if stones recur despite Phase I treatment)	
Alkalinisation of urine and citrate supplementation (K citrate or Na citrate 30 mEq × 4 day)	
Mg supplementation	May exacerbate diarrhoea
Allopurinol 300 mg/day (if stone contains uric acid)	Interaction with azathioprine/6MP

Cystitis

Lower urinary tract infection is probably the most common urological manifestation, occurring in up to 44% of patients with IBD [5–18]. Although recurrences are frequent, cystitis is usually self-limiting and does not spread upward to the kidney. Urine analysis is generally positive for *E. Coli*, *Str. Faecalis* or *Proteus*. Appropriate antibiotic therapy is the usual treatment.

Amyloidosis

IBD patients have a higher level of serum amyloid-A (SAA), an acute phase protein which is the precursor of tissue amyloid. This is probably related to chronic inflammation and to the duration and extension of the disease [32, 33], although other studies have not supported this hypothesis [34–36]. Long-term steroids therapy has also been advocated [37].

Amyloidosis may involve different organs but there is a clear predilection for renal parenchyma. This condition usually manifests with asymptomatic proteinuria, but the evolution to a nephritic syndrome is not rare, and eventually can lead to death. According to the largest reported series [33], the true incidence of amyloidosis is less than 1% in patients with CD and 0.07% in those with UC. Patients with both ileitis and colitis have the highest risk (1.3–1.6%) [32–34].

The most effective way to stop amyloidosis is resection of the affected bowel [35, 38]. However, surgery in these patients suffers from a higher rate of morbidity and mortality [32–37, 39] and is often ineffective when a nephritic syndrome has already developed [33, 34].

Success of medical treatment with colchicine (0.6–1.5 mg/day) has been reported in small series [33, 40–42], but its mechanism of action is not clear. End-stage disease can be managed with plasmapheresis and azathioprine [43], but it eventually requires a renal transplant [44].

Nephritis

Proliferative glomerulonephritis is a rare complication of IBD. There are few reports about it in the literature and most of them regard UC [45–52]. The pathogenic mechanism is not clear but there is evidence about deposition in the glomeruli of the immune complex secondary to intestinal antigens which are released from the inflamed bowel and bound to circulating antibodies [46, 53–54]. For this reason glomerulonephritis has been noticed more frequently in correlation with active inflammation of the bowel [48, 55].

Clinically, patients usually present with oliguria and analysis shows proteinuria, urinary sediment, elevated serum creatinine and a picture of severe renal disease. Immunofluorescence microscopy can demonstrate glomerular deposition of immunoglobulin and/or complement [46, 56]. Steroids are usually sufficient for improving renal function [46, 49, 57], but they should be followed by resection of the affected bowel [55].

Perirenal and Perivesical Abscesses

These complications do not exactly represent a urologic manifestation of IBD, since they are retroperitoneal or pelvic collections secondary to inflammation and perforation of the bowel. However, they can manifest with urologic symptoms and moreover they can be the intermediate step in developing a communication between the bowel and the urinary system (see section Entero-Urinary Fistula (EUF) below). Frequently the inflammatory collection causes renal displacement or bladder deformity and the development of fibrosis may result in deviation and obstruction of the ureter (see subsection) [19]. Abscesses are best diagnosed via ultrasound or CT scan (Fig. 2). Percutaneous drainage is an option, but the presence of abscesses is generally an indication for bowel resection.

Entero-Urinary Fistula (EUF)

It is well known that about one third of patients with CD have enteroenteric or enterocutaneous fistulas which are secondary to the characteristic transmural inflammation [58]. Fistulisation within the urinary system is also possible but it is much less common, occurring in 1–8% of cases [1, 3, 6, 19, 59–62].

The majority of fistulas result from direct contact between inflamed terminal ileum and the bladder dome (ileovesical fistula). Sometimes an intervening abscess is present and in this case it is not unusual to find more than one intestinal segment involved in the fistula [63, 64]. Crohn's colitis, and more rarely UC, can determine a colovesical fistula which generally involves the sigmoid colon [59]. Severe rectal disease can cause rectourethral fistulas, but this is a rare event. Other unusual fistulas are those between the terminal ileum and ureter, or urachus.

In the widest series reported in the literature [65], fistula originated from ileum in 64% of cases, colon in 21%, rectum in 8% and multiple sites in 7%, while

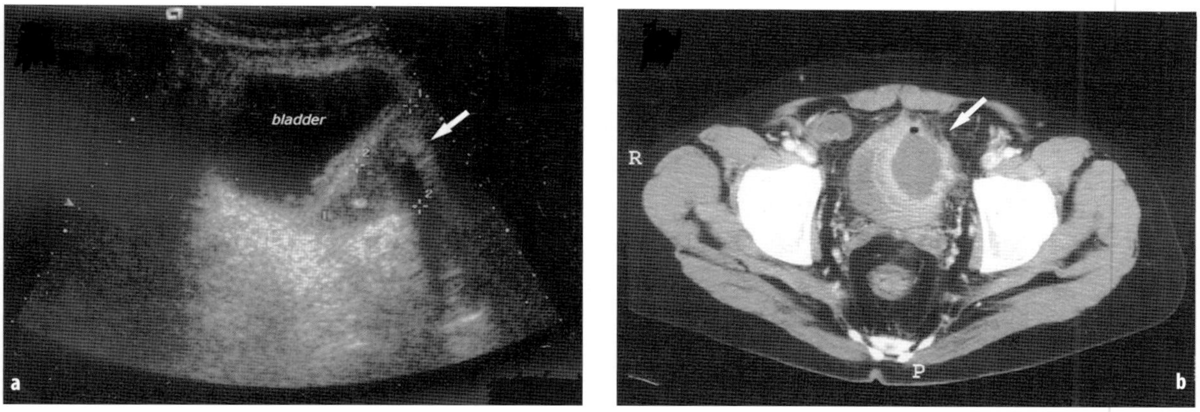

Fig. 2. Ultrasound (**a**) and CT (**b**) images of a left perivesical abscess secondary to CD

the involved urinary tract included the bladder in 88%, urethra in 6%, urachus in 3% and urether in 2%.

Entero-Urinary Fistula (EUF) are more frequent in men, with reported M:F ratio up to 9:1 [2, 59]. This fact is explained via the anatomy of the female pelvis, where the bladder and the urethra are protected by the uterus and the vagina, respectively [19]. Fistulas tend to manifest in patients with established bowel disease [3, 59, 60, 63], often within the first decade of onset [65]. Not surprisingly, the concomitance of enteroenteric or enterocutaneous fistulas arising from the same segment of bowel is frequent [59, 60, 65, 66].

However, EUF has also been reported as the presenting manifestation in patients without a previous history of CD [59]. Prodromic symptoms or signs like dysuria, urinary urgency and frequency, suprapubic discomfort, microscopic or gross hematuria, are often present in early stage, indicating a status of perivesical inflammation [3, 60, 63, 67].

When fistulisation has occurred, it usually manifests with pathognomonic signs like pneumaturia or faecaluria. Another specific but rare sign is the passage of urine through the rectum (urorrhea) [60, 67]. In a minority of cases, there is only a history of recurrent urinary tract infection (UTI) refractory to medical treatment, while very rarely the patient can be asymptomatic (Table 4) [65]. Pneumaturia has been reported with percentages varying from 38–94%. In the series from the Mayo Clinic it was present in 68% of patients (Table 4), but according to others [68], this sign is evident in more than 90% of cases and, when not noticed by the patient, air bubbles can be evident if he or she urinates while submerged in a bathtub.

The physical examination is often normal or it demonstrates symptoms and signs of the underlying pathology like tenderness in the lower abdomen, a palpable mass, enterocutaneous or perineal fistulas. Urinalysis reveals leukocytosis and microscopic hematuria in the majority of patients [65]. The culture is almost always positive for *E. Coli*, while polymicrobial infection is present in about one third of the cases [59, 63, 65]. Complications like pyelonephritis or other major infections are unusual, unless there is a direct communication with the ureter or abnormalities at the ureterovesical junctions [68].

Diagnosis of EUF can be obtained with an accuracy of 92% after oral or rectal administration of indocyanine green solution and urine examination using a colorimeter [69]. Diagnosis can be confirmed with imaging tests. A plane abdominal X-ray in erect position is sometimes sufficient for showing an air level into the bladder but this can be better demonstrated with a CT scan, which also allows the highlighting of other peculiar signs like the apposition of the thickened bowel and the bladder wall, a perivesical abscess or the presence of oral contrast into the bladder. For all these reasons, CT scan, which has an accuracy close to 100%, is considered the test of choice [70, 71].

Table 4. Presenting symptoms in 78 Crohn's disease patients with entero-urinary fistulas. (Adapted from Solem et al. [65])

Symptoms	No. of patients	%
Pneumaturia	52	68
Dysuria	49	64
Recurrent UTIs	24	32
Faecaluria	21	28
Hematuria (micro/gross)	17	22
Urorrhea	5	7
Asymptomatic	1	1

Direct identification of the fistula opening at cystoscopy is reported in 7–74% of cases [3, 60, 65, 67], although usually this exam permits the visualisation of an area of bullous edema, erythema or papillomatous hyperplasia. Other findings are the presence of feculent debris or pus in the bladder. Some authors consider cystoscopy fundamental in the work-up of this pathology [60, 65, 72, 73], while others believe that it is an invasive procedure that poses a potential risk of spreading infection and, at the end of the day, does not provide information that is any more useful than imaging exams [68]. In fact, the most important thing in planning the correct management of an enterovesical fistula is not to see its opening in the bladder but rather to identify the segment of bowel involved in the inflammatory process [68].

Other urological investigations like cystograms and excretory urograms are only occasionally useful. Small-bowel follow through, barium enema and colonoscopy are suggested because, even if the fistula is rarely demonstrated, they help to determine the extent and nature of the underlying disease and to exclude other causes of EUF such as diverticular disease or colonic malignancies [59, 67, 74, 75].

What the best management of EUF should be is still being debated. Although spontaneous closure has been described [63, 67, 76], this event is very rare and most authors agree that the presence of EUF is a sign of complicated disease that indicates surgery. The operation usually consists of disconnection of the tract, resection of the affected bowel and suture of the vesical wall. Partial cystectomy is rarely necessary and was only needed for less than 10% of the patients operated on at The Mayo Clinic [65]. Postoperative morbidity and mortality was 6.4 and 1.6% respectively in a series of 61 patients, and fistula recurrence rate was 1.6% [60].

The advances in medical therapy with the disposability of new immunosuppressive and anticorpal drugs has reinforced the opinion of those authors who believe that the fistula itself, considering its benign evolution and the low risk of ascending infection, does not require an operation and should first be managed conservatively, reserving surgery exclusively for when it is associated with intra-abdominal or pelvic abscesses or obstructive stricture of the bowel [66, 68, 77]. This is in contrast with the policy of the Mayo Clinic, where fistula alone represented the indication for surgery in 69% of their patients with EUF [65].

Medical treatment was effective in the long-term and surgery was avoided in six cases in a series of 17 patients (35%) [66]. At The Mount Sinai Medical Hospital [68], among 31 patients treated with sulphasalazine, continuous antibiotics and 6-mercaptopurine when necessary, 18 (58%) had a clinical remission and 12 of them remained well for a mean period of 8 years. Patients not responding to medical therapy were more frequently those who were already steroid dependent. In another series of 43 patients, 20 (43%) were able to avoid surgery with a combination of 6MP, antibiotics and mesalamine [77].

However, although medical treatment has shown potential promise in some small series, there have not been any prospective studies designed specifically to assess the efficacy of the medical treatment of internal fistulas [78]. At the moment, surgery is still considered to be the treatment of choice and up to 95% of patients will eventually receive it [27, 63, 65, 79]. There are still no reports on infliximab, but its well-documented benefits in healing perineal, enterocutaneous [80, 81] and also rectovaginal fistula [82] should encourage studies on it. Prospective trials to define the exact role of medical and surgical therapy are also desirable.

Ureteral Obstruction

This event is not rare and in most cases is not secondary to renal calculi. Although some signs of unilateral renal stasis have been demonstrated in almost 50% of IBD patients, who for various reasons have an intravenous pyelogram [83], the reported incidence of ureteral obstruction with associated hydronephrosis is 3.1–14.3% in patients with CD [1, 3, 6, 84–86] and 6.8% in those with UC [84]. However, these percentages might be underestimated, considering that this condition is often asymptomatic or paucisymptomatic and that not all patients with IBD are examined with a pyelogram.

In patents affected by CD, ureteral obstruction can be due to periureteral fibrosis secondary to retroperitoneal inflammation (Fig. 3), but usually it is the consequence of compression from an abscess [83]. Sometimes it is caused by an enterovesical fistula which has developed near the ureter. Over 70% of cases are right-sided and are associated with ileal or ileo-cecal disease. Left-sided obstruction has been described in 0–30% and it can be secondary to Crohn's jejunity or, more frequently, to sigmoid inflammation (Fig. 4) [2, 84]. Bilateral obstruction suggesting an extensive pelvic abscess is very rare but not impossible [19].

Ureteral obstruction in the presence of UC is much less frequent and its incidence is equally distributed between the left and right side [84]. Invasive colonic carcinoma [87] and iatrogenic complication [84] are the most common causes. The symptoms are often poor or masked by the intestinal disease. There may be a persistent right lower-quadrant pain radiat-

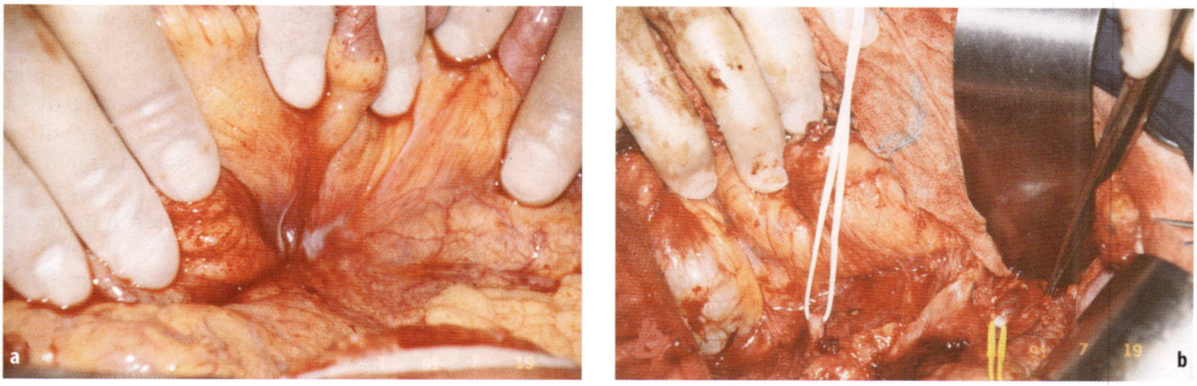

Fig. 3a. Mesenteric and retroperitoneal fibrosis due to CD of terminal ileum. **b** Identification of both ureters

ed to the hip or thigh and associated with fever and a palpable mass. Urinalysis is often negative [3, 83]. When positive for infection, an entero-urinary fistula or pyelonephritis should be suspected [88].

Any of these aspecific signs should alert the doctor and ureteral obstruction should be ruled out because, despite its paucity of symptoms, it can lead to chronic infection of the kidney which may eventually result in nephrectomy [2, 89]. Diagnosis can be usually achieved with an abdominal ultrasound demonstrating dilatation of the ureter and, if present, of the renal pelvis. CT scan is more accurate in identifying whether the cause is an abscess or periureteral fibrosis and also gives more information about the inflammatory disease. Intravenous pyelography visualises a dilated ureter with a smooth cone-shaped restriction typically located at the level of the pelvic brim (Fig. 4a).

With all these exams, differential diagnosis with calculus obstruction should not be difficult. The treatment of this condition has evolved over the last years: older reports recommended routine ureterolysis in association with bowel resection [3, 88]. However, this operation is technically difficult and frequently burdened with morbidity like pyonephrosis, ureteral fistula or nephrectomy [84, 85].

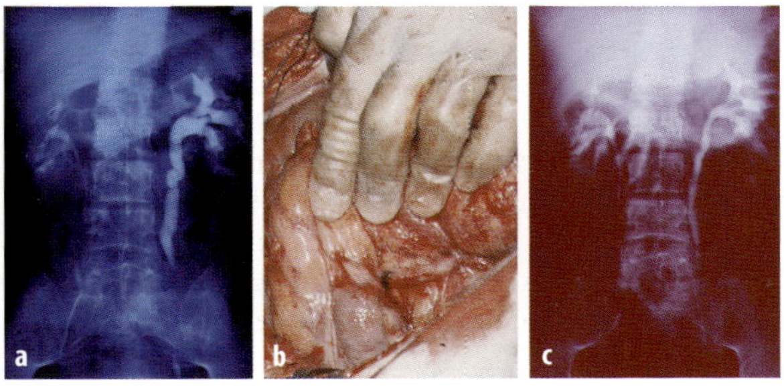

Fig. 4. Left-side ureteral obstruction secondary to Crohn's colitis. **a** Preoperative intravenous pyelography showing a dilated ureter with smooth cone-shaped restriction at the pelvic brim. **b** Intraoperative identification of the ureter after mobilization of descending and sigmoid colon. **c** iv pyelogram 6 months after resection of the affected bowel demonstrating a resolution of ureteral obstruction

It is now evident, that in many cases, the urinary stasis improves or resolves with medical treatment of the underlying bowel disease [84, 85, 90]. Significant obstruction resistant to medical therapy can be initially managed with stenting or percutaneous nephrostomy, but in these cases, surgical resection of the affected bowel and drainage of the associated abscesses should not be delayed and it is generally successful in resolving the obstruction (Fig. 4c) [3, 6, 84–86].

Nephrotoxicity from Medical Treatment

Renal toxicity is unusual with the drugs commonly utilised to treat IBD [91–95], but happens more frequently during treatment with cyclosporine, with reported incidence of up to 19% [96–98]. However, the risk of irreversible damage is very low if cyclosporine dosage does not exceed 5 mg/kg/day and if the creatinine level does not increase over 30% of the normal level [99]. Results from a review showed that a >30% increase in serum creatinine was present in 6% of patients treated with oral or intravenous cyclosporine, but the value returned within the normal range after suspension of the therapy in all of the patients except one [100]. Nephrotoxicity of cyclosporine is not related to duration of treatment but rather to its concentration [99, 101], so this drug should always be started at a low dosage and then adjusted on the basis of close monitoring of the serum creatinine level. Its use is not indicated in patients with impaired renal function and in association with other potential nephrotoxic drugs [100].

Glomerulonephritis and interstitial nephritis have also been described, although with a very low incidence, after long-term administration of aminosalicylates (ASA) [102–105]. In a series of 2 940 patients on mesalamine, only 0.3% developed mild signs of nephrotoxicity [106]. Another prospective survey among 27 European centres found that only 13 (0.8%) of 1529 patients on 5-ASA therapy, only 13 (0.8%) had renal impairment [107]. Sulphasalazine is even safer and it has been successfully given in patients who developed interstitial nephritis with mesalamine [108]. The mechanism of ASA toxicity is unknown. The fact that its occurrence is so uncommon and that it is not related to dosage or duration of treatment, has suggested that the reported cases might have been rather secondary to a hypersensitivity reaction [103, 106]. Permanent damages can be avoided with early recognition of nephropathy and prompt discontinuation of the responsible drug [103, 104].

Urinary Complications of Surgical Treatment

Urinary Tract Calculi

The increased risk of developing calcium oxalate stones after extensive ileal resection or uric acid stones after terminal ileostomy (with or without total colectomy) has been already stated (see section Urinary Tract Calculi).

Urinary Retention

This complication is seen in about 16% of proctectomies [109, 110] but fortunately when it happens it is usually transitory. Both sexes are at risk, although the highest incidence is in older men with benign prostatic enlargement [109, 110]. Other contributing factors include history of bladder over-distension, poor bladder contractility and inhibition of the micturition reflex secondary to pain. It also may be more common in long-term anti-cholinergic users [110].

Bladder dysfunction often results from direct damage to the autonomic nerve plexus during pelvic dissection. Critical areas are represented by the posterolateral ligaments, where both sympathetic and parasympathetic branches constitute the inferior hypogastric plexus, the anterolateral ligaments and anteriorly the plane of Denonvilliers' fascia, which protects the vesical and prostatic plexus [111]. A complete section of nerve trunks is less common but results in permanent lesion. More often nerves are stretched or peripheral branches are sectioned, resulting in transitory problems [112]. The most frequent abnormality is temporary loss of bladder sensation [113]. Less frequently, damage can result as detrusor hypocontractility, bladder neck incompetence, loss of bladder compliance, bladder outlet obstruction [114, 115].

A better knowledge of the pelvic anatomy and application of TME surgery and nerve sparing techniques, both for malignant and benign colorectal disease, have been essential in minimising this problem [111, 116–118]. In a Dutch series of 76 patients who received a proctocolectomy with TME followed by an ileal pouch-anal anastomosis, the incidence of severe bladder dysfunction was zero [119].

Usually retention can be prevented if the catheter is left *in situ* for at least 48–72 h postoperatively. Prophylactic administration of alpha adrenergic blockade has been effective in some series [120, 121], while the use of parasympathicomimetic drugs did not show any benefit [122].

Urological consultation and urodynamic studies are suggested when retention persists beyond a week. However, most of these cases settle after 2–4 weeks of intermittent self-catheterisation. Sometimes resolution of symptoms requires a longer period. Del Rio et al. [123] followed-up of 14 patients in whom micturition disorders were still present 3 months after the operation and noticed that 6 of them were still symptomatic after 12 months and 3 after 3 years. Patients with permanent damage are doomed to intermittent self-catheterization.

Ureteral Injury

Damage of the ureter during colorectal surgery is a known complication which fortunately happens in less than 1% of colectomies [124–126]. While in oncological patients, proximal injuries occur mainly on the left side during isolation and high ligation of the inferior mesenteric artery, in patients with IBD, these lesions are more frequent on the right side and are mainly related to ileocolic CD with extensive retroperitoneal inflammation or fibrosis [19, 64].

Distal injuries can occur on both sites during proctectomy. The more risky areas are the lateral rectal ligaments and the plane between the rectum and seminal vesicles [127]. The key to preventing injury is knowledge of the anatomy, early identification of the ureter and anterior rectal dissection preserving the Denonvillier's fascia [128]. Prophylactic catheterisation may be useful in selected cases, although it does not assure the prevention of transmural lesions and it has become associated with a risk of injury [126].

When damage is recognised at the time of surgery,

repair over a catheter is indicated. Proximal injuries can be managed with direct end-to-end anastomosis, while distal injuries often require ureteroneocystostomy. Other options like creation of an anterior bladder flap (Boari flap), transureteroureterostomy and neocreation of the ureter with a segment of ileum are rarely necessary [129]. However, up to 70% of injuries are not immediately recognised [129]. Missed lesions should be suspected postoperatively in the presence of flank pain associated with fever and paralytic ileus. In this case, initial management is provided by endoscopic positioning of ureteral stent or nephrostomy. If the patient's conditions and renal function are impaired, reconstruction may not be indicated and nephrectomy may be the procedure of choice [129, 130].

Sexual Dysfunction in IBD

There are different factors which may contribute to limiting the sexual life of an IBD patient; in fact sexual dysfunction may be related to the disease itself, and in this case it usually improves after treatment [131–134], but sometimes it is a consequence of medical or surgical therapy.

Sexual Dysfunction Related to the Disease

Sexual desire may be reduced by generalised debility or by the presence of perianal or cutaneous fistulas which alter the acceptance of his/her own body image and thus make the patient uncomfortable and embarrassed with his or her partner. More often, the constant presence of symptoms like abdominal pain and diarrhoea are the cause of reduced relational and sexual activity [9].

Besides these psychological aspects, many women suffer from dyspareunia. This can be secondary to perineal disease, severe proctitis or to the presence of an inflamed segment of bowel in the pouch of Douglas, in direct contact with the posterior fornix of the vagina [135]. In these cases symptoms generally improve after resection of the inflamed bowel [135–137]. Another possible cause of dyspareunia is vaginal candidiasis, which has been frequently noticed in women affected by CD [9].

Sexual Dysfunction Related to Medical Treatment

The various medications used to control the inflammatory process can reduce some of the problems described above. On the other hand, they have potential side effects like loss of libido, mood swings, vaginal dryness and weight gain, which may contribute to worsen the sexual activity [8].

Male impotence and infertility is another possible side effect of medical therapy, especially during treatment with sulphasalazine [138–140]. This fact has also been noticed in a survey that compared the quality of life between patients with ulcerative colitis treated medically and patients who had received a restorative proctocolectomy; utilising specific questionnaires, it emerged that 26% of patients under medical therapy suffered from impotence and another 16% reported regular failure of ejaculation, while these problems were present in only 8% of those who underwent surgery [141]. However, in most cases discontinuation or changing of the drug is sufficient to return to normality [138, 139].

Sexual Dysfunction Secondary to Surgical Treatment

Sexual dysfunction following rectal surgery for IBD has been reported in 1–27% of cases but dysfunction is often partial and transient [119, 128, 132, 133, 142–148]. This is usually due to damage of neurological structures during pelvic dissection, although psychogenic or vasculogenic factors may contribute [149].

Normal sexual function in males is under the control of both the sympathetic and parasympathetic system: erection is mainly mediated by parasympathetic fibres, while sympathetic fibres are primarily responsible for deposition of the semen in the posterior urethra and contemporaneous closure of the bladder neck during ejaculation. Damage of this mechanism will result in retrograde ejaculation.

Parasympathetic fibres from the second, third and fourth sacral foramen give rise to the nervi erigentes. They run on either site of the pelvic wall into the lateral rectal ligaments where they constitute, together with the presacral nerves, the inferior hypogastric (or pelvic) plexus. Presacral nerves start from the superior hypogastric plexus, which is the continuation of the preaortic plexus and contain sympathetic fibres from the twelfth thoracic and the first two lumbar segments. They run on the posterolateral aspect of the pelvis, protected by the presacral fascia (Waldeyer's fascia), but at the level of the mid-distal rectum, they perforate the presacral fascia and run more laterally to reach the pelvic plexus. Cavernous nerves take origin from the most caudal portion of the pelvic plexus and descend towards the penis in a plane anterior to Denonvilliers' fascia, running along the postero-lateral aspect of the prostate [149].

As already seen in the previous paragraph on urinary retention, the most critical areas are represented by the lateral ligaments and anteriorly by the plane of Denonvilliers' fascia, where both sympathetic and parasympathetic branches can be injured. Sympathetic nerves can be also damaged near the promontory of the sacrum or during lateral dissection of the rectum. For this reason, proctectomy for benign diseases has traditionally been carried out with perimuscular dissection and possibly intersphincteric dissection [150–152] and this has resulted in a much lower incidence of sexual complications as compared to surgery for malignancy [153]. However, recent studies have argued that identification of autonomic nerves, as it happens during total mesorectal excision, is the best way to lower the incidence of urinary and sexual problems both in malignant and benign rectal surgery, provided that the anterior Denonvillier's fascia is respected [111, 116–119, 154].

There are no randomised controlled trials on this aspect and the only study that has compared results after mesorectal (111 patients) or close rectal (45 patients) dissection for IBD, did not show significant differences between the two techniques in terms of permanent impotence (4.5% *vs.* 2.2%) or minor erectile difficulties (13.5% *vs.* 13.3%) [128]. In the event of postoperative impotence, a period of observation is always indicated, because dysfunction is transitory in the majority of cases. In the mean time, other possible causes such as psychological or vascular causes should be excluded.

Problems that persist beyond 3–6 months are likely to be permanent. In these cases, the therapeutic options are injection of the cavernous corpora with vasodilatory drugs (papaverine, prostaglandin) or surgical implant of either a malleable or inflatable prosthesis [155]. The last are preferred because they give a more natural appearance to the penis [156] and a higher grade of satisfaction [155]. New drugs such as sildenafil citrate (Viagra, Pfizer, NY, USA) require an intact penile innervation to work. In practice they are only effective in patients with partial but inadequate erections [149].

Retrograde ejaculation, which is the result of isolated damage of the sympathetic nerves, may be treated with sympathomimetic drugs. If they fail and the patient desires to procreate, sperm can be drawn from the bladder for artificial insemination [157, 158]. In view of this possible complication, some authors suggested that young male patients should cryopreserve sperm before elective proctectomy [159], while others find this expedient unnecessary and expensive [160].

Rectal surgery may also have negative effects on sexual function in women: in fact dorsocaudal dislocation of the vagina after proctectomy or formation of postoperative scarring angulating the vagina may be responsible for dyspareunia and chronic infections secondary to retained secretions [161, 162]. These problems are less frequent after restorative proctocolectomy, where the presence of the ileal-pouch contributes towards maintaining the vagina in its normal position [163]. This has been confirmed in a survey that compared sexual function in women after restorative proctocolectomies or after proctocolectomy and Kock pouch: the incidence of dyspareunia was 18 and 38% respectively and none of the patients in the first group complained of vaginal discharge, compared to 18% of the second group [131].

Finally, sexuality may be negatively influenced by surgery when this results in stoma formation. In fact it has been demonstrated that the presence of stoma is a strong psychological deterrent to sexual intercourse [164, 165].

Conclusions

Urologic and sexual problems in patients with IBD are not rare and can be either the consequence of the evolution of the inflammatory process or the consequence of its treatment. Males and patients with Crohn's disease are the most exposed.

Early urinary symptoms are often missed both by the patient and doctor because they are not specific and are overshadowed by the more severe intestinal manifestations. When they become evident, renal damage may have already occurred. For these reasons people with IBD should be periodically examined with simple exams such as urinalysis, serum creatinine level and abdominal ultrasound in order to recognise these manifestation at an early stage and carry out the appropriate treatment. Some conditions can be prevented or treated with diet or medicines, while others, like fistulas and obstructive uropathy *per se* indicate an advanced intestinal disease which usually requires surgery.

Sexual alterations are quite troublesome, especially because of the young age of these patients. Again, it is very important that doctors dealing with IBD are aware of the possibility of sexual problems and investigate them appropriately. Often, counselling with a specialist is sufficient for ameliorating the situation; as psychological factors may play a major role in causing dysfunction, the patient should be reassured that a correct treatment of the inflammatory disease usually results in significant improvement not only in general conditions but also in the social and sexual life.

On the other hand, patients should be informed that surgical treatment, especially in the case of rectal resection, carries the potential risk of urinary and sexual complications that in a minority of cases are permanent and may significantly affect the quality of life.

References

1. Greenstein AJ, Janowitz HD, Sachar DB (1976) The extraintestinal complications of Crohn's disease in ulcerative colitis: a study of 700 patients. Medicine 55:401–12
2. Kyle J (1980) Urinary complications of Crohn's disease. World J Surg 4:153–160
3. Shield DE, Lytton B, Weiss RM et al (1976) Urologic complications of inflammatory bowel disease. J Urol 115:701–706
4. Oefelein MG (2003) Urologic manifestations of nonurologic diseases gastrointestinal disorders. Urol Clin North Am 30:63–72
5. Ben-Ami H, Ginesin Y, Behar DM et al (2002) Diagnosis and treatment of urinary tract complications in Crohn's disease: an experience over 15 years. Can J Gastroenterol 16:225–229
6. Sato S, Sasaki I, Naito H et al (1999) Management of urinary complications in Crohn's disease. Surg Today 29(8):713–717
7. Hyams JA, Weinberg SR, Alley JL (1943) Chronic ileitis with concomitant ureteritis: case report. AM J Surg 61:117–124
8. Erwin-Toth P (2001) Sexual adjustments and body image. In: Bayless TM, Hanauer SB (eds) Advanced Therapy of Inflammatory Bowel Disease. Decker, Hamilton, Canada
9. Moody G, Probert CS, Srivastava EM et al (1992) Sexual dysfunction amongst women with Crohn's disease: a hidden problem. Digestion 52:179–183
10. Mc Leod RS, Churchill DN (1992) Urolithiasis complicatine inflammatory bowel disease. J Urol 148:974–978
11. Caudarella R, Rizzoli E, Pironi L et al (1993) Renal stones in patients with inflammatory bowel disease. Scanning Microsc 7:371–380
12. Nightingale JM (1995) The short-bowel syndrome. Eur J Gastroenterol Hepatol 7:514–520
13. Gelzayd EA, Breuer RI, Kirsner JB (1968) Nephrolithiasis in inflammatory bowel disease. Am J Dig Dis 13:1027–1034
14. Smith LH, Fromm H, Hofmann AF (1972) Acquired hyperoxaluria, nephrolithiasis, and intestinal disease: description of a syndrome. N Engl J Med 286:1371–1375
15. Chadwick VS Modha K, Dowling RH (1973) Mechanism for hyperoxaluria in patients with ileal dysfunction. New Eng J Med 289:172–176
16. Clarke AM, McKenzie RG (1969) Ileostomy and the risk of urinary uric acid stones. Lancet 2:395–397
17. Reisner GS, Wilansky DL, Schneiderman C (1973) Uric acid lithiasis in the ileostomy patient. Br J Urol 45:340–343
18. Casula G (1992) Urologic manifestations in Crohn's disease. Chir Gastroent 26:103–108
19. Banner MP (1987) Genitourinary complications of inflammatory bowel disease. Radiol Clin North Am 25:199–209
20. Sitrin MD, Rosenberg H, Chawla K (1980) Nutritional and metabolic complications in patients with Crohn's disease and ileal resection. Gastroenterology 78:1069–1079
21. Fukushima T, Matsuda I (1982) Clinical and urinary characteristics of urolithiasis in ulcerative colitis. Am J Gastroenterol 77:238–242
22. Kirks DR (1979) John Caffey Award: Lithiasis due to interruption of the enterohepatic circulation of bile salts. Am J Roentgenol 133:383–88
23. Allison MJ, Cook HM, Milne DB et al (1986) Oxalate degradation by gastrointestinal bacteria from humans. J Nutr 116:455–460
24. Argenzio RA, Liacos JA, Allison MJ (1988) Intestinal oxalate-degrading bacteria reduce oxalate absorption and toxicity in guinea pigs. J Nutr 118:787–792
25. Kumar R, Ghoshal UC, Singh G et al (2004) Infrequency of colonization with Oxalobacter formigenes in inflammatory bowel disease: possible role in renal stone formation. J Gastroenterol Hepatol 19:1403–1409
26. McConnell N, Campbell S, Gillanders I et al (2002) Risk factors for developing renal stones in inflammatory bowel disease. BJU Int 89:835–841
27. Manganiotis AN, Banner MP, Malkowicz SB (2001) Urologic complications of Crohn's disease. Surg Clin North Am 81:197–215
28. Sakhaee K, Nicar M, Hill K (1983) Contrasting effects of potassium citrate and sodium citrate therapies on urinary chemistries and crystallization of stone-forming salts. Kidney Int 24:348–352
29. Pak CY, Waters O, Arnold L et al (1977) Mechanism of calcium urolithiasis among patients with hyperuricosuria. J Clin Invest 59:426–431
30. Pardi DS, Tremaine WJ, Sandborn WJ, McCarthy JT (1998) Renal and urologic complications of inflammatory bowel disease. Am J Surg 93:504–514
31. Barilla DE, Notz C, Kennedy D et al (1978) Renal oxalate excretion following oral oxalate loads in patients with ileal disease and with renal and absorptive hypercalciurias: effect of calcium and magnesium. Am J Med 64:579–85
32. Shovron PJ (1977) Amyloidosis and inflammatory bowel disease. Am J Dig Dis 22:209–213
33. Greenstein AJ, Sachar DB, Nannan Panday AK et al (1992) Amyloidosis and inflammatory bowel disease: a 50 year experience with 25 patients. Medicine 71:261–270
34. Mir-Madjlessi SH, Brown CH, Hawk WA (1972) Amyloidosis associated with Crohn's disease. Am J Gastroenterol 58:563–577
35. Fausa O, Nygaard K, Elgjo K (1977) Amyloidosis in Crohn's disease. Scand J Gastroenterol 12:657–662
36. Lowdel CP, Shousha S, Parkins RA (1986) The incidence of amyloidosis complicating inflammatory bowel disease. Dis Colon Rectum 29:351–354
37. Werther JL, Schapira A, Rubinstein O et al (1960) Amyloidosis in regional enteritis. Am J Med 29:416–423
38. Mandelstam P, Simmons DE, Mitchell BH (1989) Regression of amyloid in Crohn's disease after bowel resection: a 19 year follow-up. J Clin Gastroenterol 11:324–326
39. Gitkind MJ, Wright SC (1990) Amyloidosis complicating inflammatory bowel disease. Dig Dis Sci 35:906–908
40. Ravid M, Shapira J, Kedar I, Feigl D (1979) Regression

of amyloidosis secondary to granulomatous ileitis following surgical resection and colchicine administration. Acta Hepatogatroenterol 26:513–515
41. Meyers S, Janowitz HD, Gumaste VV et al (1988) Colchicine therapy of the renal amyloidosis of ulcerative colitis. Gastroenterology 94:1503–1507
42. Efstratiadis G, Mainas A, Leontsini M (1996) Renal amyloidosis complicating Crohn's disease. J Clin Gastroenterol 22:308–310
43. Steinhoff J, Schulz E, Herbst EW et al (1988) Therapy of amyloid nephrosis due to Crohn's disease: plasmapheresis plus azathioprine? Wien Med Wochenschr 138:49–54
44. Lovat LB, Madhoo S, Pepys MB, Hawkins PN (1997) Long-term survival in systemic amyloid A amyloidosis complicating Crohn's disease. Gastroenterology 112:1362–1365
45. Stokke KT, Teisberg PA, Myhre E (1976) Nephrotic syndrome in ulcerative colitis. Scand J Gastroenterol 11:571–576
46. Wilcox GM, Aretz HT, Roy MA et al (1990) Glomerulonephritis associated with inflammatory bowel disease. Gastroenterology 98:786–791
47. Thomas DM, Nicholls AJ, Feest TG (1990) Ulcerative colitis and glomerulo nephritis: is there an association? Nephrol Dial Transplant 5:628–629
48. Moayyedi P, Fletcher S, Harnden P et al (1995) Mesangiocapillary glomerulonephritis associated with ulcerative colitis: case report of two patients. Nephrol Dial Transplant 10:1923–1924
49. Presti ME, Neuschwander-Tetri BA, Vogler CA et al (1997) Sclerosing cholangitis, inflammatory bowel disease and glomerulonephritis. Dig Dis Sci 42:813–816
50. Ridder, RM, Kreth HW, Kiss E et al (2005) Membranous nephropathy associated with familial chronic ulcerative colitis in a 12-year-old girl. Pediatr Nephrol 20:1349–1351
51. Diaz Rodriguez C, Granja E, Vasquez Martul et al (2004) Association between membranous glomerulonephritis and Crohn's disease. Nefrologia 24(4):368–371
52. Ashman N, Sheaff M, Raftery MJ (2003) Mesangiocapillary glomerulonephritis associated with ulcerative colitis: a 6-year follow-up of 2 cases. Clin Nephrol 60(2):146–148
53. Fiasse R, Lurhuma AZ, Cambiaso CL (1978) Circulating immune complexes and disease activity in Crohn's disease. Gut 19:611–617
54. Trimarchi HM, Iotti A, Iotti R et al (2001) Immunoglobulin A nephropathy and ulcerative colitis: a focus on their pathogenesis. Am J Nephrol 21(5):400–405
55. Schofield PM, Williams PS (1984) Proliferative glomerulonephritis associated with Crohn's disease. BMJ 289:1039
56. Glassman M, Kaplan M, Spivak W (1986) Immune-complex glomerulonephritis in Crohn's disease. J Ped Gastroenterol Nutr 5:966–969
57. Molina-Perez, Gonzalez-Reimers E, Santolaria-Fernandez F et al (1995) Rapidly progressive glomerulonephritis and inflammatory bowel disease. Dis Colon Rectum 38:1006–1007
58. Greenstein AJ, Kark AE, Dreiling DA (1974) Crohn's disease of the colon: fistula in Crohn's disease of the colon, classification, presenting features and management in 63 patients. Am J Gastroenterol 62:419–429
59. Talamini MA, Broe PJ, Cameron JL (1982) Urinary fistulas in Crohn's disease. Surg Gyn Ob 154:553–556
60. McNamara MJ, Fazio VW, Lavery IC et al (1990) Surgical treatment of enterovesical fistula in Crohn's disease. Dis Colon Rectum 33:271–276
61. Gruner JS, Sehon JK, Johnson LW (2002) Diagnosis and management of enterovesical fistulas in patients with Crohn's disease. Am Surg 68:714–719
62. Chebli JM, Gaburri PD, Pinto JR (2004) Enterovesical fistula in Crohn's disease. Lancet 364:68
63. Greenstein AJ, Sachar DB, Tzakis A et al (1984) Course of enterovesical fistulas in Crohn's disease. Am J Surg 147:788–792
64. Rankin GB (1990) Extraintestinal and systemic manifestations of inflammatory bowel disease. Med Clin North Am 74:39–50
65. Solem CA, Loftus EV, Tremaine WJ et al (2002) Fistulas to the urinary system in Crohn's disease: clinical features and outcome. Am J Gastroenterol 97:2300–2305
66. Margolin ML, Korelitz BI (1989) Management of bladder fistulas in Crohn's disease. J Clin Gastroenterol 11:399–402
67. Karamchandani MC, West CF (1984) Vesicoenteric fistulas. Am J Surg 147:681–683
68. Present DH (2002) Urinary tract fistulas in Crohn's disease: surgery versus medical therapy. Am J Gastroenterol 97:2165–2167
69. Sou S, Yao T, Matsui T, Takemura S (1999) Preoperative detection of occult enterovesical fistulas in patients with Crohn's disease: efficacy of oral or rectal administration of indocyanine green solution. Dis Colon Rectum 42:266–270
70. Goldman SM, Fishman EK, Gatewood OMB et al (1985) Computerized tomography in the diagnosis of the enterovesical fistulas. Am J Radiol 144:1229–1233
71. Koelbel G, Schmiedl U, Majer MC et al (1989) Diagnosis of fistulas and sinus tracts in patients with Crohn's disease: value of MR imaging. Am J Radiol 152:999–1003
72. Schraut WH, Block GE (1984) Enterovesical fistula complicating Crohn's ileocolitis. Am J Gastroenterol 79:186–190
73. Daniels IR, Bekdash B, Scott HJ (2002) Diagnostic lessons learnt from a series of enterovesical fistulae. Colorectal Dis 4:459–462
74. King RM, Beart RW, McIlrath DC (1982) Colovesical and rectovesical fistulas. Arch Surg 117:680–683
75. Sarr MG, Fishman EK, Goldman SM et al (1987) Enterovesical fistulas. Surg Gyn Obs 164:41–48
76. Gorcey S, Katzka I (1989) Is operation always necessary for enterovesical fistulas in Crohn's disease? J Clin Gatroenterol 11:396–398
77. Wheeler SC, Marion JF, Present DH (2000) Medical therapy, not surgery, is the appropriate first line treatment for Crohn's enterovesical fistula. Gastroenterology 114:A1113
78. Levy C, Tremaine WJ (2002) Management of internal fistulas in Crohn's disease. 8:106–111
79. Yamamoto T, Keighley MRB (2000) Enterovesical fistulas complicating Crohn's disease: clinicopathological features in management. Int J Colorectal Dis 15:211–215

80. Present DH, Rutgeerts P, Targan S et al (1999) Infliximab for the treatment of fistulas in patients with Crohn's disease. N Engl J Med 340:1398–1405
81. Parsi MA, Lashner BA, Achkar JP et al (2004) Type of fistula determines response to infliximab in patients with fistulous Crohn's disease. Am J Gastroenterol 99:445–449
82. Sands BE, Blank MA, Patel K, van Deventer SJ, ACCENT II Study (2004) Long-term treatment of rectovaginal fistulas in Crohn's disease: response to infliximab in the ACCENT II Study. Clin Gastroenterol Hepatol 2:912–920
83. Present DH, Rabinowitz JG, Banks PA et al (1969) Obstructive hydronephrosis. A frequent but seldom recognized complication of granulomatous disease of the bowel. New Engl J Med 280:523–528
84. Fleckenstein P, Knudsen L, Pedersen EB et al (1977) Obstructive uropathy in inflammatory bowel disease. Scand J Gastroenterol 12:519–23
85. Siminovitch JMP, Fazio VW (1980) Ureteral obstruction secondary to Crohn's disease: a need for ureterolysis? Am J Surg 139:95–98
86. Shofield PF, Staff WG, Moore T (1968) Ureteral involvement in regional ileitis (Crohn's disease). J Urol 99:412–416
87. Edwards FC, Truelove SC (1964) The course and prognosis of ulcerative colitis. III. Complications. Gut 5:1–15
88. Block GE, Enker WE, Kirsner JB (1973) Significance and treatment of occult obstructive uropathy complicating Crohn's disease. Ann Surg 178:323–332
89. Kent GG, McGowan GE, Hyams JS et al (1987) Hypertension associated with unilateral hydronephrosis as a complication of Crohn's disease. J Pediatric Surg 22:1049–1050
90. Hyams JS (1994) Extraintestinal manifestation of inflammatory bowel disease in children. J Ped Gastroenterol Nutr 19:7–21
91. Kjellstrand CM (1975) Side effects of steroids and their treatment. Transplant Proc 7:123–129
92. Pearson DC, May GR, Fick GH et al (1995) Azathioprine and 6-mercaptopurine in Crohn's disease: a metanalysis. Ann Intern Med 122:132–142
93. de Jong DJ, Goullet M, Naber TH (2004) Side effects of azathioprine in patients with Crohn's disease. Eur J Gastroenterol Hepatol 16:207–212
94. Goodman TA, Polisson RP (1994) Methotrexate: adverse reactions and major toxicity. Rheumat Dis Clin NA 20:513–528
95. Falagas ME, Gorbach SL (1995) Clindamicin and metronidazole. Med Clin NA 79:845–867
96. Jewell DP, Lennard-Jones JE, and the Cyclosporine Study Group of Great Britain and Ireland (1994) Oral cyclosporine for chronic active Crohn's disease: a multicentre controlled trial. Eur J Gastroenterol Hepatol 6:499–505
97. Stange EF, Modigliani R, Pena AS et al (1995) European trial of cyclosporine in chronic active Crohn's disease: a 12-month study. Gastroenterology 109:774–782
98. Feagan BG, McDonald JW, Rochon J et al (1994) Low-dose cyclosporine for the treatment of Crohn's disease. N Engl J Med 330:1846–1851
99. Feutren G, Mihatsch MJ, for the international Kidney Biopsy Registry of Cyclosporine in Autoimmune Diseases (1992) Risk factors for cyclosporine-induced nephropathy in patients with autoimmune diseases. N Eng J Med 326:1654–1660
100. Sandborn WJ (1996) A review of immune modifier therapy for inflammatory bowel disease: azathioprine, 6-mercaptopurine, cyclosporine, and methotrexate. Am J Gastroenterol 91:423–433
101. McDonald JW, Feagan BG, Jewell D et al (2005) Cyclosporine for induction of remission in Crohn's disease. Cochrane Database Syst Rev 18:CD000297
102. Barbour VM, Williams PF (1990) Nephrotic sindrome associated with sulfasalazine. Br Med J 301:818
103. Dwarakanath AD, Michael J, Allan RN (1992) Sulfasalazine induced renal failure. Gut 33:563–564
104. Thuluvath PJ, Ninkovic M, Calam J (1994) Mesalazine induced interstitial nephritis. Gut 35:1493–1496
105. Wilcox GM, Reynolds JR, Galvanek EG (1996) Nephrotoxicity associated with olsalazine. Am J Med 100:238–240
106. Hanauer SB, Verst-Brasch C, Regali G (1997) Renal safety of long-term mesalamine therapy in inflammatory bowel disease. Gastroenterology 112:A991
107. Elseviers MM, D'Haens G, Lerebours E et al (2004) Renal impairment in patients with inflammatory bowel disease: association with aminosalicylate therapy? Clin Nephrol 61:83–89
108. Mehta RP (1990) Acute interstitial nephritis due to 5-aminosalicylic acid. Can Med Assoc J 143:1031–1032
109. Baumrucker GO, Shaw JW (1953) Urological complications following abdominoperineal resection of the rectum. Arch Surg 67:502–513
110. Tank ES, Ernst CB, Woolson ST et al (1972) Urinary tract complications of anorectal surgery. Am J Surg 123:118–122
111. Hollabaugh RS Jr, Steiner MS, Sellers KD et al (2000) Neuroanatomy of the pelvis: implications for colonic and rectal resection. Dis Colon Rectum 43:1390–1397
112. Fowler JW, Bremner DN, Moffat LE (1978) The incidence and consequences of damage to the parasympathetic nerve supply to the bladder after abdominoperineal resection of the rectum for carcinoma. Br J Urol 50:95–98
113. Gerstenberg TC, Nielsen ML, Clausen S et al (1980) Bladder function after abdominoperineal resection of the rectum for anorectal cancer. Urodynamic investigation before and after operation in a consecutive series. Ann Surg 191:81–87
114. Smith JJ (2000) Bladder dysfunction after colorectal surgery. Seminars in Colon & Rectal Surgery 3:136–140
115. Enker WE, Havenga K, Polyak T et al (1997) Abdominoperineal resection via total mesorectal excision and autonomic nerve preservation for low rectal cancer. World J Surg 21:715–720
116. Lindsey I, Guy RJ, Warren BF et al (2000) Anatomy of Denonvilliers' fascia and pelvic nerves, impotence, and implications for the colorectal surgeon. Br J Surg 87:1288–1299
117. Nesbakken A, Nygaard K, Bull-Njaa T et al (2000) Bladder and sexual dysfunction after mesorectal excision for rectal cancer. Br J Surg 87:206–210
118. Havenga K, Enker WE (2002) Autonomic nerve pre-

serving total mesorectal excision. Surg Clin North Am 82:1009–1018
119. Slors FJ, van Zuijlen PP, van Dijk GJ (2000) Sexual and bladder dysfunction after total mesorectal excision for benign diseases. Scan J Gastroenterol 232:48–51
120. Velanovich V (1992) Pharmacologic prevention and treatment of postoperative urinary retention. Infect Urol 3:87
121. Goldman G, Kahn PJ, Kashtan HJ et al (1988) Prevention and treatment of urinary retention and infection after surgical treatment of the colon and rectum with alpha adrenergic blockers. Surg Gynecol Obstet 166:447–450
122. Finkbeiner AE (1985) Is bethanechol chloride clinically effective in promoting bladder emptying? A literature review. J Urol 134:443–449
123. Del Rio C, Sanchez-Santos R, Oreja V et al (2004) Long-term urinary dysfunction after rectal cancer surgery. Colorectal Dis 6:198–202
124. Graham JW, Goligher JC (1954) The management of accidental injuries and deliberate resections of the ureter during excision of the rectum. Br J Surg 42:151–160
125. Dowling RA, Corriere JN Jr., Sandler CM (1986) Iatrogenic ureteral injury. J Urol 135:912–915
126. Bothwell WN, Bleicher RJ, Dent TL (1994) Prophylactic ureteral catheterization in colon surgery: a five-year review. Dis Colon Rectum 37:330–334
127. Beahrs JR, Beahrs OH, Beahrs MM et al (1978) Urinary tract complications with rectal surgery. Ann Surg 187:542–548
128. Lindsey I, George BD, Kettlewell MGW et al (2001) Impotence after mesorectal and close rectal dissection for inflammatory bowel disease. Dis Colon Rectum 44:831–835
129. Hamawy K, Smith JJ, Libertino JA (2000) Injuries of the distal ureter. Seminars in Colon Rectal Surgery 11:163–179
130. Block GE, Hurst RD (1995) Complications of the surgical treatment of ulcerative colitis and Crohn's disease. In: Kirsner JB, Shorter RG (eds) Inflammatory bowel disease, 4th edn. Williams, Baltimore, MD, pp 898–922
131. Metcalf AM, Dozois RR, Kelly KA (1986) Sexual function in women after proctocolectomy. Ann Surg 204:624–627
132. Damgaard B, Wettergreen A, Kirkegaard P (1995) Social and sexual function following ileal pouch-anal anasotomosis. Dis Colon Rectum 38:286–289
133. Berndtsson I, Oresland T, Hulten L (2004) Sexuality in patients with ulcerative colitis before and after restorative proctocolectomy: a prospective study. Scand J Gastroenterol 39:374–379
134. Gorgun E, Remzi FH, Montague DK et al (2005) Male sexual function improves after ileal pouch anal anastomosis. Colorectal Dis 7:545–550
135. Gruner ON, Naas R, Fretheim B et al (1977) Marital status and sexual adjustment after colectomy: results in 178 patients operated on for ulcerative colitis. Scand J Gastroenterol 12:193–197
136. Weber AM, Ziegler C, Belinson JL et al (1995) Gynecologic history of women with inflammatory bowel disease. Obstet Gynecol 86:843–847
137. Sjogren B, Poppen B (1995) Sexual life in women after colectomy-proctomucosectomy with S-pouch. Acta Obstet Gynecol Scand 74:51–55
138. Ragni G, Bianchi Porro G, Ruspa M et al (1984). Abnormal semen quality and lower serum testosterone in men with inflammatory bowel disease treated for a long time with sulfasalazine. Andro 16:162–167
139. Riley SA, Lecarpentier J, Mani V (1987) Sulfasalazine induced seminal abnormalities: results of mesalazine substitution. Gut 28:1008–1012
140. Ireland A, Jewell DP (1989) Sulfasalazine-induced impotence: a beneficial resolution with olsalazine? J Clin Gastroenterol 11:711
141. Sagar PM, Lewis W, Holdsworth PJ et al (1993) Quality of life after restorative proctocolectomy with a pelvic ileal reservoir compares favourably with that of patients with medically treated colitis. Dis Colon Rectum 36:584–592
142. Watts JM, de Dombal FT, Goligher JC (1966) Early results of surgery for ulcerative colitis. Br J Surg 53:1005–1014
143. Corman ML, Veidenheimer MC, Coller JA (1978) Impotence after proctectomy for inflammatory disease of the bowel. Dis Colon Rectum 21:418–419
144. Fazio VW, Fletcher J, Montague D (1980) Prospective study of the effect of resection of the rectum on male sexual function. World J Surg 4:149–152
145. Bauer JJ, Gelernt IM, Salky B et al (1983) Sexual dysfunction following proctocolectomy for benign disease of the colon and rectum. Ann Surg 197:363–367
146. Tiainen J, Matikainen M, Hiltunen KM (1999) Ileal J-pouch-anal anastomosis, sexual dysfunction, and fertility. Scand J Gastroenterol 34:185–188
147. Dozois RR, Nelson H, Metcalf AM (1993) Sexual function after ileo-anal anastomosis. Ann Chir 47:1009–1013
148. Michelassi F, Stella M, Block GE (1993) Prospective assessment of functional results after ileal J pouch-anal restorative proctocolectomy. Arch Surg 128:889–895
149. Sorcini A, Vereb MJ (2000) Sexual and reproductive complications after pelvic surgery. Seminars in Colon Rectal Surgery 11:141–147
150. Lee EC, Dowling BL (1972) Perimuscular excision of the rectum for Crohn's disease. Br J Surg 59:29–32
151. Bauer JJ, Gelernt IM, Salk BA et al (1986) Proctectomy for inflammatory bowel disease. Am J Surg 151:157–162
152. Little JA, Parks AG (1977) Intersphincteric excision of the rectum. Br J Surg 64:413–416
153. Yeager ES, Van Heerden JA (1980) Sexual dysfunction following proctocolectomy and abdominoperineal resection. Ann Surg 191:169–170
154. Maurer CA, Z'Graggen K, Renzulli P et al (2001) Total mesorectal excision preserves male genital function compared with conventional rectal cancer surgery. Br J Surg 88:1501–1505
155. Malloy TR, Wein AJ, Carpiniello VL (1986) Reliability of AMS 700 inflatable penile prothesis. Urology 27:385–387
156. Benson GS (1996) Male sexual dysfunction—pitfalls, pills and prostheses. J Urol 156:1636
157. Cameron MC, Gillett WR (1985) The recovery of sperm, insemination and pregnancy in the treatment

of infertility because of retrograde ejaculation. Fertil Steril 44:844–845
158. Shangold GA, Cantor B, Schreiber JR (1980) Treatment of infertility due to retrograde ejaculates: a simple, cost-effective method. Fertil Steril 34:175–177
159. Thomas AJ Jr (2004) Infertility. J Urol 172(3):829–830
160. van Duijvendijk P, Slors JF, Taat CW et al (2000) What is the benefit of preoperative sperm preservation for patients who undergo restorative proctocolectomy for benign diseases? Dis Colon Rectum 43:838–842
161. Wikland M, Jansson I, Asztely M et al (1990) Gynecological problems related to anatomical changes after conventional proctocolectomy and ileostomy. Int J Colorectal Dis 5:49–52
162. Sjodahl R, Nystrom P, Olaison G (1990) Surgical treatment of dorsocaudal dislocation of the vagina after excision of the rectum: the Kylberg operation. Dis Colon Rectum 33:762–764
163. Oresland T, Palmblad S, Ellstrom M et al (1994) Gynecological and sexual function related to anatomical changes in the female pelvis after restorative proctocolectomy. Int J Colorectal Disease 9:77–81
164. Sprangers MA, Taal BG, Aaronson NK, et al (1995). Quality of life in colorectal cancer. Stoma vs. nonstoma patients. Dis Colon Rectum 38:361–369
165. Nugent KP, Daniels P, Stewart B et al (1999) Quality of life in stoma patients. Dis Colon Rectum 42:1569–1574

Biological Approach in the Treatment of Crohn's Disease

Luca Frulloni, Laura Bernardoni, Chiara Scattolini, Italo Vantini

Introduction

Crohn's Disease (CD) is a chronic inflammatory disease of the gastrointestinal tract, with a low percentage of patients remaining in clinical remission despite the long-term use of many drugs (steroids, immunosuppressants, aminosalicylates, antibiotics). As a consequence of the limited efficacy and significant toxicity of current therapy, there is widespread interest in the development of novel drugs for the clinical management of CD.

In the early 1990s, the pathogenetic mechanisms of inflammatory bowel diseases (IBDs) were clarified. Greater knowledge of systemic and local inflammatory cascade of CD (T1-helper-driven inflammation) [1] allowed identification of key mediators of inflammation, and pharmacologic research was addressed towards specific biologic drugs interfering with this cascade. Proinflammatory cytokines play a central role in amplification of the inflammatory process, inducing release of other cytokines and increasing the expression of adhesion molecules [2]. Tumour necrosis factor (TNF)-α and interleukin (IL)-1 are released at the beginning of the inflammatory cascade and contribute to recruitment and activation of inflammatory cells (macrophages, neutrophils, monocytes) by increasing mucosal intestinal permeability and stimulating the release of adhesion molecules. Anti-inflammatory cytokines play an important role in avoidance of an abnormal immune response. In particular, IL-10 controls TNF production, major histocompatibility complex (MHC)-II expression and release of other inflammatory mediators whereas IL-12 induces the release of interferon gamma (INF-γ) by macrophages and natural-killer lymphocytes [3].

The term "biological agent" means any therapeutic agent derived from a living organism. Therefore, biological therapy may include [4]: (1) modified biological compounds (i.e. vaccine), hormones, etc.; (2) recombinant peptides or proteins (i.e. growing factors, growth hormones, etc.); (3) monoclonal antibodies or fusion proteins; (4) antisense oligonucleotides. Many molecules have been used in controlled or open trials, mainly in fistulising or steroid-dependent CD (Table 1). Monoclonal antibodies and antisense nucleotides interfering with messenger ribonucleic acid (mRNA) are the drugs most frequently tested in clinical trials.

The Present: Indications, Efficacy, Problems and Open Fields Using Infliximab in Crohn's Disease

The first drug approved by the Food and Drug Administration for the treatment of CD was infliximab (Remicade) [5], a monoclonal chimeric antibody (human 75%, murine 25%). Infliximab neutralises biological activity of TNF-α by binding with high affinity to both soluble and transmembrane forms of TNF-α, inhibiting binding of TNF-α with its receptors. Therefore, infliximab heavy reduces TNF-α plasmatic levels and induces inflammatory cell apoptosis in the gut wall [6–9], thus promoting mucosal healing at colonoscopy [10, 11].

Efficacy on Remission and Maintenance Therapy

Infliximab, administrated intravenously at a dosage of 5 mg/kg of body weight at weeks 0, 2 and 6 (induction therapy) and, later, every 8 weeks (maintenance therapy) is effective in the therapy of patients with active CD [12]. Infliximab is also a corticosteroid-sparing drug in patients with active CD [13–15]. Definite indications for induction therapy with infliximab (eligible patients) are [13]: (1) Fibrostenosing (inflammatory) disease nonrespondent or refractory to steroid and conventional therapy; (2) fistulising disease, draining enterocutaneous or perianal fistulae.

The use of infliximab as first-line treatment of patients with moderate to severe CD is still controversial. There are no studies demonstrating the efficacy of this scheduled therapy even though this approach has been suggested [16].

Table 1. Biological therapy in Crohn's disease

Proper name	Trade name	Action
Inhibitors of pro-inflammatory cytokines		
Infliximab	Remicade	Chimeric (human/mouse) anti-TNF-α monoclonal antibody (IgG1)
CDP571	Humicade	Humanized anti-TNFα monoclonal antibody (IgG4)
Certolizumab	-	Humanized anti-TNF-α monoclonal antibody (polyethylene glycolated Fab' fragment)
Adalimumab	Humira	Humanized anti-TNF-α monoclonal antibody (IgG1)
Thalidomide	Thalomid	Derivative of glutamic acid with anti-inflammatory and anti-TNF-α action
Semapimod	-	Interferes with the phosphorylation of both p38 and JNK
Etanercept	Enbrel	Genetically engineered fusion protein consisting of two identical chains of the recombinant human p75 TNF receptor linked to the Fc portion of human IgG1
Onercept	-	Recombinant form of the human soluble p55 TNF receptor
MRA	-	Humanized monoclonal antibody to IL-6 receptor
ABT-874/J695	-	Humanized anti-IL-12 p40 (IgG1)
Anti-inflammatory cytokines		
RhIL-10	Tenovil	Humanized monoclonal antibody to IL-10
RhIL-11	-	Humanized monoclonal antibody to IL-11
Inhibitors of adhesion molecules		
Alicaforsen	-	Antisense phosphorothioate oligonucleotide targeting human ICAM-1 mRNA
Natalizumab	Antegren	Humanized monoclonal antibody against α4 integrin
Immune modulators		
Tacrolimus	Prograf	Inhibits production of IL-2 by T-helper cells
Mycophenolate mofetil	CellCept	Antimetabolite strongly suppressing lymphocyte proliferation
Miscellaneous		
Sargramostim	Leukine	Yeast-derived recombinant human GM-CSF
Trichuris suis	-	Worm
Probiotics	VSL#3	Bacteria

TNF, tumor necrosis factor; *IgG*, immunoglobulin G; *JNK*, Jun N-terminal kinase; *ICAM*, intercellular adhesion molecule; *mRNA*, messenger ribonucleic acid; *IL*, interleukin; *GM-CSF*, granulocyte macrophage colony stimulating factor

Induction therapy is effective in up to 70% of cases [10, 12, 17–30]. Not responders to induction therapy do not respond to a maintenance therapy. In patients who respond to induction therapy, maintenance therapy may prolong complete clinical remission [Crohn's Disease Activity Index (CDAI) <150] after 1 year in about 40% of cases, with clinical response in 60% of cases. This implies that, after 1 year of prolonged infliximab therapy, only 25% of patients attain complete clinical remission and 35% clinical response [10, 12, 17–29]. There is evidence that an increase of infliximab dosage and/or a reduction of interval time between infusions may maintain a higher number of patients in clinical remission [21, 31–33].

Disease Type and Stage

The reported incidence of fistulae in patients with CD ranges from 17% to 50% [34]. Fistulae may be enterocutaneous (more commonly perianal), easily recognisable; or internal, enteroenteric or between gut and other organs. Internal fistulae may be asymptomatic but may be more aggressive and require urgent surgery (temporary colostomy allows the patient to heal by bypassing the inflammatory tract).

In perianal disease, induction therapy with infliximab (5 mg/kg at 0, 2 and 6 weeks) is effective on fistula healing in more than 60% of patients [28, 35]. Concomitant conventional therapy (antibiotics and immunosuppressants) is useful since 3 months' treatment with antibiotic monotherapy (metronidazole and ciprofloxacin) showed 60–70% complete remission, improved quality of life and reduced disease recurrences [20, 36, 37]. Azathioprine monotherapy is effective as well, but its full action is evident after 2–3 months of therapy. Therefore, its use in fistulising (perforating) CD is limited, at least as initial treatment. In patients intolerant to azathioprine, methotrexate at dose of 25 mg intramuscularly weekly may be a possible alternative treatment [38].

In patients with perianal fistulae, first-line treatment with antibiotics is suggested. In case of relapse, antibiotics and immunosuppressant therapy (azathioprine or methotrexate) is effective. If fistulae persist, induction therapy with infliximab is recommended, followed by maintenance therapy with immunosuppressant or infliximab (every 8 weeks) [36, 39].

In our opinion, a more appropriate first-line treatment may include induction therapy with infliximab, followed in responders by a maintenance regimen with infliximab and introduction of immunosuppressant drugs. In nonresponders or those intolerant to infliximab i.v., antibiotics, immunosuppressants and local injection of infliximab may be an alternative treatment [40]. Internal fistulae are usually associated to a more aggressive subtype of CD and more difficult to treat conservatively [41]. However, treatment with azathioprine and antibiotics or infliximab may be tried [42, 43].

In some patients, clinical onset of CD occurs with subocclusive symptoms secondary to inflammatory strictures. In naïve patients, infliximab probably induces rapid anti-inflammatory effects with symptomatic improvement, reducing the need for resective surgery. There are no studies confirming this hypothesis but a top-down therapy has been recently proposed [16] and, probably, in the near future, this may be an appropriate initial treatment [44]. However, concomitant therapy with immunomodulators increases the rate of clinical response and clinical remission, and smoking seems to be a negative predictor of response to infliximab therapy [45, 46]. Therefore, an initial therapeutic approach with steroids and immunosuppressants followed by infliximab is suggested, as well as smoking cessation.

On the contrary, infliximab is not indicated in the presence of a fibrotic stenosis [44, 47]. Clinical (long-standing disease), laboratory data [inflammatory indexes, mainly C-reactive protein [48, 49] and instrumental findings by magnetic resonance imaging (MRI) or fluorodeoxyglucose positron emission tomography (FDG-PET)] may help in discriminating an inflammatory or fibrotic process in the intestinal wall [47].

Finally, infliximab significantly improved quality of life in patients with active CD, increasing their ability to work and significantly reducing hospitalisations, surgeries and procedures compared with placebo [50–55].

Adverse Events and Side Effects

Infliximab is a drug with low side effects. Up to now, more than 300,000 patients have been treated with infliximab for rheumatoid arthritis and CD [56]. The more frequent side effects, generally mild, are headache, nausea, upper respiratory infections, skin rash and diarrhoea. However, the incidence of these side effects is similar to that observed in the placebo group, except for upper respiratory infections, which are more common in patients treated with infliximab [23, 56–58].

Adverse events include acute and delayed hypersensitivity reactions. Acute reactions (1–20%) appear during or within 2 h of infusion and are not immunoglobulin E (IgE) mediated. They include headache, nausea, dyspnea, urticaria and coercion chest perception. Treatment of acute reactions consists of temporarily stopping the infusion, administrating antihistamine drugs and/or steroids and then restart infusion at a low rate [13, 22, 23, 57–59]. If acute reactions recur, retreatment is not recommended [13]. Delayed hypersensitivity reactions occur after 3–12 days after infusion in 2–3% of patients. Generally, these reactions are serious and consist in itch, headache, swelling of hands or face, rash, myalgia, polyarteritis, fever and leucocytosis. Steroids induce complete and immediate resolution of symptoms without recurrences. When delayed hypersensitivity reaction occurs, retreatment is not recommended.

Adverse events are caused by the development of antibodies to infliximab (ATI) related to its chimeric nature as it consists of 25% murine proteins. The incidence of ATI is low (10–20%) and at low titre [12, 60, 61]. The presence of ATI reduces drug efficacy in term of percentage of active response (clinical remission) and duration of effectiveness (lower in patients who develop ATI) [12, 62]. Strategies to decrease ATI production are:

- scheduled therapy (not "on demand"): single dose or sporadic infusion causes higher incidence of ATI [30, 63, 64].
- Steroids pretreatment before infliximab infusion

(particularly in the induction phase): hydrocortisone 100 mg i.v. [60, 65].

- Two- to four-month immunosuppressant pretreatment before first infliximab infusion: azathioprine 2 mg/kg per day [57, 65, 66].

Risks: Infections, Tumours, Heart and Neurologic Diseases

TNF-α plays an essential role in the immune-mediated response against infection, especially towards intracellular pathogens [67–70]. Many data support the association between TNF-α blockers and infections [71–74]. Susceptibility to all types of infections is higher, particularly upper respiratory tract infections and bacterial skin infections [74, 75]. TNF-α antagonists should not be given to patients with active infections. Severe pulmonary and abdominal infections (pneumonia, abdominal abscess) are more frequently observed in patients treated with infliximab than placebo.

Many reactivation cases of pulmonary and extrapulmonary tuberculosis have been reported during the first 3 months of infliximab therapy [72, 76–78]. Screening for tuberculosis (skin test and chest X-ray) before anti-TNF therapy is strongly recommended [67, 76]. Some authors suggested that if the skin test is negative, treatment with infliximab may be given without prophylactic therapy. If the skin test is positive, an accurate clinical history, physical examination and chest X-ray are required to rule out active disease [67]. However, it should be considered that: (1) a concomitant use of steroids or immunosuppressant drugs may interfere with the skin test; (2) a large number of patients with IBD are anergic, with a delayed hypersensitivity reaction; (3) more than 15% of patients with active tuberculosis (TBC) infection are anergic; (4) more than 90% of patients with positive skin test have a negative chest X-ray. Therefore, an accurate clinical history, skin test and chest X-ray are mandatory before infliximab administration in all cases. In the absence of tuberculosis lesions at chest X-ray but with a clinical history suggestive for TBC and/or in patients at strong risk for TBC infection (immigrant, injection-drug users, HIV patients, diabetes mellitus, etc.) empirical isoniazid for 6–9 months is a reasonable prophylactic treatment, starting infliximab after 2 months if clinically required. In the presence of TBC lesions at chest X-ray, active therapy is mandatory for at least 2 months before infliximab therapy.

Very rare cases (less than 0.01%) of fungal infection (cryptococcosis, coccidioidomycosis, listeriosis and histoplasmosis) during infliximab therapy are reported [71, 73, 79–94]. Screening and primary prophylaxis are not recommended, but patients with a history of these infections can receive secondary prophylaxis with oral fluconazole.

Patients eligible for infliximab therapy should be tested for hepatitis B and C serological markers before treatment. It has been documented that TNF-α levels are increased in patients with viral hepatitis [95, 96]. Inhibition of TNF-α may alter host antiviral defence mechanisms and promote virological replication [97]. The safety of infliximab in hepatitis C has been demonstrated in a retrospective study on patients with rheumatoid arthritis, as well as in case reports [98–102]. In hepatitis B, reactivation of infection has been documented, as has a case of fulminating hepatitis B after one infusion of infliximab [97, 103–107]. However, definitive conclusions cannot be made regarding the use of infliximab in patients suffering from viral hepatitis. If infliximab therapy is necessary in patients with hepatitis B and C, we suggest monitoring viral replication during therapy and treating hepatitis B patients with lamivudine if serum HBV-DNA levels increase [104]. Prophylaxis with lamivudine should be considered for every carrier patient (HbsAg-positive) [104, 106].

Newly diagnosed neoplasia has occasionally been reported in trials using infliximab in CD although the possible role of infliximab in the pathogenesis of cancer is unclear [108]. However, in a recent multicentre matched-pair study, the frequency of a new diagnosis of neoplasia in CD patients treated with infliximab was comparable with CD patients never receiving infliximab [109]. In particular, the development of lymphoma seemed not to be associated with infliximab therapy but with immunosuppressive drugs, particularly azathioprine, as previously reported [110–115].

Infliximab is not indicated for patients with moderate to severe congestive heart diseases [New York Heart Association (NYHA) classification III–IV] [116, 117]. Serum levels of TNF-α are elevated in patients with heart failure and correlates with its severity [118–121], but the use of infliximab (at a dosage of 10 mg/kg) significantly increases mortality and morbidity in patients with congestive heart failure [122]. Possible pathogenic mechanisms worsening congestive heart failure in infliximab-treated patients are quite complicated and are reported in a recent review [123].

Multiple sclerosis, demyelination and optic neuritis associated with anti-TNF-α therapy are reported [124–127], but a recent study shows that demyelinating disease occurs more commonly among patients with IBD than among non-IBD patients [128]. Future studies should clarify whether treatment with infliximab results in further increased incidence of neurologic diseases among IBD patients.

In pregnant women, drug safety has not been

investigated, but some authors [129] found no difference in live birth and spontaneous abortion in an infliximab-treated group compared with healthy women. It is no clear if the drug is present in mother's milk. Patients who undergo infliximab therapy should use a contraceptive method and, in the presence of a new pregnancy, biological therapy should be stopped until the end of lactation.

Postsurgical Patients

Prophylactic therapy after resection for CD may prevent recurrence of the disease. However, no clear prophylactic drug regimens have been identified. In the last decade, endoscopic recurrence has been considered a relevant outcome in patients suffering from CD since they are strictly related to the clinical outcome. After surgery, more than 70% of patients at 1 year and more than 85% at 3 years will have an endoscopic recurrence in the neoterminal ileum [130–134]. Consequently, more than 20% of patients will already have a clinical recurrence within the first year after surgery, with a 10% increase in each subsequent year [135]. The pattern of CD remains unchanged after surgery. Fistulising disease before surgery will have the same complications after resection and early recurrent symptoms [131].

Standard therapy with steroids or 5-ASA formulations are unable to prevent development of new lesions at 1 year after resection whereas nitroimidazole antibiotics (metronidazole and ornidazole) seem to be effective in preventing endoscopic and clinical recurrences [136, 137]. However, some patients are intolerant to nitroimidazole antibiotics. The benefit of immunosuppression for preventing endoscopic and clinical recurrence is lower than expected yet still high (70% and more than 50%, respectively, at 1 year).

The role of biologic therapy in postsurgical patients is still controversial, and no controlled trials are present in literature. However, aggressive disease, young age and intolerance to standard therapies (steroid dependence; steroid-refractory or immunosuppressant side effects) may represent an indication for infliximab therapy in the postsurgery period to prevent disease recurrence, as recently suggested [131].

New Drugs: What We Expect in the Near Future

Other Anti-TNF-Blocking Strategies

Adalimumab is a humanised immunoglobulin G (IgG)1 monoclonal antibody directed against TNF-α containing only human peptide sequences. It is indistinguishable in structure and function from naturally occurring human IgG1 antibodies. This molecule binds soluble and membrane-bound TNF, fixes complement and induces macrophage and T-cell apoptosis. The recently published CLinical assessment of Adalimumab Safety and efficacy Studied as Induction therapy in Crohn's (CLASSIC-I) study seems to be superior to placebo for induction of remission in patients with moderate to severe CD naïve to anti-TNF therapy [138], confirming results of previous open-labelled studies [139–143]. TNF-α exerts proinflammatory effects by binding to two specific transmembrane receptors, p55 and p75.

Etanercept is a human recombinant p75 receptor/IgG fusion protein highly effective in rheumatoid arthritis. Etanercept was shown to be ineffective in patients with moderate to severe CD [144, 145] and at the moment does not have marketing approval for any indication in IBD. In vitro examination of T lymphocytes the lamina propria of patients with CD seems to demonstrate that etanercept can neutralise TNF-α but does not induce apoptosis of inflammatory cells, differently from infliximab [146]. This experimental evidence probably explains the differences in efficacy between the two TNF-α-neutralising drugs. However, efficacy of etanercept administration on CD activity was assessed at 8 weeks [145]. Since the biological effects of the drug begin after 4–8 weeks, further clinical trials with a longer treatment period are necessary to reach definitive results.

Onercept is a recombinant form of the human soluble p55 TNF receptor, which neutralises the effect of TNF-α. An open-labelled pilot study with onercept suggests that this agent may be effective and well tolerated in patients with active CD [147]. However, other randomised double-blind trials are necessary to make definitive conclusions.

CDP571 is a humanised monoclonal IgG4 antibody anti-TNF-α (95% human, 5% murine). The first study using a single dose of 5 mg/kg i.v. in a limited number of patients reduced disease activity in CD at 2 weeks [148]. A successive study using a higher dose of CDP571 (10 or 20 mg/kg) demonstrated a significant clinical response in patients with moderate-to-severe CD compared with placebo. In the same study, retreatment with 10 mg/kg CDP571 at dose intervals of 8 or 12 weeks seemed to be beneficial although not statistically significant, probably due to the low number of patients with long-term treatment [149]. In a later randomised double-blind placebo-controlled study, patients with steroid refractory CD in clinical remission were enrolled to verify corticosteroid sparing at weeks 8 and 16. CD patients were treated with a loading dose infusion (20 mg/kg) at week 0 followed by a maintenance dose infusion (10 mg/kg) at week 8 to ensure adequate plasma concentrations of CDP571 throughout each 8-week dosing interval. Corticosteroid sparing was achieved in a higher number of patients treated with CDP571 than in those treated with placebo at week 16 [150]. Repeated treatment (every 8 weeks up to 24 weeks) did not seem to increase drug efficacy [151]. In conclusion, CDP571 may provide an alternative option in patients with previous hypersensitivity to infliximab considering the very low risk for TBC or opportunistic infections during CDP571 therapy.

Certolizumab pegol (CDP870) is a polyethylene glycolated Fab' fragment of a humanised anti-TNF-α monoclonal antibody intended for subcutaneous administration. A phase II dose-ranging trial, enrolling patients with moderate to severe CD, was recently published. Certolizumab at 4-week intervals and dosage of 400 mg induces a rapid treatment effect (2 weeks) and is clinically effective compared with placebo [152]. Certolizumab was well tolerated and, similarly to CDP571, gives potentially more advantages in clinical practice compared with infliximab. However, a phase III trial is needed to confirm these results and to better understand the precise role of this drug in the management of CD.

Thalidomide, an old drug recalled for the teratogenic effects in pregnant women, has complex and incompletely understood immunomodulatory properties. Multiple mechanisms of action have been reported, particularly its ability to inhibit production of TNF-α, inhibiting neoangiogenesis and shifting immune response Th1 to Th2. Some recently published papers seem to demonstrate that thalidomide administered for 12 weeks is effective in patients with steroid-resistant or steroid-refractory CD [153–157]. However, about 30% of patients withdrew from the clinical studies due to the development of severe adverse events. Preliminary reports also indicate that thalidomide is effective as maintenance treatment after induction of remission with infliximab [157]. Despite side effects (teratogenicity and peripheral neuropathy) and adverse events, thalidomide may be an alternative medical treatment in a select subgroup of patients.

Anti-Inflammatory Cytokines

IL-10, discovered in 1989, has shown potent anti-inflammatory properties in in vitro and in vivo animal studies. IL-10 exerts its anti-inflammatory effects by down-regulating production of proinflammatory cytokines by dendritic cells, macrophages and monocytes. In clinical trials, a modest benefit was observed in patients treated with subcutaneous injection of humanised IL-10 [158-161]. In postsurgical CD patients, IL-10 administration did not show any effect [162]. The efficacy of IL-10 is lower than expected, probably as a consequence of the stimulation of INF-γ production [158]. Furthermore, serum levels and tissue concentrations of IL-10 are generally elevated in CD patients [5].

Recent experimental studies demonstrated that the delivery of tissutal immunoregulatory proteins, including IL-10, by gene therapy may be a potentially exciting approach to treatment of IBD [163]. Future challenges for using gene therapy in CD will be to establish safety, localisation and duration of the expression of the transduced gene, as well as to ensure that delivery of immunoregulatory proteins is therapeutic.

IL-11 has been shown to be expressed and have activity in multiple other tissues, including gut, but to date, the physiologic role of this protein remains unknown. Preliminary data on short-term treatment with humanised IL-11 demonstrated that given subcutaneously for 3 weeks (16 mg/kg per week), the drug is well tolerated in patients with active CD [164]. A recent randomised trial reported that weekly subcutaneous injection with rhIL-11 (15 mmg/kg per week) compared with placebo is effective in inducing remission in patients with active CD [165]. Potentially, IL-11 may be an alternative or sparing agent for corticosteroids in the management of CD, but its role remains unclear.

Selective Inhibition of Adhesion Molecules

Adhesion molecules, up-regulated in inflamed CD mucosa, play a role in the trafficking of leukocytes and are involved in local lymphocyte stimulation and antigen presentation. Integrins are heterodimeric receptors consisting of an α4 subunit and either a β1 or β7 subunit (α4 β1 and α4 β7 integrins). Integrins bind leukocytes in the vascular endothelium and have a role in the migration of leukocytes across the vascular endothelium. Therefore, they contribute to recruitment, activation and survival of leukocytes within the parenchyma. There is evidence that in IBDs, integrins are overexpressed on the vascular endothelium at the site of inflammation. In animal models of colitis, antibodies against the a4 integrin are able to significantly reduce gut inflammation [166].

Recent double-blind placebo-controlled studies using natalizumab, a humanised mouse monoclonal antibody anti-a4 integrin (95% human, 5% murine), in patients suffering from CD administrated at dosage of 3 mg/kg per month twice improve clinical remission and clinical response rates, as well as quality of life [167–169]. However, three cases of progressive multifocal leukoencephalopathy (PML), probably secondary to reactivation of latent JC polyomavirus infection, have been reported [170–172]. Retrospective analysis of serum samples showed that JC virus became detectable only after three injections of natalizumab monotherapy, and the serum viral load increased by a factor of ten after two additional injections. Although the large number of patients enrolled in this clinical trial (over 3,000) and, consequently, the low incidence of neurologic disease in natalizumab-treated patients, the lack of diagnosis of latent infection before natalizumab treatment limits, due to ethical concerns, its clinical use [173]. In fact, there is no specific treatment for PML at the moment. A better understanding of the risk of PML in natalizumab-treated patients and the diagnostic possibilities for a latent JC polyomavirus infection will define the role of the drug in the treatment of CD.

Immunomodulators

Tacrolimus (FK506) is a macrolide antibiotic isolated from Streptomyces tsukubaensis with greater immunomodulatory properties than cyclosporine and good oral absorption. Consequently, it has been approved for the prophylaxis of organ rejection in transplant patients. The proposed dosage in CD patients is 0.1 mg/kg administered orally, adjusted for each patient to reach a blood concentration range between 5 and 15 ng/ml. Clinical open-labelled studies suggest the effectiveness and safety of short-term and long-term oral tacrolimus therapy in patients with perianal and enterocutaneous fistulising CD [174–178]. However, side effects are numerous and frequently reported by the patients. They include gastrointestinal symptoms (abdominal pain, diarrhea, nausea), headache, insomnia, paresthesias, tremor, temporary rise of creatinine, hyperkaliemia, hypertension and opportunistic infections. Therefore, tacrolimus may be an alternative drug in fistulising CD if no success is achieved with conventional therapy, including infliximab.

Mycophenolate mofetil (MMF) is an antimetabolite that undergoes ester hydrolysis in mycophenolic acid, its active form. Mycophenolic acid inhibits an enzyme required for de novo guanosine nucleotide biosynthesis and consequently blocks production of necessary precursors for synthesis of DNA and RNA. The action of MMF is considered to be directed in particular against T and B lymphocytes, interfering with the immune system. MMF has been used as an immunosuppressant in the posttransplant patients but also in chronic inflammatory diseases, particularly in patients suffering from rheumatoid arthritis and psoriasis, as with other drugs presented in this review. Earlier studies showed a potential role of MMF in CD patients intolerant to azathioprine that was not confirmed in other studies [179–183]. However, a potential steroid-sparing effect has been suggested. A recent open-labelled long-term-treatment study in patients with complicated CD shows that MMF at dosage of 1 g/b.i.d. induces an initial response (at 6 months) in more than one half of the patients, with a significant reduction in steroid dosage. However, a large number of patients relapsed during the long-term follow-up (median 18 months). Furthermore, adverse events determined discontinuation of treatment in 20% of long-term-treated patients [184]. Therefore, we strongly believe that MMF, similarly to other immunosuppressant, has a possible therapeutic role in short-term treatment of steroid-resistant or steroid-refractory CD patients intolerant to azathioprine.

Helminths

Recent experimental and clinical evidence suggest that helminthic parasites may be considered as a therapeutic option in IBDs. CD is a result of an inappropriate immune response towards normal gut flora and, probably, helminths down-regulate the host immune response towards bacterial antigens. The high prevalence of CD in industrialised Western regions and the low incidence in developing countries may be related to the different incidence of helminthic infestation. "IBD hygiene hypothesis" has been formulated based on induction of the disease by extremely hygienic environments in genetically predisposed subjects. Data from experimental colitis seems to show that helminths reduce inflammation, probably counteracting the Th1-driven immune response [185]. In fact, experimental colitis induced in mice and rats with di- or trinitrobenzene sulfonic acid (DNBS, TNBS), develop a Th1-cytokine-driven colitis that shares features with CD [186, 187]. Exposure to Schistosoma mansoni or Trichinella spiralis attenuates DNBS-induced colitis and indicates a protective role of nematode infection in Th1-cell-driven inflammation [188]. The authors suggested the possibility of an immunological distraction with helminths as a novel therapeutic strategy in CD.

Recently, therapy with Trichuris suis eggs in patients suffering from CD has been postulated. The life cycle of T. suis begins with the ingestion of embryonated eggs. Embryonated eggs hatch in the proximal small bowel, delivering larvae that migrate aborally and attach to the mucosa of the distal small bowel and proximal colon. After several weeks, they mature and begin to spread eggs. T. suis ova are capable of colonising a human host for several weeks and are eliminated from the body without any specific therapy (self-limiting infection). In an preliminary study, a single dose of 2,500 live T. suis eggs given orally in patients suffering from active CD induced a clinical response in all patients treated and a clinical remission in the large part of cases [189]. Later, a repeated dose of 2,500 live ova given orally every 3 weeks for 24 weeks induced a clinical response in 80% of patients and a clinical remission in 70% [190]. The positive results of these preliminary open-labelled studies showed that helminth therapy is tolerated and effective in the treatment of CD. Helminths inhibit intestinal inflammation by mechanisms different from current medications, and the efficacy of T. suis therapy supports the hypothesis that helminthic exposure provides protection against CD.

Probiotics

A possible pathogenesis of IBD includes mucosal inflammation secondary to abnormal immune response against resident bacteria. The intestinal environment is a persisting stimulus in normal subjects. In CD patients, normal intestinal bacteria in genetically predisposed subjects or altered intestinal flora may induce and amplify gut inflammation. Therefore, manipulation of intestinal bacterial flora is the rationale for the use of antibiotics. In the last decade, probiotics (living micro-organisms with a beneficial effect on the host), prebiotics (dietary components that induce the growth of beneficial bacteria) and synbiotics (both the previous) have been used in the treatment of CD. Despite the lack of randomised clinical trials demonstrating efficacy of this therapeutic approach to CD patients, a number of review articles have been published during the last years outlining its efficacy in the treatment of IBD [191–193]. Based on experimental evidence, many strains are tested for maintenance of remission in CD patients.

Single-strain probiotics (Lactobacillus GG) at different dosages is not effective to maintain remission in patients suffering from CD [194–196]. Probiotics containing miscellaneous strains at high dosage may be theoretically more effective than a single strain in the treatment of CD, probably due to a synergic effect. Recently, VSL#3, containing three strains of Bifidobacterium (B. longum, B. infantis, B. breve), four strains of Lactobacillus (L. acidophilus, L. casei, L. delbrueckii, L. plantarum) and one strain of Streptococcus salivarius subsp. thermophilus has been proposed in the treatment of IBD. The postulated pathogenic mechanism of VSL#3 is induction of tissutal levels of the anti-inflammatory cytokine IL-10 and a greater expression of intestinal mucin, preventing adhesion of pathological Escherichia coli strains. Efficacy of VSL#3 is being tested in a double-blind randomised trial for maintenance of remission in recurrent chronic pouchitis.

Results of randomised double-blind clinical trials are being awaited in order to make definitive conclusions on the use of probiotics in CD patients.

Conclusions

The advent of biological therapy provides the opportunity to advance the care of patients with IBD because we have opportunities to interrupt the disease pathophysiology in a more specific way. The infliximab experience teaches that interfering with cytokine-mediated inflammation improves the clinical outcome of severe CD.

New biological drugs are coming in the near future. Can we treat severe CD by blocking more than one inflammatory mediator? The mechanism of inflammation in cytokine-mediated CD is quite complex. Cytokines are numerous, act at very low titre (potent biological activity), have many target cells and the cytokine response is mediated by specific cellular receptors. Furthermore, different cytokines produce the same effects, and large interactions among cytokines are documented. We can postulate that interfering with two or more cytokines may improve the clinical course of CD. However, we do not know yet if this approach may alter immune defence towards pathogens and immune surveillance on carcinogenesis, and we must consider that biologics are expensive drugs.

Biological drugs present a major challenge: the more effective they are, the more side effects they can produce. Therefore, biological therapy should carefully managed, with close observance for possible adverse events and provision for any complication resulting from treatment. Inappropriate management of these potent drugs will compromise their use in clinical practice.

Future clinical studies should address efficacy, safety and cost effectiveness of biologic therapies for CD and should provide the necessary information to take maximum advantage of these new therapies.

References

1. Hanauer SB (2006) Inflammatory bowel disease: epidemiology, pathogenesis, and therapeutic opportunities. Inflamm Bowel Dis 12(Suppl 1):S3–S9
2. Gustot T, Lemmers A, Louis E et al (2005) Profile of soluble cytokine receptors in Crohn's disease. Gut 54:488–495

3. Lindsay JO, Hodgson HJ (2001) Review article: the immunoregulatory cytokine interleukin-10 – a therapy for Crohn's disease? Aliment Pharmacol Ther 15:1709–1716
4. Sandborn WJ, Targan SR (2002) Biologic therapy of inflammatory bowel disease. Gastroenterology 122:1592–1608
5. Vermeire S, Rutgeerts P (2004) Novel biological strategies in inflammatory bowel diseases. Inflamm Bowel Dis 10:s44–s51
6. Papadakis KA, Targan S (2000) Tumor necrosis factor: biology and therapeutic inhibitors. Gastroenterology 119:1148–1157
7. van den Brande J, Hommes DW, Peppelenbosch MP (2005) Infliximab induced T lymphocyte apoptosis in Crohn's disease. J Rheumatol 74(Suppl):26–30
8. Sandborn WJ, Hanauer SB (1999) Antitumor necrosis factor therapy for inflammatory bowel disease: a review of agents, pharmacology, clinical results, and safety. Inflamm Bowel Dis 5:119–133
9. Ringheanu M, Daum F, Markowitz J et al (2004) Effects of infliximab on apoptosis and reverse signaling of monocytes from healthy individuals and patients with Crohn's disease. Inflamm Bowel Dis 10:801–810
10. D'Haens G, Van Deventer S, Van Hogezand R et al (1999) Endoscopic and histological healing with infliximab anti-tumor necrosis factor antibodies in Crohn's disease: a European multicenter trial. Gastroenterology 116:1029–1034
11. Geboes K, Rutgeerts P, Opdenakker G et al (2005) Endoscopic and histologic evidence of persistent mucosal healing and correlation with clinical improvement following sustained infliximab treatment of Crohn's diseas. Curr Med Res Opin 21:1741–1754
12. Hanauer SB, Feagan BG, Lichtenstein GR et al (2002) Maintenance infliximab for Crohn's disease: the ACCENT I randomised trial. Lancet 359:1541–1549
13. Sandborn WJ, Hanauer SB (2002) Infliximab in the treatment of Crohn's disease: a user's guide for clinicians. Am J Gastroenterol 97:2962–2972
14. Rutgeerts PJ (2001) Review article: the limitations of corticosteroid therapy in Crohn's disease. Aliment Pharmacol Ther 15:1515–1525
15. Laine L, Hanauer SB (2003) Considerations in the management of steroid-dependent Crohn's disease. Gastroenterology 125:906–910
16. Hanauer SB (2003) Crohn's disease: step up or top down therapy. Best Pract Res Clin Gastroenterol 17:131–137
17. Targan SR, Hanauer SB, van Deventer SJ et al (1997) A short-term study of chimeric monoclonal antibody cA2 to tumor necrosis factor alpha for Crohn's disease. Crohn's Disease cA2 Study Group. N Engl J Med 337:1029–1035
18. van Dullemen HM, van Deventer SJ, Hommes DW et al (1995) Treatment of Crohn's disease with anti-tumor necrosis factor chimeric monoclonal antibody (cA2). Gastroenterology 109:129–135
19. Baert FJ, D'Haens GR, Peeters M et al (1999) Tumor necrosis factor alpha antibody (infliximab) therapy profoundly down-regulates the inflammation in Crohn's ileocolitis. Gastroenterology 116:22–28
20. Present DH, Rutgeerts P, Targan S et al (1999) Infliximab for the treatment of fistulas in patients with Crohn's disease. N Engl J Med 340:1398–1405
21. Rutgeerts P, D'Haens G, Targan S et al (1999) Efficacy and safety of retreatment with anti-tumor necrosis factor antibody (infliximab) to maintain remission in Crohn's disease. Gastroenterology 117:761–769
22. Farrell RJ, Shah SA, Lodhavia PJ et al (2000) Clinical experience with infliximab therapy in 100 patients with Crohn's disease. Am J Gastroenterol 95:3490–3497
23. Cohen RD (2001) Efficacy and safety of repeated infliximab infusions for Crohn's disease: 1-year clinical experience. Inflamm Bowel Dis 7(Suppl 1):S17–S22
24. Arnott ID, McDonald D, Williams A, Ghosh S (2001) Clinical use of Infliximab in Crohn's disease: the Edinburgh experience. Aliment Pharmacol Ther 15:1639–1646
25. Hommes DW, van de Heisteeg BH, van der Spek M, et al (2002) Infliximab treatment for Crohn's disease: one-year experience in a Dutch academic hospital. Inflamm Bowel Dis 8:81–86
26. Ardizzone S, Colombo E, Maconi G et al (2002) Infliximab in treatment of Crohn's disease: the Milan experience. Dig Liver Dis 34:411–418
27. Arslan S, Kav T, Besisik F et al (2003) Clinical outcome of Crohn's disease treated with infliximab. Hepatogastroenterology 50:952–956
28. Sands BE, Anderson FH, Bernstein CN et al (2004) Infliximab maintenance therapy for fistulizing Crohn's disease. N Engl J Med 350:876–885
29. Wenzl HH, Reinisch W, Jahnel J et al (2004) Austrian infliximab experience in Crohn's disease: a nationwide cooperative study with long-term follow-up. Eur J Gastroenterol Hepatol 16:767–773
30. Orlando A, Colombo E, Kohn A et al (2005) Infliximab in the treatment of Crohn's disease: predictors of response in an Italian multicentric open study. Dig Liver Dis 37:577–583
31. Centocor, Inc. (2002) Remicade (infliximab) for i.v. injection. Volume Package insert. Melvern, PA
32. Rutgeerts P, Mayer L, Schreiber S (2001) Infliximab (Remicade) maintenance treatment strategy is superior to episodic treatment in patients with Crohn's disease. Am J Gastroenterol 96:S302–S303
33. Menachem Y, Avidan B, Lavy A et al (2005) Increasing the infliximab dose is beneficial in Crohn's disease patients who responded to a lower dose and relapsed. Digestion 72:124–128
34. Allan A, Keighley RB (1988) Management of perianal disease. World J Surg 12:198–202
35. Regueiro M, Mardini H (2003) Treatment of perianal fistulizing Crohn's disease with infliximab alone or as an adjunct to exam under anesthesia with seton placement. Inflamm Bowel Dis 9:98–103
36. Present DH (2003) Crohn's fistula: current concepts in management. Gastroenterology 124:1629–1635
37. Felley C, Mottet C, Juillerat P et al (2005) Fistulizing Crohn's disease. Digestion 71:26–28
38. Schroder O, Blumenstein I, Schulte-Bockholt A, Stein J (2004) Combining infliximab and methotrexate in fistulizing Crohn's disease resistant or intolerant to azathioprine. Aliment Pharmacol Ther 19:295–301
39. Talbot C, Sagar PM, Johnston MJ et al (2005) Infliximab in the surgical management of complex fistulat-

ing anal Crohn's disease. Colorectal Dis 7:164–168
40. Poggioli G, Laureati S, Pierangeli F et al (2005) Local injection of infliximab for the tratment of perianal Crohn's disease. Dis Colon Rectum 48:768–774
41. Parsi MA, Lashner BA, Achkar JP et al (2004) Type of fistula determines response to infliximab in patients with fistulous Crohn's disease. Am J Gastroenterol 99:445–449
42. Wheeler C, Marion JF, Present DH (1998) Medical therapy, not surgery, is the appropriate first line treatement of Crohn's enterovesical fistula. Gastroenterology 114A:1113
43. Sonoda T, Haull T, Piedmonte MR, Fazzi M (2002) Outcomes of primary repair of anorectal and rectovaginal fistulas using the endorectal advancement flap. Dis Colon Rectum 45:1622–1628
44. Sorrentino D, Avellini C, Beltrami CA et al (2005) Selective effect of infliximab on the inflammatory component of a colonic stricture in Crohn's disease. Int J Colorectal Dis [Epub ahead of print]
45. Parsi MA, Achkar JP, Richardson S et al (2002) Predictors of response to infliximab in patients with Crohn's disease. Gastroenterology 123:707–713
46. Arnott ID, McNeill G, Satsangi J (2003) An analysis of factors influencing short-term and sustained response to infliximab treatment for Crohn's disease. Aliment Pharmacol Ther 17:1451–1457
47. Holtmann MH, Neurath MF (2005) Anti-TNF strategies in stenosing and fistulizing Crohn's disease. Int J Colorectal Dis 20:1–8
48. Biancone L, Tosti C, Fina D et al (2003) Review article: maintenance treatment of Crohn's disease. Aliment Pharmacol Ther 17(Suppl 2):31–37
49. Boirivant M, Leoni M, Tariciotti D et al (1988) The clinical significance of serum C reactive protein levels in Crohn's disease. Results of a prospective longitudinal study. J Clin Gastroenterol 10:401–405
50. Ollendorf DA, Massarotti E, Birbara C, Burgess SM (2005) Frequency, predictors, and economic impact of upward dose adjustment of infliximab in managed care patients with rheumatoid arthritis. J Manag Care Pharm 11:383–393
51. Lichtenstein GR, Yan S, Bala M et al (2005) Infliximab maintenance treatment reduces hospitalizations, surgeries, and procedures in fistulizing Crohn's disease. Gastroenterology 128:862–869
52. Bodger K (2005) Economic implications of biological therapies for Crohn's disease: review of infliximab. Pharmacoeconomics 23:875–888
53. Cadahia V, Garcia-Carbonero A, Vivas S et al (2004) Infliximab improves quality of life in the short-term in patients with fistulizing Crohn's disease in clinical practice. Rev Esp Enferm Dig 96:369–374; 374–378
54. Clark W, Raftery J, Song F et al (2003) Systematic review and economic evaluation of the effectiveness of infliximab for the treatment of Crohn's disease. Health Technol Assess 7:1–67
55. Wicks AC, Thomas C, Curran R, Mayberry JF (2002) Infliximab and Crohn's QOL. Aliment Pharmacol Ther 16:1831–1832
56. Hommes DW, van Deventer SJ (2003) Infliximab therapy in Crohn's disease: safety issues. Neth J Med 61:100–104
57. Colombel JF, Loftus EV Jr, Tremaine WJ et al (2004) The safety profile of infliximab in patients with Crohn's disease: the Mayo clinic experience in 500 patients. Gastroenterology 126:19–31
58. Hanauer SB (1999) Review article: safety of infliximab in clinical trials. Aliment Pharmacol Ther 13(Suppl 4):16–22; discussion 38
59. Cheifetz A, Smedley M, Martin S et al (2003) The incidence and management of infusion reactions to infliximab: a large center experience. Am J Gastroenterol 98:1315–1324
60. Farrell RJ, Alsahli M, Jeen YT et al (2003) Intravenous hydrocortisone premedication reduces antibodies to infliximab in Crohn's disease: a randomized controlled trial. Gastroenterology 124:917–924
61. Sandborn WJ (2003) Preventing antibodies to infliximab in patients with Crohn's disease: optimize not immunize. Gastroenterology 124:1140–1145
62. Baert F, Noman M, Vermeire S et al (2003) Influence of immunogenicity on the long-term efficacy of infliximab in Crohn's disease. N Engl J Med 348:601–608
63. Hanauer SB, Wagner CL, Bala M et al (2004) Incidence and importance of antibody responses to infliximab after maintenance or episodic treatment in Crohn's disease. Clin Gastroenterol Hepatol 2:542–553
64. Rutgeerts P, Van Assche G, Vermeire S (2004) Optimizing anti-TNF treatment in inflammatory bowel disease. Gastroenterology 126:1593–1610
65. Han PD, Cohen RD (2004) Managing immunogenic responses to infliximab: treatment implications for patients with Crohn's disease. Drugs 64:1767–1777
66. Crandall WV, Mackner LM (2003) Infusion reactions to infliximab in children and adolescents: frequency, outcome and a predictive model. Aliment Pharmacol Ther 17:75–84
67. Gardam MA, Keystone EC, Menzies R et al (2003) Anti-tumour necrosis factor agents and tuberculosis risk: mechanisms of action and clinical management. Lancet Infect Dis 3:148–155
68. Beenhouwer D, Wallis R, Broder M, Furst DE (2004) Mechanisms of action of tumor necrosis factor antagonist and granulomatous infections. J Rheumatol 31:1888–1892
69. Wallis RS, Broder M, Wong J et al (2005) Reactivation of latent granulomatous infections by infliximab. Clin Infect Dis 41(Suppl 3):S194–S198
70. Wallis RS, Broder MS, Wong JY et al (2004) Granulomatous infectious diseases associated with tumor necrosis factor antagonists. Clin Infect Dis 38:1261–1265
71. Velayos FS, Sandborn WJ (2004) Pneumocystis carinii pneumonia during maintenance anti-tumor necrosis factor-alpha therapy with infliximab for Crohn's disease. Inflamm Bowel Dis 10:657–660
72. Keane J, Gershon S, Wise RP, Mirabile-Levens E et al (2001) Tuberculosis associated with infliximab, a tumor necrosis factor alpha-neutralizing agent. N Engl J Med 345:1098–1104
73. Warris A, Bjorneklett A, Gaustad P (2001) Invasive pulmonary aspergillosis associated with infliximab therapy. N Engl J Med 344:1099–1100
74. Hamilton CD (2004) Infectious complications of treatment with biologic agents. Curr Opin Rheumatol 16:393–398

75. Listing J, Strangfeld A, Kary S et al (2005) Infections in patients with rheumatoid arthritis treated with biologic agents. Arthritis Rheum 52:3403–3412
76. Ormerod LP (2004) Tuberculosis and anti-TNF-alpha treatment. Thorax 59:921
77. De Rosa FG, Bonora S, Di Perri G (2002) Tuberculosis and treatment with infliximab. N Engl J Med 346:623–626
78. Zhang Z, Correa H, Begue RE (2002) Tuberculosis and treatment with infliximab. N Engl J Med 346:623–626
79. Morelli J, Wilson FA (2000) Does administration of infliximab increase susceptibility to listeriosis? Am J Gastroenterol 95:841–842
80. Tai TL, O'Rourke KP, McWeeney M et al (2002) Pneumocystis carinii pneumonia following a second infusion of infliximab. Rheumatology (Oxford) 41:951–952
81. Seddik M, Meliez H, Seguy D et al (2004) Pneumocystis jiroveci (carinii) pneumonia following initiation of infliximab and azathioprine therapy in a patient with Crohn's disease. Inflamm Bowel Dis 10:436–437
82. Kaur N, Mahl TC (2004) Pneumocystis carinii pneumonia with oral candidiasis after infliximab therapy for Crohn's disease. Dig Dis Sci 49:1458–1460
83. Seddik M, Melliez H, Seguy D et al (2005) Pneumocystis jiroveci (carinii) pneumonia after initiation of infliximab and azathioprine therapy in a patient with Crohn's disease. Inflamm Bowel Dis 11:618–620
84. Wood KL, Hage CA, Knox KS et al (2003) Histoplasmosis after treatment with anti-tumor necrosis factor-alpha therapy. Am J Respir Crit Care Med 167:1279–1282
85. Lee JH, Slifman NR, Gershon SK et al (2002) Life-threatening histoplasmosis complicating immunotherapy with tumor necrosis factor alpha antagonists infliximab and etanercept. Arthritis Rheum 46:2565–2570
86. Nakelchik M, Mangino JE (2002) Reactivation of histoplasmosis after treatment with infliximab. Am J Med 112:78
87. Bowie VL, Snella KA, Gopalachar AS, Bharadwaj P (2004) Listeria meningitis associated with infliximab. Ann Pharmacother 38:58–61
88. Aparicio AG, Munoz-Fernandez S, Bonilla G et al (2003) Report of an additional case of anti-tumor necrosis factor therapy and Listeria monocytogenes infection: comment on the letter by Gluck et al. Arthritis Rheum 48:1764–1765; author reply 1765–1766
89. Slifman NR, Gershon SK, Lee JH et al (2003) Listeria monocytogenes infection as a complication of treatment with tumor necrosis factor alpha-neutralizing agents. Arthritis Rheum 48:319–324
90. Kamath BM, Mamula P, Baldassano RN, Markowitz JE (2002) Listeria meningitis after treatment with infliximab. J Pediatr Gastroenterol Nutr 34:410–412
91. Gluck T, Linde HJ, Scholmerich J et al (2002) Anti-tumor necrosis factor therapy and Listeria monocytogenes infection: report of two cases. Arthritis Rheum 46:2255–2257; author reply 2257
92. Alderson JW, Van Dinter TG Jr et al (2005) Disseminated aspergillosis following infliximab therapy in an immunosuppressed patient with Crohn's disease and chronic hepatitis C: a case study and review of the literature. MedGenMed 7:7
93. van der Klooster JM, Bosman RJ, Oudemans-van Straaten HM et al (2003) Disseminated tuberculosis, pulmonary aspergillosis and cutaneous herpes simplex infection in a patient with infliximab and methotrexate. Intensive Care Med 29:2327–2329
94. De Rosa FG, Shaz D, Campagna AC et al (2003) Invasive pulmonary aspergillosis soon after therapy with infliximab, a tumor necrosis factor-alpha-neutralizing antibody: a possible healthcare-associated case? Infect Control Hosp Epidemiol 24:477–482
95. Marinos G, Naoumov NV, Rossol S et al (1995) Tumor necrosis factor receptors in patients with chronic hepatitis B virus infection. Gastroenterology 108:1453–1463
96. Tilg H (1997) New insights into the mechanisms of interferon alfa: an immunoregulatory and anti-inflammatory cytokine. Gastroenterology 112:1017–1021
97. del Valle Garcia-Sanchez M, Gomez-Camacho F et al (2004) Infliximab therapy in a patient with Crohn's disease and chronic hepatitis B virus infection. Inflamm Bowel Dis 10:701–702
98. Campbell S, Ghosh S (2001) Infliximab therapy for Crohn's disease in the presence of chronic hepatitis C infection. Eur J Gastroenterol Hepatol 13:191–192
99. Peterson JR, Hsu FC, Simkin PA, Wener MH (2003) Effect of tumour necrosis factor alpha antagonists on serum transaminases and viraemia in patients with rheumatoid arthritis and chronic hepatitis C infection. Ann Rheum Dis 62:1078–1082
100. Biancone L, Pavia M, Del Vecchio Blanco G et al (2001) Hepatitis B and C virus infection in Crohn's disease. Inflamm Bowel Dis 7:287–294
101. Holtmann MH, Galle PR, Neurath MF (2003) Treatment of patients with Crohn's disease and concomitant chronic hepatitis C with a chimeric monoclonal antibody to TNF. Am J Gastroenterol 98:504–505
102. Biancone L, Del Vecchio Blanco G et al (2002) Immunomodulatory drugs in Crohn's disease patients with hepatitis B or C virus infection. Gastroenterology 122:593–594
103. Wendling D, Auge B, Bettinger D et al (2005) Reactivation of a latent precore mutant hepatitis B virus related chronic hepatitis during infliximab treatment for severe spondyloarthropathy. Ann Rheum Dis 64:788–789
104. Ueno Y, Tanaka S, Shimamoto M et al (2005) Infliximab therapy for Crohn's disease in a patient with chronic hepatitis B. Dig Dis Sci 50:163–166
105. Esteve M, Saro C, Gonzalez-Huix F et al (2004) Chronic hepatitis B reactivation following infliximab therapy in Crohn's disease patients: need for primary prophylaxis. Gut 53:1363–1365
106. Ostuni P, Botsios C, Punzi L et al (2003) Hepatitis B reactivation in a chronic hepatitis B surface antigen carrier with rheumatoid arthritis treated with infliximab and low dose methotrexate. Ann Rheum Dis 62:686–687
107. Michel M, Duvoux C, Hezode C, Cherqui D (2003) Fulminant hepatitis after infliximab in a patient with hepatitis B virus treated for an adult onset still's disease. J Rheumatol 30:1624–1625
108. Sandborn WJ, Loftus EV (2004) Balancing the risks and benefits of infliximab in the treatment of inflammatory bowel disease. Gut 53:780–782
109. Biancone L, Orlando A, Kohn A et al (2006) Infliximab

and newly diagnosed neoplasia in Crohn's disease: a multicentre matched pair study. Gut 55:228–233
110. Kandiel A, Fraser AG, Korelitz BI et al (2005) Increased risk of lymphoma among inflammatory bowel disease patients treated with azathioprine and 6-mercaptopurine. Gut 54:1121–1125
111. Tan CW, Wilson GE, Howat JM, Shreeve DR (2001) Rectal lymphoma in ulcerative colitis treated with azathioprine. Eur J Gastroenterol Hepatol 13:989–992
112. Lewis JD, Schwartz JS, Lichtenstein GR (2000) Azathioprine for maintenance of remission in Crohn's disease: benefits outweigh the risk of lymphoma. Gastroenterology 118:1018–1024
113. Phillips T, Salisbury J, Leigh I, Baker H (1987) Non-Hodgkin's lymphoma associated with long-term azathioprine therapy. Clin Exp Dermatol 12:444–445
114. McGovern DP, Jewell DP (2005) Risks and benefits of azathioprine therapy. Gut 54:1055–1059
115. Connell WR, Kamm MA, Dickson M et al (1994) Long-term neoplasia risk after azathioprine treatment in inflammatory bowel disease. Lancet 343:1249–1252
116. Behnam SM, Behnam SE, Koo JY (2005) TNF-alpha inhibitors and congestive heart failure. Skinmed 4:363–368
117. Gupta S, Tripathi CD (2005) Current status of TNF blocking therapy in heart failure. Indian J Med Sci 59:363–366
118. Levine B, Kalman J, Mayer L et al (1990) Elevated circulating levels of tumor necrosis factor in severe chronic heart failure. N Engl J Med 323:236–241
119. Rauchhaus M, Doehner W, Francis DP et al (2000) Plasma cytokine parameters and mortality in patients with chronic heart failure. Circulation 102:3060–3067
120. Torre-Amione G, Vooletich MT, Farmer JA (2000) Role of tumour necrosis factor-alpha in the progression of heart failure: therapeutic implications. Drugs 59:745–751
121. Torre-Amione G, Kapadia S, Benedict C et al (1996) Proinflammatory cytokine levels in patients with depressed left ventricular ejection fraction: a report from the Studies of Left Ventricular Dysfunction (SOLVD). J Am Coll Cardiol 27:1201–1206
122. Chung ES, Packer M, Lo KH, Fasanmade AA, Willerson JT (2003). Randomized, double-blind, placebo-controlled, pilot trial of infliximab, a chimeric monoclonal antibody to tumor necrosis factor-alpha, in patients with moderate-to-severe heart failure: results of the anti-TNF Therapy Against Congestive Heart Failure (ATTACH) trial. Circulation 107:3133–140
123. Khanna D, McMahon M, Furst DE (2004) Anti-tumor necrosis factor alpha therapy and heart failure: what have we learned and where do we go from here? Arthritis Rheum 50:1040–1050
124. Tanno M, Nakamura I, Kobayashi S et al (2005) New-onset demyelination induced by infliximab therapy in two rheumatoid arthritis patients. Clin Rheumatol 23:1–5
125. Freeman HJ, Flak B (2005) Demyelination-like syndrome in Crohn's disease after infliximab therapy. Can J Gastroenterol 19:313–316
126. Enayati PJ, Papadakis KA (2005). Association of anti-tumor necrosis factor therapy with the development of multiple sclerosis. J Clin Gastroenterol 39:303–306
127. Thomas CW Jr, Weinshenker BG, Sandborn WJ (2004) Demyelination during anti-tumor necrosis factor alpha therapy with infliximab for Crohn's disease. Inflamm Bowel Dis 10:28–31
128. Gupta G, Gelfand JM, Lewis JD (2005) Increased risk for demyelinating diseases in patients with inflammatory bowel disease. Gastroenterology 129:819–826
129. Katz JA (2004) Pregnancy and inflammatory bowel disease. Curr Opin Gastroenterol 20:328–332
130. Froehlich F, Juillerat P, Felley C et al (2005) Treatment of postoperative Crohn's disease. Digestion 71:49–53
131. Rutgeerts P (2001) Strategies in the prevention of post-operative recurrence in Crohn's disease. Best Pract Res Clin Gastroenterol 17:63–73
132. Rutgeerts P, Geboes K, Vantrappen G et al (1990) Predictability of the postoperative course of Crohn's disease. Gastroenterology 99:956–963
133. Rutgeerts P (1994) Recurrence of Crohn's disease in the neoterminal ileum after ileal resection: is prevention therapy possible? Neth J Med 45:60–64
134. Olaison G, Smedh K, Sjodahl R (1992) Natural course of Crohn's disease after ileocolic resection: endoscopically visualised ileal ulcers preceding symptoms. Gut 33:331–335
135. Becker JM (1999) Surgical therapy for ulcerative colitis and Crohn's disease. Gastroenterol Clin North Am 28:371–90, viii–ix
136. Rutgeerts P, Van Assche G, Vermeire S et al (2005) Ornidazole for prophylaxis of postoperative Crohn's disease recurrence: a randomized, double-blind, placebo-controlled trial. Gastroenterology 128:856–861
137. Rutgeerts P, Hiele M, Geboes K et al (1995) Controlled trial of metronidazole treatment for prevention of Crohn's recurrence after ileal resection. Gastroenterology 108:1617–1621
138. Hanauer S, Sandborn W, Rutgeerts P et al (2006) Human anti-tumor necrosis factor monoclonal antibody (adalimumab) in Crohn's disease: the CLASSIC-I trial. Gastroenterology 130:323–333
139. Papadakis KA, Shaye OA, Vasiliauskas EA et al (2005) Safety and efficacy of adalimumab (D2E7) in Crohn's disease patients with an attenuated response to infliximab. Am J Gastroenterol 100:75–79
140. Hanauer SB (2004) Efficacy and safety of tumor necrosis factor antagonists in Crohn's disease: overview of randomized clinical studies. Rev Gastroenterol Disord 4(Suppl 3):S18–S24
141. Youdim A, Vasiliauskas EA, Targan SR et al (2004) A pilot study of adalimumab in infliximab-allergic patients. Inflamm Bowel Dis 10:333–338
142. Sandborn WJ, Hanauer S, Loftus EV Jr et al (2004) An open-label study of the human anti-TNF monoclonal antibody adalimumab in subjects with prior loss of response or intolerance to infliximab for Crohn's disease. Am J Gastroenterol 99:1984–1989
143. Stallmach A, Giese T, Schmidt C (2004) Severe anaphylactic reaction to infliximab: successful treatment with adalimumab – report of a case. Eur J Gastroenterol Hepatol 16:627–630
144. D'Haens G, Swijsen C, Noman M et al (2001) Etanercept in the treatment of active refractory Crohn's disease: a single-center pilot trial. Am J Gastroenterol 96:2564–2568

145. Sandborn WJ, Hanauer SB, Katz S et al (2001) Etanercept for active Crohn's disease: a randomized, double-blind, placebo-controlled trial. Gastroenterology 121:1088–1094
146. Van den Brande JM, Braat H, van den Brink GR et al (2003) Infliximab but not etanercept induces apoptosis in lamina propria T-lymphocytes from patients with Crohn's disease. Gastroenterology 124:1774–1785
147. Rutgeerts P, Lemmens L, Van Assche G et al (2003) Treatment of active Crohn's disease with onercept (recombinant human soluble p55 tumour necrosis factor receptor): results of a randomized, open-label, pilot study. Aliment Pharmacol Ther 17:185–192
148. Stack WA, Mann SD, Roy AJ et al (1997) Randomised controlled trial of CDP571 antibody to tumour necrosis factor-alpha in Crohn's disease. Lancet 349:521–524
149. Sandborn WJ, Feagan BG, Hanauer SB et al (2001) An engineered human antibody to TNF (CDP571) for active Crohn's disease: a randomized double-blind placebo-controlled trial. Gastroenterology 120:1330–1338
150. Feagan BG, Sandborn WJ, Baker JP et al (2005) A randomized, double-blind, placebo-controlled trial of CDP571, a humanized monoclonal antibody to tumour necrosis factor-alpha, in patients with corticosteroid-dependent Crohn's disease. Aliment Pharmacol Ther 21:373–384
151. Sandborn WJ, Feagan BG, Radford-Smith G et al (2004) CDP571, a humanised monoclonal antibody to tumour necrosis factor alpha, for moderate to severe Crohn's disease: a randomised, double blind, placebo controlled trial. Gut 53:1485–1493
152. Schreiber S, Rutgeerts P, Fedorak RN et al (2005) A randomized, placebo-controlled trial of Certolizumab pegol (CDP870) for treatment of Crohn's disease. Gastroenterology 129:807–818
153. Bauditz J, Wedel S, Lochs H (2002) Thalidomide reduces tumour necrosis factor alpha and interleukin 12 production in patients with chronic active Crohn's disease. Gut 50:196–200
154. Vasiliauskas EA, Kam LY, Abreu-Martin MT et al (1999) An open-label pilot study of low-dose thalidomide in chronically active, steroid-dependent Crohn's disease. Gastroenterology 117:1278–1287
155. Ehrenpreis ED, Kane SV, Cohen LB et al (1999) Thalidomide therapy for patients with refractory Crohn's disease: an open-label trial. Gastroenterology 117:1271–1277
156. Bariol C, Meagher AP, Vickers CR et al (2002) Early studies on the safety and efficacy of thalidomide for symptomatic inflammatory bowel disease. J Gastroenterol Hepatol 17:135–139
157. Sabate JM, Villarejo J, Lemann M et al (2002) An open-label study of thalidomide for maintenance therapy in responders to infliximab in chronically active and fistulizing refractory Crohn's disease. Aliment Pharmacol Ther 16:1117–1124
158. Tilg H, van Montfrans C, van den Ende A et al (2002) Treatment of Crohn's disease with recombinant human interleukin 10 induces the proinflammatory cytokine interferon gamma. Gut 50:191–195
159. Fedorak RN, Gangl A, Elson CO et al (2000) Recombinant human interleukin 10 in the treatment of patients with mild to moderately active Crohn's disease. The Interleukin 10 Inflammatory Bowel Disease Cooperative Study Group. Gastroenterology 119:1473–1482
160. Schreiber S, Fedorak RN, Nielsen OH et al (2000) Safety and efficacy of recombinant human interleukin 10 in chronic active Crohn's disease. Crohn's Disease IL-10 Cooperative Study Group. Gastroenterology 119:1461–1472
161. van Deventer SJ, Elson CO, Fedorak RN (1997) Multiple doses of intravenous interleukin 10 in steroid-refractory Crohn's disease. Crohn's Disease Study Group. Gastroenterology 113:383–389
162. Colombel JF, Rutgeerts P, Malchow H et al (2001) Interleukin 10 (Tenovil) in the prevention of postoperative recurrence of Crohn's disease. Gut 49:42–46
163. Lindsay JO, Ciesielski CJ, Scheinin T et al (2003) Local delivery of adenoviral vectors encoding murine interleukin 10 induces colonic interleukin 10 production and is therapeutic for murine colitis. Gut 52:363–369
164. Sands BE, Bank S, Sninsky CA et al (1999) Preliminary evaluation of safety and activity of recombinant human interleukin 11 in patients with active Crohn's disease. Gastroenterology 117:58–64
165. Sands BE, Winston BD, Salzberg B et al (2002) Randomized, controlled trial of recombinant human interleukin-11 in patients with active Crohn's disease. Aliment Pharmacol Ther 16:399–406
166. Sandborn WJ, Yednock TA (2003) Novel approaches to treating inflammatory bowel disease: targeting alpha-4 integrin. Am J Gastroenterol 98:2372–2382
167. Ghosh S, Goldin E, Gordon FH et al (2003) Natalizumab for active Crohn's disease. N Engl J Med 348:24–32
168. Sandborn WJ, Colombel JF, Enns R et al (2005) Natalizumab induction and maintenance therapy for Crohn's disease. N Engl J Med 353:1912–1925
169. Gordon FH, Lai CW, Hamilton MI et al (2001) A randomized placebo-controlled trial of a humanized monoclonal antibody to alpha4 integrin in active Crohn's disease. Gastroenterology 121:268–274
170. Berger T, Deisenhammer F (2005) Progressive multifocal leukoencephalopathy, natalizumab, and multiple sclerosis. N Engl J Med 353:1744–1746; author reply 1744–1746
171. Langer-Gould A, Atlas SW, Green AJ et al (2005) Progressive multifocal leukoencephalopathy in a patient treated with natalizumab. N Engl J Med 353:375–381
172. Van Assche G, Van Ranst M, Sciot R et al (2005) Progressive multifocal leukoencephalopathy after natalizumab therapy for Crohn's disease. N Engl J Med 353:362–368
173. Berger JR, Koralnik IJ (2005) Progressive multifocal leukoencephalopathy and natalizumab--unforeseen consequences. N Engl J Med 353:414–416
174. Sandborn WJ (1997) Preliminary report on the use of oral tacrolimus (FK506) in the treatment of complicated proximal small bowel and fistulizing Crohn's disease. Am J Gastroenterol 92:876–879
175. Ierardi E, Principi M, Francavilla R et al (2001) Oral tacrolimus long-term therapy in patients with Crohn's disease and steroid resistance. Aliment Pharmacol Ther 15:371–377
176. Sandborn WJ, Present DH, Isaacs KL et al (2003) Tacrolimus for the treatment of fistulas in patients with Crohn's disease: a randomized, placebo-con-

trolled trial. Gastroenterology 125:380–388

177. Gonzalez-Lama Y, Abreu L, Vera MI et al (2005) Long-term oral tacrolimus therapy in refractory to infliximab fistulizing Crohn's disease: a pilot study. Inflamm Bowel Dis 11:8–15
178. Fukuda A, Nakase H, Seno H et al (2005) Refractory enterovesical and duodenocolic fistulas in Crohn's disease successfully managed with tacrolimus. J Gastroenterol 40:433–435
179. Miehsler W, Reinisch W, Moser G et al (2001) Is mycophenolate mofetil an effective alternative in azathioprine-intolerant patients with chronic active Crohn's disease? Am J Gastroenterol 96:782–787
180. Neurath MF, Wanitschke R, Peters M et al (1999) Randomised trial of mycophenolate mofetil versus azathioprine for treatment of chronic active Crohn's disease. Gut 44:625–628
181. Ford AC, Towler RJ, Moayyedi P et al (2003) Mycophenolate mofetil in refractory inflammatory bowel disease. Aliment Pharmacol Ther 17:1365–1369
182. Fickert P, Hinterleitner TA, Wenzl HH et al (1998) Mycophenolate mofetil in patients with Crohn's disease. Am J Gastroenterol ;93:2529–2532
183. Fellermann K, Steffen M, Stein J et al (2000) Mycophenolate mofetil: lack of efficacy in chronic active inflammatory bowel disease. Aliment Pharmacol Ther 14:171–176
184. Wenzl HH, Hinterleitner TA, Aichbichler BW et al (2004) Mycophenolate mofetil for Crohn's disease: short-term efficacy and long-term outcome. Aliment Pharmacol Ther 19:427–434
185. Moreels TG, Pelckmans PA (2005) Gastrointestinal parasites: potential therapy for refractory inflammatory bowel diseases. Inflamm Bowel Dis 11:178–184
186. Elliott DE, Li J, Blum A et al (2003) Exposure to schistosome eggs protects mice from TNBS-induced colitis. Am J Physiol Gastrointest Liver Physiol 284:G385–391
187. Moreels TG, Nieuwendijk RJ, De Man JG et al (2004) Concurrent infection with Schistosoma mansoni attenuates inflammation induced changes in colonic morphology, cytokine levels, and smooth muscle contractility of trinitrobenzene sulphonic acid induced colitis in rats. Gut 53:99–107
188. Khan WI, Blennerhasset PA, Varghese AK et al (2002) Intestinal nematode infection ameliorates experimental colitis in mice. Infect Immun 70:5931–5937
189. Summers RW, Elliott DE, Qadir K et al (2003) Trichuris suis seems to be safe and possibly effective in the treatment of inflammatory bowel disease. Am J Gastroenterol 98:2034–2041
190. Summers RW, Elliott DE, Urban JF Jr et al (2005) Trichuris suis therapy in Crohn's disease. Gut 54:87–90
191. Sartor RB (2004) Therapeutic manipulation of the enteric microflora in inflammatory bowel diseases: antibiotics, probiotics, and prebiotics. Gastroenterology 126:1620–1633
192. Fedorak RN, Madsen KL (2004) Probiotics and the management of inflammatory bowel disease. Inflamm Bowel Dis 10:286–299
193. Egan LJ, Sandborn WJ (2005) Positioning novel biologic, probiotic, and apheresis therapies for Crohn's disease and ulcerative colitis. Curr Gastroenterol Rep 7:485–491
194. Schultz M, Timmer A, Herfarth HH et al (2004) Lactobacillus GG in inducing and maintaining remission of Crohn's disease. BMC Gastroenterol 4:5
195. Bousvaros A, Guandalini S, Baldassano RN et al (2005) A randomized, double-blind trial of Lactobacillus GG versus placebo in addition to standard maintenance therapy for children with Crohn's disease. Inflamm Bowel Dis 11:833–839
196. Prantera C, Scribano ML, Falasco G et al (2002) Ineffectiveness of probiotics in preventing recurrence after curative resection for Crohn's disease: a randomised controlled trial with Lactobacillus GG. Gut 51:405–409

Medical Therapy of Fistulizing Crohn's Disease

Luigi Benini, Fosca De Iorio, Naika Tacchella, Italo Vantini

Introduction

The development of fistulae is a common complication of Crohn's disease (CD). The lifetime risk of fistula development in patients with CD has typically been reported to range from 20 to 40%. The reported incidence of fistulizing CD from referral-based case series ranged from 17% to as much as 85% [1–3]. The probability of internal fistulae was particularly high in patients with perianal disease who presented a relative risk of 3.4 compared to patients with different localizations [4].

Over time, many fistulae tend to heal. As for example, in a cohort of 87 patients [5] with external fistulae, from the time of first presentation (involvement ileocolonic or colonic in 85% of cases, rectal in 65% of cases), after a median follow-up of 5.9 years, 68% showed healing of all fistulae, whereas in the remaining patients, partial or no healing was evident. Ninety-four percent of simple perianal fistulae were healed by the final visit compared with 70% of the complex perianal fistulae. Rectovaginal (median 26 months), enteroenteric (9.4 months) and abdominal wall (6.3 months) took a significantly shorter time to heal compared to perianal fistulae, either simple (44 months) or complex (42.8 months); there was no difference in healing time among complex and simple perianal fistulae.

Table 1 shows the outcome of current medical and surgical treatment in patients with different types of fistulae. It appears that medical treatment only has marginal efficacy with a failure rate of almost 90%. Even surgery has a high rate of effectiveness only in perianal disorders, whereas in the remaining locations, most patients do not respond and therefore require complex procedures (resection, defunctionating stoma, proctectomy).

In a longitudinal study of fistulizing CD in patients from Olmestead County, at least one fistula occurred in 35% of the patients, and at least one perianal fistula occurred in 20% [6]. The fistula developed before the diagnosis in 20% of cases and at the diagnosis in 29% of cases; in the remaining patients, the onset of fistulae was delayed (median time from the diagnosis to the first fistula was 5.5 years). The risk of fistulae was very high in the first year, and then it progressively increased over the following 20 years to a value of 50% for all locations and 26% for perianal lesions [7].

The clinical consequences of the fistulous tract depend on the nature of the adjacent tissues, the origin and the terminus of the fistula and the infectious process resulting from transit of enteric microorganisms through the fistula. In perianal fistulae, identification of specific routes created by fistula tracts informs prognostic and therapeutic options.

Patients with painful perianal fistula and associated abscess formations require surgical drainage, seton placement, and, in severe cases, proctectomy (Fig. 1). In contrast, patients with asymptomatic internal fistula require no intervention.

A variety of surgical and medical measures to induce healing of external fistulae has been proposed, but a comparison of their relative merits is difficult. This is due in part to different criteria used

Table 1. Efficacy of standard medical and of routine surgical treatments in different types of Crohn's disease fistulae, and the percent of patients requiring more complex surgical intervention [5]

	Perianal		Rectovaginal	Internal	Abdominal wall
	Simple	Complex			
Efficacy of medical treatment	9	13	13.5	8	7
Efficacy of simple surgery	82	47	13.5	8	13
Need of complex surgery	6	38	13.5	84	12

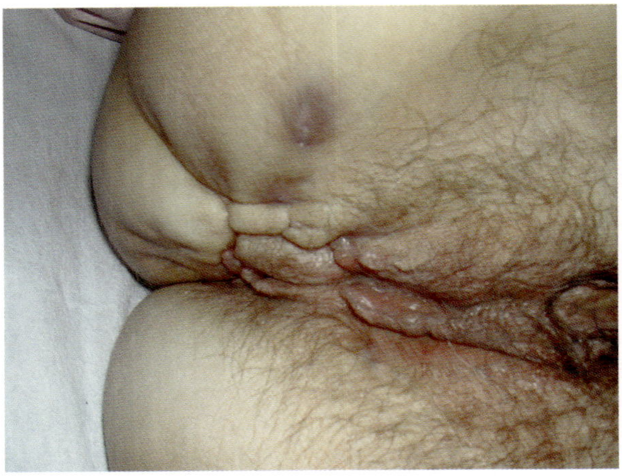

Fig. 1. Severe perineal involvement in a young female patient with complex perianal and vaginal fistula (note the discharge of stools from the vagina). All medical therapies proved uneffective, and the patient eventually required a proctocolectomy

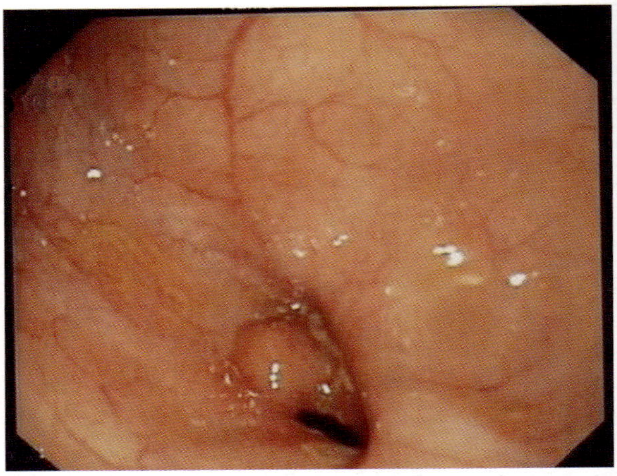

Fig. 2. Fibrotic stenosis of the colon in a patient with a colocutaneous fistula, unresponsive to all medical and endoscopic treatments. The fistula healed only with resection of the stenotic tract

to define a success. Some studies rely on an improvement of symptoms, which requires the validation of fistula-specific symptom activity indexes (Table 2), which is only effective in the research setting [8].

More recently, an attempt has been made to identify more objective parameters of success, which are, in any case, prone to criticism. For example, the absence of drainage on gentle compression of the external fistula orifice for at least 1 month has been defined as complete healing, and the reduction by at least 50% of the number of external orifices is seen as a significant improvement. Clearly, the relationship of these endpoints with a real clinical improvement is doubtful, since they don't rule out the possibility of a persistent deep abscess.

Another source of variation is represented by the definition of stenosis. A stenosis caudal to the fistula (Fig. 2) may represent the reason for medical failures,

Table 2. Parameters used for the evaluation of fistula-specific activity index in Crohn's disease

Discharge	No discharge	0
	Minimal mucous	1
	Moderate mucous or purulent	2
	Substantial	3
	Gross soiling	4
Pain/restriction of activities	No restriction	0
	Mild discomfort, no restriction	1
	Moderate discomfort, some limitation	2
	Marked discomfort, marked limitation	3
	Severe pain, severe limitation	4
Restriction of sexual activity	No	0
	Slight	1
	Moderate	2
	Marked	3
	Unable to engage in sexual activity	4
Degree of induration	No	0
	Minimal	1
	Moderate	2
	Substantial	3
	Gross fluctuance/abscess	4

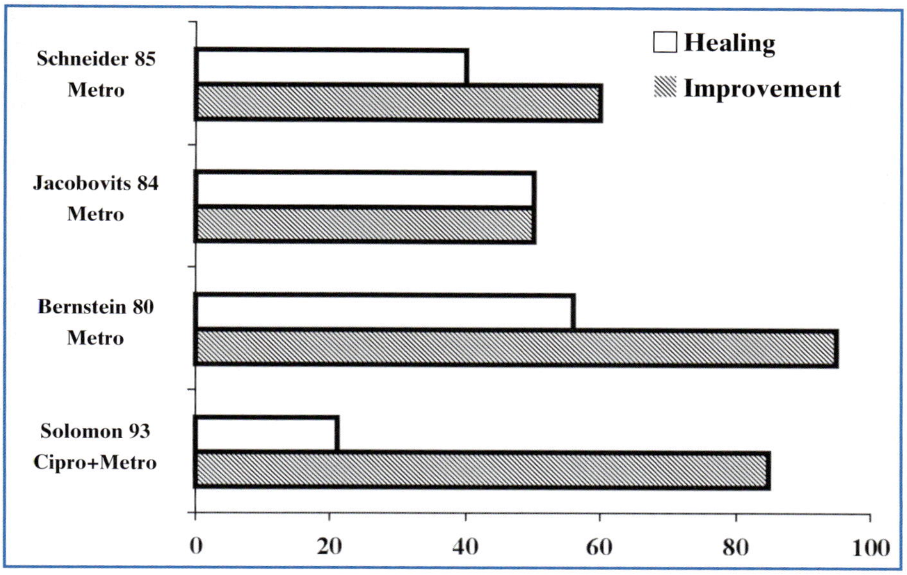

Fig. 3. Studies available on the effects of metronidazole on fistula healing or improvement

but, if considered fibrotic in nature, it also represents an exclusion criterion from most medical trials. We will review the evidence supporting the use of traditional or biological therapies in these severe, often frustrating forms of the disease.

Standard Medical Therapy

Anti-Inflammatory Medications

Several studies demonstrated that sulphasalazine and mesalazine are efficacious at high dose (3 g or more) for CD, but there is no evidence that these drugs are effective in fistula healing. Also corticosteroids have no proven efficacy in the treatment of fistulizing Crohn's disease. In most of the studies on steroid efficacy, patients were not randomized for fistulae [9]. A recent review [10] has associated in patients with fistulizing CD, the use of corticosteroids with deleterious outcome, including an increased incidence of surgery in two large uncontrolled clinical trials [11, 12]. In the European Cooperative Crohn's Disease study, three out of five CD-related deaths were in patients with a palpable abdominal mass receiving 6-methylprednisolone. Corticosteroids may mask clinical signs of an abdominal abscess with the attendant risk of delayed drainage [13, 14]. Patients with enterovesical fistulae failed to heal when on steroids [15].

Antibiotics

After an initial report that metronidazole "closed" perianal fistulae in three patients [16], the drug was frequently used in the management of fistulizing CD. However, most studies on its efficacy were on small numbers of patients and were uncontrolled (Fig. 3).

Bernstein et al. [17], in an open study with metronidazole 20 mg/kg/day on patients with longstanding perianal fistulae, observed an initial clinical response in 20/21, with complete healing at 8 weeks in 56% of cases. However, at follow-up, 78% of these patients recurred 4 months after discontinuation and only 5 of 18 patients could discontinue the metronidazole [18]. Other open studies with metronidazole confirmed closure rates of perianal Crohn's fistula of 35–50% [19–21]. Clinical improvement is usually seen within the first 6–8 weeks. So far, no controlled trials have been performed on the short and long-term efficacy of metronidazole on fistulae healing. Based on a cost-utility analysis [21], metronidazole in combination with an immunomodulatory medication, such as azathioprine (AZA), may be the most cost-effective initial therapy for fistulizing CD. Metronidazole is often poorly tolerated because of adverse effects including paresthesias, dyspepsia, a metallic-taste and a disulfiram-like response to alcohol. Peripheral neurological dysfunction has been demonstrated by physical examination and nerve conduction studies in 85% of patients, although almost 55% were asymptomatic. Peripheral neuropathy improved or resolved in 90% after antibiotic discontinuation [22].

Because of the toxicity of metronidazole, ciprofloxacin is often used, even though no controlled trial of this drug for fistulizing CD has been reported. Turunen et al. [23] first reported the use of ciprofloxacin in eight patients with perineal CD refractory to metronidazole. All patients improved with 1–1.5 g/day of ciprofloxacin for 3–12 months; however, four of eight had persistent perianal drainage and several required surgery. Recurrences of fistulae were frequent but usually responded to the restarting of ciprofloxacin.

A retrospective analysis of combination of ciprofloxacin (1 000–1 500 mg/day) and metronidazole (500–1 500 mg/day) on 14 patients, produced a clinical improvement in nine and fistula closure in three. Again, prompt recurrence of the disease was seen after cessation of therapy [24].

Immunomodulators

6-Mercaptopurine and Azathioprine

These drugs are among the few agents that have demonstrated efficacy in fistulizing CD in controlled clinical trials. Although these agents are discussed interchangeably, there have been uncontrolled trials directly comparing these medications in the treatment of inflammatory bowel disease.

The effect of 6-MP on fistulizing CD was first evaluated by Present [25] in a randomized, placebo-controlled trial (2 years with a crossover after 1 year). The superiority of the drug over the placebo in fistula healing (31% *vs.* 6%) was not significant because of the small number of patients.

An uncontrolled follow-up extended the study of 6-MP (1.5 mg/kg/day) to a total of 34 patients with fistulae (perirectal 18, abdominal wall 8, enteroenteric 7, rectovaginal 6, vulvar 2). Complete closure was observed in 39% of patients, a partial response in 26% and no response in 35%. Response was slow and required more than 3 months in 32% of the patients. Six out of the 13 with complete healing continued therapy and all maintained the response; 5 out of the 7 who discontinued therapy had a relapse and healed again when the therapy was restarted [26].

A meta-analysis of five controlled trials of AZA and 6-MP in CD confirmed these results: 54% of 41 patients receiving the active drug responded compared with 21% of 29 patients receiving placebo [27], resulting in a pooled odds ratio for fistula healing of 4.4. These results must be interpreted with some caution, since 66% of the 70 studied patients came from a single study [25]. Dosing and administration of AZA and 6-MP has not been standardized. Controlled trials indicate that AZA at doses of 2–3 mg/kg/day and 6-MP at a dose of 1.5 mg/kg/day are effective for the treatment of CD. Although titration of either drug to a specified blood 6-thioguanine nucleotide metabolite concentration (6-thioguanine >235 pM/10^8 erytrocytes) has been suggested for improving therapeutic efficacy, this has not been demonstrated convincingly in the treatment of Crohn's fistulae [28].

We can conclude that AZA/6-mercaptopurine is effective both in healing and maintaining fistula closure. Furthermore, there is evidence of long-term safety in terms of neoplasia of super-infections. Adverse events are reported to occur in 9–15% of patients receiving AZA or 6-MP for inflammatory bowel disease. The most serious adverse events are pancreatitis (3%), allergic reactions (2%) and drug induced hepatitis (0.3%). A small percentage of patients who are thiopurine methyltransferase deficient may also develop leukopenia (2%) [29]. These drugs have also been proven to be safe when taken during pregnancy, since they did not increase the number of fetal damage or abortions [30].

Methotrexate

Two recent uncontrolled studies have examined the efficacy of parenteral methotrexate in fistulizing CD. In the first, treatment with intramuscular methotrexate (25 mg/week), in 16 patients produced fistula closure in 4 and a partial response in 5, with an overall response of 56%. All the patients who achieved remission failed or were intolerant to AZA and 25% also failed to respond to CyA. However, fistulae recurred when methotrexate was reduced or was switched to an oral form [31]. In the second, a study of 20 patients with active CD who were AZA-resistant or intolerant and steroid dependent (8 with a fistula), a response was obtained in 14/20 at 12 weeks, in 10/20 at 6 months, and 4/14 at 12 months. Patients with fistulizing disease were not analyzed separately [32]. Adverse events have been reported in 50% of patients treated with parenteral methotrexate for more than 6 months and include elevation of transaminases (5–20% of patients), nausea (4–12%), bone marrow suppression (10–20%), and require discontinuation of the drug in 10% of patients [33].

Hepatic fibrosis was observed in 0–5% of patients who have undergone liver biopsy after a cumulative methotrexate dose of more than 1 500 mg [34]. A potentially life-threatening interstitial pneumonitis has been observed in 3–12% of long-term treated patients. Furthermore, methotrexate has a known toxicity on the fetus. In conclusion, MTX in a dose of 25 mg/week should be tried in AZA/6-mercaptopurine resistant or intolerant patients.

Cyclosporine A

Ten uncontrolled studies, some published only in abstract form and comprising altogether only 64 patients, examined the effect of intravenous CyA for the treatment of fistulizing CD with an overall initial response of 83% [35–44].

Present and Lichtiger [38] treated 16 patients with Crohn's fistulae (10 perirectal, 4 enterocutaneous, 2 rectovaginal) with cyclosporine A, starting with a continuous intravenous infusion (4 mg/kg/day), switched to the oral route (6–8 mg/kg/day). Fourteen responded to parenteral CyA (7 complete closure, 7 moderate improvement) and discontinued the steroids, with a mean time for response of 7.4 days. When switched to the oral route, 64% remained in remission, 36% relapsed.

These results have been supplemented by a review of literature including 39 patients with fistulizing Crohn's disease who have been treated with CyA [43]. Within this group, 90% responded to intravenous cyclosporine, but 82% relapsed with CyA suspension.

A modest reduction in fistula recurrence has been produced with combined use of CyA, AZA and a tapering schedule of prednisolone over 3 months before cessation of CyA therapy [45]. All nine patients responded to intravenous cyclosporine with no recurrences after its discontinuation. CyA was terminated after 3 months, while AZA and low-dose prednisolone were continued: four patients did not deteriorate, three deteriorated slightly and two had a recurrence.

Adverse events of high dose CyA include paresthesias, hypertrichosis, hypertension, tremor, renal insufficiency, hepatotoxicity, headache, opportunistic infections, gingival hyperplasia and seizures [46].

On the base of these studies, it is reasonable to use CyA in fistulizing Crohn's disease in the acute phase; as it will not achieve long-term response, all patients should be treated with concurrent AZA/6-mercaptopurine for maintenance or, if the patient is allergic/intolerant to AZA/6-MP, with parenteral MTX.

Tacrolimus

Tacrolimus is a potent immunosuppressant agent that inhibits the transcription of IL-2 in T-helper cells, used mainly for the prevention of allograft rejection. Uncontrolled retrospective series suggest its efficacy for treatment of fistulizing CD [47–49]. In the only randomized, double-blind, placebo-controlled trial, Sandborn et al. [50] randomized 48 patients with actively draining Crohn's fistulae to placebo or oral tacrolimus (initial dosage of 0.20 mg/kg/day for 10 weeks). A clinical response (closure of at least 50% of fistulae maintained for at least 4 weeks) occurred in 43% of tacrolimus-treated patients and 8% of placebo (p=0.004). However, there was no difference in the complete closure of fistulae, (10% of tacrolimus *vs.* 8% placebo). Adverse events observed in patients treated with tacrolimus include renal insufficiency, tremor, headaches, paresthesias, leg cramps and tremor.

In a subsequent study, ten patients with fistulae refractory to medical therapy (including infliximab) and on long-term steroids or immunosuppressors, were treated with oral tacrolimus (0.05 mg/kg every 12 hours) with 6–24 months follow-up. Four achieved a complete response and five achieved a partial response and could discontinue or reduce steroids and immunosuppressors with no serious side effect [51].

Mycophenolate mofetil

Mycophenolate mofetil (MFF) is a potent immunosuppressant that inhibits lymphocyte proliferation through a blockade of guanosine nucleotide synthesis. In a study comparing the efficacy of AZA plus steroids *vs.* MMF plus steroids, MMF produced a more rapid improvement in the activity index in cases with severe activity and a similar response in cases with moderate activity [52].

Uncontrolled case series have suggested the efficacy of mycophenolate in long-term maintenance of remission [53–56]. Wenzl et al. [56] observed that almost 55% of patients with complicated CD responded, but 64% of the initial responders relapsed within 18 months. Well-designed placebo-controlled trials are necessary to establish the role of this drug.

Anti-Tumor Necrosis Factor-Alfa Therapy

Infliximab

Cytokines including TNF-α are critical in the inflammatory processes that characterize CD. Mucosal biopsy specimens and mononuclear cells isolated from the lamina propria of a patient with CD express high levels of TNF-α. Infliximab is a chimeric monoclonal antibody that binds to and neutralizes human TNF-α. Its infusion results in a significant reduction in inflammation, as confirmed in many randomized placebo-controlled trials.

Present et al. [57] demonstrated the efficacy of infliximab in the treatment of fistulizing CD in a placebo-controlled multicentered study in which 94 patients with active abdominal or perianal fistulae received either infliximab 5 mg/kg, infliximab 10 mg/kg, or placebo. Treatments were administrated at weeks 0, 2 and 6. The primary goal was a reduction of 50% or more in the number of draining fistulae observed at two or more consecutive visits; a secondary goal was fistula-closure. Sixty-eight percent of patients on infliximab 5 mg/kg and 56% on infliximab 10 mg/kg achieved the primary goal compared to 26% on placebo. Much more notably, complete fistula healing was obtained in 55% of patients on infliximab 5 mg/kg and in 38% 10 mg/kg. The majority of fistulae closed before the third infusion and the median duration of remission was 3 months. No differences were noted with regards to duration, extent of disease, prior surgery, number of fistulae or concomitant medications.

Infliximab has also proved to maintain its efficacy in the long term. In a randomized controlled trial of 573 patients with active Crohn's disease (CDAI score of at least 220), responders to a 5 mg/kg i.v. of infliximab (335 patients) were randomly assigned to repeat infusions of placebo at weeks 2 and 6 and then every 8 weeks until week 46 (group I), or 5 mg/kg infliximab at the same timepoints (group II), or 5 mg/kg infliximab at weeks 2 and 6 followed by infliximab 10 mg/kg (group III). At week 30, 21% of the patients of group I were in remission, compared to 39% of group II and 45% of group III [58].

Sands et al. performed a multicenter randomized double-blind placebo-controlled trial to evaluate the efficacy of infliximab maintenance therapy in 306 CD patients and one or more fistulae. Initially patients received 5 mg/kg infliximab i.v. at week 0, 2 and 6. A total of 195 patients who responded at week 14 were randomized to receive infliximab or placebo. The remaining 87 patients who didn't achieve an initial response were also randomly assigned to placebo or infliximab maintenance therapy. Among the responders, those assigned to maintenance infliximab had a longer time to the loss of response than those on placebo (median 40 *vs.* 14 weeks). At week 54, 36% of the infliximab group had a complete absence of draining fistulae, compared with 19% in the placebo group. There was no difference in response between infliximab and placebo among initial non-responders [59].

No consensus has been reached on the best infliximab regimen for the long-term treatment of CD between short-term courses and retreatment of relapses *vs.* maintenance therapy. Some authors sustain that infliximab should be used as a bridge therapy while awaiting the onset of effects of conventional immunosuppressive therapy [60].

In a recent analysis of Crohn's disease, patients treated with infliximab in ACCENT I, episodic and scheduled treatment strategies were compared under conditions that simulate clinical practice. Patients treated with scheduled infliximab, particularly in the 10 mg/kg group, had better symptomatic responses than those treated on demand. Both scheduled groups had fewer hospitalizations, higher rates of mucosal healing, and lower rates of antibody positivity, with no increase in side effects, than those treated on demand [61].

The main argument in favour of long-term scheduled infliximab is represented by the reduced prevalence of anti-infliximab antibodies during scheduled therapy rather than during episodic therapy, and by the association of these antibodies with decreased serum infliximab concentrations, decreased clinical responsiveness, and increased risk of allergic reactions [62].

The long-term use of infliximab for fistulizing CD is still under investigation in terms both of a limited efficacy and cost-effectiveness. As for the first problem, Poritz et al found that, if clinical improvement was obtained in 18 out of 26 patients with fistulizing CD, with complete fistula closure in 6, surgery was ultimately required in 14 patients and 6 continued to have draining fistulae [63]. The problem of the cost-effectiveness of infliximab therapy has been raised by a recent cost-utility analysis [64] in which infliximab proved to be more effective then either metronidazole or AZA, but also far more expensive. However, these results are outweighed by the consideration that patients with fistulizing Crohn's disease in the ACCENT II study who received maintenance infliximab had significantly fewer days of hospitalization, number of hospitalizations, surgical procedures in total, and fewer major surgical procedures compared to those who received placebo [65].

Adverse events observed in patients treated with infliximab include infusion reactions such as delayed hypersensitivity, formation of anti-chimeric antibodies and anti-dsDNA autoantibodies and, in rare cases, onset of drug-induced lupus. Approximately 3% of patients in the ACCENT I trial developed delayed hypersensitivity reactions manifested by serum-sickness-like symptoms. This may be due to the fact that a proportion of the molecule is still of murine origin and therefore potentially immunogenic. Attempts are therefore being made to produce less immunogenic biologic agents, thereby increasing their "human" proportion (Fig. 4).

The efficacy of a humanized chimeric antibody (CDP-571) against human TNF-α in fistula closure has been assessed in a randomized placebo-controlled trial on 37 patients with actively draining fistulae [66]. Closure of at least 50% of fistulae was obtained in 12 of 24 patients on CDP-571 and in 2 of 23 on placebo. Other agents that inhibit TNF-α activity such as pen-

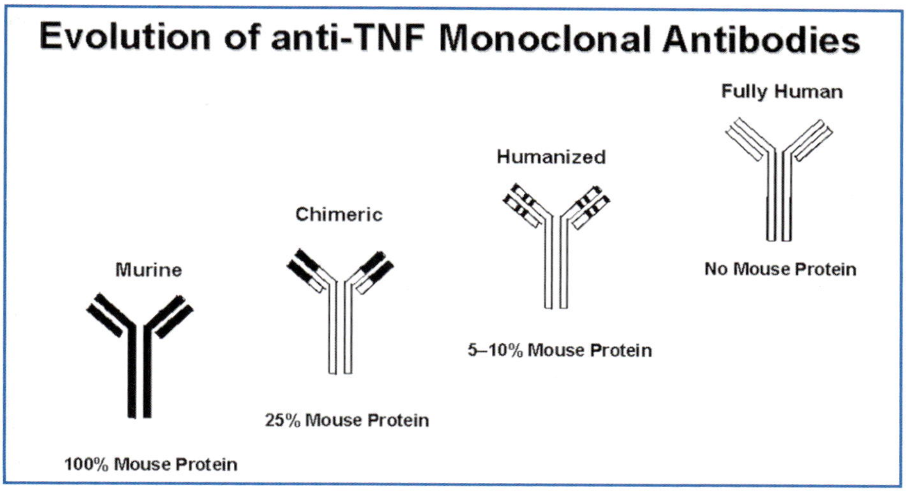

Fig. 4. Ideal progression in the development of engineered monoclonal antibodies from wholly-murine to wholly humane, in an attempt to reduce the immunogenicity of the molecules. In *black*, components of murine origin; in *white*, components of human origin.

toxifylline and etanercept failed to demonstrate their efficacy in CD. Moreover, some of these agents are only active in a subset of patients with highly active disease, as identified by elevated C-reactive protein. Possible explanations for the different activity of biological drugs sharing the same target may be found in their different biological actions (binding to soluble or to membrane-bound TNF, capacity to produce T-cell apoptosis, fixation of complement, induction of antibody-dependent cytotoxicity).

Two open-label studies of thalidomide, a potent inhibitor of TNF alfa, have shown some degree of efficacy in fistulizing CD [67, 68]. Together, these studies support a strategy of TNF-α inhibition as a basis for healing fistulizing CD. In addition to its well-known teratogenic effects, thalidomide has been complicated by marked somnolence and peripheral neuropathy.

Novel Therapies

A number of novel therapies have been suggested for the treatment of fistulizing CD. The use of fibrin glue and plasma factor XIII concentrates have been advanced as adjunctive therapies in the management of perianal fistulae. Hyperbaric oxygen has also been suggested as an adjunctive therapy in healing fistulizing CD. Although case reports have documented successful healing during therapy, no randomized placebo-controlled studies have been performed to confirm these findings. Further studies are necessary to assess the role of these therapies in the management of fistulizing CD [69].

Elemental Diet, Bowel Rest and Parenteral Nutrition

Only anecdotal experience exists on the use of elemental diets and total parenteral nutrition in fistulizing CD. Calam et al. [69] reported on six patients in whom an elemental diet was used specifically to treat perianal fistulae in Crohn's disease. Four improved with an elemental diet, but fistulae only healed completely in one patient. No studies specifically examined total parenteral nutrition in perianal CD. The use of elemental diets or total parenteral nutrition for fistulizing CD is therefore not recommended.

Conclusion

Treatment of CD fistulizing Crohn's disease requires a close collaboration between the gastroenterologist and the surgeon. Antibiotics and immunomodulators such as azathioprine/6-mercaptopurine or methotrexate, if the patient is AZA-6MP intolerant/resistant, should be given early in the disease. In the case of resistance to immunomodulators, infliximab is the treatment of choice. Short-term cyclosporine A or tacrolimus may be tried in patients who fail to respond to infliximab. Abscesses should always be drained by an expert surgeon.

References

1. Steinberg DM (1973) Abscess and fistulae in Crohn disease. Gut 14:865–869
2. Rankin GB (1979) National cooperative Crohn's disease study: extraintestinal manifestations and perianal complications. Gastroenterology 77:914–20
3. Farmer RG (1975) Clinical patterns in Crohn's disease:

a statistical study of 615 patients. Gastroenterology 68:627–635
4. Sachar DB, Bodian CA, Goldstein ES et al (2005) Is perianal Crohn's disease associated with intestinal fistulization? Am J Gastroenterol 100(7):1547–1549
5. Bell SJ, Williams AB, Wiesel P, Wilkinson K, Cohen RCG, Kamm MA (2003) The clinical course of fistulating Crohn's disease. Aliment Pharmacol Ther 17:1145–1151
6. Schwartz DA (2002) The Natural history of fistulizing Crohn's disease in Olmsted County, Minnesota. Gastroenterology 122:875–880
7. Gray BK, Lockhartmummery HE, Morson BC (1965) Crohn's disease of the anal region. Gut 6:515–524
8. Hellers G, Bergstrand O, Ewerth S, Holmstrom B (1980) Occurrence in outcome after primary treatment of anal fistulae in Crohn's disease. Gut 21:525–527
9. Present DH (2000) How to do without steroids in inflammatory bowel disease. Inflamm Bowel Dis 6:48–57
10. Judge TA, Lichtenstein GR (2004) Treatment of fistulizing Crohn's disease. Gastroenterol Clin N Am 33:421–454
11. Sparberg M, Kirsner JB (1966) Long-term corticosteroid therapy for enteritis: an analysis of 58 courses in 54 patients. Am J Dig Dis 11:865–880
12. Jones JH, Lennard-Jones JF (1966) Corticosteroids and corticotrophin in the treatment of Crohn's disease. Gut 7:181–187
13. Malchow H, Ewe J, Brandes W et al (1984) European cooperative Crohn's disease study (ECCDS): results of drug treatment. Gastroenterology 86:249–266
14. Agrawal A, Durrani S, Leiper K et al (2005) Effect of systemic corticosteroid therapy on risk for intra-abdominal or pelvic abscess in non-operated Crohn's disease. Clin Gastroenterol Hepatol 3:1215–1220
15. Present DH (2002) Urinary tract fistulae in Crohn's disease: surgery versus medical therapy. Am J Gastroenterol 97:2165–2167
16. Ursing B, Kamme C (1975) Metronidazole for Crohn's disease. Lancet 1:775–777
17. Bernstein LH, Frank MS, Brandt LJ, Boley SJ (1980) Metronidazole therapy for perineal Crohn's disease with metronidazole. Gastroenterology 79:357–365
18. Brandt LJ, Bernstein LH, Boley SJ, Frank MS (1982) Metronidazole therapy for perineal Crohn's disease: a follow-up study. Gastroenterology 83:383–387
19. Jakobovits J, Schuster MM (1984) Metronidazole therapy for Crohn's disease and associated fistulae. Am J Gastroenterol 79:533–540
20. Schneider MU, Laudage G, Guggenmoos-Holzma I, Riemann JF (1985) Metronidazol in der behandlung des morbus Crohn. Dtsch Med Wochenschr 110:1724–1930
21. Arseneau KO, Cohn SM, Cominelli F, Connors AF Jr (2001) Cost-utility of initial medical management for Crohn's disease perianal fistulae. Gastroenterology 120:1640–1656
22. Duffy LF, Daum F, Fisher SE et al (1985) Peripheral neuropathy in Crohn's disease patients treated with metronidazole. Gastroenterology 88:681–684
23. Turunen U, Farkkila M, Seppala K (1989) Long-term treatment of peri-anal or fistulous Crohn's disease with ciprofloxacin. Scan J Gastroenterol 24:144–148
24. Solomon M, McLeod R, O'Connor B et al (1993) Combination ciprofloxacin and medronidazole in severe perianal Crohn's disease. Can J Gastroenterol 7:571–573
25. Present DH, Korelitz BI, Wisch N et al (1980) Treatment of Crohn's disease with 6-mercaptopurine: a long-term, randomized, double-blind study. N Engl J Med 302:981–987
26. Korelitz BI, Present DH (1985) Favorable effect of 6-mercaptopurine on fistulae of Crohn's disease. Dig Dis Sci 30:58–64
27. Pearson DC, May GR, Fick GH, Sutherland LR (1995) Azathioprine and 6-mercaptopurine in Crohn's disease: a meta-analysis. Ann Intern Med 123:132–142
28. Cuffari C, Hunt S, Bayless T (2001) Utilization of 6-thioguanine metabolite levels to optimise azathioprine therapy in patients with inflammatory bowel disease. Gut 48:642–646
29. Present DH, Meltzer SJ, Krumholtz MP et al (1989) 6-mercaptopurine in the management of inflammatory bowel disease: short and long-term toxicity. Ann Intern Med 111:641–649
30. Mahadevan U, Marion JF, Present DH (2003) Fistula response to methotrexate in Crohn's disease: a case series. Aliment Pharmacol Ther 18:1003–1008
31. Vandeputte L, D'Haens G, Baert F, Rutgeerts P (1999) Methotrexate in refractory Crohn's disease. Inflamm Bowel Dis 5:11–15
32. Lemann M, Zenjari T, Bouhnik Y et al (2000) Methotrexate in Crohn's disease: long-term efficacy and toxicity. Am J Gastroenterol 95:1730–1734
33. Te HS, Schiano TD, Kuan SF et al (2000) Hepatic effect of long-term methotrexate use in treatment of inflammatory bowel disease. Am J Gastroenterol 95:3150–3156
34. Fukushima T, Sugita A, Masuzawa S et al (1989) Effects of cyclosporine A on active Crohn's disease. Gastroenterol JPN 24:12–15
35. Lichtiger S (1990) Cyclosporine therapy in inflammatory bowel disease: open-label experience. Mt Sinai J Med 57:315–319
36. Hanauer SB, Smith MB (1993) Rapid closure of Crohn's disease fistulae with continuous intravenous cyclosporine A. Am J Gastroenterol 88:646–649
37. Present DH, Lichtiger S (1994) Efficacy of cyclosporine in treatment of fistula of Crohn's disease. Dig Dis Sci 39:374–380
38. Markowitz J, Rosa J, Grancher K et al (1990) Long-term 6-mercaptopurine treatment in adolescents with Crohn's disease. Gastroenterology 99:1347–1351
39. Abreu-Martin M, Vasiliauskas E, Gaiennie J (1996) Continuous infusion cyclosporine is effective for severe acute Crohn's disease: but for how long? Gastroenterology 110:A851
40. O'Neill J, Pathhmakanthan S, Goh J (1997) Cyclosporine A induces remission in fistulous Crohn's disease but relapse occurs upon cessation of treatment. Gastroenterology 112:A1056
41. Hinterleitner TA, Petritsch W, Aichbichler B et al (1997) Combination of cyclosporine, azathioprine and prednisolone for perianal fistulae in Crohn's disease. Z Gastroenterol 35:603–608

42. Egan LJ, Sandborn WJ, Tremaine WJ (1998) Clinical outcome following treatment of refractory inflammatory and fistulizing Crohn's disease with intravenous cyclosporine. Am J Gastroenterol 93:442–448
43. Gurudu SR, Griffel LH, Gialanella RJ, Das KM (1999) Cyclosporine therapy in inflammatory bowel disease: short-term and long-term results. J Clin Gastroenterol 29:151–154
44. Hinterleitner TA, Petritsch W, Aichbichler B, Fickert P, ranner G, Krejs GJ (1997) Combination of cyclosporine, azathioprine and prednisolone for perianal fistulae in Crohn's disease. Z Gastroenterol 35:603–608
45. Sandborn W (1995) A critical review of cyclosporine therapy in inflammatory bowel disease. Inflamm Bowel Dis 1:48–63
46. Lowry PW, Weaver AL, Tremaine WJ, Sandborn WJ (1999) Combination therapy with oral tacrolimus (FK506) and azathioprine or 6-mercaptopurine for treatment-refractory Crohn's disease perianal fistulae. Inflamm Bowel Dis 5:239–245
47. Sandborn WJ (1997) Preliminary report on the use of oral tacrolimus (FK506) in the treatment of complicated proximal small bowel and fistulizing Crohn's disease. Am J Gastroenterol 92:876–879
48. Fellermman K, Ludwig D, Stahl M et al (1998) Steroid-unresponsive acute attacks of inflammatory bowel disease: immunomodulation by tacrolimus (FK506). Am J Gastroenterol 93:1860–1866
49. Sandborn WJ, Present DH, Isaacs KL et al (2003) Tacrolimus for the treatment of fistulae with Crohn's disease: a randomized, placebo-controlled trial. Gastroenterology 126:942–943
50. Gonzalez-Lama Y, Abreu L, Vera MI et al (2005) Long-term tacrolimus therapy in refractory to infliximab fistulizing Crohn's disease: a pilot study. Inflamm Bowel Dis 11:8–15
51. Neurath MF, Wanitschke R, Peters M et al (1999) Randomized trial of mycophenolate mofetil versus azathioprine for treatment of chronic active Crohn's disease. Gut 44:625–628
52. Fickert P, Hinterleitner TA, Wenzl HH et al (1998) Mycophenolate mofetil in patients with Crohn's disease. Am J Gastroenterol 93:2529–2532
53. Miehsler W, Reinisch W, Moser G et al (2001) Is mycophenolate mofetil an effective alternative in azathioprine-intolerant patients with active Crohn's disease? Am J Gastroenterol 96:782–787
54. Fellermann K, Steffen M, Steinn J et al (2000) Mycophenolate mofetil: lack of efficacy in chronic active inflammatory bowel disease. Aliment Pharmacol Ther 14:171–176
55. Wenzl HH, Hinterleitneir TA, Aichbichler BW et al (2005) Mycophenolate mofetil for Crohn's disease: short-term efficacy and long-term outcome. Aliment Pharmacol Ther 19:427–434
56. Present DH, Rutgeerts P, Targann S et al (1999) Infliximab for the treatment of fistulae in patients with Crohn's disease. N Engl J Med 340:1398–1405
57. Hanauer SB, Feagan BG, Lichtenstein GR et al (2002) Maintenance infliximab for Crohn's disease: the ACCENT I randomised trial. Lancet 359:1541–1549
58. Sands E, Anderson FH, Bernstein CN, Chey WY et al (2004) Infliximab maintenance therapy for fistulizing Crohn's disease. N Eng J Med 350:876–885
59. Hanauer SB (2005) Infliximab: lifetime use for maintenance is appropriate in Chron's disease. CON: "lifetime use" is an awfully long time. Am J Gastroenterol 100:1435–1437
60. Rutgeerts P, Feagna BG, Lichtenstein GR et al (2004) Comparison of scheduled and episodic treatment strategies of infliximab in Crohn's disease. Gastroenterology 126:598–601
61. Lichtenstein GR (2005) Infliximab: lifetime use for maintenance is appropriate in Crohn's disease. Pro: maintenance therapy is superior to episodic therapy. Am J Gastroenterol 100:1433–1435
62. Poritz LS, Rowe WA, Koltun WA (2002) Remicade does not abolish the need for surgery in fistulizing Crohn's disease. Dis Colon Rectum 45:771–775
63. Arseneau KO, Cohn SM, Cominelli F, Connors AF Jr (2001) Cost-utility of initial medical management for Crohn's disease perianal fistulae. Gastroenterology 120:1640–1656
64. Lichtenstein GR, Yan S, Bala M et al (2005) Infliximab maintenance treatment reduces hospitalizations, surgeries, and procedures in fistulizing Crohn's disease. Gastroenterology 128:862–869
65. Sandborn WJ, Feagan BG, Hanauer SB et al (2001) An engineered human antibody to TNF (CDP571) for active Crohn's disease: a randomized double-blind placebo-controlled trial. Gastroenterology 120:1330–1338
66. Eherenpreis ED, Kane SV, Cohen LB et al (1999) Thalidomide therapy for patients with refractory Crohn's disease: an open-label trial. Gastroenterology 117:1271–1277
67. Vasiliauskas EA, Kam Ly, Abreu-Martin MT et al (1999) An open-label pilot study of low-dose thalidomide in chronically active, steroid-dependent Crohn's disease. Gastroenterology 117:1278–1287
68. Present DH (2003) Crohn's fistula: current concepts in management. Gastroenterology 124:1629–1635
69. Calam J, Crooks PE, Walker RJ (1980) Elemental diets in the management of Crohn's perianal fistulae. JPEN 4:4–8

Surgical Options in Small-Bowel Disease

Gian Gaetano Delaini, Gianluca Colucci, Filippo Nifosì

Introduction

In his landmark article titled "Regional Ileitis: A Pathologic and Clinical Entity" [1], Crohn wrote: "Medical treatment is purely palliative and supportive. . . . THE PROPER APPROACH TO A COMPLETE CURE IS BY SURGICAL RESECTION of the diseased segment of the small intestine and of the ileocecal valve with its contiguous cecum".

The enthusiasm aroused by considering surgical therapy as a decisive treatment for Crohn's disease (CD) faded away. Knowledge acquired over time revealed the peculiar inclination of this disease to affect the entire intestine tract ubiquitously and to be connected with frequent extra-intestinal manifestations. Medical treatment has then become the mainstay of therapy for patients with CD. Introduction of new classes of drugs, such as immunosuppressants/immunomodulators, led by recognition of the role of the immune system in the disease pathogenesis, increased the success both in controlling the disease in its acute phase and in maintaining the quiescent phase. Regardless, approximately 70–80% of patients suffering from CD requires surgical treatment during the course of the disease; this percentage has been constant over the last 40 years according to data given by the literature [2, 3]. While intestinal perforation, sepsis, intestinal obstruction, continuous bleeding, fistulae and abscesses are clear and unambiguous conditions indicating the need of surgical treatment, on the contrary, there is a considerable percentage of patients falling into a "grey area" that, in clinical practice, foments the age-old argument between gastroenterologists and surgeons regarding timing of the surgical operation [4]. It is therefore clear that the therapeutical trend is to try to identify patients with a higher risk of complications to be then surgically treated [5] in order to delay surgical treatment as long as possible through more and more aggressive medical therapies [6, 7] or mini-invasive therapeutical approaches, such as percutaneous draining of abscesses or, more rarely, dilation of stenoses or haemolysation in the case of haemorrhagic events [8]. However, the risk connected with too conservative an approach is leading compromised patients towards surgical treatment with the resulting complications.

As Delaney recently pointed out [9], the absence of complications leads to a fast improvement of patients' quality of life after surgical treatment (in his study quality of life was assessed both preoperatively and 30 days postoperatively). Patients not only judged surgical therapy positively, but they even suggested applying it earlier and proposing it as a primary option in the case of disease relapse.

Application of the principle stated by the Birmingham group (as recurrence is almost inevitable, the main aim being to save as much intestinal tissue as possible [10]), certainly made surgical treatment increasingly conservative, emphasising the importance of attempting to avoid intestinal resection or at least reduce the width used in the past

From all this, we now understand that an appropriate multidisciplinary approach is essential when treating CD, a disease that, despite much enthusiasm and new therapeutical options, seems to have a clinical history that has changed very little over the last 40 years if, as Wolters concluded in a recent systematic review of the literature [11]: "structured literature review provides no hard evidence for change in disease outcome in Crohn's disease during the last four decades".

The aim of this chapter is to analyse the state of the art of surgical options in the treatment of CD, attempting to especially emphasise correct indications, surgical techniques and correct surgical timing.

Surgical Indications in Crohn's Disease and Preoperative Preparation

Table 1 summarises indications for surgical treatment in Crohn's disease [4, 12, 13]. Surgery may be either scheduled or urgent. The subdivision into absolute and relative indications is partly arbitrary. Regardless of CD, intestinal perforation is considered to require urgent surgical treatment, but determining

Table 1. Indication for surgical therapy

Absolute indication	
Fulminant form of the disease	
	Intestinal obstruction (especially terminal ileum) Intestinal perforation
Complication of the disease process	Intestinal bleeding Recalcitrant sepsis Fistulae (?) Abscess (?)
Failure of medical therapy Complications of steroids or other medical therapy	Growth failure
Controversial indications	
Series of subileus Recurrences subsiding after conservative treatment	

where the therapy failed is sometimes very difficult. Many cases also require careful consideration by the gastroenterologist. A recurring event in clinical practice that is a common experience for many individuals treating this type of patients is to define, in some cases, clear definition between a pattern of subocclusion due to inflammatory oedema (that can respond to therapy) or to fibrosis (that cannot respond to therapy but to surgery only). Some preoperative care and attention, if permitted by the clinical situation, should always be used.

The patient should be operated only after a thorough study [14]. The single-contrast gastrointestinal (GI) series with small-bowel follow-through represents, presently, an examination with a good cost/benefit ratio and that, in many important cases, gives information regarding intestinal transit and the presence of stenosis [15]. On many occasions, in urgent cases especially, enteroclysis with computed tomography (CT] and double-contrast evaluation provides information on the presence of peritoneal abscesses or on fistulae. Ultrasonography with or without Doppler as well as magnetic resonance imaging (MRI) [16] can be used for monitoring disease activity and response to therapy or when the use of ionising radiation is contraindicated (e.g. pregnancy or childhood). Even if surgical exploration allows visualisation of the intra-abdominal state, the possibility of planning the surgical approach is essential and supportive in the search for any fistulous tracts, which are often difficult to find.

An essential aspect, which is often overlooked, is preoperative marking the stoma. Creation of a temporary stoma takes place frequently, especially during urgent surgery. The most frequent indications are postoperative dehiscences, presence of major perianal fistulae, intra-abdominal sepsis (which makes creation of the anastomosis unsafe) or a serious colonic disease. Proper positioning of the stoma allows patients to not only manage it easily but to accept it [17]. It must remembered, moreover, that, as Post [18] wrote, approximately 20% of "temporary" stomas become definitive if the indication is postoperative complications; this percentage increases up to 60% if the indication is rectal stenosis or perianal fistulae.

Appropriate treatment during the postoperative period must include an antithrombotic prophylaxis and antibiotic administration. The latter will need to be broad spectrum for some days in the case of abscesses, fistulae or perforations, or just a single dose given within 30 min of skin incision (repeated if the operation lasts longer than 3 h) in the case of noncontaminated operations (the so-called short-term prophylaxis).

Another important aspect is nutritional support. A state of malnutrition is rather frequent in these patients, and it may be worsened by poor control of the disease or by the presence of infection or fistulae. Restoring electrolyte balance is essential. Caloric support may be achieved through a total parenteral nutrition or, if possible and the patient tolerates it, through enteral nutrition, which has lower costs and complications.

From Extended to Minor Resections: Evolution in the Approach to CD

In the past, CD surgery entailed resection of all diseased segments and the creation of anastomosis on the healthy tissue. Major intestinal resections were then carried out, all with a radical intent. At the beginning of the 1980s, Krause, reporting results achieved in a retrospective study with a long follow-up in which he compared minor and extended resections [19], stated that it was necessary to extend resection margins up to 10–20 cm from the margins of the diseased segment. In time, though, it became obvious that this principle was not only wrong, because the rate of CD relapses was not at all influenced by extension of the resection, but it exposed patients to a high risk of malabsorption comparable with short-bowel syndrome.

The first data proving how inappropriate wide resections were came from a study showing that the presence of disease at the resection margins (macroscopically healthy) did not affect the rate of relapse [20]. Another study proved that the use of intraoperative frozen section did not allow reduction of resection extension [21]. In 1996, Fazio published a prospective randomised study with a good sample where he compared patients operated with resection performed 2 or 12 cm from the apparently healthy margin [22]. In this study, the main outcome was defined as the need to perform surgery again. The results (median follow-up 56 months) showed a rate of relapse not statistically significant between the two groups (25% in the group with a 2-cm margin, 18% in the group with a 12-cm margin). This work definitively proved how the approach toward minor resections, with margins a few centimetres from the diseased segment, is the appropriate one.

What are the indications for resective surgery? Using Wien's classification [23], Poggioli [24] suggests that, schematically, penetrating manifestations are likely to undergo resective surgery whereas fibrostenotic manifestations (with the exception of that involving the terminal ileum) are an indication for stricturoplasty only in the case of a non-active disease. This division, even if partly overcome by Poggioli himself (as we will see when addressing stricturoplasty), is a good starting point. Fistulous tracts certainly are a high risk for non-resective surgery. Resections in this case must be minor. It must be remembered that resective surgery and stricturoplasty can and must integrate with each other. The presence of localised areas of peritonitis away from other injuries susceptible of stricturoplasty seems to be not an absolute contraindication even if there is still an agreement yet. They certainly are difficult situations, however, in which there is no consensus as yet and the surgeon's expertise is essential. Other rather difficult cases are active and diffused diseases, which are always difficult to approach. From the surgeon's point of view, wide resections give greater safety in comparison with stricturoplasty on inflammatory tissues; however, we must take into account the problems connected with absorption. In these patients, considering the inflammatory processes, absorption ability is not exclusively connected with the length of intestine left but also with the structural and functional features.

"Classic" CD, terminal ileitis, has always represented the most common indication for a resection, especially in the case of initial manifestation of the disease. This operation can be mostly performed with laparoscopy.

In literature, there are several studies comparing the results of end-to-end or end-to-side anastomosis or comparing the methodology for performing the anastomosis (either conventional or stapled). The theoretic premise was the hypothesis that the cul-de-sac ensuing from an end-to-side anastomosis could make relapse of the disease easier. The results obtained were not univocal [25–27].

Our experience suggests that anastomosis must be wide and tension free. We believe that the best alternatives are the conventional sutured end-to-end anastomosis with a longitudinal excision along the antimesenteric margin of the ileum (to allow enlargement plasty) (Fig. 1) or the use of a stapled functional end-to-end anastomosis.

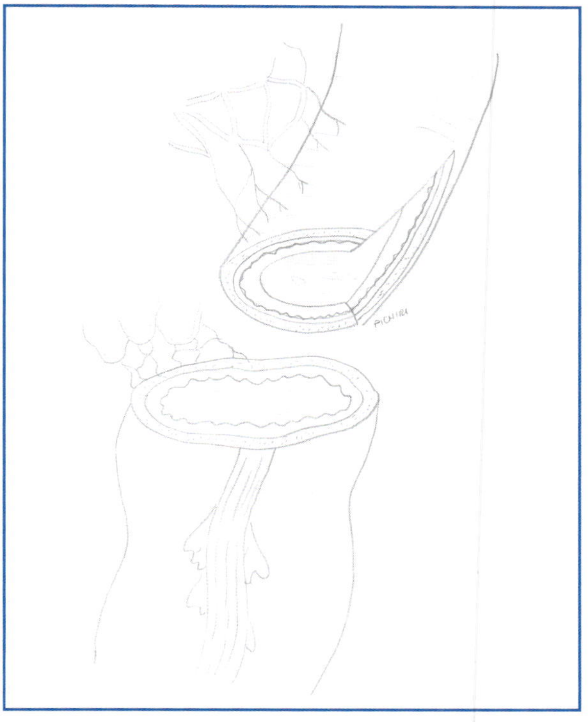

Fig. 1. Ileo-colic anastomosis with single layer suture

Laparoscopic Approach

As we will explain in another chapter, the use of the laparoscopic approach in CD surgery seems to be very convenient, both for its minor surgical impact and for reduction in hospitalisation time. After laparoscopic techniques spread and technical skill increased, surgeons could not only create diverting ileostomies but also ileal or ileocolic resections. In the literature, results of the laparoscopic approach is controversial, but it seems to reduce hospitalisation, morbility, and the need for analgesics, as pointed out in a recent study regarding open versus laparoscopic resections [28]. However, we must report the experience of Kehlet the pioneer of "fast-track surgery". In a recent work [29], he reported excellent results in 29 consecutive patients operated for CD. Using a multimodal approach (peridural anaesthesia, early mobilisation, alimentation), the average postoperative hospitalisation was 3 days and complications were extremely low. In the light of this experience, we must once more emphasise the importance of appropriate and intensive management of the patient during the perioperative stage.

Stricturoplasties: Indications and Results

Stricturoplasties certainly constituted a basic turning point for the surgical treatment of CD strictures. They allow correction of the occlusion of the tract, preserving the intestinal tissue without reducing (or at least only partly reducing) the absorption surface. In a recent and comprehensive review, Roy and Kumar [30] conducted a meta-analysis on the studies that appeared in the literature addressing both indications and results. As already described in the previous paragraph, the indications accepted in the literature regarding the use of stricturoplasties are: multiple serrated stenoses, stenosis in absence of an active disease (especially in the presence of former extensive resections or short-bowel syndrome), a disease with a fast relapse and occlusive syndromes and treatment of anastomotic stenoses already created during resections. A clear contraindication to stricturoplasty is the presence of active disease. The risk of fistulisation appears to be high, with very dangerous consequences for the patient. In a recent study, the same authors [31] published a retrospective work reporting the results achieved with 14 patients (73 stricturoplasties) with active CD (disease activity was both histologically and clinically defined). The perioperative complication rate due to the procedure was limited (one fistula needing a second surgery). These results, even if positive, must be carefully evaluated. They certainly need further confirmation, due not only to the kind of study (retrospective) but also to the poor number of samples. However, they certainly constitute an essential point for further studies. Other contraindications reported in this meta-analysis were the very poor general condition of the patients (serum albumin <2g/dl), tension on closure of strictureplasty and a segment requiring resection before a stricture suitable for plasty. The presence of fistulae or abscesses near the stenosis is another contraindication.

The treatment of the terminal ileitis (especially as first manifestation) is still at issue. While some authors, such as Poggioli [32], propose the use of stricturoplasty in this case as well, no agreement has been reached. Moreover, as already written, if it is performed in a few excellent centres, the laparoscopic approach may reduce hospitalisation periods and morbity of this operation, even if not all authors agree on this fact.

Roy and Kuman [31] analysed long-term results of stricturoplasties reported by seven studies published since 2000 (a total of 461 patients with an average follow-up of 68.8 months) comparing them with Tichansky's review published that same year [33]. Results of these meta-analyses are comparable, with a rate of reoperations after 5 years of about 26% and an overall perioperative complication incidence of 11% (slightly reduced in comparison with 13% reported by Tichansky). In the light of these data, it is clear that, even if it is not without complications, stricturoplasty in selected patients suffering from CD is a very good therapeutical option.

The use of long stricturoplasties has always been surrounded by skepticism because of the likely complications and of a hypothetical risk of stenosis or major disease relapse. In a recent work, Shatari [34] compared long-term results between long and short stricturoplasties, showing the former to give very good functional results over time, with complications and relapse rates absolutely similar with those of short stricturoplasties.

Stricturoplasties: Notes on Surgical Technique

The first description of the use of stricturoplasty dates back to 1977 when Katariya, an Indian surgeon, published its use for the treatment of multiple tubercular stenoses in a series of nine patients [35]. In 1982, Lee and Papaioannou published the first results about the use of the stricturoplasty technique in nine patients with CD [36]. Since then, many techniques were proposed on how to perform stricturoplasties.

Surgical technique for this kind of operation must be very strict. After laparotomy and accurate lysis of any adhesions, the entire small bowel must be explored for stenoses. Observation and palpation allow detection of stenotic tracts. The presence of more stenoses may be assessed after doing an enterotomy on the already identified stricture by introducing the index finger into the lumen and passing the gut over the finger in a concertina fashion or by the pull-through technique using an 18-Fr Foley catheter [30]. Exploration must, obviously, reach the duodenum proximally and the ileocecal valve distally. Besides the stenoses site, it is essential to evaluate its extension and any coexistence of fistulous tracts. Even if indications for some of these techniques are similar, many have their technical limitation in the length of the stenoses. Regardless of the kind of stricturoplasty, it is important to have a precise technique. Tissues of the diseased segments are thickened, inflamed and oedematous whereas the mesentery may be retracted. The loops must not be under tension, especially after long plasties. Moreover, control of bowel vascularisation before longitudinal incision is essential to avoid ischaemia with an inevitable dehiscence and consequent fistula. It is very delicate surgery requiring expert and dedicated surgeons in reference centres.

Heineke-Mikulicz stricturoplasty: this technique was originally used to treat hypertrophic stenosis of the pylorus [37]. It allows treatment of small stenotic tracts (8–10 cm). After the insertion of a stay suture, the antimesenteric side of the bowel is opened along the structure, and the longitudinal incision is transversely closed using seromuscular interrupted absorbable sutures (Fig. 2).

Finney stricturoplasy: this technique allows treatment of longer stenoses (from 10 to 20 cm). The antimesenteric side of the bowel is longitudinally opened along the structure and bent into a U shape. The posterior wall is first closed by a continuos, full thickness, running suture, as is the anterior one (Fig. 3).

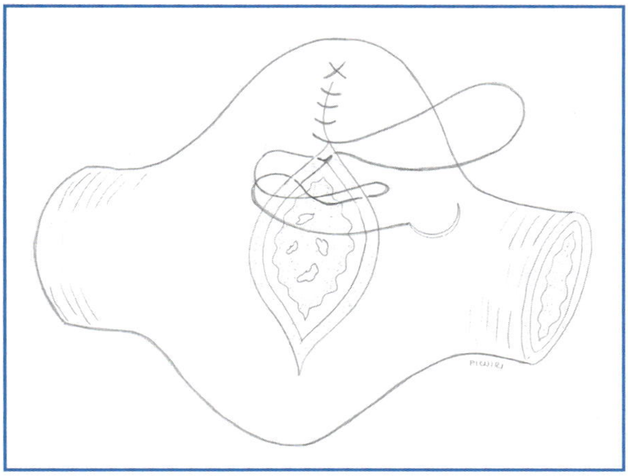

Fig. 2. Heineke-Mikulicz stricturoplasty

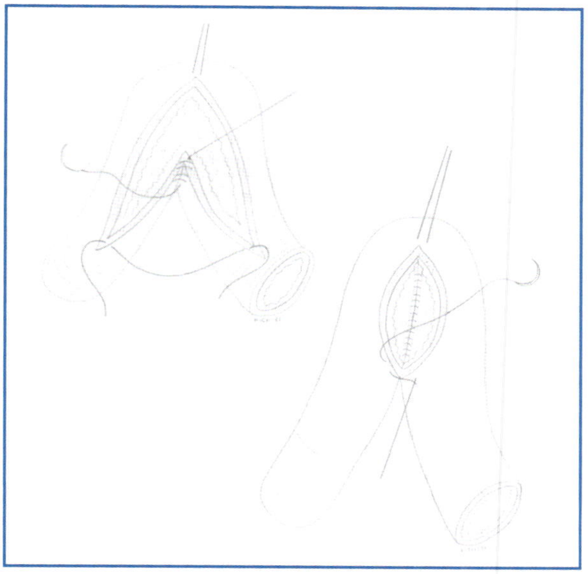

Fig. 3. Finney stricturoplasty

Fazio technique: Fazio and Tjandra [38] developed a method to treat two closed strictures by mixing the two techniques described above. Both strictures are opened with a long incision and then closed in a Heineke-Mikulicz fashion.

Michelassi technique: this is a side-to-side isoperistaltic stricturoplasty [39], which can be used to treat long strictures. It is performed by transecting the diseased segment and its mesentery at the midpoint and longitudinally opening and then suturing the proximal loop over the distal one by an interrupted or running suture. In the first description, this methodology allowed treatment of strictures up to 90 cm long in three patients with severe jejunal-ileal disease (Fig. 4).

Poggioli technique: this is a side-to-side, disease-to-disease-free anastomosis [40]. The first step involves division of the bowel and its mesentery at the beginning of the stricture. Then, the diseased segment is opened in order to be anastomise it to the proximal normal small bowel.

The literature describes many variations of the above techniques, such as the plasties according to Jaboulary, Judd, Moskel-Walske-Neuman [30] and that recently proposed by Sasaki for reconstruction following intestinal resection [41]. Every surgeon dealing with inflammatory intestinal diseases must know these techniques as well; Tichansky [32] pointed out, in a meta-analysis that stricturoplasty according to Heineke-Mikulicz is surely the most used (85%), followed by Finney's (13%). We must emphasise that this meta-analysis refers to a historical sam-

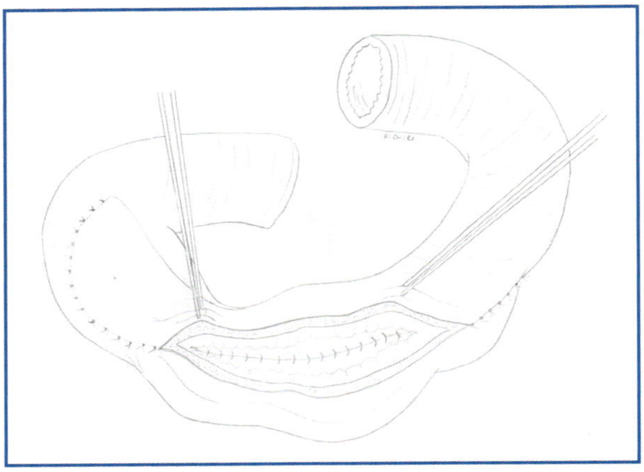

Fig. 4. Michelassi technique

ple and that, in the past, "long" plasties were not yet validated for this; even if they were already known and used [42], they had little approval.

Recently, the indication for conservative treatment extended to the treatment of terminal ileitis. Poggioli proposed a "side-to-side entero-colic anastomosis [32]", contemplating the section of the terminal loop, of the ileocecal valve and the colon along the tenia and a Finney-fashion suture. Taschieri [43] described an analogous technique to be applied in the case of important narrowing of the ileocecal valve requiring resection of the cecum and the ileocolic junction. The anastomosis is between the ileum and the right colon.

Cancer and Stricturoplasties

Appearance in the literature of reports about neoplasia in the site of a previous stricturoplasty was reason for concern [44–46]. From a theoretical point of view, the fact that an area with chronic inflammation remains in site can cause the development of neoplastic degeneration. Scarcity of patients who developed this complication (in comparison with the thousands of stricturoplasties performed with follow-up now over 5 years but that in some cases refer to patients operated even 20 years ago), must be comforting. Moreover, as pointed out by several studies, CD in and of itself is associated with an increased risk of neoplastic degeneration of the small bowel [relative risk: 15.6 (95% CI: 4.2–40.6) according to Persson [47]; 66.7 (95% CI: 18.1–170.7) according to Jess [48] and probably of the colon as well, even if data in this case are not univocal [11].

Gastroduodenal CD

Mottet [49], in a recent study, shows the presence of CD at a gastroduodenal level is rather common in patients suffering from CD of other areas of the small bowel. In cases such as this, lesions ascribable to CD may be found in 20% of patients after endoscopic examination and in 40% in biopsies. On the contrary, the presence of gastroduodenal CD as a single manifestation is very rare. Yamamoto [50], indeed, found that 96% of patients suffering from gastrointestinal CD present a second site of the disease at the intestinal level. However, fewer than 4% of patients show symptoms and signs that may be clinically detectable. Surgical treatment applied in the past in the case of stenosis was the bypass procedure (usually gastrojejunostomy) generally associated with a vagotomy to prevent ulcer. Long-term results for this procedure are excellent, as shown by two works with rather long follow-ups (average 12.3 years for Murray [51]; 11 years for Nugent [52]). Resection, on the contrary, showed its limits, which were connected with a high rate of major surgical complications (up to 78% according to Murray [53]).

New pharmacologic therapies have considerably changed the fate of many patients, given the good responses achieved. The few cases still needing surgery have also been treated with stricturoplasties, which is a procedure also recognised by many surgeons in the case of stenoses from duodenal CD [54–56]. Worsey [57] pointed out the advantages of this approach, which does not require vagotomy, mobilisation or use of the jejunum and, especially, creation of a blind loop. Long-term results of this kind of procedure are not yet known, especially considering, as observed by Hirata [58], the poor number of surgeries performed in each centre. Longer follow-ups and a larger sample population are required before definitive conclusions are available.

Another therapeutical option that may be used is endoscopic balloon dilatation, even if experience is still very limited [49].

The Future: Will Genetics Indicate the Appropriate Therapy?

As already described, CD manifestations may be subdivided into two main categories: penetrating Crohn's disease and non-penetrating or fibrostenotic Crohn's disease [23]. This subdivision, now formalised, was known and reported in many works [59], even if it was not univocally accepted [60]. What is interesting is that the manifestations of the disease tend not to change, even in the case of postsurgical relapse.

A recent study finally correlated the clinical manifestation with a genetic substratum (the stenosing form with the *Nod2/CARD15* gene). The future might enable subdivision of CD not on the basis of clinical manifestations but on the basis of genetic features. Clinical–therapeutical implications are, theoretically, very interesting because they would allow both medical and surgical tailored therapy on the basis of the patient's individual features in an attempt to verify which groups may achieve better results from a particular determined therapeutical approach.

Disease Recurrence and Postoperative Maintenance Therapy

Even though this subject will be described in more detail in another chapter, it is necessary to address it here. It must be made clear that disease recovery from a histological point of view does not automatically coincide with development of a symptomatology, which may be clinically detectable. If the former was found in over 85% of patients after 3 years, the latter may be detected in only 34% of patients [61]. Regardless, it is always appropriate to assess with the gastroenterologist the most suitable maintenance therapy for the patient and to include him or her in the follow-up programme.

Conclusions

Treatment of chronic intestinal inflammatory diseases, CD in particular, requires from disease onset a multidisciplinary approach involving pathologist, gastroenterologist, nutritionist, radiologist, surgeon and psychologist. Availability of increasingly efficient medical therapies has made it possible to take a pharmacological approach giving good results. However, due to this approach, surgeons tend to see more patients who are considerably weakened from a general and psychological point of view. Extensive use of mini-invasive techniques (laparoscopic approach, stricturoplasties or minor resections), have reduced mortality and morbility associated with surgical procedures. Even recognising the high rate of disease relapses after surgery, the appropriate surgical timing may allow the patient a better life style and a more appropriate use of the pharmacologic therapy with a better response. If treatment of complications falls clearly into the surgeon's area of competence, this therapeutic option can be used not only in "extreme" conditions but, more appropriately, in the case of poor response to medical therapy. Close cooperation among the various professional figures is increasingly important in order to assess the various therapeutical options and offer each patient tailored therapy and a high degree of professionalism, which may be assured only by referenced centres with a high number of cases treated.

References

1. Crohn BB, Ginzburg L, Oppenheimer GD (1932) Regional ileitis: a pathologic and clinical entity. JAMA 99:1323–1329
2. Binder V, Both H, Hansen PK et al (1978) Incidence and prevalence of ulcerative colitis and Crohn's disease in the country of Copenhagen 1962 to 1978. Gastroenterology 83:563–568
3. Penner R, Madsen K, Fedorak R (2005) Postoperative Crohn's disease. Inflamm Bowel Dis 11:765–777
4. Dziki A, Galbfach P (2004) Crohn's disease – when to operate? Acta Chir Iugosl 51:61–68
5. Sands BE, Arsenault JE, Rosen MJ et al (2003) Risk of early surgery for Crohn's disease: implications for early treatment strategies. Am J Gastroenterol 98:2712–2718
6. Mendoza JL, Garcia-Paredes J, Cruz Santamaria DM et al (2002) Infliximab treatment and prognostic factors for response in patients with Crohn's disease. Rev Esp Enferm Dig 94:269–279
7. Sandborn WJ, Targan SR (2002) Biologic therapy of inflammatory bowel disease. Gastroenterology 122:1592–1608
8. Krolak C, Rock C, Reiser M (2003) Radiological interventions in inflammatory bowel disease. Radiologe 43:59–65, 96
9. Delaney CP, Kiran RP, Senagore AJ et al (2003) Quality of life improves within 30 days of surgery for Crohn's disease. J Am Coll Surg 196:714–721
10. Sharif H, Alexander-Williams J (1992) The role of stricturoplasty in Crohn's disease. Int Surg 77:15–18
11. Wolters FL, Russel MG, Stockbrugger RW (2004) Systematic review: has disease outcome in Crohn's disease changed during the last four decades? Aliment Pharmacol Ther 20:483–496
12. Fazio VW (1990) Crohn's disease or the small bowel. Operative tactics and technique. Hepatogastroenterology 37:56–62
13. Hulten L (1992) Surgical management and strategy in classical Crohn's disease. Int Surg 77:2–8
14. Scotiniotis I, Rubensin SE, Ginsberg GG (1999) Imaging modalities in inflammatory bowel disease. Gastroenterol Clin North Am 28:391–421
15. Levine MS, Rubensin SE, Laufer I (2002) Barium studies. Gastrointest Endosc 55:S16–S24
16. Koh DM, Miao Y, Chinn RJ (2001) MR imaging evaluation of the activity of Crohn's disease. AJR Am J Roentgenol 177:1325–1332
17. McLeod RS, Lavery IC, Leatherman JR (1986) Factors affecting quality of life with a conventional ileostomy. World J Surg 10:474–480
18. Post S, Herfarth C, Schumacher H et al (1995) Experience with ileostomy and colostomy in Crohn's disease. Br J Surg 82:1629–1633
19. Krause U, Ejerblad S, Bergman L (1985) Crohn's dis-

ease: a long-term study of clinical course in 186 patients. Scand J Gastroenterol 20:516–524
20. Heuman R, Boeryd B, Bolin T, Sjodahl R (1983) The influence of disease at the margin of resection on the outcome of Crohn's disease. Br J Surg 70:519–521
21. Le Blanc I, Teniere P, Bokobza B et al (1990) Resections intestinales pour maladies de Crohn. Facteures predictifs de recedive postoperatoire precoce Lyon. Chir 86:226–228
22. Fazio VW, Marchetti F, Church J et al (1996) Effect of resection margins on the recurrence of Crohn's disease in small bowel. Ann Surg 224:563–573
23. Gasche C (2000) A simple classification of Crohn's disease: report of the Working Party for the World Congress of Gastroenterology, Vienna 1998. Inflamm Bowel Dis 6:8–15
24. Poggioli G, Pierangeli F, Laureti S, Ugolini, F (2002) Review article: indication and type of surgery in Crohn's disease. Aliment Pharmacol Ther 16(Suppl 4):59–64
25. Munoz-Juarez M, Yamamoto T, Wolff BG, Keighley MR (2001) Wide-lumen stapled anastomosis vs conventional end-to-end anastomosis in the treatment of Crohn's disease. Dis Colon Rectum 44:20–25
26. Scott NA, Sue-Ling HM, Hughes L E (1995) Anastomotic configuration does not affect recurrence of Crohn's disease after ileocolonic resection. Int J Colorectal Dis 10:67–69
27. Moskovicz D, McLeod RS, Greenberg GR, Cohen R (1999) Operative and environment risk factors for recurrence of Crohn's disease. Int J Colorectal Dis 14:224–226
28. Lauro A, Hamel C, Cirocchi R et al (2004) Laparoscopic treatment for Crohn's disease. Minerva Chir 59:537–545
29. Andersen J, Kehlet H (2005) Fast track open ileo-colic resections for Crohn's disease. Colorectal Dis 7:394–397
30. Roy P, Kumar D (2004) Strictureplasty. Br J Surg 91:1428–1437
31. Roy P, Kumar D (2005) Strictureplasty for active Crohn's disease. Int J Colorectal Dis 30:1–6
32. Poggioli G, Stocchi L, Laureti S et al (1997) Conservative surgical management of terminal ileitis: side to side enterocolic anastomosis. Dis Colon Rectum 40:234–237
33. Tichansky D, Cagi B, Yoo E et al (2000) Strictureplasty for Crohn disease: meta-analysis. Dis Colon Rectum 43:911–919
34. Shatari T, Clark MA, Yamamoto T et al (2003) Long strictureplasty is a safe and effective as short strictureplasty in small bowel Crohn's disease. Curr Opin Gastroenterol 6:438–441
35. Katariya RN, Sood S, Rao PL (1977) Stricture-plasty for tubercular strictures of gastrointestinal tract. Br J Surg 64:496–498
36. Lee EC, Papaioannou N (1982) Minimal surgery for chronic obstruction in patients with extensive or universal Crohn's disease. Ann R Coll Surg Engl 64:229–233
37. Mikulicz J (1888) Zur operativen Behandlung des stenosirenden Magengeschwures, Arch Klin Chir 37:79
38. Fazio VW, Tjandra JJ (1993) Strictureplasty for Crohn's disease with multiple long strictures. Dis Colon Rectum 36:71–72
39. Michelassi F (1996) Side-to-side isoperistaltic strictureplasty for multiple Crohn's disease. Dis Colon Rectum 40:342–344
40. Poggioli G, Laureti S, Pierangeli F (2003) A new model of stricturoplasty for multiple and long stenoses in Crohn's ileitis: side-to-side diseased to disease-free anastomosis. Dis Colon Rectum 46:127–130
41. Sasaki I, Shibata C, Funayama Y et al (2004) New reconstructive procedure after intestinal resection for Crohn's disease: modified side to side isoperistaltic anastomosis with double Heineke-Mikulicz procedure. Dis Colon Rectum 47:940–943
42. Alexander-Williams J, Fornaro M (1982) Strictureplasty in Crohn's disease. Chirurg 53:799–801
43. Taschieri A, Cristaldi M, Elli M et al (1997) Description of new "bowel-sparing" techniques for long strictures of Crohn's disease. Am J Surg 173:509–512
44. Marchetti F, Fazio VW, Ozuner G (1996) Adenocarcinoma arising from a strictureplasty site in Crohn's disease. Report of a case. Dis Colon Rectum 39:1315–1321
45. Jaskowiak NT, Michelassi F (2001) Adenocarcinoma at strictureplasty site in Crohn's disease: report of a case. Dis Colon Rectum 44:284–287
46. Ribeiro MB, Greenstein AJ, Heimann T et al (1991) Adenocarcinoma of the small intestine in Crohn's disease. Surg Gynecol Obstet 173:343–349
47. Persson PG, Karlen P, Bernell O (1994) Crohn's disease and cancer: a population based study. Gastroenterology 107:1675–1679
48. Jess T, Winther KV, Munkholm P et al (2004) Intestinal and extraintestinal Cancer in Crohn's disease: follow-up of a population-based cohort in Copenhagen County, Denmark. Aliment Pharmacol Ther 19:287–293
49. Mottet C, Juillerat P, Gonvers JJ et al (2005) Treatment of gastroduodenal Crohn's disease. Digestion 71:37–40
50. Yamamoto T, Allan RN, Keighley MR (1999) An audit of gastroduodenal Crohn's disease: clinicopathologic features and management. Scand J Gastroenterol 34:1019–1024
51. Murray JJ, Schoetz DJ Jr, Nugent FW et al (1984) Surgical management of Crohn's disease involving the duodenum. Am J Surg 147:58–65
52. Nugent FW, Roy MA (1989) Duodenal Crohn's disease: an analysis of 89 cases. Am J Gastroenterol 84:249–254
53. Murray JJ, Schoetz DJ Jr, Nugent FW et al (1984) Surgical management of Crohn's disease involving the duodenum. Am J Surg 147:58–65
54. Yamamoto T, Allan RN, Keighley MR (1999) An audit of gastroduodenal Crohn disease: clinicopathologic features and management. Scand J Gastroenterol 34:1019–1024
55. Poggioli G, Stocchi L, Laureti S et al (1997) Duodenal involvement of Crohn's disease Three different clinicopathologic features and management. Dis Colon Rectum 40:179–183
56. Takesue Y, Yokoyama T, Akagi S, Ohge H et al (2000) Strictureplasty for short duodenal stenosis in Crohn's disease Gastroenterology 35:929–932
57. Worsey MJ, Hull TL, Ryland L, Fazio VW (1999) Strictuloplasty is an effective option in the operative man-

agement of duodenal Crohn's disease. Dis Colon Rectum 42:596–600
58. Hirata K (2000) Is strictureplasty a safe and efficacious procedure for duodenal Crohn's disease? J Gastroenterol 35:953–954
59. Greenstein AJ, Lachman P, Sachar DB et al (1988) Perforating and non-perforating indications for repeated operations in Crohn's disease: evidence for two clinical forms. Gut 29:588–592
60. McDonald PJ, Fazio VW, Farmer RG et al (1989) Perforating and nonperforating Crohn's disease An unpredictable guide to recurrence after surgery. Dis Colon Rectum 32:117–120
61. Rutgeerts P, Geboes K, Vantrappen G et al (1990) Predictability of the postoperative course of Crohn's disease. Gastroenterology 99:956–963

Crohn's Disease of the Colon

Adam Dziki

Introduction

Crohn's disease is most frequently found in the terminal section of the small intestine, however in half of the cases, the disease affects both the small and large bowel. Pathological changes limited exclusively to the large bowel can be seen in approximately 25% of cases. We also have to remember that among patients operated on for indeterminate colitis, in almost 40% of cases the diagnosis of Crohn's disease (CD) is made postoperatively [1]. Despite the fact that Crohn's disease affects mostly the small bowel, there is a high risk of large-bowel involvement.

Symptoms

The symptoms of Crohn's disease largely depend on the intensity and localisation of the pathological changes in the GI tract. In the case of small-bowel involvement, the symptoms of malabsorption predominate along with diarrhoea, abdominal pain, loss of appetite, decrease in body mass and compromised growth in children. Bloody, mucous diarrhoea, crampy abdominal pain and faecal urgency are more characteristic for large-bowel CD [2]. Because of the variety of possible symptoms including chronic or night diarrhoea, abdominal pain, ileus, body mass loss and fever, patients at risk of Crohn's disease can present with any of those or a combination of them [3]. Cramping, intermittent abdominal pain frequently is a predominant symptom of the disease. With the progress of the disease it turns into permanent, dull pain of the abdomen. Diarrhoea occurs in 85% of patients [4].

Some patients with Crohn's disease present with extra-intestinal symptoms that may appear right at the beginning or in more advanced stages of the disease. Some 25% of patients complain of pain in the joints or develop osteoarthritis. Dermal involvement can be seen in 15% of patients who may suffer from erythema nodosum, pyoderma gangrenosum and aphthous changes in the oral cavity. Ocular symptoms develop in 5% of patients and include scleritis, choroiditis and recurring iritis [3].

Diagnosis

Diagnosis of CD is complex and has to be based on the careful evaluation of clinical symptoms as well as laboratory testing, radiological studies, endoscopy and histological evaluation of mucosa biopsies. It is important to remember that there is no laboratory finding which would be characteristic for the disease; in some cases, however, anaemia and leukocytosis with decreased concentration of serum proteins and albumins may lead to such a suspicion. The mainstream diagnosis is colonoscopy. Segmental inflammatory changes, irregular ulcerations of the mucosa surrounded by swollen, protruded or normal mucosa are typical. Pathological changes in the small bowel can be seen in X-ray examinations. Contrast studies show segmental stenosis, linear ulcerations and fistulae. Radiological studies can also have some value in diagnosis of the ascending colon involvement but are less specific in evaluation of the rectal changes. CT scans aid in identification of intra-abdominal abscess and other complications of the disease.

Differential Diagnosis

Crohn's disease has to be differentiated from [4, 5]:

1. Appendicitis
2. Small-intestine obstruction
3. Ulcerative colitis
4. Irritable-bowel syndrome
5. Malabsorption syndrome
6. Infective enteritis
7. Ischemic enteritis
8. Colorectal carcinoma
9. Diverticulosis of the intestine
10. Haemorrhoids
11. Postradiation inflammation of the large intestine
12. Anal fissure
13. Solitary rectal ulcer

Conservative Treatment of Crohn's Disease

Despite advances in medical sciences, the etiopathogenesis of Crohn's disease is still unknown; therefore, there is no effective causative treatment.

Pharmacological Treatment

Salicylates (5 ASA)

Non-steroid anti-inflammatory drugs (NSAID) have been used for over 50 years in the treatment of Crohn's disease and still are the mainstream of the conservative treatment. Sulphasalazine is a combination of 5-aminosalicylic acid (5-ASA) and sulfapyridine. 5-ASA has strong anti-inflammatory properties; it decreases synthesis of inflammatory mediators including leukotriens (LT4), prostaglandins and PAF. Sulphasalazine is indicated for mild to moderate forms of CD and also in cases with large-bowel involvement. Active inflammatory changes in the small bowel and right colon respond better to mesalazine, which is characterised by the delayed release of the active drug right in the small intestine. National Cooperative Crohn's Disease Study (1979) showed the effectiveness of sulphasalazine in doses of 1 g/15 kg/day in patients with a colonic type of the disease. Regression of symptoms was observed in 38% of patients, while in the placebo group this was only true for 20% [6]. The effectiveness of 5-ASA in the treatment of active CD was further documented in the nineties with a dose of >4.5 g/day and sustaining remission, with a dose of >2.0 g/day [7]. One of the side effects of the sulphasalazine treatment is impaired absorption of the folic acid; therefore, its supplementation is indicated during the therapy. Mesalazine has less, and milder side effects.

Glucocorticoids

Glucocorticoids have anti-inflammatory, anti-effusive, and anti-allergic properties. They decrease the effects of early inflammation including mediator release and leukocyte migration and later fibroblast activation. They also decrease histamine release [8].

Prednisone, prednisolone and methylprednisolone are most frequently used orally for 3–6 weeks for exacerbations of mild and moderate CD, and then the dose is decreased for 2–3 months. Severe cases of the disease require intravenous steroids application with hydrocortisone or methylprednisolone being the most frequently used. An NCCDS study showed that prednisone treatment in a dose of 0.25–0.75 mg/kg/day was effective in 60% of patients compared to 20% in a placebo group [6]. Eighty-two percent effectiveness of methylprednisolone in a dose of 48 mg/kg in severe cases and 8 mg/kg in maintenance treatment was described in the European study ECCDS. It confirmed glucocorticoid induced remission of the active CD from 60 to 80% [9]. In patients with pathological changes located in ileal and ileocecal regions, oral budesonide at a dose of 9 mg/day is recommended. Comparative studies of 9 mg/day of budesonide and 40 mg/day of prednisolone showed similar effectiveness of both drugs at 53 and 66% respectively, with fewer side effects from budesonide [10]. Thomson's comparative study of 2x2 g/day of mesalazine and 9 g/day of budesonide in mild and moderate CD, showed higher effectiveness of budesonide in decreasing symptoms of the active disease along with improved quality of life in that group [11]. With a steroid treatment, approximately 20–36% of patients develop steroid dependency and thus require constant steroid dosage while approximately 20% develop steroid resistance.

Immunosuppressive Treatment

Immunosuppressive drugs are not the first line of treatment and usually are used in patients who cannot be treated with steroids.

Purine Analogues (Azathioprine and 6-Mercaptopurine)

Purine analogues are indicated in fistulae, severe perianal changes, extensive pathological changes of the small and large intestine not responsive to other drugs and when there is a necessity to decrease the dosage of steroids.

A basic effect of purine analogues is a decrease in cellular cell response [8]. The effects of these drugs can be seen after 3–6 months of therapy; therefore, they are mainly used as a supportive treatment. They can be beneficial in fistula healing and decrease the need for glucocorticoids use. Suggested dosage of azathioprine is from 2 to 2.5 mg/kg/day, 6-mercaptopurine is from 1 to 1.5 mg/kg/day.

Azathioprine was effective in 67% of patients compared to 8% in the placebo group, it was successful in fistula closing in 31% of patients vs. 6% in the control group, and led to a decrease of steroid dosage in 75% of patients (32% in the placebo group) [12].

Methotrexate

Methotrexate is an immunosuppressive and antitumour drug. It helps in decreasing the dose or stopping steroid treatment. The drug is not widely used in therapy [8]. Indications are steroid dependency, active disease resistant to other treatment. Dosage: 25 mg/week in active disease, 15 mg/week in supporting treatment.

Cyclosporine A

Cyclosporine has effect mostly on lymphocytes, decreasing T-lymphocyte activity as well as decreasing lymphokine synthesis [8]. Cyclosporine A is indicated in when purine analogue treatment is not sufficient. The only study which showed effectiveness of cyclosporine A in the treatment of active CD was that of Brynskov's, which described remission in 59% of patients treated with cyclosporine vs. 38% of patients in the placebo group. Decreasing the dose of a drug and its use as a supportive treatment did not result in further improvement [13]. Another study showed direct short-term improvement in 85% of patients with intestinal fistula and a long term effect of treatment in 54% of patients [14].

Antibiotics and Chemotherapeutics

Antibiotics are not routinely used in the treatment of CD with the exception of ciprofloxacin (1 g/day dose) as a monotherapy drug or in combination with metronidazole (20 mg/kg/day), although it does have some beneficial effect in perianal changes.

Biological Treatment

Biological treatment includes antibodies, receptors, inhibitors or parts of nucleic acids which decrease the concentration of pro-inflammatory agents in the organism as well as anti-inflammatory cytokines. Infliximab is the most commonly used. It is a chimeric monoclonic antibody against tumour necrosis factor alpha (TNF-alpha, major proinflammatory cytokine). Infliximab binds TNF molecule, neutralises it and thus increases the activated T lymphocytes apoptosis [8]. Infliximab is indicated in the active severe course of disease which does not respond to other types of treatment; in non-healing fistulae and in extra-intestinal complications (skin, eyes, joints).

Patients with active disease without fistula formation should be administered a single, 2-h intravenous infusion of infliximab at a dose of 5 mg/kg. Patients with concomitant fistulae should get triple intravenous infusion (0, 2, 6 weeks) followed by the intravenous injection of 5 mg/kg every 8 weeks to sustain the effects of therapy. Side effects include increased risk for infection, especially of the respiratory tract including the activation of quiescent TB. Treatment should be preceded by chest X-ray, and TB tests [15].

There are a number of trials on the effectiveness and safety of infliximab treatment. One of the better ones is the prospective ACCENT (a Crohn's disease clinical trial evaluating infliximab in a new long-term treatment regimen). The study included CD patients from North America, Europe and Israel.

In the first phase of the trial, ACCENT I, 335 patients with active CD were enrolled and received the initial dose of infliximab (5 mg/kg/day). The results showed higher remission rates in groups receiving the consequent doses of infliximab at 2, 6 and every 8 weeks (5 mg/kg/day and 10 mg/kg/day respectively), but did not reach statistical significance between study groups. Steroids treatment however could have been stopped in both groups, and the disease-free time and time to surgical intervention was longer in both groups compared to placebo [16].

The second phase of the trial, ACCENT II, investigated the effects of infliximab in supportive treatment of patients with fistulous CD. Intravenous injections were performed every 8 weeks. After 14 weeks, almost two-thirds of the patients demonstrated significant improvement in fistula healing, and in the 54th week a complete closing of the fistula was demonstrated in 38% of patients receiving infliximab compared to 22% of patients in a control group. Patients of the study group experienced a longer positive effect of treatment lasting 40 weeks, while in the placebo group it was only 14 weeks. The trial also showed that patients undergoing supportive treatment are less likely to be hospitalised and have a lower chance for surgical intervention [17].

Symptomatic Treatment

Some of the most frequent symptoms include abdominal pain, diarrhoea, nausea and vomiting. Spasmolytic, analgesics, and anti-diarrhoeal drugs (anti-cholinergics and loperamide) can be used to control the symptoms. Conservative treatment is aimed to alleviate the symptoms, replace nutritional deficits, improve quality of life and postpone surgical intervention. The choice of treatment depends on the disease activity, location of pathological changes and complications. It has to be modified in accordance to the patient's clinical condition.

Non-Pharmacological Treatment

General and Dietary Advice

There are a few factors such as infection (upper respiratory and digestive tract), cigarette smoking and

NSAID intake, which can aggravate the symptoms of CD. The role of stress in the exacerbations of the disease symptoms has not been proven but most patients believe stress can be a factor. General recommendations therefore include elimination of stress, quitting smoking and avoiding other exacerbating factors.

There is no evidence of the impact of the diet on the development and course of CD; however, to the perception of most patients, some foods cause or worsen the symptoms of a disease. Elimination of milk and processed milk products from the diet is sometimes recommended. A CD patient's diet should be similar or identical to the general population. Diet modification can be tailored to the individual needs based on the disease symptoms. An interesting observation is that an increasing number of CD patients come from developed countries, which is related to the impact of environmental factors including diet. Dietary recommendations include frequent and small quantity meals 5–6 times per day, high calorie and diversified diet, fluid intake of 2–2.5 L/day, vitamin and microelement supplementation and elimination of alcohol and carbonated beverages.

Nutritional Therapy

Enteral and the parenteral nutrition are important and effective aspects of the therapy, especially concerning exacerbations and remission induction, malnutrition and complications of CD. Malnutrition is a common factor which affects 25–85% of hospitalised patients, and up to 23% of ambulatory patients. Malnutrition in CD is characterised by protein-caloric depletion as a result of loss of appetite, vomiting, bleeding, compromised digestion and absorption, diarrhoea, increased metabolism, and as a result of starvation as a commonly employed method of treatment at times of disease exacerbations [18]. Malnutrition leads to anaemia, hypoproteinemia, hypoalbuminemia and vitamin and microelement deficiency.

Total parenteral nutrition used to be a gold standard in the treatment of exacerbated CD. The Greenberg study showed no difference between the polymorphic diet and the total parenteral nutrition method. The authors concluded that the previously recommended "resting of the intestine" has no effect on remission induction [19]. The advantages of early enteric nutrition (tube, orally) are lower costs, less complications, positive impact on intestinal mucosa and an overall nourishment improvement. Early enteric nutrition can induce remission at a level comparable to steroid therapy.

Enteric nutrition is a first-line therapy in the nutritional treatment of CD. It should be started at 3–5 days from the onset of acute symptoms to eliminate malnutrition and malnutrition-associated complications as well as to aid steroid therapy.

Total parenteral nutrition must be reserved for patients who do not tolerate enteric feeding, who are cachectic or present with a kwashiorkor type of malnutrition after resection surgery, and in situations when enteric feeding is not efficient in satisfying calorie requirements [18].

Psychotherapy

Given that CD is incurable, affects mostly young people, has a high rate of recurrences and low effectiveness of conservative therapy with serious side effects and requires frequent hospitalisations and repeated surgeries, it is very important that patients remain under clinical psychological supervision.

Elective Procedures in Crohn's Disease of the Colon

Throughout their lifespan, 70–80% of patients suffering form CD require surgical intervention. In 10–15 years from the first surgery, approximately 40–50% of patients require the next operation due to recurrence [20, 21].

Elective surgical strategy for Crohn's disease of the colon is somehow different from the strategy for CD of the small intestine. Due to the role of the small intestine, surgical procedures must aim to minimise the risk of "short bowel" syndrome. The large bowel is mainly responsible for the fluid-electrolyte balance. Surgical procedure performed in colonic Crohn's disease should minimise the risk of recurrence and also improve the quality of the patient's life [22]. Symptoms of colonic Crohn's disease depend on the location and extensiveness of pathological changes. Right colon and ileocecal involvement with concomitant obstruction require surgery in 90% of cases. Crohn's disease affecting the left colon requires surgical procedure in 60% of patients, and usually occurs in older patients. However, only 30% of patients with rectal CD require operation.

More than a half of the patients with Crohn's disease located in the left colon and rectum will require a stoma, but their quality of life remains good during the rest of life. More than 70% of those patients live just like before the onset of the disease [23].

Indications for Surgery

The majority of patients with inflammatory changes limited to the right colon are subject to surgery due to obstruction, intra-abdominal abscesses, internal fistulae; and less frequently due to chronic increasing anaemia or bleeding from digestive tract [24]. When the descending or sigmoid colon is affected, symptoms are similar to diverticulitis with the subsequent obstruction and pericolonic abscess. Indications for elective surgery may also include stenosis after failure of endoscopic dilatation, persistent diarrhoea resistant to conservative treatment and bleeding [25]. According to the course of the disease indications for the operation can be divided into urgent and elective.

Indications for emergency surgery:

- Toxic colitis (toxic megacolon);
- Intestinal perforation;
- Peritoneal abscess;
- Extensive haemorrhage;
- Obstruction.

Types of surgical procedures performed in emergency cases:

- Colectomy with ileostomy;
- Restorative proctocolectomy;
- Segmental resection of the colon.

Despite the fact that colectomy with ileostomy is the most frequently performed type of procedure, restorative proctocolectomy finds increasingly more advocates. In a selected group of patients with no changes in the rectum, this type of surgery offers the chance of avoiding intestinal diversion. In severe stages of Crohn's disease, the risk of performing restorative proctocolectomy is very high with a complication rate reaching 56% of patients. Fisher et al. [22] reported that 64% of patients who have undergone restorative proctocolectomy had complications of a fistula, pouch stenosis and/or pelvic abscess. The same complications occurred only in 22% of patients with ulcerative colitis treated with this surgical modality. Pouch failure was reported in 56% of Crohn's disease patients, and was dramatically lower in a group of patients with ulcerative colitis, reaching only 6%. The major goal of the ileo-rectal anastomosis is to preserve the continuity of the physiological tract but may not be connected with the high risk of complications. Additionally results of the studies on the quality of life of patients who have undergone proctocolectomy with ileostomy show a good adaptation to a stoma [26]. In the case of large-bowel bleeding that cannot be managed with the use of endoscopy or in cases when pathological changes affect only a short part of the large bowel, segmental resection seems to be a good alternative to more extensive procedures. Colectomy with ileostomy remains the gold standard in surgical treatment of severe Crohn's disease of the large bowel.

Indications for elective surgical treatment of Crohn's disease of the large bowel:

- Surgical treatment of intestinal, intestinovesical, intestinovaginal, and intestinocutaneal fistulae
- Treatment of stenosis after endoscopic failure
- Disease refractory to medical management.

Options of Elective Surgery

Proctocolectomy with Ileostomy

This surgical procedure seems to be the procedure of choice in the cases of extensive pathological changes in the entire large bowel. Perioperative mortality ranges from 1.5 to 4%. The risk for recurrence in the small intestine ranges from 3 to 46%, and an important risk factor of recurrence is the time from the first operation. After one year, the chance of recurrence is 5% and rises to 20% after 20 years from surgery. In 90% of patients who have undergone proctocolectomy with ileostomy, the recurrence will localise in the terminal 25-cm segment of the ileum [22]. In a group of patients that have been treated with steroids and immunosuppressive drugs or in patients with a steroid resistant type of the disease, proctocolectomy with ileostomy may enable the withdrawal of those medications. This is a very important factor for women who are planning for pregnancy [22].

Restorative Proctocolectomy

Proctocolectomy with pouch is possible in selected group of patients with Crohn's disease. It is not appropriate to perform in cases of rectal, anal and small intestinal disease. If above excluding criteria are respected, it is possible to achieve satisfactory long-term results. It has to be remembered that complications may lead to the necessity of pouch excision and diversion. Mylonakis [29] reported that during 10.2 years of follow-up, 47% of patients experienced complications leading to the excision of the pouch. There is also a report of only 19% of complications in a selected group of patients with no pathological changes in rectum, and in distant part of ileum [30]. Despite that fact, restorative proctocolectomy is not a preferred type of surgery in patients with Crohn's disease.

Colectomy with Ileo-Rectal Anastomosis

In 25–50% of patients, pathological symptoms are limited to the colon, not affecting the rectum and/or perianal area. If a length of affected large bowel exceeds 20 cm, subtotal or total colectomy should be performed [22]. Colectomy with ileo-rectal anastomosis is considered to be the procedure of choice in patients with pathological changes widespread in the colon, but without any changes in the rectum. This method is especially suggested in the treatment of younger patients. It allows them to complete their education, start their career and family life without possible disturbances resulting from a stoma or perineal wound after proctocolectomy. Colectomy with ileo-rectal anastomosis is not recommended for patients with impaired sphincter muscles (e.g. after surgery) or with severe inflammation of the perianal area. In the case of coexisting inflammation in a distant part of the small intestine, the percentage of the recurrence may be high. Recurrences range from 34 to 58% after 5 years, and 49–83% after 10 years from the surgery. Well functioning ileo-rectal anastomosis after five years from the surgery has been reported in 74–88% of patients, and 10 years following surgery in 48–86% of patients. The procedure is connected with the risk of recurrence that requires resection after 10 years following the first procedure, and ranges from 37 to 74% in previously operated patients.

Segmental Resection of the Large Bowel

In some patients with Crohn's disease of the large bowel limited to isolated segments, a partial resection of the colon may be a reasonable solution. This method maintains the macroscopically unchanged segments of the colon and their activity regarding fluid-electrolyte balance, and also decreases the risk of episodes of gas and faecal incontinence in contrast to patients after colectomy with anastomosis. Following resection, the number of stools is approximately 2 per day, and the number of stools following colectomy with ileo-rectal anastomosis are 5 per day [32]. Segmental resection is a surgical procedure that can be allowed only in certain, selected groups of patients. Partial resection of the large bowel has a therapeutic value (low recurrence) in patients with the changes in the large bowel not exceeding 20 cm of bowel length. Patients avoid diversion, but unfortunately a risk of reoperation still exists. The risk of another resection involves 25–72% of patients. Longo et al. [33] reported that a risk of recurrence and repeated surgery corresponds to 62% of patients after 5 years following the initial surgery. A necessity of diversion in recurrences reaches only 14% of patients after a 14-year follow-up period. It the case of Crohn's disease limited to an isolated, proximal segment of large bowel, a partial resection may be a recommended surgical procedure due to a long-term disease-free and resection-free period. Numerous studies confirm the high safety of the method due to a low rate of complications [22, 23]. As a guideline for the choice of effective surgical treatment: location (right or left disease), extensiveness of the disease, patient's age, and a strength of a sphincter muscles should be considered.

How Much Bowel to Resect

Unlike in large-bowel involvement, in the case of Crohn's disease affecting the small intestine, surgical procedure is standardised. The role of surgery in CD is limited to the treatment of complications which do not respond to conservative therapy. In contrast to ulcerative colitis, CD is incurable. The high percentage of recurrences after surgery in this group is the reason for limitations in surgical procedures. The percentage of recurrences is estimated to be 55% during the 15-year period after the first surgical procedure [27]. Short-bowel syndrome is one of the most serious complications after surgery of CD with the localisation in the small intestine. Multiple laparotomies and intestinal resections result in a decrease of the total length of the small intestine. When the length of the intestine falls below 2 m, serious clinical problems appear. The introduction of new operating techniques—strictureplasty—has limited this complication considerably [34]. The strategy of surgical intervention in the treatment of complications of CD related to small intestine is clear—one should strive for the most sparing operation possible.

The fundamental question which should be asked before elective surgery relates to the possibility of preserving the continuity of the digestive tract, which mainly depends on the presence of rectal manifestations, the type of complication, location and duration of the disease as well as the general state of the patient [29]. The range of intervention options on the large bowel is not as limited as that of the small bowel. There is no risk of systemic disturbances even in vast resections of the colon. When changes affect short fragments of the large intestine, simple resection of the affected part of the intestine is an alternative to colectomy. This kind of intervention is less debilitating for the patient and the physiology of large intestine can also be kept. The limitation of this method is the high risk of recurrence, which is estimated at about 60% after 5 years from the first intervention [33]. Recurrence is more frequent in patients with changes in the distal part of colon [22]. Hence this group should qualify for proctocolectomy with ileostomy. Colectomy with ileo-rectal anastomosis is, however, preferable for young patients with no involvement of the sigmoid colon and/or rectum; the majority of these patients have normal bowel motions even after 10 years.

Balloon Dilatation

The stenosis of the small intestine is one of the typical symptoms of CD. The standard treatment should be strictureplasty or resection of the affected part [34]. The less common clinical manifestation is large-intestine stricture, which is diagnosed when a colonoscope of a standard diameter (13–13.6 mm) cannot be inserted through the affected part of the intestine. The clinical manifestations of the stricture include flatulence, tenesmus (when the stricture is localised near the rectum), constipation, abdominal pain, ileus or subileus [34]. The exacerbation and severity of symptoms depend on the diameter of the narrowing. An intestinal diameter greater than 13 mm usually suffices for correct passage. When the diameter of the stricture falls below 9 mm, it leads to increased symptoms of obstruction [35]. This type of changes is observed usually in neoplastic tumours of the large intestine. When neoplastic etiology is excluded, the most frequent causes are the healing complications of the anastomosis, inflammatory bowel disease, the ischaemia as well as postradiotherapy changes. Segmental resection is the most common procedure in treating strictures. The alternative to the surgical procedure is dilation of the narrowed fragment with an endoscopic balloon. It should be performed under endoscopic visualisation as well as/or X-ray scopy. After direct visualisation of a stricture the wire guide of the balloon is passed through the narrowing. The balloon is then filled with iodine contrast medium under pressure of 1.5–3 atm. The visualisation of the stricture with the balloon in X-ray scopy allows accurate assessment of the effectiveness of the operation. The pressure in the balloon is maintained for about 2 min and can be repeated 2–3 times [35, 36].

Endoscopic dilatation is an effective method. The improvement in the clinical picture after 3 months was observed for 50–94% of patients depending on the centre and the patient's profile [37, 38]. The effectiveness of the operation depends on the diameter of the balloon used, the applied pressure and the initial cause of the stenosis and the level of inflammatory process at the site of stenosis. More severe inflammatory changes in the affected intestine, which are typical for CD are not a contraindication for the procedure. Some authors recommend local steroid injections if severe inflammation is present [39]. Despite the coexistence of the inflammatory process, long-term results are encouraging for CD patients. In about two thirds of cases, patients in this group may avoid the necessity of surgical operation [37]. According to Sabate [37], the probability of surgery for stenosis following endoscope dilatation is 26% in the first year.

In the 5 years following endoscopic balloon dilatation, the probability grows to 46%. Couckuyt [40] achieved long-term clinical improvement in 34 of 55 patients who underwent endoscopic balloon dilatation (62%) in 33.6 months during follow-up, but also notes a high risk of perforation in this group. This complication was observed in six patients (11%). In four cases conservative treatment was sufficient while two patients underwent resection of the affected intestine. The rate of complications was not connected with the higher mortality. Results of other studies show a smaller rate of perforation (0–4.7%) [41].

The endoscopic treatment of large-intestine stenosis in patients with CD is a valuable alternative to classic surgical methods. These methods are characterised by a high effectiveness in reducing the subjective manifestations. Endoscopic methods decrease the frequency of surgical intervention and lower the risk of complications. Endoscope balloon dilatation is a method of choice for treatment of large-intestine stenosis in the course of Crohn's disease.

Colocutaneous Fistulae

Fistulae are a very frequent manifestation of CD, affecting 35% of patients. They is one of the sub-phenotypes of the disease manifesting as intestinal perforation, abscess formation and fistulae formation. Perineal fistulae make up most of cases and affect 20% [42]. Fistulae can be divided into internal and external, of which internal fistulae emerge in 5–10% of patients, while external fistulae emerging in the rest [43]. Colocutaneous fistulae are a type of external fistulae with an internal opening located anywhere in the inflamed large intestine. The fistula tract begins at the abdominal wall, and continues until it ends as an external opening on the skin. The symptoms include a constant or periodical flow of intestinal, festering, or a combination of intestinal and festering contents from the external opening of the fistula tract. Certain fistulae lack manifestation.

Treatment of colocutaneous fistulae depend on the clinical manifestations, symptoms and complications. Conservative treatment of choice is 5-ASA (mesalazine), metronidazole and ciprofloxacin. Colocutaneous fistulae are not related to any absorption disturbances and do not cause severe symptoms, therefore the first-line treatment should be a conservative one [27]. Initial treatment with 5-ASA, metronidazole and ciprofloxacin has a beneficial effect, and despite the fact that in the majority of cases it does not lead to complete healing, it considerably decreases the symptoms and improves the quality of the patient's life [44]. Increasing evidence shows that corticosteroids should not be used in fistulous CD. When patients are non-responsive to 5-ASA, metronidazole and ciprofloxacin therapy, the immunomodulators (6-mercaptopurine or azathioprine) should be considered. This line of therapy was effective in 54–65% of cases, and was followed by complete fistula closing in 31–39% of patients [45–47]. Chimeric monoclonal antibody anti-TNF (infliximab) is new and promising type of therapy that shows high effectiveness in fistulae resistant to 5-ASA, antibiotics and immunomodulators. Complete healing of fistulae has been observed in 24–55% with a simultaneous slight risk for side effects [48–52]. The external fistulae show better responsiveness to infliximab (69%) when compared to the internal fistulae (13%) [22]. External fistulae including perianal fistulae respond best to the therapy (78%), while 38% of abdominal-wall fistulae respond well to infliximab [53]. Infliximab should be recommended in the treatment of both external and internal asymptomatic fistulae that are unresponsive to the application of other medications due to low toxicity and safety of usage [54].

Septic complications of the colocutaneous fistulae are indications for immediate surgical intervention. A decision to undertake surgical treatment should also be made in the case of those fistulae resistant to conservative treatment, and when the outflow of intestinal contents causes maceration of the skin creating discomfort and lowering the patient's quality of life. The type of surgical procedure depends mostly on the image obtained after laparotomy. The aim of the procedure should always be resection of the fistula and the involved portion of intestine along with the removal of the entire fistula tract and external opening. Elective procedures should be conducted possibly at the time of remission and not sooner than 3–6 months from the time of severe onset of symptoms [27]. Some authors point out a high rate of recurrence following segmental resection [55], some present satisfactory results with only 13% of recurrences and with an average time of 27 months until recurrence.

Risk of Recurrence

The risk of recurrence following surgery is much higher in the case of small-bowel involvement [56]. The frequency of surgical recurrences following segmental resection in Crohn's disease is believed to be at 24–64% [51, 52, 57, 58, 59]. Discrepancies result because the length of observations varies, as does the criteria setting related to the surgeries.

A surveillance period that lasted 5.5 years showed a 62% chance for recurrence following segment resection of the large intestine caused by Crohn's disease [52], whereas a surveillance period that lasted 10 years showed a 66% chance [60], and a surveillance period of 14 years showed an 86% chance for recurrence [60]. The types of surgical procedures performed on the large intestine include segmental resection, left and right hemicolectomy, sigmoid resection and anterior rectal resection, colectomy with ileo-rectal anastomosis, colectomy with ileostomy and proctocolectomy. Interpretation of the results can be difficult because inclusion criteria in some trials are not homogenous; therefore, patients with segmental resection are enrolled in the same group with those who underwent subtotal colectomy with ileostomy or just stoma formation (61–63). The latest reports show that recurrence following segmental resection required repeated surgical treatment in 30–49% of patients [21, 61, 64]. The lowest level of recurrence at 15% has been noted for patients after right-sided hemicolectomies [61]. Recurrence following subtotal colectomy with ileostomy has been recorded as being between 41 and 64% [64–66]. Recurrence following subtotal colectomy with ileostomy is much lower and has been recorded at 18.5% [64] and 30% [67], respectively. The best results have been noted for the cases of stapled end-to-end anastomoses, which have reduced the rate of recurrence to as low as 3% [68], and side-to-side anastomosis with a recurrence level at 2% [69].

The most important factor creating the risk of postoperative recurrence is found to be cigarette smoking [70, 71]. Quitting smoking after the surgery decreases the risk of recurrence [72]. Another independent factor influencing recurrence is the sub-phenotype of the disease. The sub-phenotype connected with perforation and fistula creation, is believed to be at a higher risk of recurrence following resection [73]. It has been proven that the application of 5-ASA (mesalazine) as well as metronidazole and ornidazole influences the lowering of risk for early recurrence [70, 74]. Wide stapled anastomoses may also reduce recurrences following surgery, but it requires further evaluation and additional randomised trials [70].

Risk of Carcinoma

Similar to ulcerative colitis, CD is a risk factor for development of colorectal cancer [75, 76]. The risk is higher than in general population, and increases with time [77]. Patients with early Crohn's disease who are younger than 25 years of age are at the higher risk for tumour development [78]. Dysplasia precedes development of the colorectal cancer [79] which in a majority of cases shows a clear tendency to develop at the site of the inflammation. In one third of all cases, it has been recorded as developing at the site of the macroscopically unaffected part of the intestine [80]. A spreading infiltration to the digestive tract wall [81] with multiple focus points of the cancer [82] has also been observed.

The first case of a large intestine tumour connected with Crohn's disease was described in 1948 [83]. Since then, publications have recorded a couple of hundred similar cases. Patients with intense and intensifying inflammatory changes of the intestine, forming a background for basic long-lasting disease, are at a significantly increased risk of cancer. This is also true for those who have not had surgery for a pathologically affected segment that had been deemed necessary to remove [80, 83, 84]. It is believed that, due to the above deciding factors, the risk for development of cancer in Crohn's disease is 10 times higher than in the general population [85].

There are three characteristics of cancer in the course of Crohn's disease. As compared to de novo, cancer in Crohn's disease emerges at a much lower age (48 vs. 70 years of age), is much more often located in the right part of the colon (45%) and more frequently presents as a multiple-focus point [81, 82]. Multifocal development of cancer in Crohn's disease has been recorded in 14–40% of cases, while in de novo, developed cancer has only been reported in 4% of the cases [86]. It has also been recorded that a higher likelihood for development of cancer is associated with large-intestine stenosis. Crohn's disease large intestine stenosis has been recorded in 5–17% of cases. The chance for development of cancer when stenosis is present is 6.8%, and when stenosis is absent it is at 0.7% [87]. Colorectal cancer may also emerge in a distant segment of the intestine or in association to chronic fistulae between the large intestine and bladder [88], vagina [89] or skin [88, 90].

Toxic-Fulminant Colitis

Toxic colitis is a severe, life threatening complication manifested as a sudden, and deteriorating clinical condition, bloody diarrhoea, peristaltic abdominal pain, development of toxaemia, emaciation and high fever. Previously believed to be more common in the case of ulcerative colitis, it is now currently proven, based on conducted studies, to be the case in up to 50% of Crohn's disease. When toxic colitis is accompanied by a dilatation of the large intestine, toxic megacolon develops. Fibrosis and stenosis of intestinal walls in Crohn's disease may result in an X-ray without intestinal dilatation that is so characteristic for toxic megacolon. Treatment of toxic colitis should be carried out in an intensive care unit and include aggressive fluid transfusions, intravenous steroids and antibiotic administration, total parenteral nutrition and metabolic monitoring. A lack of response to the treatment for 5–7 days is an indication for surgical treatment. Operative treatment is taken up earlier when symptoms of perforation, massive bleeding and toxic colitis complicated by toxic megacolon are present. Surgical procedures indicated in such cases are colectomy with ileostomy, proctocolectomy with ileostomy, and loop ileostomy. Presently, the golden standard in toxic colitis surgical treatment is colectomy with ileostomy [91–93]. Patients undergoing this operation are at lower risk of complication and a lower mortality rate postoperatively compared to proctocolectomy. That publications report that an initial clinical diagnosis of the disease resulting eventually in toxic colitis, confirms itself in a later histopathological evaluation in 65–70%, which leads to the conclusion that colectomy with preservation of the rectum allows later reconstructive surgeries. Proctocolectomy is no longer a recommended surgical procedure in the treatment of toxic colitis because it creates the risk of a large amount of intraoperative blood loss, makes the time of the surgery longer, increases the likelihood for pelvic infection and slows down the healing of the perineal wound, which is the most frequently occurring complication of the operation [94].

Massive Bleeding

Massive bleeding from the large intestine that requires immediate surgical treatment is very rare in Crohn's disease. It affects 1.3–1.9% of all patients [91, 95], and 12% of all cases of bleeding from a digestive tract in patients with Crohn's disease [96]. Massive bleeding occurs in states of severe exacerbations, or a severe form of the disease such as toxic/fulminant colitis. It is necessary to locate the site of massive bleeding because as opposed to ulcerative colitis, its location is well defined. The site of bleeding in most cases in the affected part of the intestine is most frequently the ulceration in the left part of colon [97]. Identification of the bleeding site may be done with the use of colonoscopy; at the time of the procedure, the surgeon may attempt to stop bleeding using endoscopic methods. If the bleeding site has not been identified with the use of colonoscopy, lower mesenteric artery angiography should be considered. It is also necessary to execute the endoscopy of the upper digestive tract in order to exclude the bleeding from that part. Similar to other types of gastrointestinal bleeding, the first line of treatment is a conservative therapy consisting of anti-haemorrhagic drugs as well as blood and plasma transfusions. An example of a successful treatment of the bleeding ileocolic anastomosis with infliximab transfusion can be found in the literature [98].

Massive bleeding resistant to conservative treatment or lacking in the possibility of such treatment, recurring bleeding that follows previous conservative treatment, as well as other clinical reasons may be considered to be an indication for surgical treatment. A colectomy with ileostomy is to be performed if pathological changes affect the rectum, and a colectomy with ileo-rectal anastomosis is to be performed if the rectum is free of pathological changes [91].

Free Perforation

Large intestine perforation rarely takes place in Crohn's disease. The frequency of large-intestine perforation in patients with Crohn's disease has reached 1.8–2.4% [99, 100], making up 20–50% of all digestive tract perforations in Crohn's disease. Typical symptoms of perforation may be hidden behind the effects of high dosages of steroids, thereby delaying early diagnosis. Perforation takes place most often during the course of toxic colitis (with or without toxic megacolon) or during a severe exacerbation of inflammation especially if accompanied by stenosis below the site of perforation. Iatrogenic damage of the inflamed colon during colonoscopy may also be the cause of perforation. Due to the frequent occurrence of intraperitoneal adhesions, some perforations are covered. Surgical treatment depends on the general condition of the patient, the site of the perforation, and the circumstances that caused it. In toxic colitis perforations, colectomy with ileostomy is a recommended surgical procedure. Proctocolectomy, which used to be a recommended procedure in the past, is no longer a preferred method in a toxic colitis accompanied by a toxic megacolon. This is because of the prolonged time of the surgery, which has a dramatic impact on the risk of perioperative mortality. In the case of perforation without active toxic colitis, the affected segment should be resected and a primary anastomosis created. When iatrogenic perforation resulting from colonoscopy takes place, the type of surgical procedure depends on the general condition of the patient, location of the perforation (is it located in an affected or in unaffected fragment?), and a level of intestinal preparation. When perforation is located in the affected part of the intestine, resection of the perforated segment should be performed, and depending on the state of the patient as well as other risk factors, Hartmann's procedure, or a resection with anastomosis should be done [26, 13]. If perforation is located in healthy part of the intestine the alternative treatment includes partial resection or a local suture of perforation.

Emergency Surgery

The indication for emergency surgery occurs in 1.6–10.4% of all cases of the disease, and carries a perioperative mortality rate of 2–40% [91, 101–103].

Intraperitoneal abscess in Crohn's disease in most instances results from perforation or intestinal fistulae located in the small intestine. A large intestinal cause of abscess is most often a complication resulting from previous surgical procedure. In the case of elective procedures, the most likely cause lies in leakage of the anastomosis; in the case of emergency procedures, it results from peritonitis. Current advancement in invasive radiology makes transdermal drainage, in addition to traditional surgical drainage, possible. Transdermal drainage allows for the attainment of clinical improvement before indications for necessary surgical treatment arise. The disadvantages of transdermal drainage include the risk of fistulae and recurrent abscess; additional limitations come from technical inability in the transdermal drainage of some areas.

Obstruction in Crohn's disease is a frequent occurrence, but only 5–17% is caused by the pathological changes in a large intestine [104]. Obstruction may be caused by intra-abdominal abscess, intraperitoneal adhesions, postinflammatory stenosis, or neoplasmatic changes. It is necessary to perform diagnostic tests to search for the presence of tumours. Publications state that up to 7% of large-intestine obstruction in Crohn's disease is caused by cancer [104].

References

1. Guindi M, Riddell RH (2004) Indeterminate colitis. J Clin Pathol 57(12):1233–1244
2. Leichtner AM, Jackson WD, Grand RJ (1996) Crohn's disease. In: Walker WA, Durie PR, Hamilton JR et al (eds) Pediatric Gastroentestinal Disease. St. Louis, Mosby, pp 692–711
3. Hanauer SB, Sandborn W (2001) Management of Crohn's disease in adults. Am J Gastroenterol 96:635–643
4. Glickman RM (1998) Inflammatory bowel disease: ulcerative colitis and Crohn's disease. In: Fauci AS et al (eds) Harrison's textbook of internal medicine, 14th edn. McGraw-Hill, New York, pp 1633–1645
5. Hyams JS (1996) Crohn's disease in children. Pediat Clin N Am 100:235–254
6. Summers RW, Switz DM, Sessions JT Jr, and National Cooperative Crohn's Disease Study (1979) Results of drug treatment. Gastroenterology 77:847–869
7. Hanauer SB, Krawitt EL, Robinson M, Pentasa Crohn's Disease Compassionate Use Study Group (1993) Long-term management of Crohn's disease with mesalamine capsules (Pentasa). Am J Gastroenterol 88:1343–1451
8. Wojciechowski K, Jarosz M (2001) Conservative treat-

ment of Crohn's disease: possibilities and limitations. Proktologia 3(2):226–239
9. Malchov H, Ewe K, Brandes JW (1984) European Cooperative Crohn's Disease Study: results of drug treatment. Gastroenerology 86:249–266
10. Stange EF (1996) Steroid dependent and steroid refractory Crohn's disease: definition by indices. Abstract of invited lectures. Falk Symposium No. 96, Oct. 1996, Freiburg
11. Thomsen OO (2002) Budesonide and masalazine in active Crohn's disease: a comparison of the effects on quality of life. Am J Gastroenterol 97:649–653
12. Salemans J, Hoitsma AJ, De Abreu RA (1987) Pharmacokinetics of azathioprine and 6-mercaptopurine after oral administration of azathioprine. Clin Transplant 1:217–221
13. Brynskov J, Freund L, Rasmunssen SN (1991) A final report on placebo-controlled double blind, randomized trial of cyclosporine treatment in active Crohn's Disease. Scan J Gastroenterol 26:689–695
14. Sandborn WJ (1995) A critical review of cyclosporine therapy in inflammatory bowel disease. Inflam Bowel Dis (CCFA) 1:48–95
15. Rutgeerts P, van Assche G, Vermeire S (2004) Optimizing anti-TNF treatment in inflammatory bowel disease. Gastroenterology 126:1593–1610
16. Hanauer SB (2002) Maintenance infliximab for Crohn's disease: the ACCENT I randomized trial. Lancet 359:1541–1549
17. Hanauer SB (2002) Maintenance infliximab for Crohn's disease: the ACCENT II in patients with fistulizing Crohn's disease. Lancet 359:1541–1549
18. Szczygieł B (2001) Nutritional treatment in Crohn's disease. Proctology 2(3):240–246
19. Greenberg GR, Fleming CR, Jeejeebhoy JW (1988) Controlled trial on bowel rest and nutritional support in the management of Crohn's disease. Gut 29:1309
20. Borley NR, Mortensen NJ, Jewell DP (1997) Preventing postoperative recurrence of Crohn's disease. Br J Surg 84:1493–1502
21. Bernell O, Lapidus A, Hellers G (2000) Risk factors for surgery and recurrence in 907 patients with primary ileocecal Crohn's disease. Br J Surg 87:1697–1701
22. Fichera A, McCormack R, Rubin MA et al (2005) Long-term outcome of surgically treated Crohn's colitis: a prospective study. Dis Colon Rectum 48(5):963–969
23. Andrews HA, Lewis P, Allan RN (1989) Prognosis after surgery for colonic Crohn's disease. Br J Surg 76:1184–1190
24. Andrews HA, Keighley MR, Alexander-Williams J, Allan RN (1991) Strategy for management of distal ileal Crohn's disease. Br J Surg 78:79–82
25. Venkatesh KS, Ramanujan PS, McGee S (1992) Hydrostatic balloon dilatation of benign colonic anastomotic strictures. Dis Colon Rectum 35:789–791
26. Kennedy HK (2004) Quality of life in patients with an ileostomy. Int Disibil Stud 59(1):23–29
27. Dziki A, Galbfach P (2004) Crohn's disease: when to operate? Acta Chir Iugosl 51(2):61–68
28. Hyman NH, Cataldo P, Osler T (2005) Urgent subtotal colectomy for severe inflammatory bowel disease. Dis Colon Rectum 48(1):70–73
29. Mylonakis E, Allan RN, Keighley MR (2001) How does pouch construction for a final diagnosis of Crohn's disease compare with ileoproctostomy for established Crohn's proctocolitis? Dis Colon Rectum 44(8):1137–1142
30. Panis Y, Poupard B, Nementh J (1996) Ileal pouch/anal anastomosis for Crohn's disease. Lancet 347:854–857
31. Cattan P, Bonhomme N, Panis Y (2002) Fate of rectum in patients undergoing total colectomy for Crohn's disease. Br J Surg 89:454–459
32. Anderson P, Olaison G, Hallbook O, Sjodahl R (2002) Segmental resection or subtotal colectomy in Crohn's colitis? Dis Colon Rectum 45:47–53
33. Longo WE, Ballantyne GH, Cahow CE (1988) Treatment of Crohn's colitis: segmental or total colectomy? Arch Surg 123(5):588–590
34. Roy P, Kumar D (2005) Strictureplasty for active Crohn's disease. Int J Colorectal Dis 30:1–6
35. Lange de EF, Shaffer HA Jr (1991) Rectal strictures: treatment with fluoroscopically guided balloon dilation. Radiology 178(2):475–479
36. Solt JU, Hertelendy A, Szilagyi K (2004) Long-term results of balloon catheter dilation of lower gastrointestinal tract stenoses. Dis Colon Rectum 47(9):1499–1505
37. Sabate JM, Villarejo J, Bouhnik Y et al (2003) Hydrostatic balloon dilatation of Crohn's strictures. Alimet Pharmacol Ther 18(4):409–413
38. Skreden K, Wiig JN, Myrvold HE (1987) Balloon dilation of rectal strictures. Acta Chir Scand 153(10):615–617
39. Legnani PE, Krnbluth A (2002) Therapeutic options in the management of strictures in Crohn's disease. Gastrointest Endosc Clin N Am 12(3):589-603
40. Couckuyt H, Geveres AM, Corenmans G et al (1995) Efficacy and safety of hydrostatic balloon dilatation of ileocolonic Crohn's strictures: a prospective long-term analysis. Gut 36(4):577–580
41. Virgilio C, Cosentino S, Favara C at al (1995) Endoscopic treatment of postoperative colonic strictures using an achalasia dilator: short-term and long-term results. Endoscopy 27(3):219–222
42. Schwartz DA, Loftus EV Jr, Tremaine WJ et al (2002) The natural history of fistulizing Crohn's disease in Olmstead County, Minnesota. Gastroenterology 122:875–880
43. Levy C, Tremaine WJ (2002) Management of internal fistulas in Crohn's disease. Inflamm Bowel Dis 8:106–111
44. Present DH (2003) Crohn's fistula: current concepts in Management. Gastroenterology 124:1629–1635
45. Present DH, Korelitz BI, Wisch N et al (1980) Treatment of Crohn's disease with 6 Mercaptopurine: a long term randomized double blind study. N Engl J Med 302:981–987
46. Korelitz BI, Present DH (1985) The favorable effects of 6 mercaptopurine in the fistulous Crohn's disease. Dig Dis Sci 30:58–64
47. Pearson DC, May GR, Fick GH, Sutherland LR (1995) Azathioprine and 6 mercaptopurine in Crohn's disease: a meta-analysis. Ann Intern Med 123:132–142
48. Sample C, Bailey RJ, Todoruk D et al (2002) Clinical experience with infliximab for Crohn's disease: the first 100 patients in Edmonton, Alberta. Can J Gastroenterol 16:165–170
49. Arnott ID, McDonald D, Wiliams A, Ghosh S (2001)

Clinical use of Infliximab in Crohn's disease: the Edinburgh experience. Aliment Pharmacol Ther 15:1639–1646
50. Ricart E, Panaccione R, Loftus EV et al (2001) Infliximab for Crohn's disease in clinical practice at the Mayo Clinic: the first 100 patients. Am J Gastroenterol 96:722–729
51. Goligher JC (1985) The long-term results of excisional surgery for primary and recurrent Crohn's disease of the large intestine. Dis Colon Rectum 28:51–55
52. Longo WE, Ballantyne GH, Cahow CE (1988) Treatment of Crohn's colitis: segmental or total colectomy? Arch Surg 123:588-590
53. Parsi MA, Lashner BA, Achkar JP et al (2004) Type of fistula determines response to infliximab in patients with fistulous Crohn's disease. Am J Gastroenterol 99:445–449
54. Colombel J-F, Loftus EV Jr, Tremaine WJ et al (2004) The safety profile of infliximab in patients with Crohn's disease: the Mayo Clinic experience in 500 patients. Gastroenterology 126:19–31
55. Whelan G, Farmer RG, Fazio VW, Goormastic M (1985) Recurrence after surgery in Crohn's disease. Gastroenterology 88:1826–1833
56. Basilisco G, Campanini M, Cesana B et al (1989) Risk factors for first operation in Crohn's disease. Am J Gastroenterol 84:749–752
57. Andersson P, Olaison G, Hallbook O, Sjodahl R (2002) Segmental resection or subtotal colectomy in Crohn's colitis? Dis Colon Rectum 45:47–53
58. Bernell O, Lapidus A, Hellers G (2000) Risk factors for surgery and postoperative recurrence in Crohn's disease. Ann Surg 231:38–45
59. Allan A, Andrews H, Hilton CJ et al (1989) Segmental colonic resection is an appropriate operation for short skip lesions due to Crohn's disease in the colon. Word J Surg 13:611-616
60. Goligher JC (1988) Surgical treatment of inflammatory bowel disease-introduction. World J Surg 12:139-141
61. Polle SW, Slors JFM, Weverling GJ et al (2005) Recurrence after segmental resection for colonic Crohn's disease. Br J Surg 92:1143–1149
62. Prabhakar LP, Laramee C, Nelson H, Dozois RR (1997) Avoiding a stoma: role for segmental or abdominal colectomy in Crohn's colitis. Dis Colon Rectum 40:71–78
63. Stern HS, Goldberg SM, Rothenberger DA (1984) Segmental versus total colectomy for large bowel Crohn's disease. World J Surg 8:118–122
64. Bernell O, Lapidus A, Hellers G (2001) Recurrence after colectomy in Crohn's colitis. Dis Colon Rectum 44: 647–654
65. Ambrose NS, Keighley MR (1984) Clinical impact of colectomy and ileorectal anastomosis in the management of Crohn's disease. Gut 25:223–227
66. Flint G, Strauss R (1977) Ileorectal anastomosis in patients with Crohn's disease of the colon. Gut 18:236–239
67. Lock MR, Fazio VW, Farmer RG (1981) Proximal recurrence and the fate of the rectum following excisional surgery for Crohn's disease of the large bowel. Ann Surg 194:754–760
68. Yamamoto T, Bain IM, Mylonakis E et al (1993) Stapled functional end-to-end anastomosis versus sutured end-to-end anastomosis after ileocolonic resection in Crohn's disease. Scand J Gastroenterol 34:708–713
69. Hashemi M, Novell JR, Lewis AAM (1988) Side-to-side stapled anastomosis may delay recurrence in Crohn's disease. Dis Colon Rectum 41:1293–1296
70. Yamamoto T (2005) Factors affecting recurrence after surgery for Crohn's disease. World J Gastroenterol 11:3971–3979
71. Cosnes J, Beaugerie L, Carbonnel F, Gendre JP (2001) Smoking cessation and the course of Crohn's disease: an intervention study. Gastroenterology 120:1093–1099
72. Ryan WR, Allan RN, Yamamoto T, Keighley MR (2004) Crohn's disease patients who quit smoking have a reduced risk of reoperation for recurrence. Am J Surg 187: 219–225
73. Lautenbach E, Berlin JA, Lichtenstein GR (1998) Risk factors for early postoperative recurrence of Crohn's disease. Gastroenterology 115:256–267
74. Cottone M, Orlando A, Viscido A (2003) Review article: prevention of postsurgical relapse and recurrence in Crohn's disease. Aliment Pharmacol Ther 17:(Suppl 2):38–42
75. Bernstein CN, Blanchard JF, Kliewer E, Wajda A (2001) Cancer risk in patients with inflammatory bowel disease: a population-based study. Cancer 15:854–862
76. Mpofu C, Watson AJ, Rhodes JM (2004) Strategies for detecting colon cancer and/or dysplasia in patients with inflammatory bowel disease. Cochrane Database Syst Rev 2:CD000279
77. Shanahan F (2003) Colitis-associated cancer: time for new strategies. Aliment Pharmacol Ther 18(Suppl 2):6–9
78. Gillen CD, Andrews HA, Prior P, Allan RN (1994) Crohn's disease and colorectal cancer. Gut 35:651–656
79. Greenstein AJ (2000) Cancer in inflammatory bowel disease. Mt Sinai J Med 67:227–240
80. Greenstein AJ, Sachar DB, Smith H et al (1981) A comparison of cancer risk in Crohn's disease and ulcerative colitis. Cancer 48:2742–2745
81. Clemmens T, Johansen A (1972) A case of Crohn's disease of the colon associated with adenocarcinoma extending from cardia to the anus. Acta Pathol Microbiol Scand 80:5–8
82. Keighley MRB, Thompson H, Alexander-Williams J (1975) Multifocal colonic carcinoma and Crohn's disease. Surgery 78:534–537
83. Gillen CD, Andrews HA, Prior P, Allan RN (1994) Ulcerative colitis and Crohn's disease: a comparison of the colorectal cancer risk in extensive colitis. Gut 35:1590–1592
84. Eckbom A, Helmick C, Zack M, Adami HO (1990) Increased risk of large bowel cancer in Crohn's disease with colonic involvement. Lancet 336:357–359
85. Sachar DB (1994) Cancer in Crohn's disease: dispelling the myths. Gut 35:1507–1508
86. Greenstein AJ, Slater G, Heimann TM et al (1986) A comparison of multiple synchronous colorectal cancer in ulcerative colitis, familial polyposis coli, and de novo cancer. Ann Surg 203:123–128

87. Yamazuki Y, Ribeiro MB, Sachar DB et al (1991) Malignant colorectal strictures in Crohn's disease. Am J Gastroenterol 86:882–885
88. Greenstein AJ, Sachar D, Pucillo A et al (1978) Cancer in Crohn's disease after diversionary surgery: a report of seven carcinomas occurring in excluded bowel. Am J Surg 135:86–90
89. Sher ME, Bauer JJ, Gelernt I (1991) Surgical repair of rectovaginal fistulas in patients with Crohn's disease: transvaginal approach. Dis Colon Rectum 34:641–648
90. Church JM, Weakley FI, Fazio VW et al (1985) The relationship between fistulas in Crohn's disease and associated carcinoma: report of four cases and review of the literature. Dis Colon Rectum 28:361–366
91. Berg DF, Bahadursingh AM, Kamiński DL, Longo WE (2002) Acute surgical emergencies in inflammatory bowel disease. Am J Surg 184:45–51
92. Hyman NH, Cataldo P, Mosler T (2005) Urgent subtotal colectomy for severe inflammatory bowel disease. Dis Colon Rectum 48:70–73
93. Katz JA (2000) Medical and surgical management of severe colitis. Semin Gastrointest Dis 11:18–32
94. Yamamoto T, Allan RN, Keighley RB (2000) Audit of single-stage proctocolectomy for Crohn's disease: postoperative complications and recurrence. Dis Colon Rectum 43:249–256
95. Parc YR, Radice E, Dozois RR (1999) Burgery for ulcerative colitis: historical perspective: a century of surgical innovations and refinements. Dis Colon Rectum 42:299–306
96. Sirocco WC, Reilly JC, Rusin LC (1995) Life threatening hemorrhage and exsanguination from Crohn's disease. Dis Colon Rectum 38:85–95
97. Balaiche J, Louis E, D'Haens G et al (1999) Acute lower gastrointestinal bleeding in Crohn's disease: characteristics of a unique series of 34 patients: Belgia IBD Research Group. Am J Gastroenterol 94:2177–2181
98. Tsujikawa T, Nezu R, Andoh A et al (2004) Infliximab as a possible treatment for the hemorrhagic type of Crohn's disease. J Gastroenterol 39:284–287
99. Veroux M, Angriman I, Ruffolo C et al (2003) A rare surgical complication of Crohn's disease: free peritoneal perforation. Minerva Chir 58:351–354
100. Greenstein AJ, Aufses AH Jr (1985) Differences in pathogenesis, incidence and outcome of perforation in inflammatory bowel disease. Surg Gynecol Obstet 160:63–69
101. Bortnik M, Lukas M (2001) Toxic megacolon. Cas Lek Cesk 140:619–623
102. Levine CD (1999) Toxic megacolon: diagnosis and treatment challenges. AACN Clin Issues 10:492–499
103. Gsell O, Loew E (1960) Toxic megacolon in ulcerative colitis. Gastroenterol 94:29–47
104. Yamazaki Y, Ribeiro MB, Sachar DB et al (1991) Malignant strictures in Crohn's disease. Am J Gastrenterol 86:882–885

Laparoscopy for the Treatment of Crohn's Disease

Annibale D'Annibale, Emilio Morpurgo

Introduction

Crohn's disease is a complex disease with a complicated natural history that differs greatly from the majority of common diseases of the gut. It is a panenteric, incurable disease. It has a peak incidence in young people and onset in childhood is not uncommon. The majority of patients will need surgery within 10 years from diagnosis and 50% of them will undergo additional operations for recurrent disease, with 8–10% of patients recurring every year. Many patients will undergo surgery after long periods of steroid or immunosuppressive treatment and therefore their immunological status is poor. In addition, these individuals have a high risk of receiving a stoma, either permanent or temporary (41 and 14% respectively) [1].

For all these reasons, the laparoscopic approach, which has the theoretical advantage of preserving the abdominal wall, reducing intra-abdominal manipulation and thus adhesion formation and helping to reduce immunological stress, when compared to the open surgery, could be the approach of choice for the treatment of such patients.

The comparison of laparoscopy and an open approach for the surgical treatment of Crohn's disease is difficult to make, due to the difficulty of stratifying patients in homogenous groups, in particular those with complicated disease. The only randomised trial available so far is elective ileocolic resectioning for refractory non-complicated disease of the terminal ileum [2]. Studies on laparoscopic treatment of complicated disease so far have been cohort, or case series studies. This understandably categorises them as grade 3–4 evidence and therefore rate low in terms of recommendation (Table 1). The results and the recommendations about the use of laparoscopy for the treatment of Crohn's disease vary according to the type and the severity of the disease, and therefore must be described separately in brief.

Ileocolic Non-Complicated Disease

The ideal patients who may benefit from laparoscopy are those undergoing elective ileocolic resection. These patients are young and often are attracted by the advantage of smaller abdominal scars [3]. The minimally invasive nature of the laparoscopic approach has a favourable impact, as patients undergoing this approach may require further surgery in the future. The outcomes of the randomised trial [2] and of several cohort comparison studies [4–8], show that after laparoscopic ileocolic resection there is a shorter hospital stay, with a faster recovery of pulmonary function, possibly a reduced postoperative ileus and better cosmesis. Three reports conclude that the cost of laparoscopic resection is globally less than open resection [5, 7, 8]. Due to the less extensive intra-abdominal manipulation and consequent less adhesion formation, laparoscopy seems to have decreased long-term small-bowel obstruction non-related to recurrence [4].

Flogistic and Fistulous Disease

Flogistic mass is a frequent finding in Crohn's patients, in particular in recurrent disease. Large palpable mass per se, especially if associated with complex fistulous disease or with a frozen abdomen, are often considered to be a contraindication to laparoscopy [4, 7, 9 10], whereas a mininvasive approach is considered possible even after previous multiple surgeries [11, 12]. When a flogistic mass is present with thickened mesentery, the size of the minilaparotomy depends on the size of the inflamed specimen to be removed. Due to the friability of the inflamed tissue, care has to be taken in order to avoid bleeding during the extraction manoeuvres of the thickened mesentery and the mesentery has to be divided outside the abdominal cavity [6, 8, 13]. On the other hand, severe disease with large inflammatory masses is cause for conversion to open surgery in up to 40% of cases,

Table 1. Studies on laparoscopic treatment of complicated disease

Author	Study	Procedure	Exclusion / inclusion criteria	Conversion (%)	Blood loss (cc)	Op time (min)	Hosp stay (day)	Diet (day)	Complications (%)	Conclusions
Reissmann 1996	CS	ICR 32 Colect 7 Loop ileost 6 Other 6	Exclusion for obstruction, short bowel, perforation, peritonitis, toxic colitis	14 (mass, bleeding)			5.1		14 Stoma obstr Abscess Enterotomy bleeding	Feasible
Canin Enders 1999	CS	ICR 70 SBR 13 R HEM 3 Colect 3 Ant/sigm res 5	Elective procedure	1.2 (mass)	168	183	4.2	1		Feasible in complicated disease and reoperation
Bemelman 2000	CCC	ICR	Elective primary ICR	6	130 vs 204 (Ns)	130 vs 104	5.7 vs 10.2	2.8 vs 3.3		Similar morbidity Longer operation Reduced stay Better cosmesis
Hamel 2001	CS	ICR 109 Colect 21	Elective ICR and colectomy			ICR 167 Colect 231	8.8		ICR 20% (5 leaks) Colect 18% (2 leaks)	ICR and colectomy are feasible with comparable post-op compl; compl; colect has more operat complic
Milsom 2001	PR	31 ICR lap 29 ICR open	Elective cases; TI +/- cecum, single site disease; BMI<32	6.3% (adhesions, mass)	133 vs 173	140 vs 85	5 vs 6		Minor: 13% lap, 26% open Major: 3% la, 3% open	Better pulmonary function Shorter stay Less minor complications Longer operation

continue

Author	Study	Procedure	Exclusion / inclusion criteria	Conversion (%)	Blood loss (cc)	Op time (min)	Hosp stay (day)	Diet (day)	Complications (%)	Conclusions
Young Fadok 2001	CCC	ICR	Elective ICR	5.9		147 vs 124	4 vs 7	0 vs 3		Feasible Longer operation Reduced ileus
Watanabe 2002	CS	8 SBR 12 ICR	Fistulous disease; Obvious mass or multiple previous surgeries excluded	16% (adhesions)		180	8	1	16%	Reduced stay Reduced cost Laparoscopy feasible in fistulous Crohn's
Evans 2002	CS	84 ICR	Exclusion for >2 previous surgeries, bowel obstruction, complex fistulas	18% (adhesions, mass)		145	5.6		6%	Laparoscopy is possible even in presence of mass of fistulous disease
Duepree 2002	CCC	21 ICR lap 24 ICR op	Only elective initial ICR	5%	50 vs 100		3 vs 5	0 vs 2	10 (abscess, leak)	Shorter stay Less blood loss Lower cost
Bergamaschi 2003	HNCC C	39 ICR lap 53 ICR op	Exclusion for: frozen abdomen, recurrent dis, emergency	0		185 vs 105	5.6 vs 11.2			Lap has less long term bowel obstruction (11.1 vs 35.4%) Longer op.
Shore 2003	NRCR	20 lap (14 TI, 6 TI+right colon) 20 open (8 TI, 12 TI+right col)	Exclusion for previous resections for Crohn's	5% (adhesions)	77 vs 265	145 vs 133	4.2 vs 8.2	1.3 vs 2.7		Feasible. Longer operation

CCC, concurrent cohort comparison (matched, non randomised); *CS*, case series; *HNCC*, historic non concurrent cohort case study; *NRCR*, non randomised comparative retrospective; *PR*, prospective randomised; *Lap*, laparoscopic; *Op*, open surgery; *ICR*, ileo-colic resection; *TI*, terminal ileum together with extensive abdominal adhesions in unselected groups of patients [9, 11, 14–19]. Nevertheless, many patients requiring conversion benefit from a preliminary laparoscopic dissection that can render the subsequent laparotomy smaller in size and more targeted [18]

In order to facilitate laparoscopic dissection, preoperative drainage of abscesses should be performed percutaneously and is suggested in several reports [10, 13]. During laparoscopic lysis of adhesions, tears of the bowel may occur and therefore all the intestinal loops have to be carefully inspected, probably via minilaparotomy at the end of the procedure [15, 16]. Fistulas can be approached laparoscopically in many cases and the fistula track can be divided with laparoscopic linear staplers [11].

Skip Lesions

Skip lesions are a frequent feature of Crohn's disease and with laparoscopy there is the theoretical risk of overlooking them due to less precise tactile sensation compared to open surgery [8, 13]. Preoperative studies (small-bowel follow through and CT scans) can be done pre-operatively, but the small bowel has to be thoroughly run from the ligament of Treitz to the caecum, if necessary, through the minilaparotomy.

Perianal and Colonic Crohn's Disease

When isolated perianal Crohn's disease is present, loop ileostomy is often offered to patients as a temporary or definitive solution. Laparoscopic ileostomy construction is easily performed [20] and at the same time it gives the possibility of performing a complete abdominal exploration in order to detect additional sites of disease. Bowel obstruction due to bowel twisting is a possible complication and therefore particular care has to be taken to mark the bowel in order to exteriorise it in the proper manner and with the proper orientation. As a general rule, during surgery for Crohn's disease, all the scars and all the port sites must be positioned in areas distant from possible sites that may have to be used in the future for stoma creation.

Conclusions

From the data currently available, firm and absolute recommendations cannot be drawn for the use of laparoscopy in the surgical treatment of Crohn's disease, due to the heterogeneous features of the disease.

For elective ileocolic resections, laparoscopy offers better immediate post-operative results possibly at a lower global cost and with potentially less incidence of small-bowel obstructions due to adhesions in the long-term. For complex disease, laparoscopy can be offered as a trial to all patients. Inflammatory masses, presence of fistulas and reoperation for recurrence are not absolute contraindications for this approach, even though they are the most significant cause of conversion. Pre-operative percutaneous drainage of abscesses together with accurate pre-operative medical therapy can be used to render surgery less demanding. For isolated perianal Crohn's disease, laparoscopy can be considered the approach of choice for stoma construction.

References

1. Gordon P, Nivatvongs S (1999) Principles and practice of surgery for the colon, rectum, and anus. Quality Medical, St. Louis, MO, USA
2. Milsom JW, Hammerhofer KA, Böhm B et al (2001) Prospective, randomised trial comparing laparoscopic vs. conventional surgery for refractory ileocolic Crohn's disease. Dis Colon Rectum 44:1–9
3. Dunker MS, Stiggelbout AM, van Hogezand RA et al (1998) Cosmesis and body image after laparoscopic-assisted and open ileocolic resection for Crohn's disease. Surg Endosc 12:1334–1340
4. Bergamaschi R, Pessaux P, Arnaud JP (2003) Comparison of conventional and laparoscopic ileocolic resection for Crohn's disease. Dis Colon Rectum 46:1129–1133
5. Young-Fadok TM, Hall Long K, MvConnell EJ et al (2001) Advantages of laparoscopic resection for ileocolic Crohn's disease: improved outcomes and reduced costs. Surg Endosc 15:450-454
6. Bemelman WA, Slors JFM, Dunker MS et al (2000) Laparoscopic assisted vs. open resection for Crohn's disease: a comparative study. Surg Endosc 14:721–725
7. Shore G, Gonzalez QH, Bondora A et al (2003) laparoscopic vs. conventional ileocolectomy for primary Crohn's disease. Arch Surg 138:76–79
8. Duepree H-J, Senagore AJ, Delaney CP et al (2002) Advantages of laparoscopic resection for ileocecal Crohn's disease. Dis Colon Rectum 45: 605-610
9. Watanabe M, Hasegawa H, Yamamoto S et al (2002) Successful application of laparoscopic surgery to the treatment of Crohn's disease with fistulas. Dis Colon Rectum 45:1057–1061
10. Evans J, Poritz L, Mac Bade H (2002) Influence of experience on laparoscopic ileocolic resection for Crohn's disease. Dis Colon Rectum 45:1595–1600
11. Canin-Endres J, Salky B, Gattorno F et al (1999) Laparoscopically assisted intestinal resection in 88 patients with Crohn's disease. Surg Endosc 13:595–599
12. Hasegawa H, Watanabe M, Nishibori H et al (2003) Laparoscopic surgery for recurrent Crohn's disease. Br J Surg 90:970–973
13. Hamel CT, Hildebrandt U, Weiss EG et al (2001)

Laparoscopic surgery for inflammatory bowel disease. Surg Endosc 15:642–645
14. Schmidt CM, Talamini M, Kaufman HS et al (2001) Laparoscopic surgery for Crohn's disease: reasons for conversion. Ann Surg 233:733–739
15. Reissmann P, Salky BA, Edye M et al (1996) Laparoscopic surgery in Crohn's disease. Surg Endosc 10:1201–1204
16. Wexner SD, Moscovitz ID (2000) Laparoscopic colectomy in diverticular and Crohn's disease. Surg Clin North Am 80:1299–1319
17. Kishi D, Nezu R, Ito T et al (2000) Laparoscopic-assisted surgery for Crohn's disease: reduced surgical stress following ileocolectomy. Surg Today 30:219–222
18. Moorthy K, Shaul T, Hons BS et al (2004) Factors that predict conversion in patients undergoing laparoscopic surgery for Crohn's disease. Am J Surg 187:47–51
19. Bauer JJ, Harris MT, Grumbach NM et al (1996) Laparoscopic-assisted intestinal resection for Crohn's disease. J Clin Gastroenterol 23:44–46
20. Oliveira L, Reissman P, Nogueras J et al (1997) Laparoscopic creation of stomas. Surg Endosc 11:19–23

Postoperative Prevention of Relapse in Crohn's Disease

Anil Keshava, David C.C. Bartolo

Introduction

Crohn's disease (CD) is a chronic inflammatory bowel disease with no known cure. Since its first description, its nature has remained relapsing [1], and continues to be a clinical challenge due to the variability of its presentation and complex pathophysiology. Its prevalence is affected by the distance from the equator and its incidence has slowly increased. [2]. Crohn's disease has an incidence of 2–5/1 000, and causes significant morbidity and health care expense for Western countries [3].

One unanswered dilemma in the management of patients with CD, is the role of treatment in the postoperative period. When followed up long-term, more than three quarters of patients with CD will require surgery [4] Postoperatively, disease recurrence is common and a high proportion of those patients will require reoperation [3–5]. Despite the availability of newer therapies and the fact that up to 57% of patients may require further surgery within 10 years, there is a lack of evidence to show that medical therapy can reduce relapse.

Research into the maintenance of remission has been hampered by many factors. Firstly, there is not a universal definition for disease recurrence, and although there are studies reporting on histological, clinical, radiological and endoscopic criteria in an effort to define recurrence, their correlation is often imperfect [6–8]. Secondly, validated CD assessment tools are often not appropriate for use in the postoperative period. Thirdly, disease incidence can vary due to the geography of large units around the world and also differing patient-care pathways, and finally animal models in examining the postoperative period can be labour intensive and expensive and therefore often not feasible [4].

The purpose of this chapter is to review the literature on the various influences on the postoperative recurrence of CD.

Surgery for Crohn's Disease

Surgical intervention is required for CD for urgent and elective reasons. Surgical emergencies such as bleeding, perforation and obstruction can be life threatening whilst elective situations are required for failure of medical therapy, fistulous disease and strictures. The Cleveland clinic foundation followed 615 patients from the time of diagnosis for a mean of 13 years and found that 438 (71%) required intestinal surgery [9]. In this study, those with ileocolonic disease had a cumulative probability of resection of 91.5% after a mean of 13 years compared to 66% of patients with CD limited to the small intestine and 58% of patients with only colonic disease [10].

Postoperative Recurrence

Recurrence of CD is extremely common and usually occurs proximal to the site of the surgical anastomosis [4]. Endoscopic recurrence has been shown to occur in 73% at 1 year and in 85 % at 3 years. Clinical relapse rates, however, were only 20 and 34% respectively [11]. Similarly, evidence of histological recurrence has not been shown to correlate with clinical recurrence nor has early endoscopic recurrence with the need for later surgical intervention [12].

The most pertinent clinical outcome in the postoperative period is the requirement for reoperation. The need for surgical reintervention follows a similar prevalence relating to the site of disease and mirrors that for the first operation. Thus, ileocolic disease at 53% is generally associated with higher rates of reoperation than isolated colonic (45%) or small bowel disease (44%) [10]. In the National Cooperative Crohn's Disease Study, more than 70% of patients who underwent resection for ileocolitis required a second intervention within 15 years, and the median time to reoperation was between 5 and 10 years [6]. Stricturing jejunoileal disease is much less common but is recognized as having the highest relapse rates [13, 14]

Risk Factors for Crohn's Disease Recurrence

Numerous factors have been studied to see if they can predict disease recurrence. In a retrospective analysis of 1 379 patients, Michalessi et al. identified the number of intestinal sites involved as an independent risk factor associated with reoperation, and re-operation also seems to be more likely with a greater extent of preoperative disease.[13, 14]. Other studies have shown that factors such as smoking, the presence of granulomas and perianal disease are predictors of disease recurrence [15–17].

Surgical Technique

With the growing knowledge of the recurrent nature of CD, surgical treatment has evolved with the goal of preserving as much bowel length as possible. The application of a "bowel-sparing policy", in which only grossly diseased tissue was resected, was found to be reasonable in CD colitis as well as ileitis [18]. In small bowel stricturing disease, the technique of strictureplasty is preferred to resection and it has been shown not to impact on recurrence or postoperative complications [19, 20].

The effect of the anastomotic technique and CD recurrence has been studied. Clinical studies have had variable results. Retrospective studies have shown lower recurrence rates in both stapled and hand-sewn anastomoses when compared with one another [21, 22]. One non-randomised prospective study found a lower rate of recurrence in patients with stapled anastomoses [23]. As there is no randomised trial of anastomotic technique, at present there is no conclusive evidence that one anastomotic technique is superior to another.

Medical Prophylaxis Against Postoperative Recurrence

5-Aminosalicylate

Sulfasalazine was the agent used in most of the early trials of 5-aminosalicylate (5-ASA) for maintenance of surgically induced remission in CD. Since then, trials have included other preparations in which the active agent is 5-ASA. In the past 10 years, these 5 ASA preparations have been more frequently used as they are better tolerated than sulfasalazine. The earlier data on sulfasalazine when pooled, suggested a slight improvement in 1-year relapse rates, which was statistically significant [4].

Several studies have now examined other 5-ASA-containing preparations for medical prophylaxis against postoperative recurrence. The largest was conducted as part of the European Cooperative Crohn's Disease Study [25]. A total of 318 postoperative patients were randomized to receive mesalamine (Pentasa; 4 g/day) or placebo, and were followed for 18 months. Clinical recurrence occurred in 24.5% of treated patients and 31.4% in the placebo group. This trend was not statistically significant (P=0.10) in the group as a whole but was significant in those patients with isolated small-bowel disease.

Another randomized controlled trial of mesalamine in this setting compared 163 patients randomized to mesalamine (3 g/day) or placebo. They found a risk ratio for recurrence of 0.628 favouring the treated group and, strangely, found the greatest treatment effect in patients with isolated colonic disease [26]. More recently, a RCT evaluated mesalamine at a dose of 4 g/day compared with a dose of 2.4 g/day and found no difference in rates of clinical recurrence at 12 months [27]. Another recent randomized controlled trial, designed primarily for the evaluation of 6-mercaptopurine, evaluated mesalamine compared with 6-mercaptopurine or placebo, but did not show any significant difference between groups in terms of clinical recurrence at 2 years after surgery [28]. A meta-analysis of all randomized trials fully published up until 1997 suggested that mesalamine decreases the risk of postoperative recurrence by approximately 13% [29].

The main benefits appear to be for prevention of colonic disease site recurrence, whereas following ileocecal resection, the benefits appear to be minimal. Definite conclusions cannot be drawn as different studies used different preparations with varying regimens. Overall, the beneficial effect of mesalamine is likely to be small.

Steroids

Corticosteroids have no benefit as a maintenance therapy [31]. Over the past 10 years, a newer steroid, budesonide, which showed several features that made it particularly suitable for study as a long-term anti-inflammatory agent in Crohn's disease, has generated interest. It has a high first-pass hepatic metabolism and high steroid receptor affinity. Controlled release preparations were developed that delivered high ileal concentrations of the drug taken orally to produce considerable topical anti-inflammatory activity with a decreased systemic effect [31].

The theoretical benefits of budesonide seem to be at a dose of 6 mg or greater for those who underwent resection for active ileocecal disease rather than fibro-stenotic disease. Despite this, a recent RCT has shown no benefit of therapy. In summary, corticosteroid use is not indicated for postoperative patients to prevent recurrence.

Antibiotics

Antibiotics have been widely used in the treatment of active CD, but only two randomized controlled trials are available to support their use for maintenance of postoperative remission. Rutgeerts et al. assigned postoperative patients to 20 mg/kg per day of metronidazole for a total of 12 weeks. One-year recurrence rates were 25% for the placebo group and only 4% for the treated group, a difference that was statistically significant. After 3 years, however, the endoscopic recurrence rates were the same between the two groups, and clinical recurrence rates showed only a non-significant trend favouring therapy [33].

In a second study by Rutgeerts et al. assessing the use of nitroimidazole antibiotics in this setting, 80 postoperative patients were randomized to placebo or ornidazole 500 mg (Tiberal; Roche, Basel, Switzerland) twice daily for 1 year. The primary endpoint was clinical recurrence 1 year after surgery. A significantly lower rate was found in the treated group compared to those receiving placebo (37.5% *vs.* 7.9%). Ornidazole was used because it was thought to have side effects which were similar to those of metronidazole, but of a lesser severity. Unfortunately, in this study, more than 30% of patients in the ornidazole group dropped out as a result of side effects, the most common being nausea, vomiting, and metallic taste. This is also a major problem with long-term use of metronidazole [34].

These two well-designed studies support the effectiveness of nitroimidazole antibiotics in the maintenance of surgically induced remission of CD, however, there is a lack of clarity with regards to the dosing and duration of therapy given the significant side-effect profile.

Immunomodulators

Although immunosuppressive drugs such as azathioprine (AZA) have been shown to be effective in preventing relapse after medically induced remission, there remains little data available for prevention of postoperative recurrence [35]. Recent studies have suggested possible benefits from immunomodulation. Hanauer et al. assessed 131 postoperative patients randomized to either placebo, mesalamine 3 g/day, or 6-MP 50 mg/day and followed for 2 years. Rates of endoscopic and clinical recurrence at multiple time-points were assessed and generally showed non-significant trends favouring 6-MP. For example, clinical recurrence rates at 2 years were 77% for placebo, 58% for mesalamine, and 50% for 6-MP. The 95% confidence intervals overlapped for all groups, but further analysis showed a difference between 6-MP and placebo (P=0.045). The authors felt the study showed the efficacy of 6-MP compared with placebo. It should also be noted that the dose of 6-MP they used was relatively low compared with doses known to be effective in other clinical settings [38].

The second study, by Ardizzone et al. compared AZA at a dose of 2 mg/kg per day to mesalamine or placebo in an unblinded, prospective randomized study of 142 patients lasting 2 years. Two-year clinical recurrence rates were 28% for mesalamine and 17% for AZA, a difference that did not reach statistical significance but showed a beneficial trend towards immunomodulation [39].

A retrospective analysis published in 2001 in France examined 38 patients who were treated with azathioprine between 1987 and 1996 to prevent postoperative CD [37]. The median duration of postoperative follow-up was 29 months. Probabilities of clinical recurrence were 9, 16 and 28% at 1, 2 and 3 years, respectively. The authors concluded that in patients treated with AZA, the rate of postoperative endoscopic recurrence was lower than that previously reported in untreated patients.

In summary, the few trials conducted on the role of immunomodulation tend to support the maintenance efficacy of AZA or 6-MP in the postoperative setting. Because of the stronger evidence supporting the use of AZA or 6-MP in the setting of medically induced remission, even authors highly critical of the existing data acknowledge that the use of thiopurines is likely warranted in high-risk postoperative patients [40].

Blood Transfusion

Blood transfusion has been known to have an important immunosuppressive effect in certain settings and this led this led to the hypothesis that perioperative blood transfusion might decrease the later possibility of relapse after resection. When data from numerous trials are combined, this theoretical benefit has not been shown [24].

Probiotics

The role of intestinal bacteria in the pathophysiology of CD has led to the use of beneficial enteric bacteria as therapeutic agents. This area requires further study and may prove beneficial in the postoperative use for CD.

Conclusion

The goal of reducing recurrence after surgery for Crohn's disease is a challenging one. Despite numerous studies, we do not have conclusive evidence of predictors of recurrence; however, data on the risks associated with smoking, particularly in females, have accumulated and it is appropriate to advise patients that smoking increases the risk not only of developing Crohn's disease but also of disease recurrence.

Recent studies suggest that 5-ASA confers only a small benefit at doses between 2.4 and 3 g/day in patients undergoing ileocolic resection; the long-term role of this drug is uncertain. The oral steroid budesonide shows some promise in preventing the development of new lesions. Its side-effect profile makes it a candidate for further study but, as yet, there is no firm evidence of its worth in standard preventive management regimens.

We feel that RCTs need to be conducted to examine the role of immunomodulator therapy. The limited data available suggests a small therapeutic benefit for this class of drug and further studies are required to validate this.

References

1. Crohn BB, Ginzburg L, Oppenheimer GD (1932) Regional ileitis: a pathologic and clinical entity. JAMA 99:1323–1329
2. Sonnenberg A, McCarty DJ, Jacobsen SJ (1991) Geographic variation of inflammatory bowel disease within the United States. Gastroenterology 100:143–149
3. Wolters FL, Russel MG, Stockbrugger RW (2004) Systematic review: has disease outcome in Crohn's disease changed during the last four decades? Aliment Pharmacol Ther 20:483–496
4. Penner R, Madsen K Fedorak R (2005) Postoperative Crohn's disease. Inflamm Bowel Dis 11:765–777
5. Cuillerier E, Lemann M, Bouhnik Y et al (2001) Azathioprine for prevention of postoperative recurrence in Crohn's disease: a retrospective study. Eur Gastroenterol Hepatol 13:1291–1296
6. Mekhjian HS, Switz DM, Watts HD et al (1979) National Cooperative Crohn's Disease Study: factors determining recurrence of Crohn's disease after surgery. Gastroenterology 77:907–913
7. Kotanagi H, Kramer K, Fazio VW et al (1991) Do microscopic abnormalities at resection margins correlate with increased anastomotic recurrence in Crohn's disease? Retrospective analysis of 100 cases. Dis Colon Rectum 34:909–916
8. McLeod RS, Wolff BG, Steinhart AH et al (1997) Risk and significance of endoscopic/radiological evidence of recurrent Crohn's disease. Gastroenterology 113:1823–1827
9. Whelan G, Farmer RG, Fazio VW et al (1985) Recurrence after surgery in Crohn's disease. Relationship to location of disease (clinical pattern) and surgical indication. Gastroenterology 88:1826–1833
10. Farmer RG, Whelan G, Fazio VW (1985) Long-term follow-up of patients with Crohn's disease: relationship between the clinical pattern and prognosis. Gastroenterology 88:1818–1825
11. Rutgeerts P, Geboes K, Vantrappen G et al (1990) Predictability of the postoperative course of Crohn's disease. Gastroenterology 99:956–963
12. De Jong E, van Dullemen HM, Slors JF et al (1996) Correlation between early recurrence and reoperation after ileocolonic resection in Crohn's disease: a prospective study. J Am Coll Surg 182:503–508
13. Michelassi F, Balestracci T, Chappell R et al (1991) Primary and recurrent Crohn's disease: experience with 1379 patients. Ann Surg 214:230–240
14. Bernell O, Lapidus A, Hellers G (2000) Risk factors for surgery and postoperative recurrence in Crohn's disease. Ann Surg 231:38–45
15. Ryan WR, Allan RN, Yamamoto T et al (2004) Crohn's disease patients who quit smoking have a reduced risk of reoperation for recurrence. Am J Surg 187:219–225
16. Anseline PF, Wlodarczyk J, Murugasu R (1997) Presence of granulomas is associated with recurrence after surgery for Crohn's disease: experience of a surgical unit. Br J Surg 84:78–82
17. Greenway SE, Buckmire MA, Marroquin C et al (1999) Clinical subtypes of Crohn's disease according to surgical outcome. J Gastrointest Surg 3:145–151
18. Fazio VW, Marchetti F, Church M et al (1996) Effect of resection margins on the recurrence of Crohn's disease in the small bowel: a randomized controlled trial. Ann Surg 224:563–557
19. Dietz DW, Laureti S, Strong SA et al (2001) Safety and long-term efficacy of strictureplasty in 314 patients with obstructing small-bowel Crohn's disease. J Am Coll Surg 192:330–338
20. Yamamoto T, Bain IM, Allan RN et al (1999) An audit of strictureplasty for small-bowel Crohn's disease. Dis Colon Rectum 42:797–803
21. Munoz-Juarez M, Yamamoto T, Wolff BG et al (2001) Wide-lumen stapled anastomosis vs. conventional end-to-end anastomosis in the treatment of Crohn's disease. Dis Colon Rectum 44:20–26
22. Kusunoki M, Ikeuchi H, Yanagi H et al (1998) A comparison of stapled and hand-sewn anastomoses in Crohn's disease. Dig Surg 15:679–682
23. Tersigni R, Alessandroni L, Barreca M et al (2003) Does stapled functional end-to-end anastomosis affect recurrence of Crohn's disease after ileocolonic resection? Hepatogastroenterology 50:1422–1425
24. Hollaar GL, Gooszen HG, Post S et al (1995) Perioperative blood transfusion does not prevent recurrence in Crohn's disease: a pooled analysis. J Clin Gastroenterol 21:134–138
25. Lochs H, Mayer M, Fleig WE et al (2000) Prophylaxis of postoperative relapse in Crohn's disease with mesalamine: European Cooperative Crohn's Disease Study VI. Gastroenterology 118:264–273
26. McLeod RS, Wolff BG, Steinhart AH et al (1995) Prophylactic mesalamine treatment decreases postoperative recurrence of Crohn's disease. Gastroenterology 109:404–413

27. Caprilli R, Cottone M, Tonelli F et al (2003) Two mesalazine regimens in the prevention of the postoperative recurrence of Crohn's disease: a pragmatic, double-blind randomized controlled trial. Aliment Pharmacol Ther 17:517–523
28. Hanauer SB, Korelitz BI, Rutgeerts P et al (2004) Postoperative maintenance of Crohn's disease remission with 6-mercaptopurine, mesalamine, or placebo: a 2-year trial. Gastroenterology 127:723–729
29. Camma C, Giunta M, Rosselli M et al (1997) Mesalamine in the maintenance treatment of Crohn's disease: a meta-analysis adjusted for confounding variables. Gastroenterology 113:1465–1473
30. Steinhart AH, Ewe K, Griffiths AM et al (2003) Corticosteroids for maintenance of remission in Crohn's disease. Cochrane Database Syst Rev 4:CD000301
31. Brattsand R (1990) Overview of newer glucocorticoid preparations for inflammatory bowel disease. Can J Gastroenterol 4:407–414
32. Hellers G, Cortot A, Jewell D et al (1999) Oral budesonide for prevention of postsurgical recurrence in Crohn's disease: the IOIBD Budesonide Study Group. Gastroenterology 116:294–300
33. Rutgeerts P, Hiele M, Geboes K et al (1995) Controlled trial of metronidazole treatment for prevention of Crohn's recurrence after ileal resection. Gastroenterology 108:1617–1621
34. Rutgeerts P, Van Assche G, Vermeire S et al (2005) Ornidazole for prophylaxis of postoperative Crohn's disease recurrence: a randomized, double-blind, placebo-controlled trial. Gastroenterology 128:856–861
35. Pearson DC, May GR, Fick G et al (2000) Azathioprine for maintaining remission of Crohn's disease. Cochrane Database Syst Rev 2:CD000067
36. Domenech E, Scala L, Bernal I et al (2004) Azathioprine and mesalazine in the prevention of postsurgical recurrence of Crohn's disease: a retrospective study. Gastroenterol Hepatol 27:563–567
37. Cuillerier E, Lemann M, Bouhnik Y et al (2001) Azathioprine for prevention of postoperative recurrence in Crohn's disease: a retrospective study. Eur J Gastroenterol Hepatol 13:1291–1296
38. Hanauer SB, Korelitz BI, Rutgeerts P et al (2004) Postoperative maintenance of Crohn's disease remission with 6-mercaptopurine, mesalamine, or placebo: a 2-year trial. Gastroenterology 127:723–729
39. Ardizzone S, Maconi G, Sampietro GM et al (2004) Azathioprine and mesalamine for prevention of relapse after conservative surgery for Crohn's disease. Gastroenterology 127:730–740
40. Sandborn WJ, Feagan BG (2004) The efficacy of azathioprine and 6-mercaptopurine for the prevention of postoperative recurrence in patients with Crohn's disease remains uncertain. Gastroenterology 127:990–993

Surgical Treatment of Perineal Crohn's Disease

Bruno Roche, Joan Robert-Yap

Introduction

Crohn's disease, a chronic inflammatory condition, may involve the entire alimentary tract from the mouth to the anus. The three major locations of the disease are:

1. Ileocolic (41–55% of cases).
2. Small bowel (30–40%).
3. Colon (14–26%) [1].

Perianal or anorectal Crohn's disease affects the patient as a primary feature with a prevalence of 8–90%. Approximately one in three patients are afflicted [2–5] and it is rarely the only site of disease. The prevalence of perianal disease has been found to be greater in blacks than in whites [2]. More than 50% of patients with colon involvement will have anal complications, whereas less than 20% of patients with small-bowel disease will develop anal symptoms [6].

Clinical Presentation

Most patients with Crohn's disease present with weight loss, abdominal pain and diarrhoea. An isolated anal lesion is the first manifestation in 5% of patients. Most will develop intestinal symptoms, sometimes many years later [1]. The spectrum of anal complaints is great. Fissures and oedematous skin tags are most common. In the general population most anal fissures are located in the posterior midline. In patients with Crohn's disease, fissures may occur eccentrically. They are deep, indolent and rarely painful unless an abscess is present. Skin tags are usually asymptomatic, but if they become painful or interfere with anal hygiene, they can be excised. They also are an excellent source for biopsy specimens for the presence of granulomata. Other common clinical manifestations include anal stricture, ulceration, complex fistulae, abscesses and finally faecal incontinence. Haemorrhoids are not a common feature of anal Crohn's disease. Management of these varied clinical manifestations is discussed.

Diagnosis

Physical and rectal examinations are often sufficient for diagnosing and staging most perianal conditions in patients with Crohn's disease. Some patients must be examined under general anaesthesia, especially if perianal suppuration and tenderness are present. In addition, examination under general anaesthesia is considered an extension of the physical examination in patients with painful anorectal disease. For more complex presentations, additional modalities are needed including CT scanning with rectal contrast, endorectal sonography, endoscopies and MR imaging. Each test has specific advantages as already described in a previous chapter.

Endorectal ultrasonography is the easiest test for detection of abscesses and fistulae. Anal-wall thickness may be measured as an indicator of disease activity [4]. MR imaging greatly facilitates the detection of fistulous tracts that extend into the supralevator space. Rectal-wall thickening and perirectal inflammation are clearly shown [7]. In a prospective study from St. Mark's Hospital in which 35 patients with fistula-in-ano were evaluated by examination under anaesthesia and MR imaging, four patients had occult fistulae identified on MR imaging that were not seen during the physical examination [8]. Overall, studies suggest that 4–9% of cases may benefit from the increased diagnostic accuracy offered by MR imaging [9].

Treatment

Many patients with anorectal Crohn's disease present other intestinal locations of the disease, requiring an evaluation of the colon and small bowel. The presence of proximal disease poses a therapeutic dilemma: early reports suggest that perianal conditions persist in the presence of proximal disease and improve only if proximal disease is resected [10, 11]; however, other reports refute these findings and show no improvement in perianal disease after treatment of proximal disease [12].

Thus, the proximal intestinal tract should be evaluated but does not necessarily require surgery before treatment of perianal manifestations unless they are symptomatic. Surgical management of the perianal area is a challenge. Historically, surgeons were reluctant to perform surgery because of delayed wound healing and the risk of compromising sphincter competence. Alexander-Williams expressed a prevailing sentiment in 1974: "Faecal incontinence is the result of aggressive surgeons and not progressive disease." Advocates of this non-invasive approach, which included medicinal and hygienic management, considered that aggressive surgical procedures only created more complex problems [13, 14].

In the late eighties, investigators found that a more aggressive but still limited surgical approach to perianal disease was possible [15, 16]. Two resolutions were adopted:

1. the management of a septic focus is an indication for surgery.
2. The sphincter should be preserved if a patient is continent [15].

One multicentre study reviewing treatment of patients with perianal Crohn's disease shows medical treatment to be curative in only a few patients, whereas surgical procedures were curative in more than half of the patients [17]. A role for both approaches exists and success is attributed to careful patient selection, limited surgical intervention, and improved perioperative medical management [18, 19].

Specific Clinical Manifestations

Abscess

Infection may spread and seek the path of least resistance (Fig. 1). It may extend downwards into the intersphincteric space resulting in a perianal abscess (A), upwards inside the longitudinal muscle layer within the gut wall causing an intermuscular abscess, or upwards outside the gut wall resulting in a supralevator abscess (E). It may spread across the external sphincter (B) at any level resulting in an ischiorectal abscess which may also extend upwards or downwards (C). Furthermore, circumferential spread is possible at any level within the intersphincteric space, the ischiorectal space or the supralevator space. It may extend from one ischiorectal fossa to the contra lateral one via the intersphincteric space of Courtney or deep postanal space [20] resulting in a so-called horseshoe abscess.

The main symptoms of an abscess are discomfort, perianal pain and swelling. The symptoms develop more or less rapidly within hours or days. The clinical presentation can include swelling, tenderness, induration at palpation, asymmetry of the buttocks, redness, superficial cellulitis, or even gangrenous skin. Inguinal lymph nodes may be enlarged. Systemic symptoms such as fever, chills, malaise, and tachycardia occur more frequently with high or deep abscesses than with more superficial ones. Only a careful rectal examination reveals the development of a high anorectal abscess.

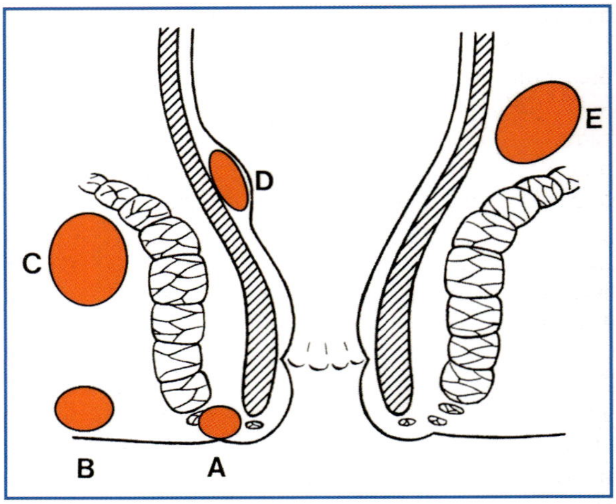

Fig. 1. Location of the abscess in the perineal spaces: **A**, perianal abscess (intersphincteric). **B**, perianal abscess (transsphincteric). **C**, ischiorectal abscess. **D**, submucosal or high intramuscular abscess. **E**, supralevator abscess (pelvirectal)

Treatment of Anorectal Suppuration

To treat anorectal abscesses, some guidelines must be followed. Spontaneous healing and complete resolution of perianal cellulitis is very rare and should not be expected. Broad-spectrum antibiotics without drainage delay the need for surgery and create more complex lesions. Microbiological investigations may be useful for obtaining evidence of some specific infection or of an anal venereal disease. Incision should not be delayed and should allow optimal drainage without pocketing. A lay-open or one-stage operation should not be performed in cases of Crohn's disease.

Surgical Treatment of Superficial Abscesses

A superficial abscess can almost always be drained under local anaesthesia in the office. The skin must not be shaved but disinfected with antiseptics; lidocaine with epinephrine 0.5% mixed with 10% sodium bicarbonate 8.4 mEq are injected intradermally at the level of the most tender point. The incision must be radial and long enough to allow free drainage of the pus. Packing to control bleeding should be reduced to a minimum as it interferes with drainage.

Surgical Treatment of Ischiorectal Abscesses and Pelvirectal Abscesses

These lesions are too deep to be treated under local anaesthesia; therefore caudal, loco-regional or general anaesthesia is required. A radial incision is made in the perianal tissue and continued into the ischiorectal space. If the internal opening is clearly identified and if the underlying fistulous tract may be catheterised easily, a seton drainage should be placed. A probe should never be introduced forcefully to avoid creation of a false tract. After gentle curettage, the wounds are loosely packed with a mesh dressing for 24-48 h. A perianal fistula with a pelvic abscess extending from the anal canal should never be drained into the rectum as it could result in an extra-sphincteric fistula which is a much more complex problem to treat.

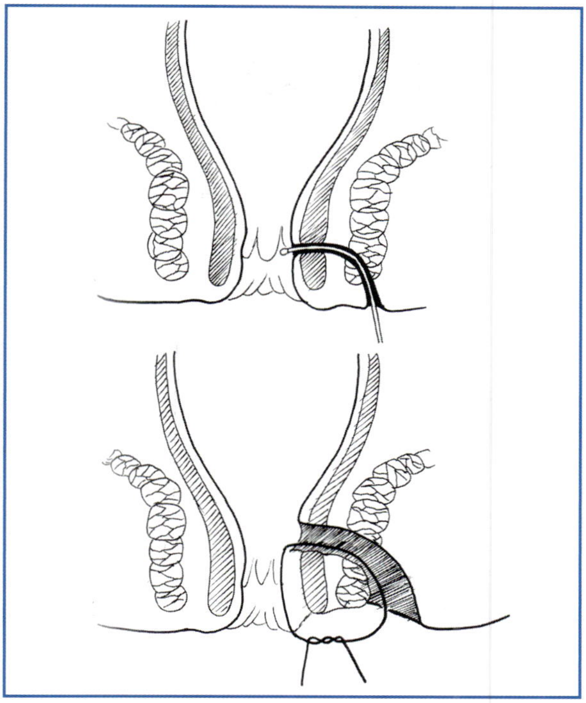

Fig. 2. Seton drainage. *Superior*: introduction of a probe in the fistula tract. *Inferior*: two nylon stitches 4/0 are tied separately

Are Antibiotics Necessary?

As antibiotics do not remove the cause of anorectal infection, they have very little place in the management of anorectal abscesses. They are useful in cases of extensive cellulitis to prevent bacteriologic dissemination due to the surgical procedure. They must be given if the patient is diabetic, immunosuppressed, suffering from valvular lesions of the heart, or wearing prosthetic material. They should also be prescribed in cases of specific infection.

One or Two-Stage Operation: the Value of Seton Drainage

After the abscess is incised and drained as previously described, the fistulous tract should be drained using a seton drainage [21]. Two or three 4-0 or 5-0 non-absorbable monofilament sutures are placed from the incision of the abscess along the tract to the primary orifice (Fig. 2). They are then tied separately and loosely without tension to avoid pain and skin damage. The seton will allow drainage and promote fibrosis around the fistulous tract. In cases of Crohn's disease, setons can be used for months or years. The prevalence of abscesses in patients with perianal Crohn's disease is approximately 50% [5, 22, 23]. Abscesses in these patients may be complex and multiple requiring complementary investigations such as sonography and/or MR Imaging.

The cause of Crohn's abscesses (Fig. 3) is not completely understood. Following Park's theory, which states that an infection begins in the anal gland in the intersphincteric space and all other tracts and collections are secondary [24, 25], many investigators believe that Crohn's abscesses are no different than crypto glandular abscesses. Other investigators believe that the abscess is secondary to a cavitating ulcer that penetrates the anorectal wall, spreading sepsis to the perirectal tissue [7]. This distinction may not affect treatment. Abscesses must be drained urgently to prevent spread into adjacent tissue.

Fissure or Ulcers

Anal fissures in perineal Crohn's disease are classically deep, indolent, relatively painless and eccentrically located (Fig. 4) but most Crohn's related fissures are in the midline.

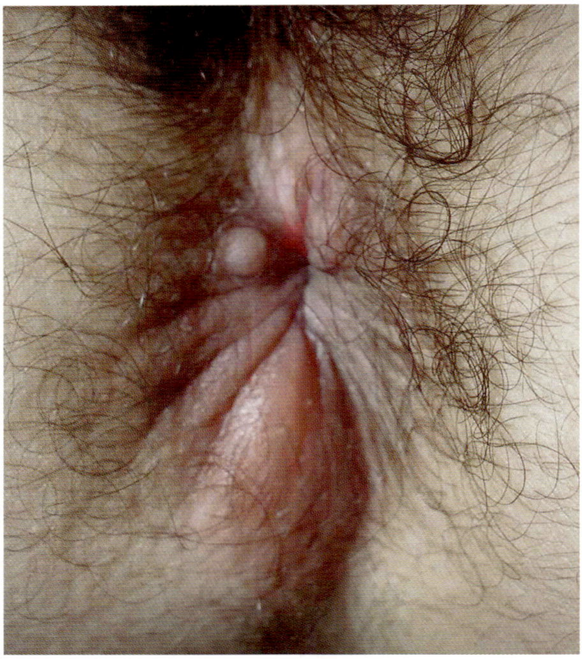

Fig. 3. Abscess in perineal Crohn's disease

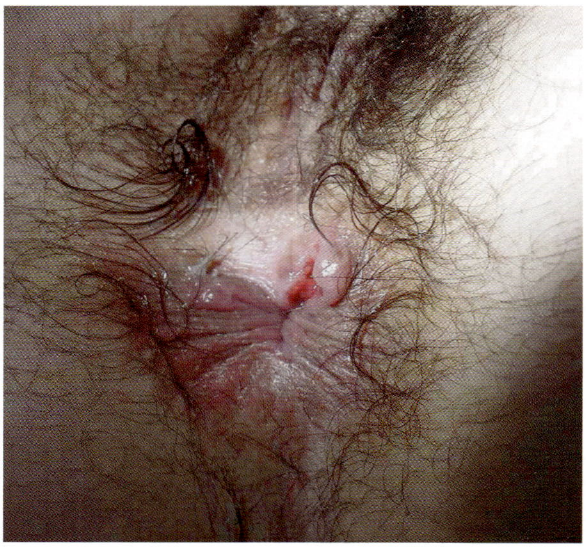

Fig. 4. Ulceration located at 1 o'clock lithotomy position with granulation tissue

Crohn's Disease Fissure

If a midline fissure appears abnormal or fails to heal with conventional therapy, Crohn's disease should be suspected [26]. Spontaneous healing is observed in 80% of patients with Crohn's fissures followed for 10 years [12]. For this reason, the majority of the fissures may be treated medically. The Lahey Clinic found that only 15% of 56 patients with fissures required surgical treatment, despite 88% presenting with symptoms [27]. A painful fissure is generally associated with an underlying abscess and may require an examination of the patient under general anaesthesia. If an abscess is found, simple drainage as described in the previous paragraph can provide relief without incontinence [25]. If no abscess is found, medical management is appropriate, using local agents such as topical glyceryl nitrate or isosorbide dinitrate, nifedipine or symptomatic measures such as topical steroids or anaesthetic creams. In cases of persistent pain, the fissure may be treated as a classical anal fissure with careful internal sphincterotomy which may provide relief. The Ferguson Clinic reported healing without incontinence in 22 of 25 patients treated for anal fissure by internal sphincterotomy with a rectum free of disease and an anal fissure as presentation [28]. In the Lahey Clinic experience, internal sphincterotomy was successful in 87% of patients without proximal disease, compared to a 42% healing rate if the proximal intestine was involved [27]. Anal dilatation has not been successful and is discouraged as therapy. Some Crohn's ulcers may be large and acute with erosion into the sphincters compromising the continence. Intralesional injection of steroids may be effective if the ulcer is not too extensive. The natural evolution of these fissures and ulcerations result in strictures of the anal canal. Unfortunately, many of these patients will eventually require a proctectomy.

Anorectal Stricture

Chronic anorectal abscesses, fistulae, ulcers or inflammation may lead to an anorectal stricture. Three varieties have been described:

1. Short, annular strictures less than 2 cm in length, resulting in diaphragmatic deformity.
2. Longer, tubular strictures.
3. Strictures secondary to "dysfunction" atrophy.

In a series of 44 patients, Linares et al. [29] reported approximately 50% of the strictures as being located in the rectum, 33% in the anus, and the remainder in the anorectum. They also found that most of these patients had coexisting proctitis or perianal disease. The majority of strictures are asymptomatic or well tolerated. If they become symptomatic, they may be incapacitating because of urgency, incontinence, tenesmus and difficulty with defecation. Mild disease may respond to medical treatment such as topical steroids, 5-aminosalicylic

Table 1. Stoma and proctectomy rate in Crohn's disease

Reference	No. of patients	No. of operations	Stoma rate	Proctectomy
Shivananda et al. (1989) [44]	210	118 (56%)	15 (7%)	18 (15%)
Harper and Fazio (1987) [45]		139	65 (47%)	44 (32%)
Allan and Keighley (1988) [46]	171	171	-61 (36%)	20 (12%)
Galandiuk et al (2005) [42]	356	344	65 (47%)	44 (32%)

acid or systemic metronidazole. Non-invasive surgical management using gentle dilatation may be successful, particularly in cases of short diaphragmatic lesions. Repeat dilatations may be necessary until disease remission. Most symptomatic strictures are not cured with simple dilatation and may require faecal diversion or proctectomy [29, 30].

Anal Skin Tags and Haemorrhoids

Anal skin tags are typically asymptomatic and present problems only when they interfere with perianal hygiene (Fig. 5). They are more prominent with active intestinal disease. Approximately 25% resolve spontaneously, generally after remission of concomitant bowel disease. These tags should not be removed because that may result in an unhealed wound, a chronic ulcer or perianal sepsis [22]. Exceptions to this are in cases of severe haemorrhage or suspected malignancy.

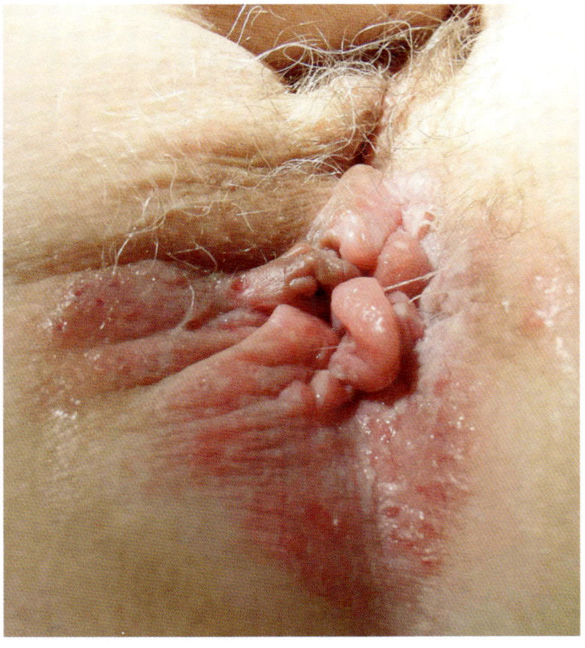

Fig. 5. Anal tags with ulceration and tissue inflammation

Haemorrhoids are uncommon in patients with Crohn's disease. They usually become symptomatic when accompanied by diarrhoea. Conservative treatment must include control of bowel function, warm sitz-baths, and topical medications. Usually these non-invasive measures are successful. If symptoms persist, rubber-band ligation might be helpful. In rare cases, if symptoms are severe, and the rectum is spared from illness, selective surgical haemorrhoidectomy may be successful [28].

Most surgeons believe that surgery should be avoided in the treatment of haemorrhoid diseases in Crohn's patients. In a publication, Jeffery et al [31] reported the results of 21 patients with Crohn's disease presenting with active haemorrhoids that were treated surgically. Postsurgical complications, including sepsis, strictures, fistulae and unhealed wounds, occurred in ten patients, and six patients ultimately required a proctectomy.

Incontinence

Faecal incontinence in patients with perianal Crohn's disease is common, occurring in 39% of patients [32]. Management of this condition is challenging because the cause is often multifactorial. The incontinence may be secondary to severe perineal Crohn's disease associated with chronic fibrosis and scarring of the anorectum resulting in loss of reservoir function. In this situation, faecal diversion or proctectomy is indicated. If the patient suffers from severe Crohn's-related muscle destruction, a colostomy is indicated. Diarrhoea from colonic disease or short-bowel syndrome also may lead to incontinence and may require a colostomy if diarrhoea and stool consistency cannot be controlled.

On the other hand, incontinence may be unrelated to Crohn's disease and may be caused by obstetric injury or an overly aggressive surgery such as fistulotomy. The cause may become evident based on medical history and physical examination. Complementary examinations such as anal manometry, electromyography, and transrectal ultrasonography will help in the choice of treatment. Some of these patients may benefit from sphincter repair when the Crohn's disease is in remission. Scott et al. [33] successfully treated five of six patients with this type of surgery. Keighley and Williams [34] reported a 100% success rate in eight patients who underwent sphincter repair. In all of these patients, a proximal covering stoma was used.

Anorectal Cancer

The risk for squamous-cell carcinoma of the anus is not increased in patients with perianal Crohn's disease [15, 35]. The presence of inflammation may delay the diagnosis of cancer, so in any patients with persistent perineal ulcers or fissures that fail to heal, a biopsy of the lesion should be considered. An association exists between colorectal cancer and Crohn's disease. [36]. A long duration of illness and the presence of chronic perianal disease may increase the risk for rectal malignancy [15, 37–39]. The risk for colorectal cancer is not confined just to areas of inflammation; in addition the risk for rectal cancer may be increased if the rectum has been excluded from intestinal flow or placed out of intestinal continuity. This is similar to the increased cancer risk in bypassed segments of small bowel [38, 40]. Lavery and Jagelman [41] identified two cases of cancer that developed in the out-of-circuit rectum after subtotal colectomy and colostomy for Crohn's disease. Because of this risk, such patients require cancer surveillance or proctectomy.

Role for Proctectomy

Devastating perianal complications such as severe recurrent abscesses and fistulae, incontinence and anal stenosis, may lead to proctectomy if local procedures are unsuccessful. Fortunately, less than 20% of patients with a history of anorectal Crohn's disease require permanent diversion and/or proctectomy [5, 42]. It is important to consider that the timing of proctectomy must be dictated by the patient. It is at this point when they believe that all other medical and surgical interventions have been exhausted. Patients need to be psychologically prepared because this surgical procedure creates a permanent and definitive stoma. Proctectomy is the last surgical procedure for perianal Crohn's disease and gives patients the best chance for success. It may be curative in 5% of patients with Crohn's disease localised to this region [43].

Anal Fistulae

M.L. Corman observed that, "More surgeons' reputations have been impugned because of problems with fistula operations than from any other operative procedure" [47]. In general, anal fistulae present symptomatically (Fig. 6). In Crohn's disease, they have the reputation of being difficult to treat with a high rate of recurrence.

Patients are more concerned with postoperative incontinence, even if minor. Many authors advise the most cautious attitude in regards to surgical treatment [12, 18, 22, 47]. Many of these assertions are rooted in the surgical practices of the fifties and sixties and have been accepted without much challenge, particularly in the Anglo-Saxon literature. Anal disease should not be considered simply as a complication of intestinal Crohn's disease. It should be considered, in the same way as terminal ileal and colonic Crohn's disease, as a localisation of the disease to an anatomical site within the gastrointestinal tract. Taking this into account, diverse surgical treatment options can be proposed for the management of anal fistulae in Crohn's disease.

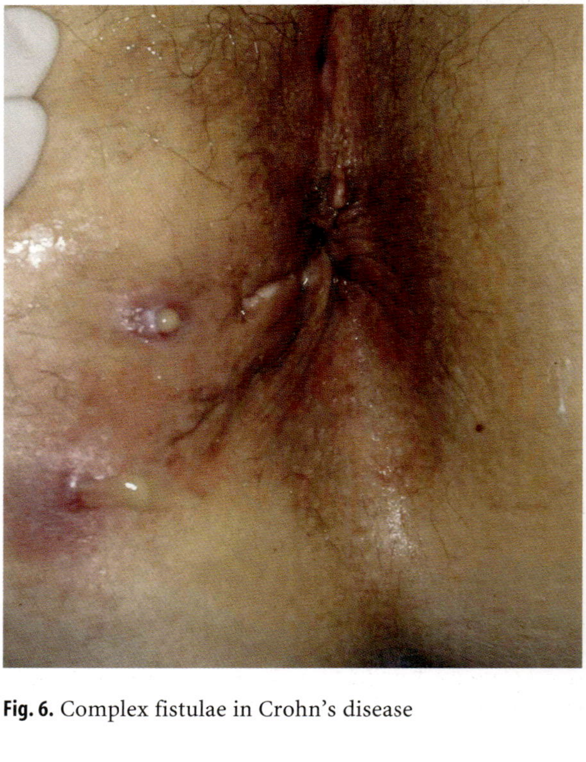

Fig. 6. Complex fistulae in Crohn's disease

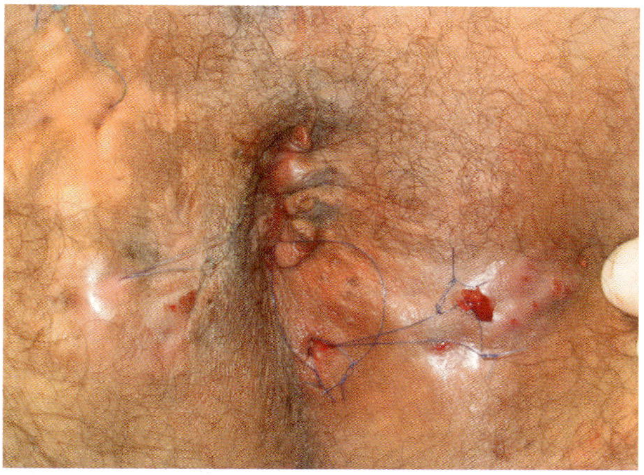

Fig. 7. Crohn's disease fistulae with multiple seton drainage

In the presence of active rectal Crohn's disease, proctitis may complicate the clinical situation and lower the rate of healing. On the other hand, patients with simple fistulae may experience higher rates of improvement and/or healing compared to a complex fistulising disease [48]. Fistulae decrease the quality of life, increase the likelihood of total colectomy and frequently require surgery [49]. Surgery may consist of:

1. Fistulotomy: laying open the fistula tract through a 1 or 2-stage procedure (in case of low fistulae).
2. Non-cutting setons: used in high fistulae involving a significant portion of the external anal sphincter (Fig. 7).
3. Endorectal advancement flap: as an alternative to fistulotomy in patients with low fistulae or an alternative to non-cutting setons in patients with high fistulae who do not have macroscopic evidence of rectal inflammation.

Sanitising the Perineum

Abscesses must be drained and necrotic tissues excised. Any granulation tissue should be curetted, and sinuses must be deroofed. Simple fistulae should be laid open, more complex fistulae should be drained and the primary track marked by a loose seton. The intention is to end up with a healthy surgical wound from which to use as a starting point. Medical treatments are discussed in a previous chapter and are always considered as the first choice in perineal Crohn's disease treatment. In cases of failure or recurrence, new procedures such as local injection of antibody tumour necrotising factor (TNF) or glue sealing treatment are the second option in fistulae treatment. Finally, if none of these therapies are successful, then quite complicated surgical procedures can be attempted with a reasonable chance of healing. All these procedures and the results will be discussed; the sequence is summarised in an algorithm for treatment of perineal Crohn's disease.

Local Injection of Antibody Tumour Necrotising Factor (TNF)

The TNF blocker infliximab has been proven to be safe and effective in the treatment of both luminal and fistulising Crohn's disease, particularly when used as maintenance therapy with infusions at fixed intervals [50, 51]. This treatment is described in the medical treatment chapter. Further advantages of infliximab therapy include the steroid-sparing effect, the decrease in concomitant anti-inflammatory medication use (mesalazine, sulfadiazine), as well as the reduction in hospitalisations and surgeries and the improved quality of life. Some recent pilot studies have reported the potential benefit of local injection of infliximab for the treatment of perianal fistulae in Crohn's disease [52–54]. It seems that this method of administration minimises the adverse effects associated with the systemic use of infliximab [55].

The treatment consists of a three-step procedure:

1. Removal of the seton.
2. Injection of anaesthetic (5 ml of lidocaine 1% mixed with 3 ml of 8.4% bicarbonate solution).
3. Injection of infliximab (20 mg diluted in 10 ml of physiologic solution) along the fistula tract and around both orifices.

These injections are repeated every 4 weeks until complete remission is reached and maintained. Lichtiger reported nine patients with mild to moderate perianal disease refractory to antibiotics, 6-mercaptopurine or systemic infliximab. They were subsequently treated with circumferential and intrafistulae injections of infliximab at 1, 2 and 4 weeks. Within 4 weeks, complete healing of fistulae was observed in 4/9 patients and a partial response in 3/9 patients, whereas no response was observed in the remaining 2 patients [53]. Poggioli et al. [54] modified the technique by injecting infliximab at the internal and external orifices and along the fistula tract in order to allow the closure of the entire tract. Fifteen patients in whom sepsis was not manageable using surgical or medical therapy, were included in the study. Efficacy was obtained in ten of fifteen patients after 3 to 12 injections and no major adverse effects were reported. Local infliximab injection seems to be effective, safe and feasible for the treatment of selected cases of perianal Crohn's disease. This treatment can thus represent an alternative to either medical or surgical therapies.

Glue Sealing Treatment

More recently, fibrin glue injection has also been proposed as an alternative to classical methods of surgical treatment for obtaining long-term healing of Crohn's anal fistulae [56]. The use of fibrin glues in the treatment of fistulae-in-ano has been described over the last 12 years. The results published on this subject report success rates of up to 85% (Table 2) [57, 63]. The series studied in the literature so far have included only a very small number of patients suffering from inflammatory diseases where this type of treatment gives rather poor success rates [58, 60–63]. Several authors have therefore concluded that the existence of a fistula complicating CD is a predictive factor for failure of fibrin glue injection treatment. Vitton et al. included only CD patients with anoperineal fistula tracts in an original study [56]. After a long follow-up period of nearly 2 years, their report shows that more than half (57%) of the 14 patients treated with this method were still asymptomatic. The local fibrin glue injection method has the obvious advantage of avoiding sphincter complications. They concluded that, partly because autologous fibrin glue was used, which seems to be less effective than the heterologous form, the results published to date on this method have not been very encouraging when the patients were suffering from a chronic inflammatory intestinal disease.

One-Stage Fistulotomy and Fistulectomy

Fistulotomy involves the deroofing or the laying open of a fistulous tract along a probe. Fistulectomy means excision of all the fistulous tract, granulation, and dense fibrous tissue, creating larger wounds and a greater separation of the ends of the sphincter, which results in a longer healing time and increased risk of incontinence. Fistulectomy and fistulotomy are easy to perform in cases of perineal, intersphincteric and low trans-sphincteric fistulae. If the fistulous tract crosses the external sphincter, a lay-open technique or fistulotomy results in some sphincter damage, depending on the amount of sphincter which is divided [64, 65].

After excision or incision of a fistulous tract, the wound can be left open for healing by second intention. In some cases, a partial suture at the level of the pectineal line and anoderm may achieve haemostasis, speed up healing time and prevent an anal key-hole deformity. The outer part of the excision is left open to ensure drainage. The wide inter-study variability in success rates of surgery probably depends on the non-homogeneity of the sample of patients treated, but might also depend on the type of fistula treated. Makowiec et al. [66] found the healing rates after surgical treatment of low perianal, transsphincteric and high perianal fistulae to be 64, 40 and 33%, respectively. Moreover, absence of active rectal Crohn's disease decreased the recurrence rate and increased the probability of complete healing. Due to the high incontinence rate and key-hole deformity generated by these procedures, we prefer to use the advancing flap technique in cases of Crohn's perineal fistulae, unless the fistulous tract is quite distal.

Excision and Advancement Flap

When there is a high fistula, the primary tract across the sphincters is excised and an advancement flap is performed. This procedure consists of a conventional fistulectomy, an opening of the intersphincteric space through a partial excision of the internal sphincter, occlusion of the former primary orifice of the fistula and an advancement mucosal flap [67, 68].

Table 2. Use of biological glues in fistulae-in-ano

Reference	N. of patients/ follow-up (months)	Success rate (%)	N. of CD patients	N. of successfully treated CD patients
Hjortrup et al. [57]	23/31	74	0	–
Abel et al. [58]	10/12	60	3	0
Cintron et al. [59]	53/12	64	2	1
Venkatesh and Ramanujam [60]	30/12	60	6	0 but 50% improvement
Patrlj et al. [61]	69/28	74	0	–
Park et al. [62]	29/12	68	2	1
Sentovich [63]	20/10	85	4	3

Technique

The first step consists of coring out the entire fistulous tract from the external to the internal opening (Fig. 8a). The intersphincteric space is curetted. The gap through the external and internal sphincters is closed by separate stitches of absorbable material starting from the anal lumen (Fig. 8c). The mucosa and anoderm, depending on the level of the tract, are excised around the internal opening. A flap of mucosa is undermined (Fig. 8b). The size of the flap must have a base which is twice the width of the apex, but the length should be as short as possible to reduce the risk of ischemia. The flap is sutured to the lower edge of the mucosa (Fig. 8d). The suture line must lie distal to the previous muscle closure. The external wound is left open. If the wound below the pectineal line cannot be totally closed, the flap is sutured to the muscles below the previous opening [69]. No stoma is necessary. The external wound should be cleaned at least twice daily with saline and some disinfectant solution. This technique preserves a greater amount of sphincter than any other: it minimises scar formation, avoids anatomic deformity such as keyhole deformity and does not require any intestinal diversion. If a recurrence of the fistula occurs, the procedure can be repeated later. When the anorectal mucosa is minimally inflamed and the Crohn's disease is under control, with or without a reduced amount of steroids, success rates from 40–60% can be expected [70–72]. In our experience of 42 patients treated with advancing flap technique, 23 patients (54.7%) were free of fistula 1 year after the procedure. Functional results confirm that this technique does not change the median maximal resting pressure nor the resting pressure profile of the anal canal because the external sphincter is preserved and no keyhole deformity is created [73]. After severe prior inflammation, extensive submucosal and even transmural fibrosis can make construction of an advancement flap difficult. In some complicated fistulae, the technique should not be the primary treatment used. The situation should be simplified by earlier surgery so that there is only a single tract remaining. Finally, a previously drained supralevator fistula extending close to the rectal wall will not leave enough residual tissue to support an advancement flap. Using the flap technique in this situation would lead to leakage at the suture and a recurrence of the fistula.

Rectovaginal Fistulae

Rectovaginal fistulae occur in 3–10% of women with Crohn's disease [74, 75]. Most of these fistulae originate from an anterior rectal ulcer eroding into the vagina, which usually occurs in the midportion of the rectovaginal septum. These fistulae are the most difficult to treat and have a poor prognosis [76–78]. Less commonly, these fistulae may arise from an infected anal gland and they may travel superficially, through, or above the sphincters. Bartholin's abscesses may also fistulise to the anorectum. This type of fistula carries a poor prognosis [79]. Patients with rectovaginal

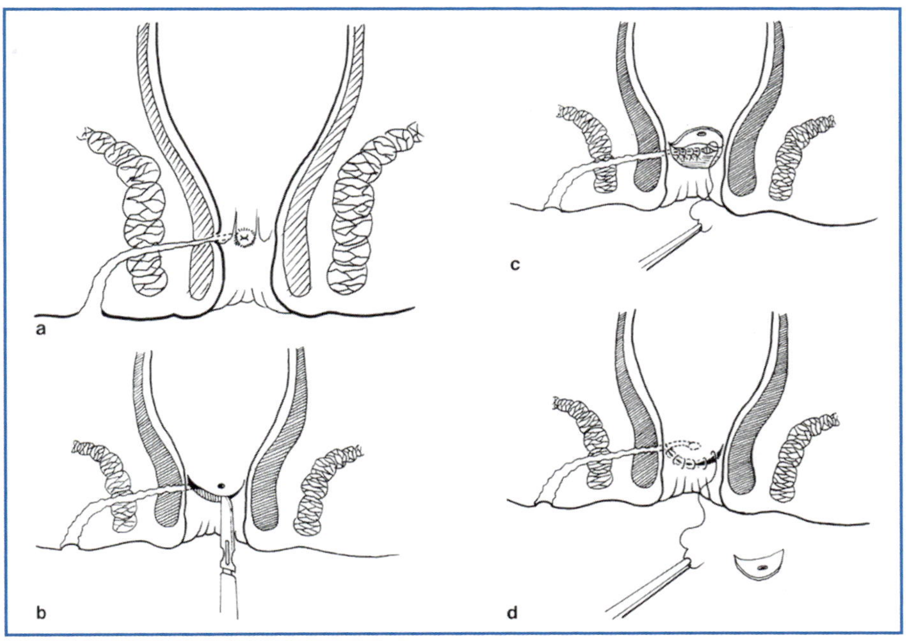

Fig. 8. Advancing flap technique. **a** Fistula tract is cored out without sphincter division. **b** Excision of the primary orifice and removal of the entire tract. **c** Liberation of a mucosal flap and suture of the muscular space. **d** Suture of the mucosal flap

fistulae typically present with benign symptoms and severe incontinence and excoriation are rare. Instead, these patients complain of intermittent vaginal discharge or the passage of gas through the vagina [76]. The diagnosis of these fistulae may be difficult. The best test can be done during rectoscopy by injecting air into the rectum and verifying its passage into the vagina. In some cases, examination should be done under anaesthesia. The treatment options in these cases are reduced, in our point of view, to the advancing flap technique described previously.

Results

From 1994 to 2004 we treated 672 patients with anal fistulae, of whom 59 (8.8%) had Crohn's disease. The male-to-female ratio was found to be 0.31 in Crohn's disease and 2.48 in idiopathic fistulae. The mean age of the Crohn's patients was 34 and 45 years for the idiopathic fistula patients. On average, the Crohn's patients had twice as many fistulae and they were generally more complex and the proportion of recto-vaginal fistulae was higher at 14.2% *vs.* 2%. The most frequent operations used in idiopathic fistulae were fistulotomy or fistulectomy (71.8%), advancing flap (27.7%) and glue sealant (0.5%). In Crohn's disease the respective proportions of these three techniques were fistulotomy (10.2%), advancing flap (71.2%) and glue sealant (18.6%). The median failure rates were quite different: idiopathic fistulae (8.7%) and Crohn's fistulae (40.5%). One must always be aware that early success may be followed by later recurrence, so scrupulous follow-up is necessary. The main reason for using the advancing flap technique is to preserve the anal profile and to maintain continence. However, even if there is a recurrence, the potentially long intervals without perineal sepsis are a benefit to the patient in their own right. As a summary of our work in this chapter we propose a non-exhaustive algorithm for the treatment of perineal Crohn's disease (Fig. 9).

Summary

Anorectal disorders affect many patients with Crohn's disease. Clinical manifestations range from asymptomatic skin tags to severe, debilitating perineal destruction and sepsis. Surgical management must be conservative and must focus on draining septic foci if present, preserving sphincter function and palliating symptoms. Medical management has shown some success in improving symptoms but has not yet been

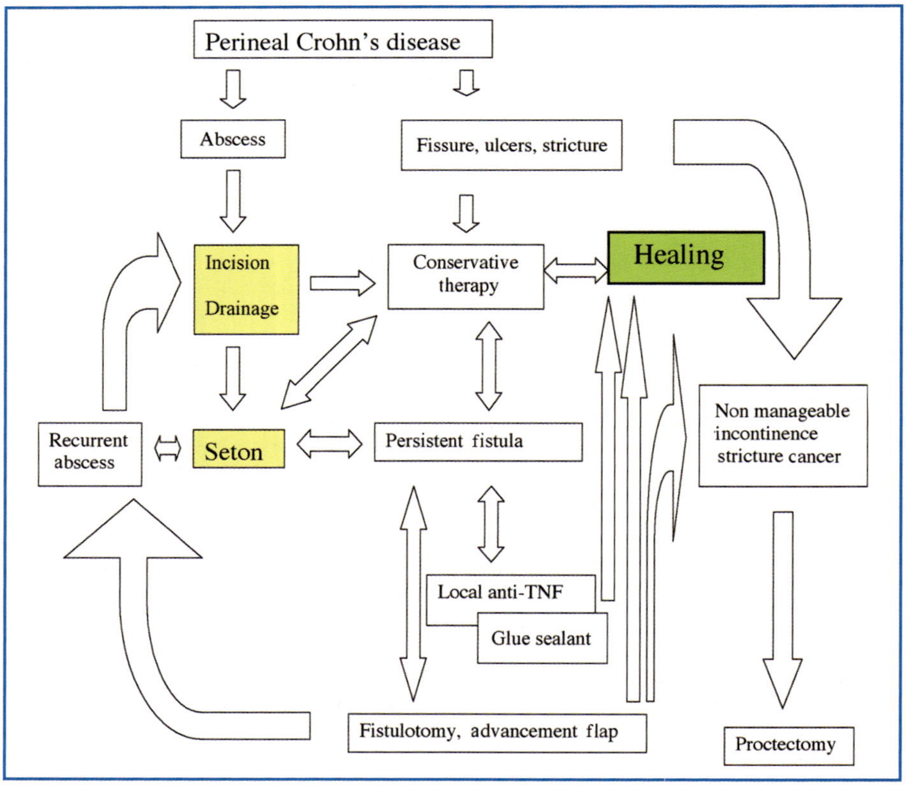

Fig. 9. Algorithm for treatment of perineal Crohn's disease

able to ameliorate most perineal complaints quickly with long lasting effects. Many new and exciting treatment modalities are being investigated, and it is hoped that more effective approaches to these complex and difficult problems will be found.

References

1. Schraut WH, Medich DS (1997) Crohn's disease. In: Greenfield LJ, Mulholland M, Oldham KT et al (eds) Surgery scientific principles and practice, 2nd edn. Lippincott, Philadelphia
2. Kodner IJ (1997) Perianal Crohn's disease. In: Allan RN, Rhodes JM, Hanauer SB et al (eds) Inflammatory bowel diseases, 3rd edn. Churchill Livingstone, New York, p 863
3. Platell C, Mackay J, Collopy B et al (1996) Anal pathology in patients with Crohn's disease. Aust N Z J Surg 66:5–7
4. Solomon MJ (1996) Fistulae and abscesses in symptomatic perianal Crohn's. Int J Colorectal Dis 11:222–224
5. Williamson PR, Hellinger MD, Larach SW et al (1995) Twenty-year review of the surgical management of perianal Crohn's disease. Dis Colon Rectum 38:389–391
6. Williams DR, Collier JA, Corman ML et al (1981) Anal complications in Crohn's disease. Dis Colon Rectum 24:22–24
7. Allan A, Keighley MR (1988) Management of perianal Crohn's disease. World J Surg 12:198–201
8. Lunniss PJ, Barker PG, Sultan AH et al (1994) Magnetic resonance imaging of fistula-in-ano (comments). Dis Colon Rectum 37:708–711
9. Borley NR, Mortensen NJ, Jewell DP (1999) MRI scanning in perianal Crohn's disease: an important diagnostic adjunct. Inflamm Bowel Dis 5:231–233
10. Hellers G, Bergstrand O, Ewerth S et al (1980) Occurrence and outcome after primary treatment of anal fistulae in Crohn's disease. Gut 21:525–527
11. Heuman R, Bolin T, Sjodahl R et al (1981) The incidence and course of perianal complications and arthralgia after intestinal resection with restoration of continuity for Crohn's disease. Br J Surg 68:528–530
12. Buchmann P, Keighley MRB, Allan RN et al (1980) Natural history of perianal Crohn's disease. Ten year follow-up: a plea for conservatism. Am J Surg 140:642–644
13. Fry RD, Shemesh EI, Kodner IJ et al (1989) Techniques and results in the management of anal and perianal Crohn's disease. Surg Gynecol Obstet 168:42–48
14. Wolff BG, Culp CE, Beart RW et al (1985) Anorectal Crohn's disease: a long-term perspective. Dis Colon Rectum 28:709–711
15. Kosinski L, Welton ML (1998) Surgical options in the management of perianal Crohn's disease. Semin Gastrointest Dis 9:15–20
16. Williams JG, Rothenberger DA, Nemer FD et al (1991) Fistula-in-ano in Crohn's disease Results of aggressive surgical treatment. Dis Colon Rectum 34:378–384
17. Pescatori M, Interisano A, Basso L et al (1995) Management of perianal Crohn's disease: results of a multicenter study in Italy. Dis Colon Rectum 38:121–124
18. Buchmann P, Alexander-Williams J (1980) Classification of perianal Crohn's disease. Clin Gastroenterol 9:323–330
19. Irvine EJ (1995) Usual therapy improves perianal Crohn's disease as measured by a new disease activity index. J Clin Gastroenterol 20:27–32
20. Hamilton CH (1975) Anorectal problems: the deep postanal space: surgical significance in horseshoe fistula and abscess. Dis Colon Rectum 18:642–645
21. Ramanujam P, Prasad ML, Abcarian H (1983) The role of seton in fistulotomy of the anus. Surg Gynecol Obstet 57:419–422
22. Keighley MR, Allan RN (1986) Current status and influence of operation on perianal Crohn's disease. Int J Colorectal Dis 1:104–107
23. Makowiec F, Jehl EC, Becker H et al (1997) Perianal abscess in Crohn's disease. Dis Colon Rectum 40:443–450
24. Fuhrman GM, Larach SW (1989) Experience with perirectal fistulas in patients with Crohn's disease. Dis Colon Rectum 32:847–848
25. Sohn N, Korelitz BI, Weinstein MA (1980) Anorectal Crohn's disease: definitive surgery for fistulas and recurrent abscesses. Am J Surg 139:394–397
26. Levien DH, Gross EL, Auriemma WS (1995) Anal Crohn's disease. In: Mazier WP, Levien DH et al (eds) Surgery of the colon, rectum, and anus. Saunders, Philadelphia, p 971
27. Fleshner P, Schoetz D, Roberts P et al (1995) Anal fissure in Crohn's disease: a plea for aggressive management. Dis Colon Rectum 38:1137–1143
28. Wolkomir AF, Luchtefeld MA (1993) Surgery for symptomatic hemorrhoids and anal fissures in Crohn's disease. Dis Colon Rectum 36:545–547
29. Linares L, Moreira LF, Andrews H et al (1988) Natural history and treatment of anorectal strictures complicating Crohn's disease. Br J Surg 75:653–655
30. Homan WP, Tang C, Thorbjarnarson B (1976) Anal lesions complicating Crohn's disease. Arch Surg 111:1333–1335
31. Jeffery PJ, Ritchie JK, Parks AG (1977) Treatment of haemorrhoids in patients with inflammatory bowel disease. Lancet 1:1084–1085
32. Felt-Bersma R, Poen AC, Cuesta MA et al (1999) Anal lesions and anorectal function in perianal Crohn's disease (abstract). Gastroenterology 116:714
33. Scott A, Hawley PR, Phillips RKS (1989) Results of external sphincter repair in Crohn's disease. Br J Surg 76:959–960
34. Keighley MR, Williams NS (1999) Surgical treatment of perianal Crohn's disease. In: Keighley MR, Williams NS (eds) Surgery of the Anus, Rectum, and Colon. 2nd edn. Saunders, Philadelphia, p 2135
35. Buchman AL, Ament ME, Doty J (1991) Development of squamous cell carcinoma in chronic perineal sinus and wounds in Crohn's disease. Am J Gastroenterol 86:1829–1832
36. Bernstein D, Rogers A (1996) Malignancy in Crohn's disease. Am J Gastroenterol 91:434–440
37. Gyde SN, Prior P, Macartney JC et al (1980) Malignancy in Crohn's disease. Gut 21:1024–1029
38. Nikias G, Eisner T, Katz S et al (1995) Crohn's disease and colorectal carcinoma: rectal cancer complicating

longstanding active perianal disease. Am J Gastroenterol 90:216–219
39. Richards ME, Rickert RR, Nance FC (1989) Crohn's disease associated carcinoma: a poorly recognized complication of inflammatory bowel disease. Ann Surg 209:764–773
40. Hawker PC, Gyde SN, Thompson H et al (1980) Adenocarcinoma of the small intestine complicating Crohn's disease. Gut 23:188–193
41. Lavery IC, Jagelman DG (1982) Cancer in the excluded rectum following surgery for inflammatory bowel disease. Dis Colon Rectum 25:522–524
42. Galandiuk S, Kimberling J, Al-Mishalb TG, Stromberg AJ (2005) Perianal Crohn disease: predictors of need for permanent diversion. Ann Surg 241:796–801
43. Lockhart-Mummery HE (1975) Crohn's disease: anal lesions. Dis Colon Rectum 18:200–202
44. Shivananda S, Hordijk ML, Pena AS, Mayberry JF (1989) Crohn's disease: risk of recurrence and reoperation in a defined population. Gut 30:990
45. Harper PH, Fazio VW et al (1987) Long-term outcome in Crohn's disease. Dis Col Rectum 30:174–177
46. Allan A, Keighley MRB (1988) Management of perianal Crohn's disease. World J Surg 12:198–201
47. Corman ML (1989) Colon and rectal surgery, 2nd edn. Lippincott, Philadelphia
48. Bell SJ, Williams AB, Wiesel Pilkinson K et al (2003) The clinical course of fistulating Crohn's disease. Aliment Pharmacol Ther 17:1145–1151
49. Lapidus A, Bernell O, Hellers G, Löfberg R (1998) Clinical course of colorectal Crohn's disease: a 35-year follow-up study of 507 patients. Gastroenterology 114:1151–1160
50. Targan SR, Hanauer SB, van Deventer SJ et al (1997) A short-term study of chimeric monoclonal antibody cA2 to tumor necrosis factor alpha for Crohn's disease: Crohn's Disease cA2 Study Group. N Engl J Med 337:1029–1035
51. Sands BE, Anderson FH, Bernstein CN et al (2004) Infliximab maintenance therapy for fistulising Crohn's disease. N Engl J Med 350:876–885
52. Sandborn WJ, Hanauer SB (1999) Antitumor necrosis factor therapy for inflammatory bowel disease: a review of agents, pharmacology, clinical results, and safety. Inflamm Bowel Dis 5:119–133
53. Lichtiger S (2001) Healing of perianal fistulae by local injection of antibody to TNF. Gastroenterology 120(Suppl l):A3154
54. Poggioli G, Laureti S, Pierangeli F et al (2005) Local injection of Infliximab for the treatment of perianal Crohn's disease. Dis Colon Rectum 48:768–774
55. Fiocchi C (2004) Closing fistulas in Crohn's disease: should the accent be on maintenance or safety? N Engl J Med 350:934–936
56. Vitton V et al (2005) Long term healing of Crohn's anal fistulas with fibrin glue injection. Aliment Pharmacol Ther 21:1453–1457
57. Hjortrup A, Moesgaard F, Kjaergard J (1991) Fibrin adhesive in the treatment of perineal fistulas. Dis Colon Rectum 34:752–754
58. Abel ME, Chiu YS, Russell TR, Volpe PA (1993) Autologous fibrin glue in the treatment of rectovaginal and complex fistulas. Dis Colon Rectum 36:447–449
59. Cintron JR, Park JJ, Orsay CP et al (2000) Repair of fistulas-in-ano using fibrin adhesive: long-term follow-up. Dis Colon Rectum 43:944-949
60. Venkatesh KS, Ramanujam P (1999) Fibrin glue application in the treatment of recurrent anorectal fistulas. Dis Colon Rectum 42:1136–1139
61. Patrlj L, Kocman B, Martinac M et al (2000) Fibrin glue-antibiotic mixture in the treatment of anal fistulae: experience with 69 cases. Dig Surg 17:77–80
62. Park JJ, Cintron JR, Orsay CP et al (2000) Repair of chronic anorectal fistulae using commercial fibrin sealant. Arch Surg 135:166–169
63. Sentovich SM (2003) Fibrin glue for anal fistulas: long-term results. Dis Colon Rectum 46:498–502
64. Sainio P, Husa A (1985) Fistula-in-ano: clinical features and long-term results of surgery in 199 adults. Acta Chir Scand 151:169–176
65. Van Tets W F, Kuijpers HC (1994) Continence disorders after anal fistulotomy. Dis Colon Rectum 37:1194–1197
66. Makowiec F, Jahle EC, Starlinger M (1995) Clinical course of perianal fistulas in Crohn's disease. Gut 37:696–701
67. Athanasiadis S, Lux N, Fischbach N et al (1991) One-stage surgery of high trans- and supra-sphincter anal fistula using primary fistulectomy and occlusion of the internal fistula ostium: a prospective study of 169 patients. Chirurg 62:608–613
68. Athanasiadis S, Köhler A, Nafe M (1994) Treatment of high anal fistulae by primary occlusion of the internal ostium, drainage of the intersphincteric space and mucosal advancement flap. Int J Colorect Dis 9:153–157
69. Girona J, Denkers D (1996) Fistula, fissure, abscess [in German]. Chirurg 67:222–228
70. Jones IT, Fazio VW, Jagelman DG (1987) The use of transanal rectal advancement flaps in the management of fistulas involving the anorectum. Dis Colon Rectum 30:919–923
71. Makowiec F, Jehle EC, Becker HD et al (1995) Clinical course after transanal advancement flap repair of perianal fistula in patients with Crohn's disease. Br J Surg 82:603–606
72. Ozuner G, Hull TL, Cartmill J et al (1996) Long-term analysis of the use of transanal rectal advancement flaps for complicated anorectal/vaginal fistulas. Dis Colon Rectum 39:10–14
73. Finan PJ (1996) Management by advancement flap technique. In: Phillips RKS, Luniss PJ (eds) Anal fistula. Chapman, London pp 107–115
74. Goodsall DH, Miles WE (1900) Diseases of the anus and rectum. Longmans, London, pp 92–173
75. Oh C (1983) Management of high recurrent anal fistula. Surgery 93:330–332
76. Dukes CE, Galvin C (1956) Colloid carcinoma arising within fistulae in the anorectal region. Ann R Coll Surg Engl 18:246–261
77. Parks AG, Thomson JPS (1973) Intersphincteric abscess. Br Med J 2:537–539
78. Hull TL (1996) rectovaginal fistula in Crohn's disease. In: Phillips RKS, Luniss PJ (eds) Anal fistula. Chapman, London, pp 143–1162
79. Contou JF (1993) Imagerie et suppurations anopérinéales. Gastroenterol Clin Biol 17:159–161

Medical Treatment of Ulcerative Colitis

Fosca De Iorio, Luigi Benini, Naika Tacchella, Italo Vantini

Introduction

Ulcerative colitis (UC) is a chronic inflammatory disease of the colon affecting mainly young people, with a peak incidence between the ages of 10 and 40 years; 15% of patients are over the age of 60 at diagnosis. Its incidence is approximately 10–20 per 100 000 per year with a reported prevalence of 100–200 per 100 000 and is stable over time. The value of prevalence is less reliable, but it is probably underestimated because it implies an average disease duration of 10 years for a condition that is known to last for life [1]. A hospital serving a population of 300 000 will typically see 45–90 new cases per year and have 500 under follow-up.

Patients find symptoms of UC and CD embarrassing and humiliating. Inflammatory bowel diseases (IBD) can result in loss of education and difficulty in gaining employment or insurance [2]. It can also cause psychological problems, growth failure or a retardation in the sexual development of young people. Medical treatments with corticosteroids or immunosuppressants may cause major health problems, and surgery may result in complications such as impotence or intestinal failure. There is only a small increase in mortality for both UC (hazard ratio 1.44) and CD (hazard ratio 1.73), largely dependent on age and extension of the disease [3]. However, even if some patients have only functional symptoms (which are not in themselves an indication to potentiate the treatment and which may benefit from symptomatic drugs such anti-diarrheals, anti-spasmodics or fibres), the impact of IBD on society is disproportionately high, as presentation often occurs at a young age and has a potential to cause lifelong illness.

These considerations explain the peculiar expectations that patients with inflammatory bowel diseases have concerning both the pharmacological treatment and the overall clinical management. These considerations and their rationale have been summarised in recent clinical guidelines by the British Society of Gastroenterology, and reported in Table 1 [4].

Therapy

The peculiar expectations of patients and the need of a complex multidisciplinary approach to these patients, support the referral of patients to units with specific competence in this field. Therapy for IBD is a rapidly evolving field with many new biological agents under investigation that are likely to change therapeutic strategies radically in the next decade. We will try to summarise recent evidence concerning the effect of the drugs and some warnings recently outlined.

Aminosalicylates

Aminosalicylates act on epithelial cells via a variety of mechanisms to moderate the release of lipid mediators, cytokines and reactive oxygen species. These drugs are available as oral tablets, sachets or suspension, liquid or foam enemas, or suppositories. Different formulations deliver millimolar concentrations to the gut lumen. Oral forms include:

- pH dependent release/resin coated mesalazine;
- time controlled release mesalazine;
- Delivery by carrier molecules, releasing 5-ASA after splitting by bacterial enzymes in the large intestine (sulfasalazine, olsalazine, balsalazide).

Mesalazine has been recommended both for inducing and for maintaining remission.

Induction of Remission

Sutherland et al. [5, 6], in a meta-analysis of controlled trials, observed that 5-ASA was superior to placebo in active colitis (OR for maintaining remission 2). The same Authors, in an update of the aforementioned meta-analysis, confirmed that 5-ASA was superior to placebo for all outcome variables (global/clinical remission, global/clinical improvement, endoscopic remission or improvement).

When 5-ASA was compared to sulfasalazine, there

Table 1. Expectations expressed by members of the British National Association of Colitis and Crohn's Disease for their medical management

Before diagnosis
– Rapid access to hospital investigation
– Referral to a hospital that has a gastroenterologist specialised in IBD
At diagnosis
Availability of suitable written information and audio-visual material
Information about patient support groups and sources of help
Opportunity to meet non-medical members of staff, such as a clinical nurse specialist or medical social worker familiar with IBD
Hospital management
Sufficient information to make a rational personal choice about treatment options
Close integration of medical and surgical management
Straightforward access to support services, including dieticians, psychological support, and social workers
Clearly stated management plans on discharge with well defined roles and responsibilities
Outpatient management
Continuity of care, both in hospital and in primary care
Patients dislike seeing different individuals at each visit
A system that allows a choice about appropriate long term follow up
Direct telephone access
Attention to physical, emotional, and quality of life issues
Help with problems related to insurance, employment, or social security

were no differences for all the endpoints, but there was a tendency for a greater efficacy and lower side effects of 5-ASA preparations over sulfasalazine [5]. It was concluded that for their higher cost, 5-ASA preparations should be reserved for selected groups such as sulfasalazine-intolerant patients or men concerned about infertility.

The best dosage of mesalazine for inducing remission remains open to debate. Higher doses seem to produce better results, doses below 2 g/day did not show any benefit over placebo [5]. Disease extension does not influence the response to therapy in that similar responses are found in pancolitis and distal colitis [7].

Few data are available on the different outcomes concerning the efficacy of various 5-ASA formulations. Only a single study suggested that balsalazide induces more rapid clinical remission with less adverse effects compared to a pH-dependent formulation of mesalazine [8], but this requires confirmation. On the other hand, olsalazine was not superior to an enteric-coated mesalazine in inducing endoscopic remissions [9].

Maintenance

Four out of six studies demonstrated that 5-ASA is superior to placebo in remission maintenance at 6–12 months [10–15]. In a meta-analysis of randomised, double-blinded, placebo-controlled trials with a duration of at least 6 months, 5-ASA was able to halve the number of relapses compared to placebo, with a number needed to treat of 6 to prevent one relapse [6]. Sulfasalazine and 5-ASA have similar efficacy in long-term maintenance remission and the choice among the drugs should be based on factors such as cost or tolerance. For maintenance therapy, doses of 5-ASA ranged between 2 to 4.4 g/day. In the acute phase, while disease extension did not influence the efficacy in maintaining remission [16], no information exists on the different effects of various ASA formulations.

Topical Therapy

Topical mesalazine is an effective alternative to steroids enemas during the acute-phases of left-sided colitis [17–24]. In two recent meta-analyses, rectal 5-ASA was superior to rectal steroids in inducing clinical, endoscopic and histologic improvement [25, 26].

Mesalazine enemas were as effective as oral sulfasalazine but with fewer adverse effects in left-sided mild/moderate UC [27]. The drug induced remission in a duration-dependent but not in a dose-dependent way [26].

In a recent comparison of the use of these old drugs according to international guidelines in IBD patients, it was concluded that (1) 64% of patients received suboptimal dosages of oral 5-ASA, despite the evidence that their efficacy is dose-related; (2) topical aminosalicylates were not used in 75% of patients with distal colitis, despite the evidence that combined oral and topical therapy is more effective than systemic therapy alone [28, 29].

Adverse Effects of Aminosalycilates

Mild side effects of sulfasalazine (mainly headache, nausea, epigastric pain, and diarrhoea) occur in 10–45% of patients, whereas serious idiosyncratic reactions (including Stevens Johnson syndrome, pancreatitis, agranulocytosis, or alveolitis) are rare. These reactions are mainly associated with the sulphonamidic part of the molecule, which explains why mesalazine or olsalazine are associated with a frequency of adverse events (diarrhoea, headache, nausea, and rash, bloody diarrhoea) similar to placebo [30, 31]. No comparison between balsalazide and placebo has been published, but adverse events are lower than with sulfasalazine [31]. A population based study found that renal derangement (interstitial nephritis and nephrotic syndrome) is associated with disease severity rather than with dosage or type of mesalazine and that, in any case, the risk is only marginally increased (OR 1.60 *vs.* normal) [32]. Patients with pre-existing renal impairment or using other potentially nephrotoxic drugs, should have renal function monitored during 5-ASA therapy.

Corticosteroids

Corticosteroids are potent anti-inflammatory agents for moderate to severe relapses of both UC and CD. They have no role in maintenance therapy for either disease. They act through inhibition of several inflammatory pathways via the suppression of interleukin transcription, induction of IkB (an inhibitor of the NFkB complex), suppression of the arachidonic acid metabolism and stimulation of apoptosis of lymphocytes within the lamina propria of the gut. Many strategies attempt to maximise their topical effects, while limiting systemic side effects. As for example, budesonide is a poorly absorbed corticosteroid with limited bioavailability and extensive first-pass metabolism which reduces its systemic toxicity in ileocecal CD or UC.

Efficacy for Active UC

Trials are all over 30 years old, but results are consistent: oral prednisolone (starting at 40 mg daily) induced remission in 77% of 118 patients with mild to moderate disease within 2 weeks, compared with 48% treated with 8 g/day sulfasalazine. A combination of oral and rectal steroids is better than either alone. Adverse events are more frequent with a dose of 60 mg/day compared with 40 mg/day, without added benefit; doses of prednisolone of 15 mg/day are ineffective for active disease. The optimal dose for "outpatient" management of acute UC appears to be 40 mg.

Efficacy should be balanced against side effects, but decisive treatment of active disease in conjunction with a strategy for complete withdrawal of steroids is often appreciated by patients suffering miserable symptoms. Regimens of steroid therapy vary among centres. A standard weaning strategy helps to identify patients who relapse rapidly or do not respond and need adjunctive therapy with thiopurines or hospital admission [4].

Adverse Effects of Steroids

Three broad groups can be identified, although 50% of patients report no adverse event. Early effects are mainly due to high doses and include cosmetic effects (acne, moon face, oedema), sleep and mood disturbance, dyspepsia, or glucose intolerance. Effects associated with prolonged use (usually 12 weeks) include posterior subcapsular cataracts, osteoporosis, osteonecrosis of the femoral head, myopathy, and susceptibility to infections. Effects during withdrawal include acute adrenal insufficiency (from sudden cessation), a syndrome of myalgia, malaise, and arthralgia (similar to recrudescence of UC), or raised intracranial pressure. Complete steroid withdrawal is facilitated by early introduction of azathioprine, adjuvant nutritional therapy, or timely surgery.

One of the most frequent mistakes in the therapy of UC is the prolonged use of steroids (effective only in inducing clinical remission but not in maintenance). There is no excuse either for using them repeatedly for either frequent relapses, either for fruitless attempts at tapering them or for continuing them at homeopathic doses to maintain remission. Steroids are neither safe nor effective in any of these situations. Corticosteroids are often used for an excessive duration even in patients with mild disease without a clear "exit" strategy, utilising alternative drugs to maintain remission. The standard of practice worldwide is currently to maintain long-term remissions with either a high-dose of 5-ASAs, antimetabolites, anti-TNF drugs, or even surgery, rather than with long-term or frequently repeated steroids [29].

Immunomodulators

Purine anti-metabolites inhibit ribonucleotide synthesis, but the mechanism of immunomodulation is carried out by inducing T-cell apoptosis. Azathioprine (AZA) is metabolised to 6-mercaptopurine (6-MP) and subsequently to 6-thioguanine nucleotides. Thioguanine has been used for treatment of IBD, but caution is appropriate because of potential hepatotoxicity.

Maintenance of Remission

Despite the general acceptance of these drugs in UC, there are few randomised controlled trials (RCT) evaluating the efficacy of AZA and 6-MP. This is mainly due to the fact that researchers must adjust the dosage of the drugs to their haematological effects, which makes the maintenance of blindness difficult. The first trials in the seventies showed a steroid-sparing effect, but not an improvement in disease activity [33–34].

In a large and long-term retrospective clinical survey, AZA was significantly more effective in inducing remissions in patients with UC compared with CD (87% *vs.* 64%) [35]. This was also true in a recent prospective, randomised, controlled study on the efficacy and safety of AZA and 5-ASA in inducing remission in steroid dependent UC [36]. Seventy-two patients were randomised to receive AZA 2 mg/kg/day or oral 5-ASA 3.2 g/day, for a 6-month period. At the beginning, all patients were taking 40 mg of prednisolone, which was gradually tapered according to the clinical improvement. Endoscopic and clinical remission was achieved in 19 of 36 AZA patients compared to 7 of 36 in the 5-ASA group. Four AZA and 3 5-ASA patients underwent colectomy. Significantly more AZA than 5-ASA patients complained of mild to moderate adverse events.

Patients with UC in whom remission was induced by AZA benefited from maintenance treatment, since withdrawal of therapy doubled the relapse rate [37]; moreover, AZA is effective in avoiding colectomy in steroid-dependent or steroid-resistant UC [38].

Pharmocodynamics

AZA is a prodrug that is rapidly cleaved in the liver by glutathione-S-transferase to 6-MP. This active component is metabolised in the liver and in the gut by one of three enzymes: (1) thiopurin-S-methyltransferase (TPMT), (2) xanthine-oxidase, (3) hypoxanthine-guanine-phosphoryl transferase.

Side Effects of Immunosuppressants

AZA and 6-MP inhibits the proliferation of T and B lymphocytes, thereby reducing cytotoxic T cells and plasma cells. During AZA or 6MP, 6-thioguanine nucleotides accumulate slowly in tissues, probably accounting for the protracted action of these drugs upon their suspension. This intracellular accumulation of 6-thioguanine nucleotides is responsible for the cytotoxic effects of these drugs by the inhibition of purine synthesis, nucleotide interconversions, DNA and RNA synthesis and chromosomal replication. Measurements of erythrocyte 6-thioguanine may be helpful in optimising the dose of AZA/6-MP for a clinical response without myelosuppressive effects.

In has been suggested that leukaemic patients deficient in TPMT are at increased risk of myelotoxicity [39], but this does not necessarily apply to IBD. In one study, 31 of 41 IBD patients with AZA-induced myelosuppression did not carry a TPMT mutation. Evidence that TPMT activity predicts other side effects or outcome is limited, and so far, it cannot be recommended as a prerequisite to therapy [40].

AZA should be introduced at a low dose, 0.5–1.5 mg/kg daily, and increased gradually within 2 weeks to 2.5 mg/kg daily. Blood monitoring (haematology and liver function tests) should be performed weekly until the maintenance dose is reached, and monthly thereafter. The equivalent dose of 6-MP is initially 0.25–0.5 mg/kg daily, increasing to 1.0–1.5 mg/kg daily. If white blood cells decrease below 3 000/mm^3 or platelets below 120 000/mm^3, the drug should be discontinued or the dose reduced until these parameters normalise. Furthermore, if liver biochemistry (and/or serum amylase) exceeds more than 50% of the upper normal limit, AZA/6MP should be discontinued, and then cautiously reintroduced.

Both AZA and 6-MP are considered slow-acting drugs, with an effect expected after 12–17 weeks. A recent study suggests that AZA works faster than previously believed, showing effects after 4 weeks [41]. In any case, for their slow onset of action, these drugs have no place as a monotherapy in acute relapses of UC. Allopurinol blocks the metabolism of 6-MP by the inhibition of xanthine-oxidase, so that patients on allopurinol should receive half doses of AZA/6-MP.

Side-effects of immunosuppressants can be categorised as (1) bone-marrow suppression, 2) short-term effects and 3) long-term effects. The side-effects occur in about 10–15% of patients with IBD and are either dose-dependent (bone marrow suppression) or idiosyncrasic (pancreatitis, allergic reactions or hepatitis).

Severe leukopenia, although rare (around 3%), may develop suddenly and unpredictably in between blood tests, even during long-term treatment. Side effects detected with short-term use often occur within the first week of treatment and include pancreatitis (3.3% of patients), allergic reactions including rash, idiosyncratic hepatitis with cytonecrosis, cholestasis or insidious onset of liver dysfunction (3.3%) and infections (7.4%). Pancreatitis resolves upon drug withdrawal but recurs on retreatment, which precludes the use of either AZA or 6MP.

Some 5–10% of patients stop treatment on their own mainly during the first month. Nausea, vomiting and malaise are the most common problems especially if the dose is increased too fast. Infections are the theoretical risk of the long-term use of these agents, but their incidence is not higher than with high-dose prednisolone.

In patients on long-term immunosuppressants one may expect an increase incidence of neoplastic diseases. Actually, a prospective study of 1 349 non-transplant patients receiving AZA, including 280 patients with IBD, showed a significant increase in non-Hodgkin's lymphoma, squamous cell carcinoma and other tumours (overall risk increased by a factor of 1.6) [42]. In contrast, reports from St Mark's Hospital (755 patients) and Oxford (2 205 patients) showed a risk of neoplasia comparable with the general population, but after a treatment of only 1 year [43, 44].

A recent meta-analysis found a fourfold increase risk of lymphoma in IBD patients on azathioprine/6-MP possibly as a result of the drugs, the severity of the disease, or a combination of the two [45]. In any case, decision analysis suggests that in IBD, the benefits of AZA outweigh the risk of lymphoma [46, 47].

The main mistake in the use of anti-metabolites is probably undertreatment [29]. Three forms of undertreatment are still rampant. The first is waiting too long to introduce these agents. One relapse noted during or soon after an attempted steroid withdrawal is an indication for the introduction of anti-metabolites. Likewise, neither cyclosporine nor infliximab should be used without a previous introduction of anti-metabolites in the expectation that they will be needed over the long-term.

The second mistake is underdosing. The habit of administering 6-MP or azathioprine at a fixed dosage of 50 mg/day should have long been abandoned. A reasonable starting dose of 6-MP is 1.5 mg/kg/day and of azathioprine 2.5–3 mg/kg/day. Even more important, is not giving up with these drugs until being sure that they have been administered at the maximal doses. By definition, the dose has been pushed up enough either when success is achieved or when mild leukopenia has occurred (WBC in the 3 000–4 000/mm^3 range). If there is uncertainty about efficacy, adsorption, or adherence, additional information can be gained by looking for a substantial increase in MCV or by measuring drug metabolites.

The last mistake is an early suspension of the drug. No "safe" number of years has been established after which these medications can be withdrawn without the risk of relapse. Moreover, it is of critical importance not to suspend 6-MP or azathioprine during pregnancy. Safety in pregnancy has been unequivocally established via published experience [48]. Indeed, the risk to pregnancy is infinitely greater from relapse of disease than from adverse effect of treatment.

Methotrexate (MTX)

Conflicting results are available on the efficacy of MTX in UC. In an early RCT, no significant differences were found between oral MTX (12.5 mg/week) and placebo at 9 months in 67 UC patients [49]. In another RCT, MTX (15 mg/week) was as effective as 6-MP (1.5 mg/kg/day) and 5-ASA (3 g/day), but less effective in maintaining remission in steroid-dependent UC patients. A dose of subcutaneous MTX at 15 and 25 mg/week showed a similar efficacy in inducing remission [50].

It is often accepted that MTX is more effective in Crohn's disease than in UC. However, in a recent retrospective study on 22 UC and 48 CD patients treated with MTX (orally or i.m.) with a mean maintenance dose of 20 mg/week, remission was achieved in 34 of 55 patients who completed more than 3 months of treatment. Treatment was equally effective for Crohn's disease and UC. Life-table analysis showed that the chances of remaining in remission at 12, 24 and 36 months of treatment were 90, 73 and 51%, respectively [51].

Side Effects

Measurement of full blood count and liver function tests are advisable before and within 4 weeks of starting therapy, then monthly thereafter. Early toxicity from methotrexate is primarily gastrointestinal (nausea, vomiting, diarrhoea, and stomatitis) and may be limited by 5 mg of folic acid the day following MTX injection. Treatment is discontinued in 10–18% of patients because of side effects. The principal concerns are hepatotoxicity and pneumonitis. A study of liver biopsies in IBD patients taking MTX showed mild histological abnormalities despite cumulative doses of up to 5.4 grams. Surveillance liver biopsy is not warranted, but if the transaminases increase to more than twice the upper normal limit, it is sensible to withhold MTX until it returns to normal before a retrial of the drug [52]. The prevalence of pneumonitis has been estimated at 2–3 cases per 100 patient years of exposure, but even large series have not reported any case. The main concern with this drug is its teratogenicity, which limits its use in fertile patients.

Cyclosporin

Cyclosporin (CyA) is an inhibitor of calcineurin, preventing clonal expansion of T-cell subsets. It has a rapid onset of action and is effective in the management of severe UC which failed to improve from the intensive steroidal therapy. Several uncontrolled studies and a few controlled studies of intravenous cyclosporine in patients with severe UC are available. Lichtiger et al. reported on 20 patients, 9 randomized to placebo and 11 to CyA, in continuous infusion, in addition to steroids for up to 14 days. Nine out of 11 patients on CyA responded after a mean period of 7 days compared with none on placebo. Responders continued on oral CyA 8 mg/kg/day and, at 6 months, 5 out of 11 maintained remission [53].

When used as a monotherapy (continuous infusion of either CyA 4 mg/kg/day or methylprednisolone 40 mg/day), a response at 8 days was obtained in 9 out of 14 of CyA *vs.* 8 out of 15 of methylprednisolone. Responders were slowly switched to AZA maintenance. At 12 months, 7 out of 9 patients initially treated with CyA maintained remission compared with 3 out of 8 with steroids. [54].

In a further study, 30 patients were randomised to monotherapy with CyA 4 mg/kg/day i.v. or CyA i.v in combination with methylprednisolone 1 mg/kg/day. At 7 days, a complete remission was obtained in 10 out of 15 on CyA *vs.* 14 out of 15 on the combination therapy [55]. While 2 and 4 mg of the drug show the same efficacy, topical treatment is not effective [56, 57].

Intravenous CyA is rapidly effective as a salvage therapy for patients with refractory colitis, who would otherwise face colectomy, but its use is controversial because of toxicity and its high long-term failure rate. There is now a trend to use CyA earlier to improve outcome. To do so, early predictors of steroid failure are needed [58–59]. For its rapid onset of action, CyA can be considered as a "bridge" to maintenance therapy with immunomodulators and only rarely should be continued for more than 3–6 months.

In a recent Cochrane Review, it was concluded that there is limited evidence that CyA is more effective than standard treatment alone in preventing colectomy in severe UC, even if its beneficial effect cannot be excluded due to the small sample size [60]. The possible efficacy of CyA in these severe cases has to be weighed against possible side effects. Minor side effects occur in 31–51%, including tremor, paresthesias, malaise, headache, abnormal liver function, gingival hyperplasia, and hirsutism. Major complications are renal insufficiency (23%), infections (20%), seizures (3%), death (2%) and anaphylaxis (1%) [61].

The risk of seizures is increased in patients on intravenous CyA with serum cholesterol less than 120 mg/dl and serum magnesium less than 1.5 mg/dl. Oral therapy is an alternative in these circumstances [62]. Using prophylaxis against *Pneumocystis carinii* pneumonia is an individual decision dependent on nutritional state, concomitant immunomodulator therapy, and duration of therapy, but other opportunistic infections (for example, *Aspergillus* sp.) may be as common.

Tacrolimus

Tacrolimus (FK 506), a macrolide immunosuppressant, acts by blocking the enzyme calcineurin which interrupts the signal transduction pathway in the T-cell. It is 10 to 100-fold more potent in inhibiting lymphocyte activation in vitro than CyA, and its intestinal absorption is more reliable even in the presence of gastrointestinal disease. This drug, which is expensive and rather toxic, may be effective in a subset of patients with severe disease, steroid resistant or intolerant [63–65].

Infliximab

Infliximab (IFX) (Remicade) is a chimeric anti-TNF monoclonal antibody with potent anti-inflammatory effects, possibly dependent on apoptosis of inflammatory cells, which has become the best choice in both active and fistulising CD unresponsive to standard therapy.

Additionally, TNA-α plays a crucial role in the inflammatory process in UC. In this disease, high levels of TNF-α are mainly found in the superficial colonic layers, as opposed to CD, where it is found deeper in the mucosa or submucosa. Normally the inflammatory response to TNF-α is counterbalanced by inhibitors, and there is evidence that the production of TNF-α inhibitors is down-regulated in IBD.

It has been shown that TNF-α blocking agents probably do not act by binding and inactivating TNF-α, but rather by inducing the apoptosis of TNF-expressing inflammatory cells, as proven by the inefficacy of etanercept. Resistance to apoptosis has been shown in both CD and UC, but with different mechanisms. The defect in CD occurs in the mitochondrial pathway of apoptosis (imbalance of mitochondrial bcl-2 bax), whereas in UC it derives from the overexpression of FLICE-inhibitory protein (FLIP) and impairment of the caspase mediated apoptosis.

These data support the use of IFX in UC, mainly in steroid-refractory or severely ill patients. Open trials on such patients suggested an effect in 50–75% of cases, which was maintained long-term in 25% of cases [66–68]. Concomitant use of anti-metabolites was associated with a lower rate of relapse.

Recently, two large multicentre placebo-controlled studies—Active Ulcerative Colitis 1 and 2 (ACT 1 and 2)—evaluated the efficacy of IFX for induction and maintenance of remission in UC patients [69]. Three hundred and sixty-four patients with moderate to severe active UC according to the Mayo Index despite concurrent medications (corticosteroids alone or in combination with AZA/6-MP, in ACT 1, or with AZA/6-MP and 5-ASA in ACT 2), were randomised to receive placebo or IFX 5 mg/kg or 10 mg/kg intravenously at weeks 0, 2 and then every 8 weeks through week 46 (in ACT 1) or week 22 (in ACT2). In both studies, a clinical response was obtained in 69% of IFX 5 mg and 61–69% IFX 10 mg, compared to 29–37% in the placebo group, with no difference between patients who are or are not steroid-refractory. At week 30 in both studies, IFX patients were more likely to have a clinical response than controls, and showed a clear steroid-sparing effect. In fact, while at baseline, 56% of patients were on steroids, by week 30, 22% of them discontinued steroids while maintaining remission. Long-term studies will clarify whether these promising results and the cost-effectiveness of this medical approach in avoiding colectomy will be maintained over the years.

Other Approaches

Interferon-β

Immunomodulatory therapy with interferon-beta (IFN-β) might represent a new strategy in UC due to the divergent effects of this cytokine on the immunological and inflammatory process. IFN-β produces an anti-inflammatory effect by inhibiting the production of IFN-γ and TNF-α and by antagonising early events in the IFN-γ signalling pathway. In addition, IFN-β increases the expression of anti-inflammatory cytokine IL-10 and enhances T suppressor and NK cell activity.

A pilot-study investigated whether IFN-β could induce clinical remission in 25 patients with steroid-refractory UC. Patients were treated with 0.5 MIU human IFN-β i.v. (n=18) or 1MIU recombinant IFN-β s.c. (n=7). Maintenance treatment was carried out for 52±78.8 weeks, 3 times a week. Twenty-two patients entered remission with a mean time to response of 3 weeks and a mean duration of remission of 13 weeks [70]. However, in two subsequent larger trials, no differences were observed between IFN-β and placebo [71–72].

Antibodies Anti-Integrin

A therapeutic approach in UC could be the inhibition of migration of leukocytes into the inflamed intestine by blocking cellular adhesion molecules. The α4β7 integrin is primarily involved in the recruitment of leukocytes in the gut; it is present on the cell surface of a small population of circulating T lymphocytes. Its major ligand is mucosal-addressin-cell adhesion molecule 1, selectively expressed on the endothelium of the intestinal vasculature especially in the inflamed bowel. MLN02 is a monoclonal antibody that specifically recognises the α4β7 heterodimer.

Its efficacy in UC was recently assessed in a multicentre double-blind placebo-controlled trial [73]. A clinical improvement was observed in 66% of patients on 0.5 mg/kg/day of MLN02, in 53% on 2 mg/kg/day of MLN02 and in 33% on placebo. The role of MLN02 in clinical practice needs to be carefully evaluated to define its safety profile. In fact, natalizumab, a similar drug that interrupts leukocyte homing through the blockade of the α4β1 integrin, reduced immune surveillance in the brain with subsequent reactivation of the JC virus. This led to progressive multifocal leuko-encephalopathy, invariably fatal, in three patients and the drug was withdrawn from the market [74].

Leukocytapheresis

Accumulating evidence suggests that an abnormal T-cell-specific immune response to host flora may be a driving force in abnormal inflammation in UC. There is also reasonable consensus that the intestinal epithelium in patients with UC is dominated by leukocytes, macrophages and CD4+ lymphocytes with a T-helper 2 phenotype. Recruitment of these inflammatory cells from the systemic circulation into the intestinal epithelium may be a critical step in the amplification of the inflammatory response. Each cell can generate pro-inflammatory mediators such as cytokines, chemokines, growth factors and nitric oxide radicals which will deteriorate inflamed epithelium. Leukocytapheresis (LCAP) is a therapy based on a selective removal of leukocytes from systemic circulation, obtained by the passage of blood either through a column or through a filter. So far, this form of therapy has mainly been studied in Japan. Recent studies demonstrated that LCAP might be useful for active Crohn's disease and UC after failure of conventional drug treatments.

In an early study, the effect of LCAP on maintaining remission was evaluated in steroid-refractory UC after induction of remission with the same therapeutic procedure. Via induction-LCAP, six patients reached complete remission and one reached partial remission and was then treated with maintenance-LCAP. Four of them were maintained in remission without steroid treatment over 12 months. Recurrence was observed in three patients 3–6 months after the beginning of maintenance, and two of them re-entered remission by re-induction. One patient then presented a second recurrence and underwent a total colectomy [75].

Sakata et al. evaluated 51 UC patients with severe or moderate disease, who failed to respond to conventional therapy. Thirty-three patients went into complete remission after the first induction therapy with significant improvement of the activity score. Ten of them relapsed, but 21 maintained remission with LCAP maintenance [76].

In another study [77], 60 UC patients on sulfasalazine for at least 8 weeks prior to the treatment received a total of 10 sessions of LCAP therapy (once or twice a week). Most patients were also on prednisolone at entry, and had steroids tapered or discontinued during the study depending on the level of improvement. Fifty patients responded to therapy, 14 by achieving a complete remission, with no serious adverse effects.

The endoscopic severity scores were markedly improved in 22 of 46 patients and 68% of steroid-dependent cases could stop steroids. The average dose of steroid after 10 sessions decreased from 15.3 to 3.6 mg/day. In terms of symptom activity, LCAP is more effective in patients who during the course of their disease had received a low cumulative dosage of steroids. There was a highly significant association between symptomatic improvement of diarrhoea, abdominal pain and rectal bleeding and duration of apheresis or number of sessions per week. Five of the non-responders to LCAP improved with conventional therapy, the other five underwent elective colectomy. No additional maintenance therapy was provided. The improvement continued for a mean duration of 199 days (range: 21–614). The time to relapse was negatively correlated with endoscopic and histologic findings and the cumulative dosage of steroids. Further studies will clarify whether this approach will also prove cost-effective in Western populations.

Conclusions

Many different and evolving approaches are available for the treatment of ulcerative colitis. A comprehensive treatment that includes not just the disease but also the patient (often severely debilitated by a lifelong disease, in a proportion of cases refractory to standard treatments) and an effective patient-doctor alliance may improve the overall results.

References

1. Loftus EV Jr (2004) Clinical epidemiology of inflammatory bowel disease: incidence, prevalence and environmental influences. Gastroenterology 126:1504–1517
2. Longobardi T, Jacobs T, Wu L et al (2003) Work losses related to inflammatory bowel disease in Canada: results from a national population health survey. Am J Gastroenterology 98:844–849
3. Card T, Hubbard R, Logan RFA (2003) Mortality in inflammatory bowel disease: a population-based cohort study. Gastroenterology 125:1583–1590
4. Carter MJ, Lobo AJ Travis SPL (2004) Guidelines for the management of inflammatory bowel disease in adults. Gut 53:v1–v16
5. Sutherland LR, May GR, Shaffer EA (1993) Sulfasalazine revisited: a meta-analysis of 5-aminosalicylic acid in the treatment of ulcerative colitis. Ann Intern Med 118:540–549
6. Sutherland L, Roth D, Beck P et al (2000) Oral 5-aminosalicylic acid for inducing remission in ulcerative colitis. Cochrane Database Syst Rev 2:CD000543
7. Hanauer S, Schwartz J, Robinson M et al (1993) Mesalamine capsules for treatment of active ulcerative colitis: results of a controlled trial: Pentasa Study Group. Am J Gastroenterol 88:1188–1197
8. Green JR, Lobo AJ, Holdsworth CD et al (1998) Balsalazide is more effective and better tolerated than mesalamine in the treatment of acute ulcerative colitis: The Abacus Investigator Group. Gastroenterology 114:15–22
9. Kruis W, Brandes JW, Schreiber S et al (1998) Olsalazine versus mesalazine in the treatment of mild to moderate ulcerative colitis. Aliment Pharmacol Ther 12:707–715
10. Miner P, Hanauer S, Robinson M et al (1995) Safety and efficacy of controlled-release mesalamine for maintenance of remission in ulcerative colitis: Pentasa UC Maintenance Study Group. Dig Dis Sci 40:296–304
11. Hawkey CJ, Dube LM, Rountree LV et al (1997) A trial of zileuton versus mesalazine or placebo in the maintenance of remission of ulcerative colitis: The European Zileuton Study Group For Ulcerative Colitis. Gastroenterology 112:718–724
12. Sandberg-Gertzen H, Jarnerot G, Kraaz W(1986) Azodisal sodium in the treatment of ulcerative colitis: a study of tolerance and relapse-prevention properties. Gastroenterology 90:1024–1030
13. Wright JP, O'Keefe EA, Cuming L, Jaskiewicz K(1993) Olsalazine in maintenance of clinical remission in

patients with ulcerative colitis. Dig Dis Sci 38:1837–1842
14. Hanauer S, Sninsky C, Robinson M et al (1996) An oral preparation of mesalamine as longterm maintenance therapy for ulcerative colitis: a randomized, placebo-controlled trial. Ann Intern Med 124:204–211
15. Ardizzone S, Petrillo M, Imbesi V et al (1999) Is maintenance therapy always necessary for patients with ulcerative colitis in remission? Aliment Pharmacol Ther 13:373–379
16. Miner P, Hanauer S, Robinson M et al (1995) Safety and efficacy of controlled-release mesalamine for maintenance of remission in ulcerative colitis: Pentasa UC Maintenance Study Group. Dig Dis Sci 40:296–304
17. Ngo Y, Gelinet JM, Ivanovic A et al (1992) Efficacy of a daily application of mesalazine (Pentasa) suppository with progressive release, in the treatment of ulcerative proctitis: a double-blind versus placebo randomized trial [In French]. Gastroenterol Clin Biol 16:782–786
18. Williams CN, Haber G, Aquino JA (1987) Double-blind, placebo-controlled evaluation of 5-ASA suppositories in active distal proctitis and measurement of extent of spread using 99mTc labeled 5-ASA suppositories. Dig Dis Sci 32:71S–75S
19. Campieri M, De Franchis R, Bianchi Porro G et al (1990) Mesalazine (5-aminosalicylic acid) suppositories in the treatment of ulcerative proctitis or distal proctosigmoiditis: a randomized controlled trial. Scand J Gastroenterol 25:663–668
20. Campieri M, Gionchetti P, Belluzzi A et al (1990) Topical treatment with 5-aminosalicylic in distal ulcerative colitis by using a new suppository preparation: a double-blind placebo controlled trial. Int J Colorectal Dis 5:79–81
21. Campieri M, Gionchetti P, Belluzzi A et al (1991) Optimum dosage of 5-aminosalicylic acid as rectal enemas in patients with active ulcerative colitis. Gut 32:929–931
22. Sutherland LR, Martin F, Greer S et al (1987) 5-Aminosalicylic acid enema in the treatment of distal ulcerative colitis, proctosigmoiditis, and proctitis. Gastroenterology 92:1894–1898
23. Campieri M, Gionchetti P, Belluzzi A (1990) Sucralfate, 5-aminosalicylic acid, and placebo enemas in the treatment of distal ulcerative colitis. Eur J Gastroenterol Hepatol 3:41–44
24. Hanauer SB (1998) Dose-ranging study of mesalamine (PENTASA) enemas in the treatment of acute ulcerative proctosigmoiditis: results of a multicentered placebo-controlled trial: The US Pentasa Enema Study Group. Inflamm Bowel Dis 4:79–83
25. Marshall JK, Irvine EJ (1995) Rectal aminosalicylate therapy for distal ulcerative colitis: a meta-analysis. Aliment Pharmacol Ther 9:293–300
26. Cohen RD, Woseth DM, Thisted RA, Hanauer SB (2000) A meta-analysis and overview of the literature on treatment options for left-sided ulcerative colitis and ulcerative proctitis. Am J Gastroenterology 95:1263–1276
27. Kam L, Cohen H, Dooley C et al (1996) A comparison of mesalamine suspension enema and oral sulfasalazine for treatment of active distal ulcerative colitis in adults. Am J Gastroenterol 91:1338–1342
28. Reddy SI, Friedmanm S, Telford JJ et al (2005) Are patients with inflammatory bowel disease receiving optimal care? Am J Gastroenterol 100:1357–1361
29. Sachar DB (2003) Ten common errors in the management of inflammatory bowel disease. Inflamm Bowel Dis 9:205–209
30. Loftus EV, Kane SV, Bjorkman D (2004) Systemic review: short-term adverse effects of 5-aminosalicylic acid agents in the treatment of ulcerative colitis. Aliment Pharmacol Ther 19:179–189
31. Ransford RAJ, Langman MJS (2002) Sulphasalazine and mesalazine: serious adverse reactions re-evaluated on the basis of suspected adverse reaction reports to the Committee on Safety of Medicines. Gut 51:536–539
32. Van Staa TP, Travis SPL, Leufkens HJM et al (2004) 5-aminosalicylic acids and the risk of renal disease: a large British epidemiological study. Gastroenterology 126:1733–1739
33. Rosenberg JL, Wall AJ, Levin B et al (1975) A controlled trial of azathioprine in the management of chronic ulcerative colitis. Gastroenterology 69:96–99
34. Kirk AP, Lennard-Jones JE (1982) Controlled trial of azathioprine in chronic ulcerative colitis. Br Med J (Clin Res Ed) 284:1291–1292
35. Fraser AG, Orchard TR, Jewell DP (2002) The efficacy of azathioprine for the treatment of inflammatory bowel disease: a 30 year review. Gut 50:485–489
36. Ardizzone S, Maconi G, Russo A et al (2006) Randomised controlled trial of azathioprine and 5-aminosalicylic acid for treatment of steroid dependent ulcerative colitis. Gut 55:47–53
37. Mantzaris GJ, Archavlis E, Kourtessas D et al (2001) Oral azathioprine for steroid refractory severe ulcerative colitis. Am J Gastroenterol 96:2797–2808
38. Ardizzone S, Molteni F, Imbesi V et al (1997) Azathioprine in steroid resistant and steroid dependant ulcerative colitis. J Clin Gastroenterol 25:330–333
39. Lennard L, Gibson BE, Nicole T (1993) Congenital thiopurine methyltransferase deficiency and 6-mercaptopurine toxicity during treatment for acute lymphoblastic leukaemia. Arch Dis Child 69:577–579
40. Colombel JF, Ferrari N, Debuysere H et al (2000) Genotypic analysis of thiopurine S-methyltransferase in patients with Crohn's disease and severe myelosuppression during azathioprine therapy. Gastroenterology 118:1025–1030
41. Sandborn WJ, Tremaine WJ, Wolf DC et al (1999) Lack of effect of intravenous administration on time to respond to azathioprine for steroid-treated Crohn's disease. Gastroenterology 117:527–535
42. The mycophenolate mofetil refractory rejection study group (1996) Mycophenolate mofetil for the treatment of refractory acute, cellular renal transplantation rejection. Transplantation 61:722–729
43. Farell RJ, Ang Y, Kileen P et al (2000) Increased incidence of non Hodgkin's lymphoma in inflammatory bowel disease patients on immunosuppressive therapy but overall risk is low. Gut 47:514–519
44. Connel WR, Kamm MA, Dickson MB et al (1994) Long-term neoplasia risk after azathioprine treatment in inflammatory bowel disease. Lancet 343:1249–1252
45. – (2005) Increased risk of lymphoma among inflam-

matory bowel disease patients treated with azathioprine and 6-mercaptopurine Gut 54:1121–1125
46. Fraser Ag, Jewell DP (2000) Long-term risk of malignancy after treatment of inflammatory bowel disease with azathioprine: a 30 years study. Gastroenterology 118:A1471
47. Lewis JD, Bilker WB, Brensinger C et al (2001) Inflammatory bowel disease is not associated with an increased risk of lymphoma. Gastroenterology 121:1080–1087
48. Francella A, Dyan A, Bodian C et al (2003) The safety of 6 mercaptopurine for childbearing patients with inflammatory bowel disease: a retrospective cohort study. Gastroenterology 124:9–17
49. Stange EF, Neurath MF (1996) Methotrexate in chronic active ulcerative colitis: a double-blind, randomized, Israeli multicenter trial. Gastroenterology 110:1416–1421
50. Mate-Jimenez J, Hermida C, Cantero-Perona J, Moreno Otero R (2000) 6-mercaptopurine or methotrexate added to prednisone induces and maintains remission in steroid-dependent inflammatory bowel disease. Eur J Gastroenterol Hepatol 12:1227–1233
51. Morton D, McGovern D, Jewell DP (2002) The efficacy of methotrexate for maintaining remission in inflammatory bowel disease Aliment Pharmacol Ther 16:693–697
52. Te HS, Schiano TD, Kuan SF et al (2000) Hepatic effects of long-term methotrexate use in the treatment of inflammatory bowel disease. Am J Gastroenterol 95:3150–3156
53. Lichtiger S, Present DH, Kornbluth A et al (1994) Cyclosporine in severe ulcerative colitis refractory to steroid therapy. N Engl J of Med 330:1841–1845
54. D'Heans G, Lemmens L, Geboes K et al (2001) Intravenous cyclosporine versus intravenous corticosteroids as single therapy for severe attacks of ulcerative colitis. Gastroenterology 120:1323–1329
55. Svanoni F, Bonassi U, Bagnolo F et al (1998) Effectiveness of cyclosporine A (CsA) in the treatment of active refractory ulcerative colitis (UC). Gastroenterology 114:A1096
56. Van Assche G, D'Haens G, Noman M et al (2003) Randomized, double-blind comparison of 4 mg/kg versus 2 mg/kg intravenous cyclosporine in severe ulcerative colitis. Gastroenterology 125:1025–1031
57. Sandborn WJ, Tremaine WJ, Schroeder KW et al (1994) A placebo-controlled trial of cyclosporine enemas for mildly-moderate active left-sided ulcerative colitis. Gastroenterology 106:1429–1435
58. Travis SP, Farrant JM, Ricketts C et al (1996) Predicting outcome in ulcerative colitis. Gut 38:905–910
59. Lindgren SC, Flood LM, Kilander AF et al (1998) Early predictors of glucocorticoids treatment failure in severe and moderately severe attacks of ulcerative colitis. Eur J Gastroenterol Hepatol 10:831–835
60. Schibolet O, Regushevskaya E, Brezis M, Soares-Weise K (2005) Cyclosporin A for induction of remission in severe ulcerative colitis. The Cochrane Database of Systematic Review Issue 4
61. Sternthal M, George J, Kornbluth A et al (1996) Toxicity associated with the use of cyclosporine in patients with inflammatory bowel disease. Gastroenterology 110:A1019
62. De Groen PC, Aksamit AJ, Rakela J et al (1987) Central nervous system toxicity after liver transplantation: the role of cyclosporine and cholesterol. N Engl J Med 317:861–866
63. Fellermann K, Ludwig D, Stahl M et al (1998) Steroid-unresponsive acute attacks of inflammatory bowel disease: immunomodulation by tacrolimus (FK506). Am J Gastroenterol 93:1860–1866
64. Baumgart DC, Wiedenmann B, Dignass AU (2003) Rescue therapy with tacrolimus is effective in patients with severe and refractory inflammatory bowel disease. Aliment Pharmacol Ther 15:1273–1281
65. Hogenauer C, Wenzl HH, Hinterleitner TA, Petritsch W (2003) Effect of oral tacrolimus on steroid-refractory moderate/severe ulcerative colitis. Aliment Pharmacol Ther 18:415–423
66. Actis GC, Bruno M, Pinna-Pintor M, Rossini FP, Rizzetto M (2002) Infliximab for treatment of steroid-refractory ulcerative colitis. Dig Liver Dis 34:631–634
67. Gornet Jm, Couve S, Hassani Z et al (2003) Infliximab for refractory ulcerative colitis or indeterminate colitis:an open-label multicentre study. Aliment Pharmacol Ther 18:175–181
68. Jarnerot G, Hertevig E, Friis-Liby I et al (2005) Infliximab as a rescue therapy in severe to moderately severe ulcerative colitis: a randomized, placebo-controlled study. Gastroenterology 128:1805–1811
69. Rutgeerts P, Sandborn WJ, Feagan BG et al (2005) Infliximab for induction and maintenance therapy for ulcerative colitis. N Engl J Med 353:2462–2476
70. Musch E, Andus T, Malek M (2002) Induction and maintenance of clinical remission by interferon-beta in patients with steroid-refractory active ulcerative colitis: an open long-term pilot trial. Aliment Pharmacol Ther 16:1233–1239
71. Nikolaus S, Rutgeerts P, Fedorak R (2003) Interferon b-1a in ulcerative colitis: a placebo-controlled, randomised, dose escalating study. Gut 52:1286–1290
72. Musch E, Andus T, Kruis W et al (2005) Interferon beta-1a for the treatment of steroid refractory ulcerative-colitis: a randomized double-blind placebo-controlled trial. Clin Gastroenterol Hepatol 3:581–586
73. Feagan BG, Greenberg GR, Wild G et al (2005) Treatment of ulcerative colitis with a humanized antibody to the a_4b_7 integrin. N Engl J Med 352:2499–2507
74. Danese S, De La Rue SA, Gasbarrini A (2005) Antibody to the $\alpha_4\beta_7$ integrin. N Engl J Med 353:1180
75. Kondo K, Shinoda T, Yoshimoto H (2001) Effective maintenance leukocytapheresis for patients with steroid dependent or resistant ulcerative colitis. Ther Apher 5:462–465
76. Sakata H, Kawamura N, Takashi H et al (2003) Successful treatment of ulcerative colitis with leukocytapheresis using non-woven polyester filter. Ther Apher Dial 7:536–539
77. Kanke K, Nakano M, Hiraishi H, Terano A (2004) Clinical evaluation of granulocyte/monocyte apheresis therapy for active ulcerative colitis. Dig Liver Dis 36:811–817

Indications for Surgical Treatment of Ulcerative Colitis

Zoran V. Krivokapic, Goran I. Barisic

Introduction

Surgery continues to play a major role in the management of ulcerative colitis because it may save the patient's life, eliminate the long-term risk of cancer, and most importantly, eradicate the disease. Surgical treatment of ulcerative colitis still remains a challenge for the surgeon despite growing knowledge about the disease and advanced surgical techniques. Optimal timing for surgery is the mainstay of a good outcome and is as important as the quality of surgery. Although as many as one third of patients with ulcerative colitis require at least one surgical procedure to address complications derived from their disease, the decision in favour of a surgical approach and its timing is rarely an easy one. It is estimated that approximately 30% of patients with ulcerative colitis will undergo colectomy during the course of the disease [1]. All indications for surgical treatment of ulcerative colitis can be divided into two major types: those requiring emergency surgery and those requiring elective operation.

Indications for Emergency Surgery

Emergency surgery in ulcerative colitis is indicated in cases when life-treating complications occur during the course of the disease. It is of paramount significance to stress the value of well-timed surgical treatment since in many cases appropriate indications (Table 1) and timely operation can save the patient's life.

Table 1. Indications for emergency surgery in ulcerative colitis

- Massive haemorrhage
- Fulminant colitis
- Toxic megacolon
- Perforation
- Obstruction

Massive Haemorrhage

Massive haemorrhage is rarely an indication for emergency colectomy. Severe, life-treating haemorrhage occurs in 0–4.5% of patients with ulcerative colitis and it accounts for approximately 10% of all emergency colectomies performed due to ulcerative colitis [2]. The clinician should recognise potentially severe, massive bleeding and undertake appropriate measures in a timely fashion because a haemorrhage is one of the indications of the disease and can be easily underestimated. It is of paramount importance to distinguish a slow but persistent haemorrhage from severe bleeding with rapidly circulating volume loss. Haemorrhage with anaemia <6 g/dl, requiring 4–6 units of packed red cells, or haemorrhage with shock resistant to resuscitation should prompt emergency colectomy.

Since the bleeding is a marker of the severity of the disease, the clinician should be aware that the patient's life is not jeopardised only by the bleeding itself but by the severe underlying disease. Massive haemorrhage is often associated with concomitant toxic megacolon [2]. Many of these patients are or were using an immunosuppressive therapy that could further increase the risk. Sometimes paramedical reasons like reserves of blood in the blood bank, surgical facilities, etc., can also influence the decision for operative treatment. In any case, the clinician, erroneously believing that the bleeding will spontaneously cease, should not prolong medical treatment indefinitely. There are some reports of successfully managed severe bleeding in ulcerative colitis using a highly selective transcatheter embolisation [3]. This procedure is suggested as an alternative therapeutic approach in selected cases. Despite this successful but sporadic attempt, emergency proctocolectomy is currently advocated as the only reliable treatment. The alternative approach could be emergency colectomy without proctectomy. This alternative has the advantages of being a more simple procedure that can be performed in emergency settings by a less experienced surgeon and is less traumatic for the patient. It should be remembered, however, that total colectomy without proctectomy may not succeed in arresting the bleeding and, due to continued haemorrhage from the preserved rectum, subsequent proctectomy may be warranted in as much as 12% of cases [2]. Severe haemorrhage is a result of intense vascular congestion, erosion and ulceration through mucosa and submucosa. During an operation, it is necessary to resect the area of ulcerated bowel. The surgeon should make the decision, taking into account his experience with colorectal procedures, the condition of the patient and the endoscopic appearance of rectal mucosa. If he has a lack of experience, or the patient is in a poor condition, he should probably choose total colectomy without proctectomy as a first-line treatment. Probably the risk of continued bleeding from the rectal stump can be minimised by ligation of the superior haemorrhoidal artery and vein during colectomy. If the bleeding persists from the rectal stump, it could be managed with rectal washouts with adrenaline chloride in saline solution [4] at 4–6°C or with rectal packings. In case of continued bleeding despite rectal washouts and packings, proctectomy should be performed without hesitation. In this circumstance, the anal canal and pelvic floor should always be preserved. Specific procedures and management of acute severe bleeding in ulcerative colitis are presented in Figura 1.

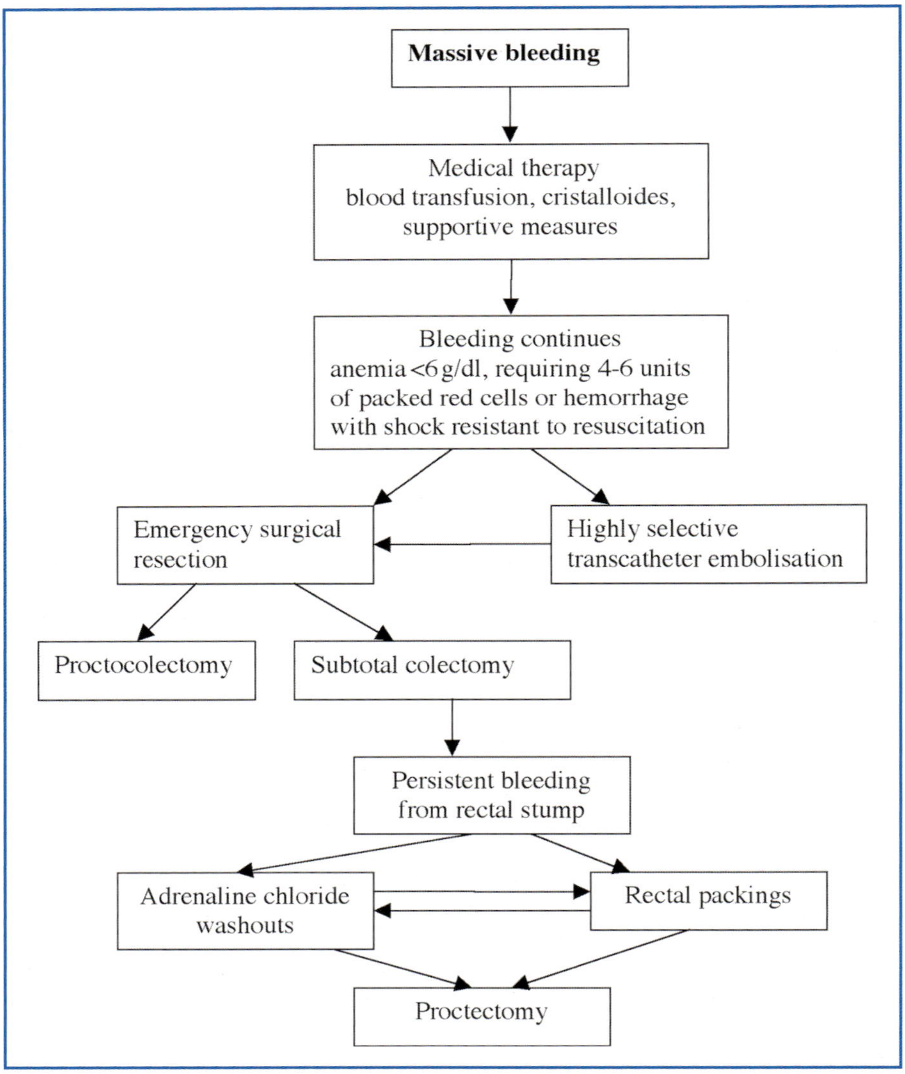

Fig. 1. Management of severe bleeding in ulcerative colitis

Fulminant Colitis

Fulminant colitis represents transmural extension of inflammation to the serosa and is manifested by abdominal tenderness in addition to systemic toxicity. Fulminant colitis with acute abdomen occurs in approximately 10% of patients with ulcerative colitis [5]. A definition of fulminant colitis is not equally accepted and lacks uniformity. To date, severity of the disease is based upon a composite of clinical and endoscopic criteria but no single system has been accepted. Truelove and Witts [6] criteria remain the most commonly used estimate of severity of the disease in clinical practice. According to this criteria, fulminant colitis is suspected when there is more than 10 stools per day, continuous rectal bleeding, anaemia requiring transfusion, temperature above 37.5 °C, pulse rate >90 min, erythrocyte sedimentation rate >30, dilated colon on X-ray and distended abdomen with decreased bowel sounds and rebound tenderness. Travis et al. [7] proposed a much more simplified predictor of the probable need for surgical treatment based on stool frequency and elevated C-reactive protein. One authority considers a patient to have fulminant colitis when evidence of at least two of the following exists: tachycardia, fever, leukocytosis greater than 10 500 cells/mm and hypoalbuminemia [8]. The advent of toxic colitis must be recognised before progression to toxic megacolon. Once the diagnosis of fulminant colitis is established, prompt aggressive medical management with intravenous steroids, antibiotics, decompressive manoeuvres (colonoscopic, patient positioning, etc.) and other supportive measures should be started. Frequent bedside and laboratory assessments together with radiologic evaluation for signs of early loss of small and large-bowel tone are mandatory. An experienced gastroenterologist and surgeon should closely monitor the patient in an intensive care unit. If there are no signs of substantial improvement within 7–10 days at most, or any signs of deterioration and threatening complications at any earlier point in the course, the patient should be offered a trial of intravenous cyclosporine or operated on immediately [9]. If there is no response to intravenous cyclosporine within 7 days or deterioration at any time during medical therapy, urgent colectomy should be performed. There is universal consensus that fulminant colitis unresponsive to medical therapy should be treated with urgent colectomy. The difficulty is that there is considerable disagreement about the definition of "unresponsive" thus making the decision for surgical treatment and especially timing for surgery unclear. An operative specimen from a patient suffering from fulminant colitis is presented in Figure 2.

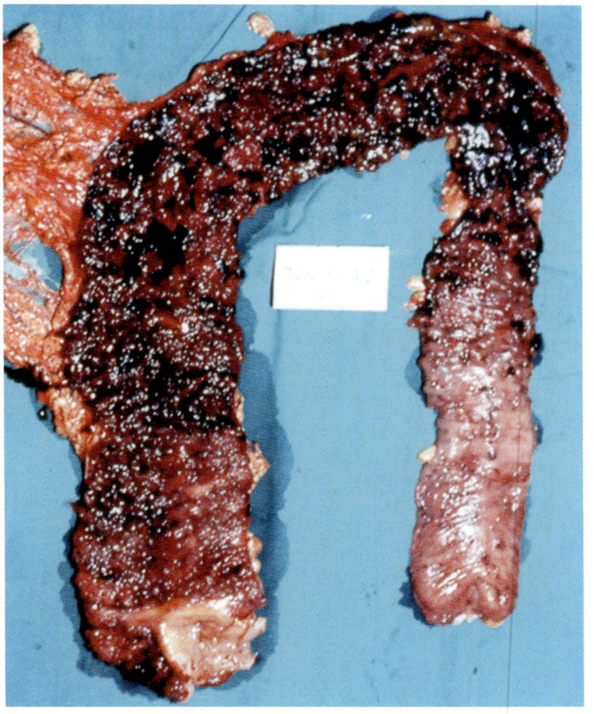

Fig. 2. Operative specimen of fulminant ulcerative colitis

Intensive medical therapy with high-dose intravenous steroids and intravenous cyclosporine for those patients whose disease proves refractory to intravenous steroids, can spare colectomy in more than 80% of patients with no serious drug-related toxicity [10, 11, 12, 13]. Anti-tumour necrosis factor alpha (infliximab) was used in the treatment of severe ulcerative colitis with satisfactory results [14, 15] but with severe toxicity and it is generally believed that off label use of infliximab in ulcerative colitis should be avoided until efficacy is proven in randomised controlled trials [16]. Despite satisfactory results with aggressive medical therapy, and the fact that more than half of the patients retain their colons over the long term, stubborn insistence on medical treatment and the delay of surgery can be very hazardous. Surgery should not be indefinitely delayed, as it is a very effective treatment with acceptable mortality and morbidity rates. There is growing and encouraging experience with laparoscopic total colectomies in acute settings. Laparoscopic colectomy allows for earlier hospital discharge, facilitates subsequent pelvic pouch construction and provides an excellent alternative to conventional surgical treatment [17, 18]. It should be stressed again that an experienced surgeon, gastroenterologist, endoscopist and radiologist should

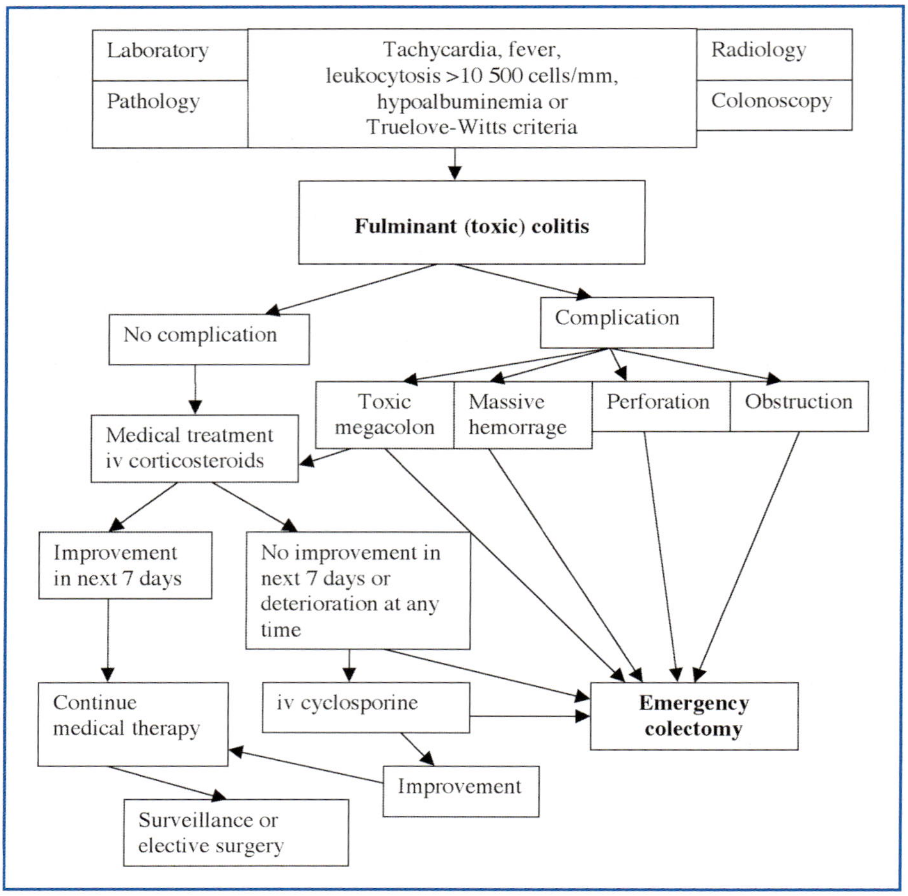

Fig. 3. Diagnosis and management of fulminant colitis

frequently monitor the patient and prompt surgical treatment in cases refractory to medical treatment before serious life-threatening complications occur. Their priorities must focus less on saving colons than on saving lives [19]. Management of fulminant colitis is presented in Figure 3.

Toxic Megacolon

Toxic megacolon is an infrequent but potentially fatal complication of ulcerative colitis. The lifetime incidence of toxic megacolon in individuals with ulcerative colitis is 1–2.5% [20], while there is a reported incidence of 7.9% in patients admitted to hospital due to ulcerative colitis [21]. In the majority of patients, toxic megacolon occurs during a relapse of the disease, but there is substantial amount of those who present with toxic megacolon during the first attack. Diagnosis of toxic megacolon is usually established by clinical exam and plain X-rays of the abdomen. Segmental or total colonic distension of >6 cm in the presence of acute colitis and signs of systemic toxicity are pathognomonic for toxic megacolon. Dilatation of the colon is not by itself an indication for immediate operation. The dilatation may increase, fluctuate or even disappear, leaving the patient still extremely ill requiring urgent surgical treatment. Clinical criteria include any three of the following: fever >38.6 °C, pulse rate >120 beats/min, white blood cell count >10.5 ($x10^9$/l) or anaemia with dehydration, mental changes, electrolyte disturbances or hypotension. In some cases, progression to toxic megacolon is clinically manifested in a decreasing number of stools per day. It is very important to notice that a decreasing number of stools do not always mean that the patient is improving and one should always be suspicious about the possibility of progression to toxic megacolon. The management of toxic megacolon is complex and includes both a medical and surgical approach. Medical and surgical treatment should be regarded as complementary, and not as a competitive treatment modality.

In the onset of toxic megacolon, initial treatment

should be medical with complete bowel rest, supportive measures, decompressive procedures and intravenous steroids. Some authorities advocate "early surgery" shortly after diagnosis in order to save the patient's life ("save the patient, not the colon"), claiming that mortality rates are reduced from 20–7% with this approach [22]. A recent study favouring surgical treatment shortly after the diagnosis of toxic megacolon without using medical therapy as the first-line treatment, showed no mortality and no major complications in patients less than 65 years old [23].

Although there is some controversy about the use of corticosteroids in patients with toxic megacolon, it is now generally agreed that they should be initiated shortly after the diagnosis is established. Aggressive medical therapy with antibiotics and corticosteroids continued up to 7 days showed to be safe and reduced the need for emergency surgery with more than 50% salvage of colons [24, 25].

Medical treatment can be continued for at least 7 days as long as there are signs of clinical improvement. In case of worsening or signs of complication during medical therapy, surgery should be performed without hesitation. Whereas there is confirmed benefit with cyclosporine in patients with fulminant colitis, little experience is available with its use in toxic megacolon and it is generally not recommended. There have been reports of the utilisation of hyperbaric oxygen [26] in the treatment of toxic megacolon and sporadic attempts of treatment with tacrolimus [27] and leukocytapheresis [28] with claims of improvement in the clinical condition; however, due to limited experience with their use, these modalities are not widely accepted and cannot be recommended for standard practice. The long-term prognosis of medically managed toxic megacolon is relatively poor since 47–57% of medically successfully treated patients require colectomy during the follow-up period with 83% of them undergoing surgery on an urgent basis. Medical therapy should be considered as a preparation for surgery and more or less as "a bridge" transforming emergency into elective surgery, thus considerably reducing mortality rates. The procedure of choice is total colectomy and ileostomy. The rectal stump is either closed or the sigmoid remnant is exteriorised as a mucous fistula.

Perforation

Perforation is an acute surgical emergency in patients with ulcerative colitis. Perforation is rare in the absence of toxic megacolon and the risk of perforation is greatest at the time of the first attack. Perforation can be free or walled off and carries a high mortality rate of up to 40% [29]. Free perforation occurs in approximately 2% of patients with UC and is usually associated with toxic colitis or toxic megacolon. If perforation occurs due the course of the disease, it is clear, but for a substantial proportion of patients, it is unfortunately an indication that is "too late" for urgent surgical treatment. The best prevention of this complication is proper, early surgical treatment in patients with fulminant colitis or toxic megacolon before perforation occurs. It should be emphasised that sometimes signs of perforation can be masked in patients receiving high-dose steroids. The patient with this complication is typically severely ill with increased abdominal or shoulder pain associated with tachycardia and fever [30]. Only early recognition of this complication can save the patient's life, necessitating multidisciplinary treatment and frequent monitoring (close cooperation between gastroenterologist, radiologist and surgeon). In the majority of patients, free perforation can easily be seen on upright films of the abdomen but evidence of confined, walled-off perforation may be more subtle. If a perforation is suspected, the patient should be transferred to the operating theatre without delay. The procedure of choice in these circumstances is subtotal colectomy with terminal ileostomy. The rectal stump should be closed in a usual manner or if there is a great risk of dehiscence, mucous fistula can be created.

Obstruction

Obstruction in a patient with long-standing ulcerative colitis results almost invariably from malignancy [31]. Usually, the obstruction is only partial and the patient can be prepared for an elective procedure. Complete acute obstruction occurs infrequently and the patient presents as an emergent case. A thorough clinical exam and upright films of the abdomen can easily establish the diagnosis. In such cases, the surgeon should act as in other cases of acute colonic obstruction and operate on the patient shortly after the diagnosis, but should always have in mind that ulcerative colitis as an underlying disease alters the operative strategy demanding total colectomy. Since the obstruction in a long-standing ulcerative colitis is highly suspicious for malignancy, the operation should be performed utilizing standard oncologic principles. If the rectum is not involved, total colectomy with a Hartmann's procedure or mucus fistula should be performed. When the rectum is involved, proctocolectomy and terminal ileostomy with preservation of anal sphincters is suggested if the oncologic procedure is not compromised. In very rare circumstances, colectomy with abdominoperineal resection of rectum is the only solution.

Indications for Elective Surgery

The indications for elective colectomy have not changed dramatically in recent years despite more effective medical management and advanced surgical procedures that reduce the functional disadvantages associated with conventional proctocolectomy and terminal ileostomy. Each treatment modality, medical and surgical, has advantages and disadvantages, different treatment potentials, complications and influence on the quality of life. Ulcerative colitis is a complex disease and medical and surgical treatment should be regarded as complementary, and not as a competitive treatment modality. Clinical decision-making should be in the hands of a well-trained and experienced team consisting of a surgeon, gastroenterologist, radiologist and pathologist. Elective operation is usually recommended to alleviate devastating consequences of chronic illness, to avoid the distressing side effects of long-term medical treatment and to prevent the development of colorectal carcinoma (Table 2).

Table 2. Indications for elective surgery in ulcerative colitis

Failure of medical treatment
Fulminant/unresponsive nature of first attack
Inadequate response to medical therapy
Side effects or complications related to medications
Noncompliance with medication
Extra-intestinal manifestations
Recurrent haemorrhage
Growth retardation in children
Presence of carcinoma
Cancer prophylaxis

Failure of Medical Treatment

Failure of medical therapy to control the symptoms of chronic, intractable disease is the most common indication for all operations in ulcerative colitis. In general, the response to medical treatment is good, with a success rate ranging from 87–92% for moderate to mild disease, but results are less favourable for severe disease [32]. Failure of medical therapy comprises as much as 75% of patients operated on due to ulcerative colitis in a large series [5]. There is no controversy that the failure of medical therapy is an indication for surgical treatment, however, the problem is in defining the failure of medical therapy. This issue is a highly individualised matter for each patient. Before advising surgery, the clinician should be convinced that medical therapy has been optimally applied including new medications, adequate dose regimens and the patient's compliance to medical therapy. Many factors such as personal, familial, economic, logistical and psychosocial should be analysed together with the patient and the proper decision made with focus on the best interest of the patient. The indication for surgery should be a balance between the severity of the disease and the symptoms despite full medical treatment and the potential disadvantages of surgery.

Fulminant or unresponsive first attack is usually an indication for emergency surgical treatment and was previously discussed. *Intractable disease* is the most common indication for surgical treatment in ulcerative colitis. Criteria of intractability are frequently difficult to define since intractable disease may have a variety of manifestations. This group includes patients with persistent symptoms and inability to achieve remission despite adequate medical treatment with anti-inflammatory or immunosuppressive medications. The stubborn insistence on medical therapy in these patients leads to further deterioration in health and performance status making impending surgical therapy more difficult and hazardous. Another group of patients with intractable disease are those who require continuous corticosteroid therapy to maintain remission. These patients are "steroid dependent" and experience a relapse of symptoms as soon as the dose of steroids is reduced or withdrawn. They should be offered a course of intravenous cyclosporine or surgical therapy. Recent developments in medical therapy with the introduction of infliximab, tacrolimus and leukocytapheresis may alter the therapeutic plan. Intravenous cyclosporine as an inductive therapy followed by oral cyclosporine or 6-mercaptopurine or azathioprine to maintain remission, has the changed indications for surgical treatment, since 78% of cyclosporine responders maintain clinical remission for 1 year. Additionally, there is a potential to use lower inductive doses of cyclosporine (2 mg/kg/day) [33] as well as tacrolimus [34] for outpatient management of steroid-refractory patients. A recent Cochrane analysis showed that the long-term benefit of cyclosporine is unclear while there is substantial risk of cyclosporine-induced nephrotoxicity. Therefore some institutions have restricted the use of cyclosporine to steroid-refractory patients due to the serious risk of toxicity and the high cost of therapy [35]. Oral tacrolimus may be an effective alternative to intravenous cyclosporine for the therapy of steroid-refractory disease. Recent trials with the use of infliximab showed promising results and infliximab appears to be an effective agent for inducing long-term remission in refractory patients with severe ulcerative colitis. In this way, patients who are steroid dependent can often be weaned from steroids. Patients who suffer from an intractable disease can be rescued and avoid colectomy in up to 70% of cases with a single infusion of infliximab [35]. There are promising results with the use of leukocytapheresis in patients with active ulcerative colitis, especially for those at higher risk of steroid-induced adverse effects and those refractory to steroid therapy [36]. Patients whose symptomatic remission is frequently interrupted with attacks of acute colitis despite adequate maintenance therapy, could benefit from surgical treatment. Patients with a chronic mildly active disease and a shortened tubular colon on radiographic examination due to chronic mucosal inflammation and scarring, probably will not benefit from anti-inflammatory agents and should be regarded as candidates for surgical treatment. An operative specimen from a patient with longstanding ulcerative colitis with pseudopolyposis is presented in Figura 4.

There are no accepted criteria for defining the limits of medical therapy in the long-term treatment of ulcerative colitis. Generally, active disease that fails to improve following 3 months of medical therapy or corticosteroid dependence for more than 12 months, should be regarded as indications for surgical treatment. Patients who have devastating symptoms and substantial impairment of quality of life despite appropriate medical therapy may benefit more from elective proctocolectomy and ileal-pouch creation than prolonged unsuccessful medical therapy.

Patients with *serious side effects or complications* during medical therapy are sometimes candidates for surgical treatment. In most cases, reducing the dose or withdrawal of medication alleviates symptoms but in some cases, elective colectomy may be warranted when remission cannot be achieved with alternative medications. This occurs most frequently in patients receiving corticosteroids. Some complications require only supportive care regarding skin lesions, edema, hypertrichosis and dysmenorrhoea while in others, dose adjustment such as steroid induced diabetes, peptic ulcer, hypertension etc. is necessary. The most serious complications of steroid therapy necessitating discontinuation of therapy are osteonecrosis, cataracts, myopathy, psychosis and growth retardation. In these circumstances, elective colectomy should be considered even when underlying colitis could be controlled with alternative medications.

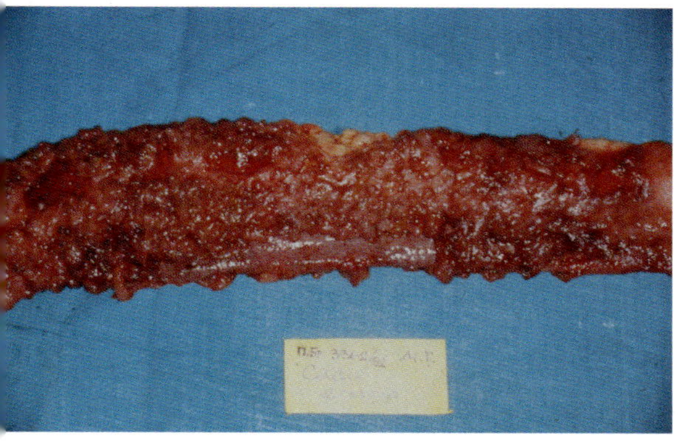

Fig. 4. Operative specimen of ulcerative colitis with pseudopolyposis

Extra-intestinal manifestations of ulcerative colitis are rarely an indication for surgical treatment; even almost 30% of patients with ulcerative colitis will have at least one manifestation that may contribute to the decision for surgery [37]. Unfortunately the most disabling manifestations do not improve after colectomy. Improvement after elective colectomy can be expected only in colitis-dependent extra-intestinal manifestations such as peripheral arthritis, erythema nodosum, thromboembolic complications and uveitis, iritis and episcleritis. Unfortunately, elective colectomy does not influence expression of colitis-independent extra-intestinal manifestations such as sclerosing cholangitis, ankylosing spondylitis, sacroiliitis and pyoderma gangrenosum.

Growth retardation is rarely the only indication for colectomy in children with ulcerative colitis. Usually, growth retardation is one of many severe manifestations of intractable disease. When growth retardation complicates ulcerative colitis, medical therapy should be abandoned and the patient referred to surgery since the best results can be achieved if colectomy is performed prior to the onset of puberty.

Presence of carcinoma in a patient with ulcerative colitis is a clear indication for surgical treatment. Cancer is an indication for surgery in 2% of all colectomies performed due to ulcerative colitis. Although colonic cancer in chronic IBD accounts for 1–2% of all cases of colorectal carcinoma, it accounts for approximately 15% of all deaths in these patients [38].

Cancer Prophylaxis

Colorectal carcinoma is the most serious long-term complication of chronic ulcerative colitis. The relation between long-standing ulcerative colitis and cancer is well documented although the risk of malignancy was overestimated in the past. It is believed that cancer develops through a sequence of

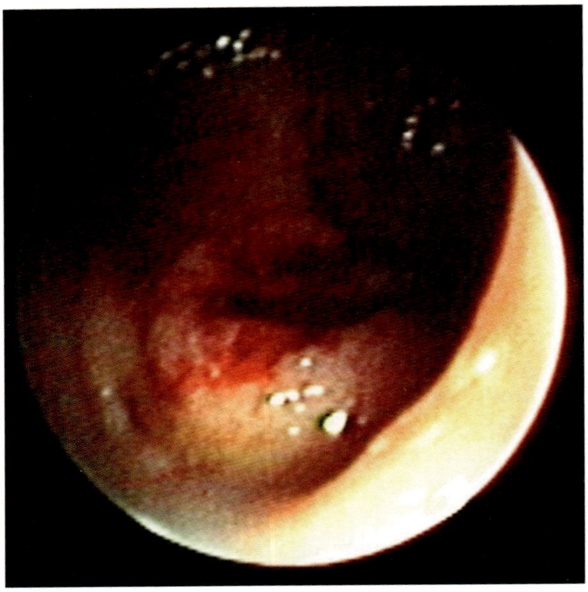

Fig. 5. Endoscopic view. Adenocarcinoma of the cecum in patient with ulcerative colitis

changes from no dysplasia to low-grade and high-grade dysplasia and finally adenocarcinoma. The endoscopic appearance of adenocarcinoma of the cecum in a patient with ulcerative colitis is presented in Figure 5.

The overall absolute risk of colorectal cancer in longstanding extensive or total ulcerative colitis is estimated to be 10–15%, which is 6–10 times higher than expected in the general population. The risk of malignant transformation is not high (0.3–1.0%), but does remain a constant threat especially after a 10-year duration of the disease, when the disease involves the entire colon and when colitis had its onset in childhood [39]. In a meta-analysis by Eaden [40], the cumulative risk of developing colorectal cancer was 8% at 20 years after the diagnosis, rising up to 18% at 30 years. In patients aged 15–39 years at onset of extensive disease, the cumulative risk of developing carcinoma after 25 years is 12% [41]. The cumulative cancer risk in patients with left-sided colitis at the time of diagnosis is less than 5% after 30 years. In recent meta-analysis, the estimated colorectal cancer risk in all patients with ulcerative colitis is 2% at 10 years, 8% at 20 years and 18% at 30 years, irrespective of the extent of the disease [40]. However, treatment of carcinoma or cancer prophylaxis is an indication for operation in 15–30% of patients who undergo elective colectomy. The risk of developing cancer is influenced by the extent and duration of disease while the age of onset of colitis as an independent factor for developing carcinoma remains controversial. Patients with extensive disease (proximal to the splenic flexure) of long duration (>8 years) have a major risk of developing colorectal carcinoma. The severity of the colitis does not correlate with the cancer risk. When cancer occurs, it is usually multicentric and poorly differentiated. Since it is generally believed that cancer in ulcerative colitis develops through a sequence of changes from dysplasia to carcinoma, the presence of low-grade dysplasia (LGD) and high-grade dysplasia (HGD) should be considered to be the particular points of the disease where preventative measures should be instituted. There are several areas of misunderstanding regarding this issue. First, the term dysplasia is a complicated concept and is not always accepted the same way. Second, there are technical hitches regarding the detection of dysplasia, problems with histopathological assessment of biopsy specimens and lastly there is considerable debate about what kind of preventive measures should be initiated-colonoscopic surveillance or total colectomy. By definition, dysplasia is an unequivocal neoplastic change confined to the epithelium [42]. Dysplasia may be patchy and unevenly distributed throughout the colon demanding many biopsies to reduce the risk of sampling errors. It has been estimated that approximately 33 biopsies are necessary to allow 90% confidence in the detection of dysplasia. In practice, biopsies taken from six to ten different sites throughout the colon and rectum have proved to be safe in detecting dysplasia and have a low risk of missing incurable carcinoma [43, 44]. The difficulty with histopathological assessment is in inter- and intraobserver variations in dysplasia assessment. Agreement in the evaluation of dysplasia among experienced pathologists has only reached 42–65% [45, 46]. Therefore, grading of dysplasia should always be evaluated by two experienced pathologists. Apart from controversies in evaluation of dysplasia in ulcerative colitis, there are more controversies concerning treatment. Some studies have suggested that LGD has a low risk of progression to HGD or colorectal carcinoma and have advocated a conservative approach with an increased surveillance schedule [47, 48]. Studies have shown that if LGD does progress to advanced lesions, it does so within 3 years. Therefore, intensive surveillance with repeated colonoscopies every 6 months with four quadrant biopsies every 10 cm should be recommended and colectomy should be performed only for those developing HGD or dysplasia associated lesion or mass (DALM). Others have estimated the risk of progression of LGD to more advanced lesions and colorectal carcinoma to be high enough and recommend prophylactic colectomy [49, 50, 51]. In some cases, flat LGD can progress to colorectal carcinoma without going through a stage of HGD [52]. This fact supports

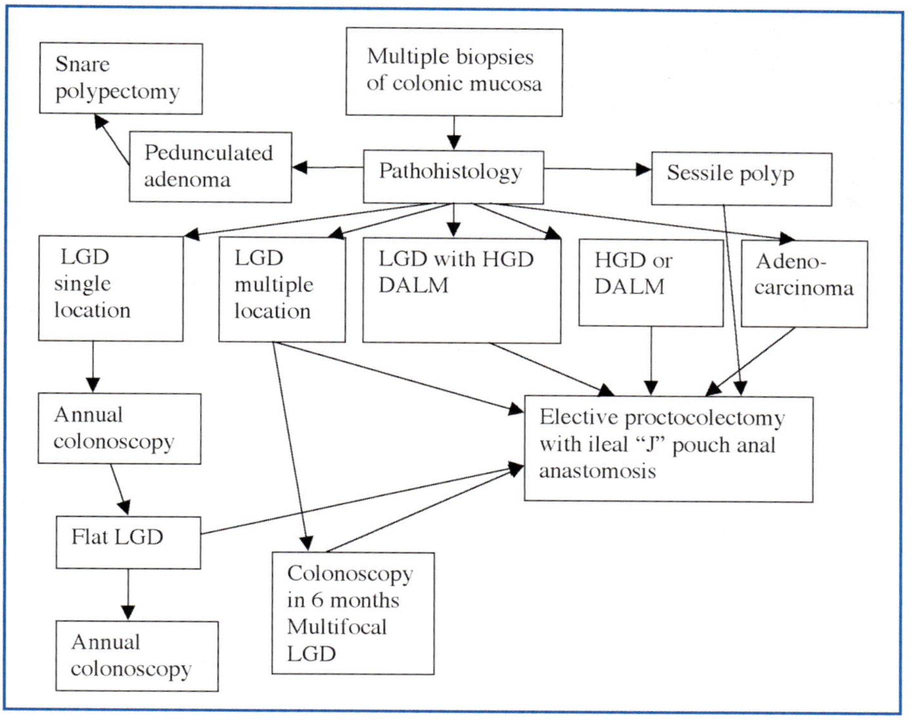

Fig. 6. Cancer prophylaxis

prophylactic colectomy in cases of flat LGD. LGD in the presence of DALM is a sensitive predictor of simultaneous colorectal cancer or progression to colorectal cancer and with the current available evidence, the presence of DALM should be an indication for colectomy. Cancer prophylaxis with the required diagnostic procedures and management are presented in Figure 6.

If LGD is found at a single location, increased vigilance regarding surveillance is advocated along with annual colonoscopy. In cases of multifocal LGD, a new examination should be performed in 6 months and if multifocal LGD is present, the patient should be advised to undergo proctocolectomy. There are wide variations in the management of LGD in ulcerative colitis compared with HGD and DALM where there seems to be more uniform agreement. Findings of dysplasia associated lesion or mass (DALM) with HGD or HGD in flat mucosa are considered as indications for surgery [53, 54]. Pedunculated adenomas in dysplasia-free mucosa should be managed with snare polypectomy as in non-colitis patients. Findings of sessile polyps should be regarded as a potential DALM and prophylactic colectomy should be discussed.

There are a lot of controversies and different and opposite opinions regarding treatment of ulcerative colitis that may lead to some confusion for the one who has to deal with this disease. A lot of knowledge has been accumulated during the past few decades, altering our view and understanding of ulcerative colitis with inevitable repercussion on treatment modalities. There is a growing tendency of conservative treatment in ulcerative colitis using new medications in order to defer or abandon surgery as much as possible. However, surgery should be considered as complementary and not competitive to medical treatment, and not as a last resort because it is a very effective treatment. An experienced gastroenterologist and surgeon, assisted by the radiologist and pathologist, should act as a team in decisions regarding the optimal treatment plan for the patient. Treatment priorities must focus less on saving colons than on saving lives.

References

1. Stewenius J, Adnerhill I, Ekelund GR et al (1996) Operations in unselected patients with ulcerative colitis and indeterminate colitis: a long term follow-up study. Eur J Surg 162:131
2. Robert JH, Sachar DB, Aufses AH Jr et al (1990) Management of severe hemorrhage in ulcerative colitis. Am J Surg 159:550
3. Mallant-Hent RCh, van Bodegraven AA, Meuwissen SG, Manoliu RA (2003) Alternative approach to massive gastrointestinal bleeding in ulcerative colitis: highly selective transcatheter embolisation. Eur J Gas-

troenterol Hepatol 15(2):189–193
4. Pesce G, Ceccarino R (1991) Treatment of severe hemorrhage from a defunctionalized rectum with adrenaline chloride in ulcerative colitis. Dis Colon Rectum 34:1139
5. Michelassi F, Finco C (1995) Indications for surgery in inflammatory bowel disease: the surgeon's perspective. In: Kirsner JB, Shorter RG (eds) Inflammatory bowel disease, 4th edn. Williams, Baltimore, pp 771–783
6. Truelove SC, Witts LJ (1995) Cortisone in ulcerative colitis: final report on a therapeutic trial. BMJ 2:1041
7. Travis SPL, Farrant JM, Ricketts C et al (1996) Predicting outcome in severe colitis. Gut 38:905
8. Fazio VW (1980) Toxic megacolon in ulcerative colitis and Crohn's colitis. Gastroenterol 9:389–407
9. Lichtiger S, Present DH, Kornbluth A et al (1994) Cyclosporine in severe ulcerative colitis refractory to steroid therapy. N Engl J Med 330:1841
10. Marion JF, Present DH (1997) The modern medical management of acute, severe ulcerative colitis. Eur J Gastroenterol Hepatol 9:831–835
11. Daperno M, Sostegni R, Scaglione N et al (2004) Outcome of a conservative approach in severe ulcerative colitis. Dig Liver Dis 36:4–6
12. Rayner CK, McCormack G, Emmanuel AV, Kamm MA (2003) Long-term results of low-dose intravenous ciclosporin for acute severe ulcerative colitis. Aliment Pharmacol Ther 18:303–308
13. D'Haens G, Lemmens L, Geboes K et al (2001) Intravenous cyclosporine versus intravenous corticosteroids as single therapy for severe attacks of ulcerative colitis. Gastroenterology 120:1323–1329
14. Kohn A, Prantera C, Pera A, Cosintino R et al (2002) Anti-tumour necrosis factor alpha (infliximab) in the treatment of severe ulcerative colitis: result of an open study on 13 patients. Dig Liver Dis 34:626–630
15. Lam EC, Bailey RJ (2003) Infliximab salvage therapy after cyclosporine in an acute flare of chronic ulcerative colitis. Can J Gastroenterol 17:198–200
16. Ljung T, Karlen P, Schmidt D et al (2004) Infliximab in inflammatory bowel disease: clinical outcome in a population based cohort from Stockholm County. Gut 53:849–853
17. Bell RL, Seymour NE (2002) Laparoscopic treatment of fulminant ulcerative colitis. Surg Endosc 16:1778–1782
18. Marohn MR, Hanly EJ, McKenna KJ, Varin CR (2005) Laparoscopic total abdominal colectomy in the acute setting. Gastrointest Surg 9:881–886
19. Sachar DB (2000) Indications for surgery in inflammatory bowel disease: a gastroenterologist's opinion. In: Kirsner JB (ed) Inflammatory bowel disease, vol 4. Saunders, Philadelphia, pp 611–615
20. Grieco MB, Bordan DL, Geiss AC et al (1980) Toxic megacolon complicating Crohn's colitis. Ann Surg 191:75–80
21. Latella G, Vernia P, Viscido A et al (2002) GI distension in severe ulcerative colitis. Am J Gastroenterol 97:169–175
22. Goligher JC, Hoffman DC, DeDombal FT et al (1970) Surgical treatment of severe attacks of ulcerative colitis, with special reference to the advantages of early operation. BMJ 4:703–706
23. Amico C, Vitale A, Angriman I et al (2005) Early surgery for the treatment of toxic megacolon. Digestion 72:146–149
24. Katzka I, Katz S, Morris E (1979) Management of toxic megacolon: the significance of early recognition in medical management. J Clin Gastroenterol 1:307–301
25. Present DH, Wolfson D, Gelernt IM et al (1988) Medical decompression of toxic megacolon by "rolling": a new technique of decompression with favorable long-term follow-up. J Clin Gastroenterol 10:485–490
26. Kuroki K, Masuda A, Uehara H, Kuroki A (1998) A new treatment for toxic megacolon. Lancet 352:782
27. Pascu M, Muller AR, Wiedenmann D, Dignass AU (2003) Rescue therapy with tacrolimus in a patient with toxic megacolon. Int J Colorectal Dis 18:271–275
28. Sawada K, Egashira A, Ohnishi K et al (2005) Leukocytapheresis (LCAP) for management of fulminant ulcerative colitis with toxic megacolon. Dig Dis Sci 50:767–773
29. Greenstein AJ, Barth JA, Sachar DB et al (1985) Outcome of toxic dilatation in ulcerative and Crohn's colitis. J Clin Gastroenterol 7:137
30. JJ Tjandra (1999) Toxic colitis and perforation. In: Michelassi F Milsom JW (eds) Operative strategies in inflammatory bowel disease. Springer, Berlin Heidelberg New York, pp 234–245
31. Dozois RR, Kelly KA (2000) The surgical management of ulcerative colitis. In: Kirsner JB (ed) Inflammatory bowel disease. Saunders, Philadelphia, pp 626–657
32. Järnerot G, Rolny P, Sandberg-Gertzen H (1985) Intensive intravenous treatment of ulcerative colitis. Gastroenterology 89:1005
33. Actis GC (2000) Cyclosporin for steroid-refractory ulcerative colitis. Am J Gastroenterology 95:830
34. Bousvaros A, Kirschner BS, Werlin SL et al (2000) Oral tacrolimus treatment of severe colitis in children. J Pediatr 137:794–799
35. D'Haens G (2005) Infliximab for ulcerative colitis: finally some answers. Gastroenterology 128:2161–2164
36. Nishioka C, Aoyama N, Maekawa S (2005) Leukocytapheresis therapy for steroid-naïve patients with active ulcerative colitis: its clinical efficacy and adverse effects compared with those of conventional steroid therapy. J Gastroenterol Hepatol 20:1567–1571
37. Britton A, Peppercorn MA (1995) Emergencies in inflamatory bowel diseases. Crit Care Clin 11:513–529
38. Choi PM, Zelig MP (1994) Similarity of colorectal cancer in CD and UC: implications for carcinogenesis and prevention. Gut 35:950–954
39. Ransohoff D (1988) Colon cancer in ulcerative colitis. Gastroenterology 94:1089
40. Eaden JA, Abrams KR, Mayberry JF (2001) The risk of colorectal cancer in ulcerative colitis: a meta analysis. Gut 48:526–535
41. Ekborn A, Helmick C, Zack M, Adami HO (1990) Ulcerative colitis and colorectal cancer: a population-based study. N Engl J Med 323:1228–1233
42. Riddell RH, Goldman H, Ransohoff DF et al (1983) Dysplasia in inflammatory bowel disease: standardised classification with provisional clinical applications. Hum Pathol 14:931–968
43. Rosenstock E, Farmer RG, Petras R et al (1990) Surveillance for colonic carcinoma in ulcerative colitis. Gastroenterology 89:1342–1346

44. Lofberg R, Brostrom O, Karlen P et al (1990) Colonoscopic surveillance in long-standing total ulcerative colitis: a 15-year follow-up study. Gastroenterology 99:1021–1031
45. Ransohoff Df, Riddell RH, Levin B (1985) Ulcerative colitis and colonic cancer: Problems in assessing the diagnostic usefulness of mucosal dysplasia. Dis Colon Rectum 28:383
46. Melville DMN, Jass JR, Morson BC et al (1998) Observer study on the grading of dysplasia in ulcerative colitis: comparison with clinical outcome. Hum Pathol 20:1990
47. Lim CH, Dixon MF, Vail A et al (2003) Ten year follow up of ulcerative colitis patients with and without low-grade dysplasia. Gut 52:127–113
48. Befrits R, Ljung T, Jaramillo E, Rubio C (2002) Low-grade dysplasia in extensive, long-standing inflammatory bowel disease: a follow-up study. Dis Colon Rectum 45:615–620
49. Ulman TA, Loftus VE, Kakar S et al (2002) The fate of low-grade dysplasia in ulcerative colitis. Am J Gastroenterol 97:922–927
50. Bernstein CN, Shanahan F, Weinstein WM (1994) Are we telling patients the truth about surveillance colonoscopy in ulcerative colitis? Lancet 8:71–74
51. Ullman TA (2003) Patients with low-grade dysplasia should be advised to undergo colectomy. Inflamm Bowel Dis 9:267–269
52. Ullman T, Croog V, Harpaz N et al (2003) Progression of flat low-grade dysplasia to advanced neoplasia in patients with ulcerative colitis. Gastroenterology 125:1311–1319
53. Blackstone MO, Riddel RH, Rogers BH, Levin B (1981) Dysplasia associated lession or mass (DALM) detected by colonoscopy in long-standing ulcerative colitis: an indication for colectomy. Gastroenterology 80:366–374
54. Connel WR, Lennard-Jones JE, Williams CB et al (1994) Factors affecting the outcome of endoscopic surveillance for cancer in ulcerative colitis. Gastroenterology 107:934–944

Surgical Management of Acute Ulcerative Colitis

Roberto Tersigni, Luciano Alessandroni, Riccardo Bertolini

Introduction

Acute ulcerative colitis is a potentiality life-threatening disorder once associated with a very high mortality. However, multidisciplinary strategies have improved dramatically to the point where today, mortality is lower than 3% [1, 2]. The Truelove and Witts classification identified clinical criteria for categorising as mild, moderate or severe the severity of ulcerative colitis [3]. The terms acute, severe, fulminant and toxic have been used to describe seriously ill patients with ulcerative colitis. In practice, they are considered almost synonymous, although an acute fulminating colitis can be considered as a toxic exacerbation of an acute, severe attack, according to the modified classification of Hanauer [4]. Outcome following an acute colitis episode depends upon severity of the attack and extent of the disease. Development of toxic colonic dilatation is one of the most serious complications that can occur in patients with severe, acute colitis. Toxic megacolon may be the initial presentation or may represent a flare-up in patients with long standing disease. Colonic perforation, with or without megacolon, and massive colon hemorrhage represent very serious complications. Usually, the main conditions calling for emergency operative treatment of ulcerative colitis are fulminating colitis, toxic megacolon, colonic perforation and massive hemorrhage.

Severe, Toxic and Fulminant Disease

Although many authors use the terms severe, toxic and fulminant interchangeably, the term fulminant ulcerative colitis describes a clinical condition associated with systemic deterioration (Fig. 1). Approximately 10% of patients initially present with severe disease [1, 2]. In the severe attack, the patient has diarrhoea frequently containing blood, with more than six bowel movements in 24 h. There will be systemic toxic effects, with a temperature of greater than 37.5°C, pulse rate over 90 beats per minute, decrease in hemoglobin below 75% of normal value and increase of erythrocyte sedimentation rate over 30 mm/h (Fig. 2). A flat abdominal X-ray usually shows colonic wall oedema. Variable abdominal tenderness can be observed on clinical examination. Fulminant colitis, as originally described by Truelove and Witts in 1955, is characterised by sudden onset of more than ten per day bloody bowel movements, high body temperature, tachycardia, anaemia requiring blood transfusions, leukocytosis sedimentation rate over 30 mm/h and hypoalbuminemia [3, 4]. Dilated colon, abdominal distension and tenderness are often described [4, 5].

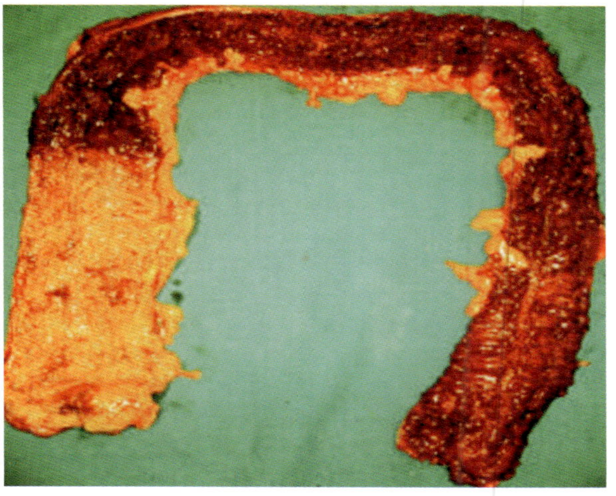

Fig. 1. Acute severe colitis: gross appearance

Toxic Megacolon

Toxic megacolon is one of the most life-threatening complications of severe ulcerative colitis. The terms of toxic colitis and toxic megacolon are often interchangeably but not correctly used. Whereas toxic colitis implies an acutely ill patient with a diseased colon, toxic megacolon is defined as total or segmental [6] nonobstructive hypotonic dilatation of the colon exceeding 6 cm in diameter in the transverse colon on plain abdominal film, with or without signs of systemic toxicity [7-10]. An overall incidence of about 8% of toxic megacolon in ulcerative colitis patients' admission is generally observed [11]. Small bowel distension may precede colonic dilatation and is reported as impending megacolon. This condition is present in about 50% of patients affected by severe ulcerative colitis and is at high risk for development of toxic megacolon. Both conditions, impeding megacolon and toxic megacolon, may be associated with development of multiple organ dysfunction syndrome (MODS), which is responsible of high mortality rates. Remarkably, mortality is similar in patients with pancolitis or with limited colitis but is significantly higher in perforated patients [12, 13]. Although an increasing number of patients is now successfully managed with medical treatment, up to 50% will require urgent or emergent colectomy [14].

The exact explanation for toxic megacolon is not known; the pathogenic mechanism driven by soluble inflammatory mediators and bacterial products, leading to downstream inhibitory effect on colonic muscle tone, could be one of the key players responsible for the and systemic inflammatory response syndrome [11, 15]. Appearance of gastrointestinal distension during the clinical course of acute ulcerative colitis attack should be considered an alarm signal for toxic megacolon or systemic multiorgan dysfunction leading, with high probability, to an emergent colectomy. A certain number of patients presents with toxic megacolon during the first bout of ulcerative colitis or within 2–3 months of diagnosis. Mean duration of disease, before the attack, has been reported to be 3–5 years [6, 16]. Many patients present in the midst of an ongoing attack of severe colitis, with a predominating clinical picture before the onset of toxic megacolon. Patients are acutely ill, with fever, chills and abdominal cramping. Toxic megacolon may be heralded by tachycardia, leukocytosis, dehydration, bloody diarrhoea, abdominal distension, pain and tenderness. Jalan's clinical criteria for diagnosis of toxic megacolon are fever >38.6°C, heart rate >120 beats/min, white blood cell count >10.500/ mm^3 and anaemia, plus one of the following criteria: dehydration, mental changes, electrolyte imbalance or hypotension [16]. Radiological findings show dilatation of transverse or ascending colon >6 cm in patients in the supine position [8], small bowel dilatation with gas shadow areas greater than 36.5 cm^2 and gastric distension with disappearance of gastric mucosal folds. Computed tomography (CT) and magnetic resonance imaging (MRI) scan findings are colonic dilatation >6 cm, abnormal haustral pattern, diffuse colonic wall thickening, submucosal oedema, pericolic stranding, ascites, perforations and adjacent abscess and ascending pyelophlebitis with septic emboli. Delaying treatment increases the risk of perforation, which raises mortality from less than 5% to nearly 30% [2, 5].

Colonic Perforation

Colonic perforation complicates ulcerative colitis in about 3–5% of cases and typically occurs in the setting of toxic megacolon [17]. Colonic perforation without megacolon should raise suspicion of Crohn's disease. However, perforation may also be seen in about 1% of acute colitis without colonic dilatation and is most commonly located in the sigmoid colon. Perforation may occur during diagnostic endoscopies performed without extreme caution. Free perforation is demonstrated on upright or lateral X-ray films. Sealed perforation, while not detected radiologically, is occasionally recognised as a palpable mass and always diagnosed at surgery. Free perforation is associated with high mortality rate [18]. Therefore, whatever the cause of perforation, the patient should immediately undergo surgical exploration.

Severe Hemorrhage

Severe bleeding resulting in haemodynamic instability is an unusual complication of acute ulcerative colitis. After excluding the possibility of gastric or duodenal ulcer bleeding, if the patient remains haemodynamically unstable after adequate resuscitation, emergency surgical procedure is indicated. If there is slow but continuing hemorrhage, in a haemodynamically stable patient, an attempt at medical management may be tried for 48–72 h, before proceeding to surgery. A number of studies have proposed clinical prognostic criteria or a predictive model that can forecast risk of recurrent bleeding, need for therapeutic treatment and outcome of patients with massive colonic bleeding [2, 18]. However, the main indications for emergency surgery for severe lower intestinal bleeding are hypotension and shock despite resuscitation, continuous bleeding (>6 U of packed red blood cells transfused) and/or recurrent bleeding after 24 h of stability, with additional transfusion and further decrease of hematocrit value.

Therapeutic Strategy and Timing of Medical and Surgical Management

The first priority of any therapeutic strategy for acute ulcerative colitis is to reduce or avoid morbidity and mortality. Mortality decreased dramatically from 30% to less than 5% after Truelove and Witts proposed in 1955 a three-step strategy [3]:

- Selection of patients with severe ulcerative colitis
- Intensive medical treatment, including high-dose intravenous steroids, for 5–7 days
- Colectomy for patients who fail to respond or who deteriorate

Initial investigations include abdominal examination focused on peritoneal signs (sometimes masked by previous corticosteroid therapy), complete blood count, serum profile, blood cultures, stool testing for *Clostridium difficile*, cytomegalovirus (CMV), *Escherichia coli*, salmonella, shield, amoeba, coagulation studies and plain abdominal and chest X-rays. A limited proctosigmoidoscopy with minimal insufflation can be helpful in previously undiagnosed patients to exclude pseudomembranous colitis or ischaemic colitis. However, barium enema and colonoscopy are usually contraindicated in the presence of acute fulminating colitis or toxic megacolon because overdistension may lead to colonic perforation. Endoscopic findings of deep ulcers can provide useful prognostic information, facilitating the decision to proceed with medical or urgent surgical treatment. Intravenous fluids are given to correct metabolic derangement, and blood products are administered for anaemia or coagulopathy. A central venous catheter is inserted for total parenteral nutrition (TPN); bowel rest and hyperalimentation have potential clinical advantage and should be maintained until the patient is receiving adequate enteral feedings. Nasogastric suction is used only in case of severe vomiting or gastrointestinal dilatation. In true fulminant colitis, the usual therapeutic scheme is shortened: 2–3 days of intense steroid therapy (methylprednisolone 40–60 mg/day i.v.), followed by surgery in case of resistance. Finally, patients with unresponsive toxic megacolon after 24–48 h of intensive intravenous treatment and patients with impending perforation, free perforation, generalised peritonitis, septic shock or massive rectal bleeding should be submitted to urgent or emergent surgery.

In patients in whom a satisfactory response is obtained with medical therapy, the intravenous corticosteroid is reduced after 5 days and gradually switched to oral prednisolone. Maintenance therapy with purine analogues or immunosalicylates is started. If a stable patient does not respond to i.v. corticosteroid therapy within 5–7 days, i.v. cyclosporine therapy (2 or 4 mg/kg per day i.v.), adjusted as necessary, is initiated. If cyclosporine therapy is contraindicated because of renal insufficiency, hypocholesterolemia, sepsis or patients refusal, surgical treatment is advised. When colitis responds to cyclosporine treatment, maintenance therapy with mercaptopurine (6-MP) or azathioprine is considered. If colitis does not respond to cyclosporine treatment within 4–5 days or complete remission is not achieved within 10–14 days, there is indication for surgery. Infliximab, heparin and tacrolimus have been studied for management of severe colitis. The role of these medications will be better clarified through future investigations [19]. Most patients with acute, severe, fulminant colitis respond to aggressive medical therapy. Care must be taken, however, not to overtreat patients because of the side effects of immunosuppressive drugs. Patients who show no signs of improvement must be referred to surgery. The decision regarding management of fulminant ulcerative colitis requires considerable experience, especially in unstable patients who do not rapidly respond to conservative treatment [20].

Surgical Strategies: Choice of Procedure

Operative strategies for treating severe ulcerative colitis are controversial. Nonresponder patients healthy enough to undergo full procedure at once can be submitted to restorative proctocolectomy. Conversely, patients with perforation, peritonitis, sepsis or massive bleeding should be submitted to a staged procedure: subtotal or total colectomy and ileostomy, followed later by ileorectal anastomosis (IRA) or by proctectomy with ileal pouch/anal anastomosis or by proctectomy with definitive ileostomy. In patients without perforation, peritonitis, sepsis or severe bleeding but not healthy enough to undergo full procedure at once, operative options include subtotal colectomy or rectum sparing total colectomy with ileostomy. Rarely, a blowhole colostomy with ileostomy may be performed. Colectomy with IRA is rarely performed in a select group of patients, namely, those who have a contraindication to a stomy (e.g., portal hypertension or ascites). In most instances, a staged approach, with subtotal colectomy or rectum sparing total colectomy with an end ileostomy, is probably the best treatment because it safely removes the majority of the diseased organ, allowing the patient to recover from the toxic disease state for a future elective full procedure (Fig. 2). Diverting loop ileostomy or segmental colectomy are unusually performed in seriously ill patients. Specific criteria to assume the decision whether to perform an extensive resection or a staged approach are not defined. It is general experience, however, that a staged procedure is mandatory in patients with perforation, peritonitis or sepsis or in patients who do not respond to best medical treatment. Although a few studies report low morbidity and mortality in patients undergoing immediate restorative proctocolectomy [21, 22],

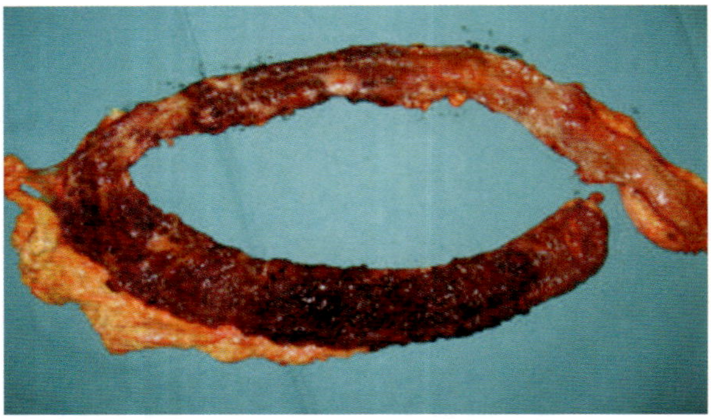

Fig. 2. Acute severe colitis in pediatric age: gross appearance

most authors noted higher incidence of anastomotic leakage (30–40%) in patients undergoing immediate reconstruction [23, 24]. Currently, the choice of surgical procedure must be individualised on the basis of underlying physical, medical, sexual, social and psychological situation [25]. Special consideration in patient selection and in operative planning must be given to age, fertility and fecundity. Advanced age is not an absolute contraindication for ileal pouch–anal anastomosis (IPAA). According to some authors [26], there are no significant functional differences between young or healthy older patients with good sphincter tone. However, a few institutions have reported poorer functional outcomes in elderly patients (>45 years) submitted to IPAA [27]. Given the deep impact of surgery on fertility and fecundity, women should be informed of the possibility of decreased fertility after IPAA. Fecundity is significantly lower in young patients submitted to IPAA than those who undergo to IRA [28–30], probably due to anatomic changes in the pelvic configuration. Patients submitted to ileorectostomy or coloproctectomy with an end ileostomy usually have a normal pregnancy and delivery. Higher rate of caesarean sections are noted in IPAA patients. Both groups often experience temporary stoma or pouch dysfunction with increase in stool frequency, incontinence and pad usage during pregnancy [29, 31, 32].

Diverting Loop Ileostomy and Decompressive "Blowhole" Colostomy

Rarely, when multiple walled-off perforations are found at laparotomy or when the patient is critically septic or with prohibitive comorbidities, in the presence of long-standing distension of the colon and in case of an inexperienced surgeon, a decompressive procedure is advocated, as described by Turnbull et al. [33]. Blowhole colostomy with loop ileostomy is also recommended during pregnancy, for high-lying splenic flexure leading to the possibility of iatrogenic perforation with diffuse faecal contamination or for sealed perforation with impending risk of disruption during bowel dissection. This surgical option can be also considered if the diagnosis has not been cleared. Turnbull's operation is contraindicated in case of free perforation, abscess or hemorrhage. This operation is essentially a temporary decompression procedure bridging to a safe, definitive procedure.

Operative Technique

A small lower midline incision is performed, and the peritoneal cavity is inspected to ensure there is not a free perforation. Through a small right transrectal incision 3- to 5-cm long in the lower quadrant of the abdomen, a loop of ileum proximal to the ileocecal valve is brought out as a loop ileostomy. The distal loop is incised for about three quarters of its circumference; the ileum is everted and sutured at skin level with absorbable interrupted sutures. Through a vertical left paramedian incision 4- to 6-cm long, an antimesenteric transverse skin-level colostomy is performed in the upper abdomen. The "blowhole" colostomy is constructed by dividing the omentum and suturing it to the peritoneum. The transverse colon is sutured to the rectus sheath and deflated by inserting a large bore needle. The colonic wall is incised and sutured to the fascia and skin with interrupted absorbable sutures. No attempt is made to evert the colonic wall, as is usually done. A sigmoidostomy is sometimes created.

Subtotal Colectomy or Total Colectomy and Ileostomy

Over recent years, the majority of reports strongly suggest that subtotal or total colectomy with Brooke ileostomy are the safest and most widely used operations in acute severe ulcerative colitis [34]. A two- or three-stage procedure can be performed. Stage I consists of subtotal or total abdominal colectomy with a sigmoid or rectal stump closure and an end ileostomy [35, 36]. Once the majority or the totality of the diseased colon is removed, the patient's clinical condition will improve, allowing the tapering off of steroids or immunosuppressive therapy. Once the patient has recovered and is clinically fit for another operation, stage II IRA or total proctectomy with end ileostomy or restorative procedure with or without diverting loop ileostomy is carried out [37]. Stage III involves reversal of the ileostomy. Occasionally, persistent bleeding from the retained rectal stump can be observed, but in most cases, it can be controlled by topical steroids application.

Operative Technique

The operation is usually performed with the patient in the Lloyd–Davies position. With the surgeon standing to the patient's left side, the abdomen is entered through a midline incision and fully explored, with particular attention paid to any signs of small-bowel Crohn's disease. Extreme care must be taken when handling the friable bowel in order to avoid colonic traction and to provide easy exposure of the colonic flexure. The entire colon is mobilised away from any retroperitoneal attachments, starting from the cecum (Fig. 3). To avoid injuries, the right spermatic vessels and the right ureter are identified through their course.

The common sites for iatrogenic perforation are the transverse colon with a thickened, highly vascularised omentum, and the splenic flexure, particularly in case of extreme colon dilatation. Since the omentum may be quite adherent to the colon, it may be easier to divide the gastrocolic ligament closer to the stomach than to the transverse colon, and a gentle decompression of the colon with a rectal tube may be helpful. Special attention is required during division of the thickened splenocolic ligament to avoid tearing the splenic capsule. Once the entire colon has been mobilised down to the sigmoid, the terminal ileum is divided adjacent to the ileocecal valve with a linear stapler (Fig. 4). The main ileocolic vessels supplying the terminal ileum are preserved for future pouch construction and mobilised to construct end ileostomy. Two to three centimetres of ileum can be

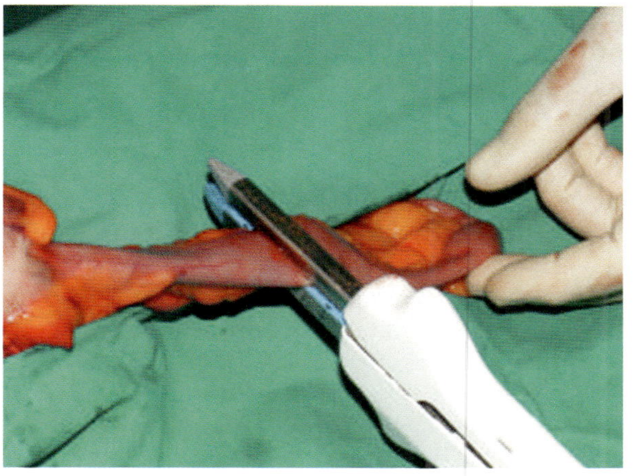

Fig. 4. Total colectomy: section of terminal ileum

denuded of blood supply in preparation of ileostomy, and the mesentery is divided up to the region of the right and middle colic vessels. Individual sigmoid branches, rather than the inferior mesenteric trunk, are isolated in order for the distal sigmoid colon to reach the anterior abdominal wall without tension (Fig. 5). Terminal branches of the inferior mesenteric artery and the superior rectal artery are preserved in order to ensure a good supply to the rectal stump. When rectum-preserving total colectomy is performed, the whole colon is excised to the point of confluence of the colonic taenia at level of the sacral promontory with a stapler loaded with 4.8-mm staples. The sutured link may be oversewn with continuous or interrupted Lembert sutures. In most cases, disease activity settles down, and the rectum heals without problems. It is mandatory to leave intact the

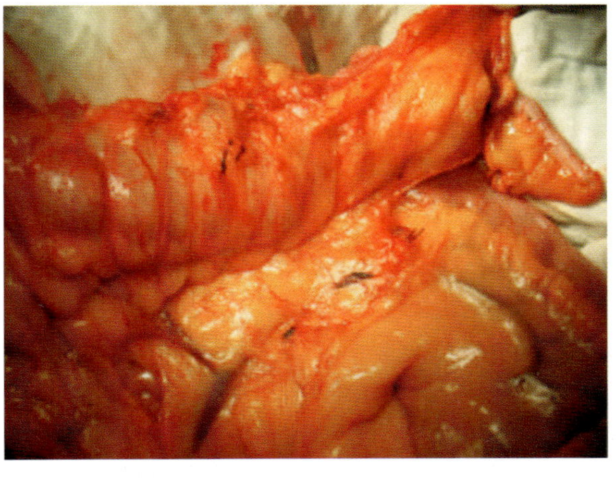

Fig. 3. Total colectomy: preparation of right colon

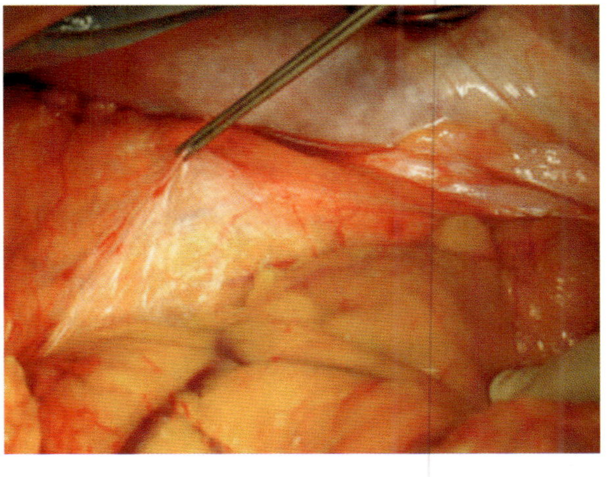

Fig. 5. Total colectomy: preparation of left colon

pelvic peritoneum and the planes of dissection in the pelvis to reduce the risk of sepsis and pelvic-nerve injuries and avoid inconvenience for other future surgical options, such as rectal excision or secondary IRA. In case of massive rectal bleeding or when the rectum is affected by deep ulceration and severe inflammation, the Hartmann pouch can be performed below the peritoneal reflection. An ultralow Hartman's closure of the rectum, at the level of the levators floor, can be performed, with future option of a delayed ileoanal reservoir or a complete proctectomy as a perineal procedure.

When subtotal colectomy is performed, the sigmoid colon is divided at a level where it can be brought out easily through a left lower quadrant incision or lie, without tension, in the subcutaneous plane at the lower end of the midline incision. The seromuscular layer of the bowel is usually sutured circumferentially to the peritoneum. The bowel is divided with a linear stapler or a two-layer suture closure. The skin over the bowel is partially left open or closed with sutures. The benefit of this procedure is that subcutaneous implantation of the stump avoids intraperitoneal abscess and troublesome discharging mucous fistulae. Less commonly, a particularly diseased friable sigmoid colon is brought out as a formal mucous fistula. The sigmoid stump is left protruding 3–5 cm to allow amputation at the skin level and maturation of the mucous fistula in 7–10 days. A long colonic stump is associated with higher risk of bleeding and a very foul odour.

Rectum-sparing total colectomy is a simple and quick procedure in emergency. The rationale for this operation has come from studies that have shown better inflammation and bleeding control, especially in case of severely diseased sigmoid colon [38, 39]. Another advantage of this procedure is that it can avoid parietal abscess, intra- or extrafascial faecal contamination, which is very common when the sigmoid colon is buried in the subcutaneous tissue. About 10% of all patients who have a relatively spared rectum are candidates for future straight end-to-end IRA [40]. Of course, regular surveillance is required for the potential risk of recurrent disease and/or malignant transformation. If the sigmoid colon and rectum are so friable that a safe stapled or sutured closure cannot be obtained, an ultralow Hartman's closure of the rectum, at the level of the levators floor, may be realised. If low rectal closure cannot be performed, the anal stump may be left open, leading a drainage pelvic tube through the anal canal.

Ileorectostomy

Many surgical procedures for acute ulcerative colitis entail a temporary or definitive stoma, with all its attending aesthetic, emotional and sexual implications. Total abdominal colectomy with temporary ileostomy and subsequent ileorectostomy is more acceptable, particularly for young people [41]. However, there are many deterring factors against routine acceptance of ileorectostomy. Although functional results are satisfactory and many patients are quite pleased with the outcome, bowel movement frequency range is between two and ten per day, with a mean of four to five per day. Approximately 50% of patients require occasional antidiarrhoeal agents. Normal continence is generally reported, but a few patients feel social limitations for leakage or soiling.

Proctitis, with progression of disease in the rectal

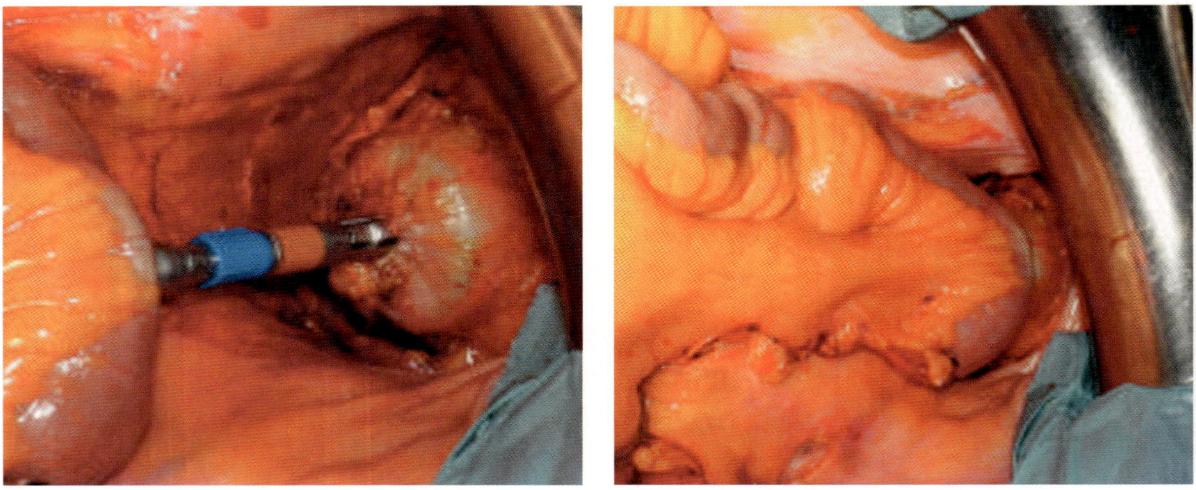

Fig. 6. Ileorectal end-to-end mechanical anastomosis

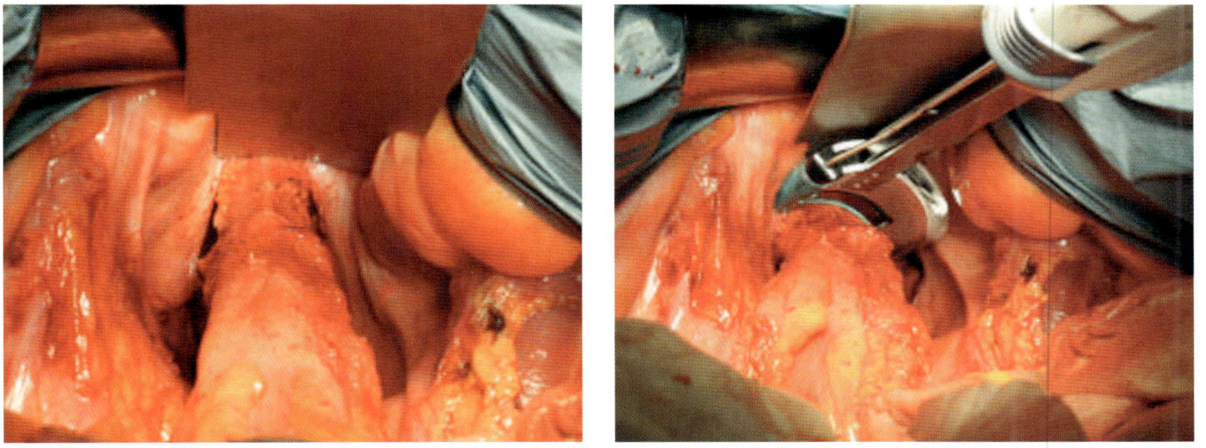

Fig. 7. Restorative proctocolectomy: preparation and closure of rectal stump

stump leading to subsequent proctectomy, is a potential disadvantage. Development of cancer in the residual rectum, with a cumulative risk of 15% at 30 years, is one of the main arguments against ileoproctostomy. Based on many observations, patients with cancer or severe dysplasia in the resected colon are not candidates for ileoproctostomy because of the potential development of cancer in the retained rectum. Therefore, if ileorectostomy is performed, the rectal stump must be kept under close endoscopic evaluation. Besides, high incidence of anastomotic leakage has been documented in many studies [42, 43]. Only patients who have none of the high risk factors should be considered for ileorectostomy; the prognostic significance of disease in the rectum at time of anastomosis, level of anastomosis and patient age at operation should be carefully evaluated (Fig. 6).

Approximately 30% of patients submitted to ileorectostomy will require a subsequent proctectomy, but quality of life is satisfactory in about 55% of patients. Young patients have higher incidence of subsequent proctectomy.

Total Proctocolectomy with Brooke End Ileostomy

Total proctocolectomy has the advantage of removing all disease, thereby obviating the risk of subsequent malignancy. Controversy exists about the role of primary total proctocolectomy in urgent cases, as the procedure is more demanding and associated with higher morbidity rate. Pelvic dissection is more difficult, risk of injury to the autonomic nerve plexuses and possibility of septic sequelae are increased in spite of improvements in bowel preparation. As a general rule, such an extensive operation should be avoided. However, current candidates for total proctocolectomy with Brooke end ileostomy include elderly patients in good condition with poor anal sphincter function, patients with massive rectal bleeding or distal rectal cancer invading the anal sphincter and patients who have a personal preference for this surgical option. Complications, such as impotence and perineal wound breakdown, can be reduced if an intersphincteric proctectomy is performed. Continent ileostomy as functioning Kock pouches [44–46], the Barnett pouch or the T-pouch [34, 47] have achieved some level of acceptance. However, these procedures are associated with numerous complications and are performed largely in referral centres where the need for reoperations is lower than 10%.

End ileostomy as described by Brooke [48] is actually the gold standard in patients not qualified for a restorative procedure. The two major complications of end ileostomy, high output and stoma stricture, were best prevented by the technique of stoma eversion that Brooke reported in 1952 [49]. Sufficient stoma length, its proper seating and its relationship to the waistline should be emphasised and are of major concern. The site for ileostomy is a little below the midway point between the umbilicus and the right anterior iliac spine. A button of skin is excised, the rectal fascia is incised and a noncrushing instrument is inserted between the lateral fibres of the right rectum muscle. The ileum is withdrawn through the ileostomy site. At least 5 or 6 cm of ileum should be brought above the skin level. The mucosa is everted and anchored with interrupted sutures to the skin. The complete ileostomy should extend upward from the skin level at least 2.5–3 cm. The mesentery of the ileum is anchored to the abdominal wall laterally, and the right lumbar gutter is closed off to avoid potential postoperative internal hernias. The chances of peristomal hernia, fistula, retraction and stenosis are minimal.

The Brooke ileostomy is the easiest and quickest type of stoma. The function of stoma begins 3–4 day after is construction. This ileostomy is always used in patients unable to manage intubations required for a continent ileostomy, such as children, the aged and the physically handicapped. It can be difficult to construct in obese patients; a loop ileostomy provides a satisfactory solution.

Despite the advantages, the Brooke ileostomy and the loop ileostomy carry some potential disadvantages. Patients are completely incontinent for gas and stool; bags are uncomfortable; and some patients develop peristomal dermatitis, obstructive ileitis and clinical backwash ileitis. Manifestations of intestinal malfunction may require vigourous replacement of fluid and electrolytes. Alteration in intestinal flora, often caused by the preoperative use of antibiotics, should be of great concern.

Restorative Total Proctocolectomy

The ileoanal pull-through procedure, also referred as restorative proctocolectomy, is rarely performed in urgent cases. This procedure can be potentially offered to patients in good clinical condition, namely, young patients with normal anal sphincter function and/or rectal adenocarcinoma or uncontrollable hemorrhage (Figs. 7, 8). The real advantages of the IPAA are avoidance of permanent stoma and maintenance of the anal route of evacuation, along with the inherent eradication of the disease and discontinuation of anti-inflammatory therapy. Disadvantages include length and complexity of the procedure, possibility of pelvic nerve injuries, pouchitis, septic complications and frequent evacuations. The most significant complications of IPAA include anastomotic and pouch suture-line leak that can lead to pelvic infection, fibrosis and poor functional outcome. Another major complication is pouch vaginal fistula that can require pouch resection. Pouchitis is an inflammatory disease with an aetiologic mechanism not yet clarified. Increasing bowel movements, fever, abdominal cramps and tenderness usually respond to rehydration and metronidazole. Repeated episodes of pouchitis may have deleterious functional effects. The two main technical controversies of the IPAA procedure regard choice of anastomosis and need for diverting ileostomy. The double-stapled pouch-anal anastomosis, 1.5–2.0 cm proximal to the dentate line, is currently considered easier to perform than a mucosectomy with hand-sewn anastomosis [50]. There is no significant difference between the two techniques with respect to functional outcome although patients with mechanical anastomosis tend to experience higher resting sphincter pressure and less nocturnal incontinence [51–53].

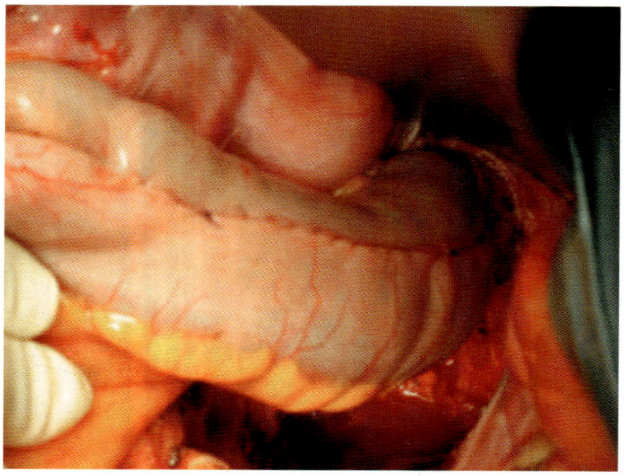

Fig. 8. Restorative proctocolectomy: J-pouch and mechanical end-to-end ileo pouch–anal anastomosis (IPAA)

Opponents of the stapled procedure without mucosectomy are concerned about leaving in place columnar epithelium with the potential risk of cancer in the transitional area. However, there is evidence of an island of residual mucosa even after mucosectomy with hand-sewn anastomosis [54, 55]. Proponents of the one-stage procedure, without diverting ileostomy, believe that a single operation lowers risk of postoperative small-bowel obstruction and reduces hospital stay and total costs. Supporters of the double-stapling technique suggest that septic complications related to pouch leakage might be more severe in patients without a diverting ileostomy [56]. A one-stage procedure, without temporary loop ileostomy, should be offered only to select patients in order to avoid ileostomy takedown and ileostomy-associated morbidity higher than 20% [57–59]. However, in patients with portal hypertension due to primary sclerosing cholangitis, an ileostomy should be discouraged to avoid peristomal varices [60]. Ileostomy closure should be delayed after 6 weeks of primary surgery. After stoma mobilisation, the ileostomy can be closed with a hand-sewn, end-to-end anastomosis, a stapled side-to-side anastomosis or a mechanical end-to-end functional anastomosis.

Operative Technique

The initial incision, abdominal exploration, mobilisation and dissection of the colon are similar to that for total colectomy. When the colon has been full mobilised and the mesentery has been divided, the patient is placed in a steep Trendelenburg position. The presacral space is entered by dividing the left and right pararectal peritoneum. The plane is developed posteriorly and laterally. Anteriorly in male patients, care is taken to identify seminal vesicles, fascia and prostate. The rectum is circumferentially dissected down to the pelvic floor and transected with an articulate linear stapler positioned 1–2 cm above the dentate line. Although various reservoir designs have been described, it was not until 1978 when Parks et al. [61], from St. Mark's Hospital of London, reported their experience with the triple-folded S-shaped reservoir that the modern era of the IPAA began. Several other reservoir designs were later proposed, including the double-folded J-shaped reservoir, the four-folded W-shaped reservoir, the later lateral reservoir of Fonkalsrud, and the U-shaped reservoir. The ileal J-pouch described by Utsunomiya et al. [62] has become the most popular because of its simplicity and functional outcome. The distal 30–40 cm of the ileum is looped approximating the antimesenteric borders of the bowel forming a "J" loop, with 15- to 18-cm limbs and a reservoir capacity of approximately 400 ml. The 75-mm or 100-mm linear cutting stapler is inserted through a stab wound into the antimesenteric border of the ileum at the apex of the lumen, thereby dividing the common wall between the two limbs. The procedure is repeated using the same opening until pouch construction is complete. The anastomotic staple line is inspected for haemostasis. The pouch will reach the pelvic floor without vascular tension if its apex can be pulled 3–5 cm below the upper aspect of the pubic symphysis. It may be necessary to score the visceral peritoneum along the superior mesenteric artery and, sometimes, to transect the ileocolic vessels or a few proximal branches. If the region of anastomosis is difficult to reach, an S-pouch may be used, avoiding too long an efferent limb with functional outlet obstruction. By transecting the rectum at the level of the levators, a short mucosectomy can be performed transanally from the dentate line, leaving a short muscular cuff. The tip of the pouch can be sewn by hand at the level of the dentate line [50, 51], sometimes after rectal eversion according to the technique published by Panis et al. [63].

To simplify the operation and with the hope of improving continence, many surgeons prefer to transect the upper anal canal as close to the dentate line as possible and perform a stapled anastomosis. A manual purse-string suture is placed around the tip of the pouch, the head of a circular stapler is inserted into the lumen of the pouch and the purse-string suture is tied. The pin of the stapler is placed upward through the anus. The instrument is closed, and the stapler is fired to anastomose the pouch to the anus [25]. If the pelvic floor is difficult to reach, a straight IAA may be rarely carried out with lower continence rate and poor patient satisfaction.

Laparoscopic Subtotal or Total Colectomy or Proctocolectomy and Ileal Pouch–Anal Anastomosis

Experience has shown favorable results in patients undergoing urgent laparoscopic colectomy for acute ulcerative colitis [64–66] followed by delayed ileoproctostomy or proctectomy and ileo pouch construction. However, the significant clinical advantages of a laparoscopic-assisted procedure remain to be determined. When compared with open colectomy, laparoscopic colectomy has been shown to be associated with improved postoperative pulmonary function, quicker return of bowel function, less postoperative pain, decreased postoperative length of hospital stay, positive body image and less small-bowel obstruction due to postoperative adhesions. Patients on immunosuppressive therapy are also exposed to minor risk of wound infections, incisional hernia and intra-abdominal abscesses. The main disadvantages of laparoscopic operation are steeper learning curve, longer operative time and increasing operative-room costs [67–70]. Toxic megacolon is usually excluded from laparoscopic procedure because of technical challenges in the management of the severely thinned walls of the dilated colon [68]. Emergency laparoscopic restorative coloproctectomy is associated with higher risk of bleeding and injury of pelvic nerves. Perforated acute ulcerative colitis and abscess formation should not be operated in a laparoscopic emergency setting. Laparoscopic-assisted procedures may therefore be considered as an option for patient with fulminant colitis. At the moment, longer procedures or technically demanding operations are a reasonable alternative only in experienced hands.

Operative Techniques

Total Colectomy

A four or five 5/10/12-mm port method in a variable-shaped pattern, a 30° angled laparoscope and an intra-abdominal insufflation of 12 mmHg are usually used with the patient in a modified lithotomic position. If a diverting ileostomy is planned, a 10- to 12-mm trocar is placed in the right lower quadrant. After abdominal exploration to assess laparoscopic feasibility, dissection is carried out in a sequential fashion from the cecum to the rectosigmoid junction a few centimetres above the anterior peritoneal reflection (Figs. 9–14). Care is taken when grasping the bowel not to injure it. The ileocolic branches, middle colic and inferior mesenteric branches are sequentially isolated and transected. Lateral colonic attachments are divided, and the omentum is dissected along with the transverse colon. The terminal ileum is transected with a linear stapler proximal to the ileocecal valve. The presacral space is not entered, and the pararectal peritoneum is not scored. The rectosigmoid junction is transected at the promontory with an articulated linear stapler. The entire colon is exteriorised through an enlarged right lower quadrant trocar incision overlying the rectus muscle. Finally, the terminal ileum is brought out through the same preoperatively marked site for port and stoma placement, and a standard Brooke ileostomy is constructed.

Restorative Proctocolectomy

After placement of trocars and survey of the abdomen, complete mobilisation of the intra-abdominal colon and terminal ileum up to the inferior border of the duodenum is accomplished. The distal ileum and mesenteric vessels are divided intracorporeally. With the patient in Trendelenburg position, the rectum is circumferentially dissected down to the pelvic floor and transected with an articulate linear stapler at a level confirmed by digital examination.

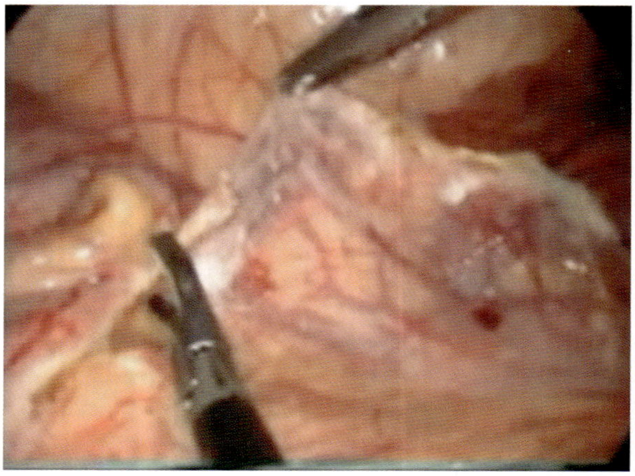

Fig. 9. Laparoscopic total colectomy: preparation of the right colon from hepatic fissure to ileocolic junction

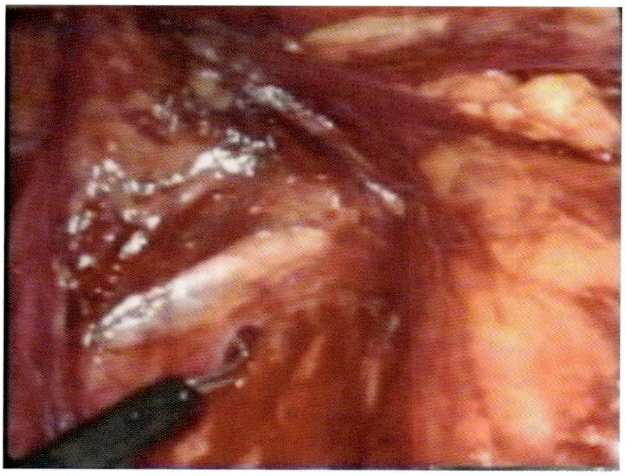

Fig. 10. Laparoscopic total colectomy: identification of right ureter

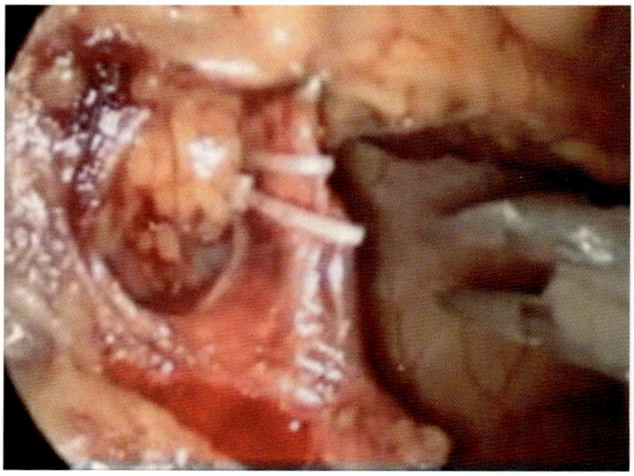

Fig. 11. Laparoscopic total colectomy: ligature and section of right colic vessels

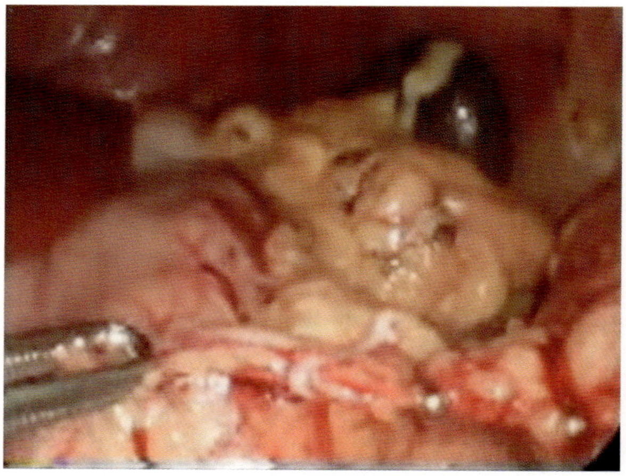

Fig. 12. Laparoscopic total colectomy: preparation of left colon (ligature and section of left colic vessels)

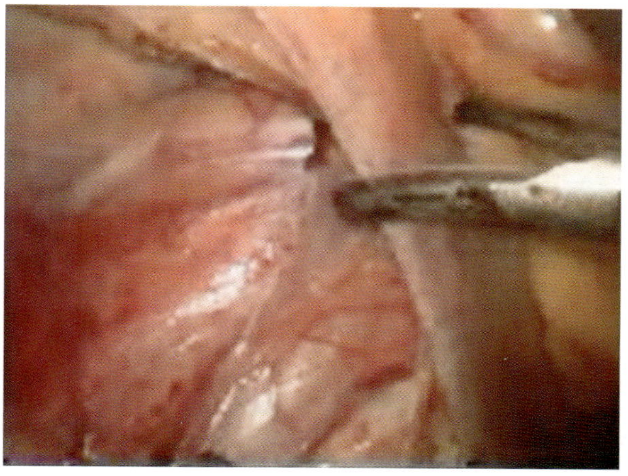

Fig. 13. Laparoscopic total colectomy: identification of left ureter

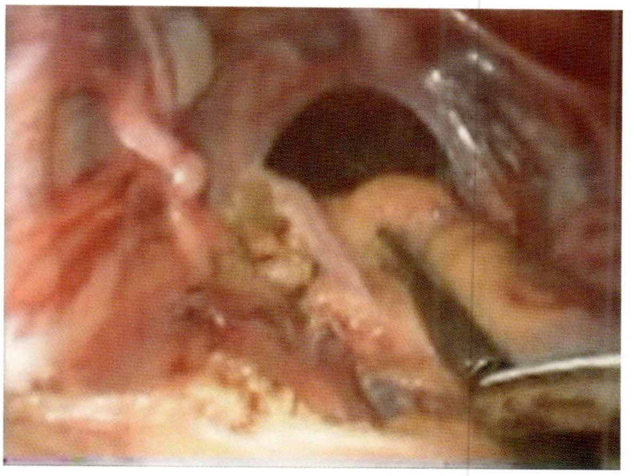

Fig. 14. Laparoscopic total colectomy: preparation of sigmoid colon

The entire specimen is exteriorised through the enlarged inferior low-quadrant incision. Alternatively, mesenteric vessels are divided outside the abdomen, closer to the colon, brought out through a periumbilical or a suprapubic incision. A standard J-pouch is constructed, the head of a circular stapler is secured in the apex of the pouch. The abdominal incision is sutured, and the pneumoperitoneum is re-established. The pouch is then brought down well oriented to the pelvic floor, the head is connected to the pin of the stapler, which is advanced through the anus and fired. A suction drain is positioned in the pelvic region behind the ileal pouch. A loop ileostomy is usually created in the enlarged right lower quadrant trocar site. All trocars sites are inspected, and the parietal incisions are sutured.

References

1. Langholz E, Munkholm P, Davidsen M et al (1994) Course of ulcerative colitis: analysis of changes in disease activity over years. Gastroenterology 107:3-11
2. Becker JM (1999) Surgical therapy for ulcerative colitis and Crohn' disease. Gastroenterol Clin North Am 28:371
3. Truelove SC, Witts LJ (1955) Cortisone in ulcerative colitis: final report on a therapeutical trial. Br Med J 2:1041-1081
4. Hanauer SB (1966) Inflammatory bowel disease. N Eng J Med 334:841-848
5. Strong SA (2002) Fulminant colitis: the case for operative treatment. Inflamm Bowel Dis 8:135-137
6. Gan SI, Beck PL (2003) A new look at toxic megacolon: an update and review of incidence, etiology, pathogenesis, and management. Am J Gastroenterol 98:2363-2371
7. Marshak RH, Lester LJ, Friedman AI (1950) Megacolon, a complication of ulcerative colitis. Gastroenterology 16:768
8. Hywel-Jones J, Chapman M (1969) Definition of megacolon in colitis. Gut 10:562-565
9. Fazio VW (1980) Toxic megacolon in ulcerative colitis and Crohn's colitis. Clin Gastroenterol 9:389-407
10. Sheth SG, LaMont JT (1998) Toxic megacolon. Lancet 351:509-513
11. Latella G, Vernia P, Viscido A et al (2002) GI distension in severe acute colitis. Am J Gastroenterol 97:1169-1175
12. Neschis M, Siegelman SS, Parker JG (1968) The megacolon and ulcerative colitis. Gastroenterology 55:251-259
13. Greenstein AJ, Sachar DB, Gibas A et al (1985) Outcome of toxic dilatation in ulcerative and Crohn's colitis. J Clin Gastroenterol 7:137-143
14. Grant CS, Dozois RR (1984) Toxic megacolon ultimate fate of patients after successful medical management. Am J Surg 147:106-110
15. Caprilli R (1992) Pathogenesis of gastrointestinal distension in severe ulcerative colitis: a hypothesis. Gastroenterol Int 268-272
16. Jalan KN, Sircus W, Card WI et al (1969) An experience in ulcerative colitis. 1. Toxic dilation in 55 cases. Gastroenterology 57:68-82
17. Greenstein AJ, Barth JA, Sachar DB, Aufses AH Jr (1986) Free colonic perforation without dilation in ulcerative colitis. Am J Surg 152:272-275
18. Kaiser AM, Beart RW Jr (2001) Surgical management of ulcerative colitis. Swiss Med Wkly 131:323-337
19. Hanauer SB (2004) Medical therapy for ulcerative colitis 2004. Gastroenterology 126:1582-1592
20. Hurst RD, Michelassi F (2005) Fulminant ulcerative colitis. ACS Surgery, Principles and Practice. Chapter 36. http://www.acssurgery.com, WebMed, Inc.
21. Ziv YM, Fazio VW, Church JM et al (1995) Safety of urgent restorative proctocolectomy with ileal pouch anal anastomosis for fulminant colitis. Dis Colon Rectum 38:345-349
22. Ilarms BA, Myers GA, Rosenfeld DJ et al (1994) Management of fulminant ulcerative colitis by primary restorative proctocolectomy. Dis Colon Rectum 37:971-978

23. Heyvaerr G, Penninekx F, Filez I et al (1994) Restorative proctocolectomy in elective and emergency cases of ulcerative colitis. Int J Colorectal Dis 9:73-76
24. Fukushima T, Sugiura A, Koganei K et al (2000) The incidence and outcome of pelvic sepsis following hand-sewn and stapled ileal pouch anal anastomoses. Surg Today 30:223-227
25. Cima RR, Young-Fadok T, Pemberton JH (2004) Procedure for ulcerative colitis. ACS Surgery, Principles and Practice, chapter 27. www.acssurgery.com. WebMed, Inc.
26. Tan HT, Connolly AB, Morton D et al (1997) Results of restorative proctocolectomy in the elderly. Int J Colorectal Dis 12:319-322
27. Farouk R, Pemberton JH, Wolff BG et al (2000) Functional outcomes after ileal pouch anal anastomosis for chronic ulcerative colitis. Ann Surg 231:919-926
28. Metcalf AM, Dozois RR, Kelly KA (1986) Sexual function after proctocolectomy. Ann Surg 204:624
29. Juhasz ES, Fozard B, Dozois RR et al (1995) Ileal pouch-anal anastomosis function following childbirth: an extended evaluation. Dis Colon Rectum 38:159-165
30. Olsen KO, Juul S, Bulow S et al (2003) Female fecundity before and after operation for familial adenomatous polyposis. Br J Surg 90:227-231
31. Gopal KA, Amshel AL, Shonberg IL et al (1985) Ostomy and pregnancy. Dis Colon Rectum 28:912
32. Nelson H, Dozois RR, Kelly KA et al (1989) The effect of pregnancy and delivery on the ileal pouch anal anastomosis functions. Dis Colon Rectum 32:384-388
33. Turnbull RB, Jr, Hawk WA, Weakley FL (1971) Surgical treatment of toxic megacolon. Ileostomy and colostomy to prepare patients for colectomy. Am J Surg 122:325-331
34. Kaiser AM, Stein JP, Beart RW Jr (2001) T-pouch: a promising new valve design for a continent ileostomy. Dis Colon Rectum 45:411-415
35. Binder S, Miller HH, Deterling RA Jr (1975) Emergency and urgent operations for ulcerative colitis. Arch Surg 110:84-289
36. Albrechtsen D, Bergan A, Mygaard K et al (1981) Urgent surgery for ulcerative colitis: early colectomy in 132 patients. World J Surg 5:607-615
37. Tersigni R, Alessandroni L, Sorgi G (2004) Trattamento chirurgico della malattia di Crohn. Principi di strategia, tattica e tecnica chirurgica. In: Croce E, Olmi S (eds) Chirurgia del colon, del retto e dell'ano. Masson, Milano, pp 195-220
38. van Duijvendijk P, Slors JF, Taat CW et al (1999) Functional outcome after colectomy and ileo-rectal anastomosis compared with proctocolectomy and ileal pouch-anal anastomosis in familial adenomatous polyposis. Ann Surg 230:648-654
39. Soravia C, O'Connor BI, Berk T et al (1999) Functional outcome of conversion of ileo-rectal anastomosis to ileal pouch-anal anastomosis in patients with familial adenomatous polyposis and ulcerative colitis. Dis Colon Rectum 42:903-908
40. Leijonmarck CE, Lofberg R, Ost A, Hellers G (1990) Long-term results of ileo-rectal anastomosis in ulcerative colitis in Stockholm County. Dis Colon Rectum 33:195-200
41. Binderow SR, Wexner SD (1994) Current surgical therapy for mucosal ulcerative colitis. Dis Colon Rectum 37:610-624
42. Fazio VW, Turnbull RB Jr, Goldsmith MG (1975) Ileorectal anastomosis: a safe surgical technique. Dis Colon Rectum 18:107-114
43. Khubchandani IT, Sandford MR, Rosen L et al (1985) Current status of ileo-rectal anastomosis for inflammatory bowel disease. Dis Colon Rectum 32:400-403
44. Kock NG (1969) Intra-abdominal reservoir in patients with permanent ileostomy. Preliminary observations on a procedure resulting in "faecal continence" in five ileostomy patients. Arch Surg 99:223-231
45. Dozois RR, Kelly KA, Ilstrup D et al (1981) Factors affecting revision rate after continent ileostomy. Arch Surg 116:610-613
46. Litle VR, Barbour S, Schrock TR, Welton ML (1999) The continent ileostomy: long-term durability and patient satisfaction. J Gastrointest Surg 3:625-632
47. Barnett WO (1984) Modified techniques for improving the continent ileostomy. Am Surg 50:66-69
48. Parc YR, Radice E, Dozois RR (1999) Surgery for ulcerative colitis: historical perspective. A century of surgical innovations and refinements. Dis Colon Rectum 42:299-306
49. Brooke BN (1952) The management of an ileostomy including its complications. Lancet 2:102-104
50. McIntyre PB, Pemberton JH, Beart RW Jr et al (1994) Double-stapled vs. hand sewn ileal pouch anal anastomosis in patients with chronic ulcerative colitis. Dis Colon Rectum 37:430-433
51. Reilly WT, Pemberton JH, Wolff BG et al (1997) Randomized prospective trial comparing ileal pouch anal anastomosis performed by excising the anal mucosa to ileal pouch-anal anastomosis performed by preserving the anal mucosa. Ann Surg 225:666-676
52. Gemlo BT, Belmonte C, Wiltz O et al (1995) Functional assessment of ileal pouch-anal anastomotic techniques. Am J Surg 169:137-142
53. Saigusa N, Kurahashi T, Nakamura T et al (2000) Functional outcome of stapled ileal pouch–anal canal anastomosis versus handsewn pouch–anal anastomosis. Surg Today 30:575-581
54. Heppell J, Weiland LH, Perrault J et al (1983) Fate of the rectal mucosa after rectal mucosectomy and ileoanal anastomosis. Dis Colon Rectum 26:768-771
55. O'Connell PR, Pemberton JH, Weiland LH et al (1987) Does rectal mucous regenerate after ileoanal anastomosis? Dis Colon Rectum 30:1-5
56. Williamson MER, Lewis WG, Sagar PM et al (1997) One-stage restorative proctocolectomy without temporary ileostomy for ulcerative colitis: a note of caution. Dis Colon Rectum 40:1019-1022
57. Galandiuk S, Wolff BG, Dozois RR, Beart RW Jr (1991) Ileal pouch-anal anastomosis without ileostomy. Dis Colon Rectum 34:870-873
58. Gorfine SR, Gelernt IM, Bauer JJ et al (1995) Restorative proctocolectomy without diverting ileostomy. Dis Colon Rectum 38:188-194
59. Dolgin SE, Shlasko E, Gorfine SR et al (1999) Restorative proctocolectomy in children with ulcerative colitis utilizing rectal mucosectomy with or without diverting ileostomy. J Ped Surg 34:837-840
60. Kartheuser AH, Dozois RR, Wiesner RH et al (1993)

Complications and risk factors after ileal pouch anal anastomosis for ulcerative colitis associated with primary sclerosing cholangitis. Ann Surg 217:314-320
61. Parks AG, Nicholls RJ, Belliveau P (1980) Proctocolectomy with ileal reservoir and anal anastomosis. Br J Surg 67:533-538
62. Utsunomiya J, Iwanna T, Imajo M et al (1980) Total colectomy, mucosal proctectomy and ileo-anal anastomosis. Dis Colon Rectum 23:459-466
63. Panis Y, Bonhomme N, Hautefeuille P, Valleur P (1996) Ileal pouch-anal anastomosis with mesorectal excision for rectal cancer complicating familial adenomatous polyposis. Eur J Surg 162:817-821
64. Hildebrandt U, Lindemann W, Kreissler Hag D et al (1998) Laparoscopically-assisted proctocolectomy with ileo-anal pouch in ulcerative colitis. Zentralbl Chir 123:403-405
65. Meijerink WJ, Eijsbouts QA, Cuesta MA et al (1999) Laparoscopically assisted bowel surgery for inflammatory bowel disease. Surg Endosc 13:882-886
66. Marcello PW, Milsom JW, Wong SK et al (2000) Laparoscopic restorative proctocolectomy: a case matched comparative study with open restorative proctocolectomy. Dis Colon Rectum 43:604-608
67. Marcello PW, Milsom JW, Wong SK et al (2001) Laparoscopic total colectomy for acute colitis. A case-control study. Dis Colon Rectum 44:1441-1445
68. Bell RL, Seymour NE (2002) Laparoscopic treatment of fulminant ulcerative colitis. Surg Endosc 16:1778-1782
69. Ky AJ, Sonoda T, Milsom JW et al (2002) One-stage laparoscopic restorative proctocolectomy: an alternative to the conventional approach? Dis Colon Rectum 45:207-210
70. Kienle P, Weitz J, Benner A et al (2003) Laparoscopically assisted colectomy and ileoanal pouch procedure with and without protective ileostomy. Surg Endosc 17:716-720

The Cancer Risk in Longstanding Ulcerative Colitis: Surveillance Colonoscopy and Prophylactic Surgery

Leif Hultén

Introduction

Colorectal cancer is far from being the most common complication of ulcerative colitis (UC), but it is the one that has been most extensively studied, and the literature on the subject exceeds that dealing with other complications of the disease. Many groups of workers have investigated the complex relationship between ulcerative proctocolitis and cancer of the large bowel.

Incidence

The colitic patient faces a higher risk of large-bowel cancer than does a member of the general population. Opinions as to how large this risk is differ greatly between different authors. This is hardly surprising, however, as there have been differences in the method of collection of materials, and the duration of the colitis has not always been taken into account [1, 2]. In facing the problem of cancer development in longstanding ulcerative colitis, many important issues have to be considered.

Are all patients subject to the same risk from large-bowel cancer, or can any one group of patients be singled out as being especially at risk? If such a group can be identified, at what stage of their disease are they particularly liable to develop the cancer? If the patient's risk group can be defined with reasonable precision, is it possible to predict the sort of cancer risk which an individual patient faces? How should these patients be followed up and how should the surveillance programme be designed? Another crucial issue is whether the risk of cancer is sufficient to warrant the use of prophylactic surgery, and if so, when should it be recommended, and with all options present today, what form should the prophylactic surgery take?

The cumulative probability of cancer for all patients with ulcerative colitis, regardless of disease extent, has been demonstrated to be 2 % at 10 years, 8% at 20 years and 18% at 30 years, while the overall prevalence of colorectal cancer in any patient has been demonstrated to be 3–4% [3]. However, there is convincing evidence that there are colitis patients who have an especially high risk of developing cancer. Investigations into the relationship between cancer and colitis have focussed upon the identification of a "high-risk" group of patients and the one single factor which does exert the most influence regarding cancer risk in colitic patients concerns the extent of the patient's colitis. It seem to be quite clear that patients who are especially at risk for development of carcinoma are those with total or near-total involvement of the colon (i.e. involvement of the whole left half of the colon and the transverse colon as well). There is indeed a remarkable unanimity of opinion on this point between the various workers who have studied the problem [4, 5, 6]. There is, additionally, convincing evidence to show that the duration of colitic symptoms has a strong impact on the incidence of cancer in those high-risk patients. In other words, the longer the history of colitis, the greater the risk of carcinoma.

An idea of the risk of cancer facing the individual patient with total involvement can be gained from the many studies that have been undertaken over the years. Remarkably little attention has been paid to the variation in the duration of the disease between different patients when the incidence of cancer in UC has been calculated. In published reports, the crude incidence is often used. However, the use of crude incidence to evaluate the risk of carcinoma in UC is misleading, as it fails to correct for differences in duration between individual patients. The figures may thus underestimate the true incidence of carcinoma in UC. The time factor is essential and by employing the life-table concept much more sophisticated and accurate results can be obtained. While there is evidence to show that the cancer risk for a patient with total involvement is low during the first 10 years of colitic symptoms, being around 0.4% per annum, the annual risk of cancer starts to rise sharply after this initial decade, and after 20 years of colitis, the individual with total involvement faces an annual risk of cancer of over 5% for the remainder of his life.

However, the yearly risks accumulate, so that the cumulative risk during a period of 5, 10, 20 or even 25 years is far higher. The cumulative risk of cancer in such patients rises slowly at first to around 4% after 10 years of colitic symptoms. However, after 10 years of colitis, the cumulative risk increases more and more sharply to reach a startling level of 41–48% after 25 years of colitic symptoms [5, 6]. Recently, similar results have been presented, while others demonstrate that those with total or extensive colitis (extending proximal to the splenic flexure), colitis of 8 years or more, a family history of colorectal cancer, primary sclerosing cholangitis and an early age of onset of colitis have the greatest risk of developing cancer [3, 7]. Primary sclerosing cholangitis (PSC) occurs in about 2.5–6% of patients with UC, adding considerable risk of cancer compared with UC in general [7]. The mean interval from diagnosis of PSC to dysplasia or cancer is only 2.9 years. Colorectal cancer associated with PSC is more likely to be proximal, to be diagnosed at a more advanced stage, and to be fatal.

While patients with extensive colitis may have an almost 20 times higher risk of cancer compared with the general population of patients, those with left-sided colitis may only have a four times higher risk, and for an individual patient with a distal proctocolitis, the risk is very small, probably about the same as that in the general population of the same age and sex [4, 8].

The age of the patient at the onset of colitis is another factor which has inspired debate. It has often been claimed that colitic patients whose disease began in childhood may have a particular tendency to develop cancer [9]. One explanation that has been put forward is that total involvement – a strong risk factor – is far more common in patients under 20 years of age than in elderly patients. Another important reason why patients who develop ulcerative colitis as children are particularly at risk from carcinoma, is that they are the only patients who will live long enough to develop cancer! Patients who develop total involvement at the age of 50 or later already have a curtailed life expectation and will probably not live long enough to develop cancer. Therefore, the main factor which undoubtedly exerts an effect upon the cancer risk for colitic patients is the extent of the patient's colitis.

Tumour Characteristics and Prognosis

Colitis carcinoma occurs as a rule at an earlier age than does ordinary large-bowel cancer, the average age incidence being 41 years, compared with about 60 years in cases of ordinary carcinoma of the colon and rectum [9]. While most writers claim that the siting of colitis carcinomas does not differ materially from that of ordinary large bowel carcinomas, others have demonstrated that while approximately three-quarters of ordinary carcinomas are concentrated in the rectum and sigmoid, only one-quarter of the colitic carcinoma occurs in the rectosigmoid segment [10]. Another notable feature of colitis carcinomas is the high incidence of multiple primary growths which is about four times greater than that found with carcinoma of the colon in general. The individual growth may exhibit the gross features of an ordinary colorectal cancer but may sometimes be quite atypical, being flat and infiltrating with an ill-defined edge or sometimes appearing rather as a relatively inconspicuous thickening of the colon wall-like fibrous strictures.

Colitic cancers differ even histologically from sporadic cancer as they are more often high grade and mucinous or of a signet-ring cell type, and usually they have spread extensively by the time the patient comes to surgery [11]. Dysplasia in non-colitic cancers is almost always polypoid. In patients with colitis, however, there are flat dysplasia (mostly invisible to an endoscopist), raised dysplasia called DALM (dysplasia-associated lesion or mass) and incidental adenomas.

Because of the active nature of these colitic growths and the delay that often attends their diagnosis, many of them may have reached an advanced inoperable or incurable stage by the time they come to surgery. In the treatment of established colitis carcinomas, if the growth is operable, the ideal is panproctocolectomy since more limited resections are very liable to be followed by the development of further carcinomas in the remaining colon or rectum [11].While reasonably good results may sometimes be achieved after surgery, the average 5-year survival rate is less than after idiopathic cancer [12].

The Justification for Prophylactic Surgery

The high cancer risk and dubious prognosis is disquieting and it automatically raises the question as to the advisability of prophylactic excisional surgery. Over the years, the opinion has been sharply divided as to the justification for this step. While some authors consider that the cancer risk does not necessarily justify an increased use of colectomy [13, 14] others advocate preventive surgery for all patients with a 10-year history of ulcerative colitis and total involvement of the colon and rectum [4, 5, 6]. Still others go even further and recommend surgery for all patients with a radiologically abnormal colon four or more years after the onset of disease [15]. However, even in patients with longstanding colitis, elective proctocolectomy, with its inherent mortality and morbidity, cannot be justified on the basis of cancer prevention in patients whose colitis is restricted to the distal half of the colon. However, in the group of patients with total or subtotal involvement of the colon with a colitic history of 10 or more years, a very strong case can clearly be argued for elective surgery on the basis of cancer prevention alone. In such patients, the risk of cancer with continued conservative treatment is so high as to completely outweigh the hazards of prophylactic surgery.

Cancer Screening and Colonoscopy Surveillance

In the past, the indication for prophylactic colectomy for patients with longstanding ulcerative colitis was mainly based on the disease history and the clinical risk factors mentioned above. Today, with the availability of colonoscopy and the recognition of the dysplasia–precancer–cancer sequence, surveillance colonoscopy with serial colonoscopic examinations and mucosal biopsies is thought to allow for a more adequate individual assessment of the cancer risk and firm recommendation for surgery before the development of cancer. Thus, it is stated that prophylactic surgery should be reserved for patients whose biopsy findings are indicative of heightened cancer risk based on the joint interpretation by the clinician and the pathologist.

Surveillance Guidelines

Guidelines have recently been published by authors from different expert centres [16–19]. Since duration and anatomic extent of the ulcerative colitis have been shown to be the two strong and independent risk factors regarding the development of cancer, special attention to these variables is crucial in the practice of surveillance. The UK guidelines for surveillance in ulcerative colitis [19] state that surveillance colonoscopy should preferably be performed in disease remission, it should be performed in all patients after 8–10 years of disease to clarify disease extent, and regular surveillance should begin after 8–10 years in those with pancolitis and after 10–15 years in those with left-sided colitis. Given that cancer risk increases with the duration of disease, the interval between colonoscopies should decrease in line with increased disease duration. In the second decade of disease, colonoscopy should be carried out every 3 years, in the third decade every 2 years and every year in the fourth decade. Based on the fact that interval cancers can develop within 2 years after an examination, patients with extensive (or left-sided) colitis who have a negative result should begin surveillance within 1–2 years. With a negative surveillance colonoscopy, subsequent examinations should be performed every 1–2 years. With two negative examinations, the next surveillance examination may be performed in 1–3 years until colitis has been present for 20 years.

To obtain 90% sensitivity for the detection of dysplasia in patients with extensive disease, a minimum of 33 biopsies is suggested, taking 4 biopsies for every 10 cm around the colon. In those with less extensive microscopic disease, four quadrant biopsies taken from the proximal extent of disease and every 10 cm distally would be satisfactory. The commonly followed guideline is that any diagnosis of high-grade dysplasia (and low-grade dysplasia when associated with a DALM) should lead to consideration of colectomy, while low-grade dysplasia in flat mucosa should not be an indication for colectomy but for continuous surveillance with colonoscopy. The issue is controversial. While DALM or cancer in such cases has been proved to occur in more than half the patients at 5 years [20] other authors [21] considered low-grade dysplasia (unrelated to a DALM) less alarming and not sufficiently reliable as a marker to justify prophylactic colectomy.

Careful comparative studies by experienced pathologists show evidence that surveillance and screening programmes may carry a significant rate of histological error due to interobserver variation between the gastrointestinal pathologists when grading dysplasia in ulcerative colitis [22].

The Efficacy of Surveillance

There is evidence showing that colonoscopic surveillance may detect precancerous dysplasia and early treatable cancer. Thus, some studies indicate that patients with cancers detected by surveillance tend to be at a curable stage while patients not adhering to surveillance are most likely to die from cancer [23]. Other studies, however, are less convincing [24], showing evidence that only very few of the malignancies found were treatable cancers detected by true surveillance colonoscopy and with only a marginally better success rate. There seems in fact to be no direct evidence that endoscopic surveillance reduces cancer mortality in inflammatory bowel disease [25], and a review reported on in the Cochrane Central Register of Controlled Trials presents a similar message [18]. Although cancers tend to be detected at an earlier stage and has a correspondingly better prognosis in patients who are undergoing surveillance, lead-time bias seems to contribute substantially to this apparent benefit; and there is no clear evidence that surveillance colonoscopy prolongs survival in patients with extensive colitis. Nevertheless, there seems to be consensus that a surveillance programme should offer colonoscopy to patients with extensive ulcerative colitis of 8 years duration and to those with less extensive disease of 15 years duration. Surveillance colonoscopy should be performed every 3 years for 10 years, every 2 years for 10 and then annually including at least four biopsies taken every 10 cm around the colon with careful biopsy of any macroscopic lesion.

Surveillance and its Limitations

Mucosal dysplasia documented by surveillance colonoscopy used clinically to identify the "high risk" patients has proven to have significant limitations. Sampling error, presence of acute mucosal inflammation, differences in pathological interpretation (observer variations) and variable patient compliance are factors that might interfere with the diagnostic accuracy.

The reliability of dysplasia as a precursor of cancer is poor [22]. The histological interpretation is often subjective and of doubtful diagnostic value and the decision making resulting from its discovery will, therefore, often be doubtful. The grading of dysplasia, differentiation between true dysplastic changes and active inflammatory changes and differentiation between DALM and "sporadic" adenomas constitute the dilemma for the pathologist. Moreover, an important obstacle to an accurate assessment of dysplasia is an active mucosal inflammation that may result in cytological changes that are hard to distinguish from dysplasia.

Because dysplasia is focal and patchy, it may not even be detected by extensive colonoscopic biopsies, and established cancers may be missed entirely. Thus, there is evidence showing that a significant fraction of patients may have colorectal cancer in the absence of dysplasia at the colonoscopic surveillance, although this may at least in part be attributable to inadequate surveillance [26]. Based on such observations, the authors claimed that if proctocolectomy is recommended only upon detection of either high-grade dysplasia or dysplasia of any grade, a large proportion of patients may already have an established cancer at the time of surgery. It is obvious that there are practical limitations to the theoretical concept that dysplasia surveillance can reliably serve as a marker for malignant degeneration. The authors also emphasised that failure to operate on high-risk patients – i.e. those with pancolitis, those with duration of disease more than 10 years and those with disease presenting during childhood – while waiting for dysplasia to be discovered by surveillance colonoscopy will invite a high risk of developing concomitant colorectal cancer.

How Can Diagnostic Accuracy be Improved?

It is possible that new molecular markers in conjunction with histologic dysplasia will improve the sensitivity of the surveillance and biopsy approach. Cancer surveillance may also be improved by better selection of patients for inclusion in surveillance programmes, using markers other than dysplasia to predict cancer. Molecular genetic research may produce better ways of selecting patients at greatest risk [27]. It may also produce a better premalignant marker than dysplasia and it can help in distinguishing colitic dysplasia from other entities. Chromoendoscopy can improve the detection of dysplasia and may also be helpful in distinguishing colitic neoplasia from non-colitic neoplasia. Dye spraying of the colonic mucosa during colonoscopy (chromoendoscopy) combined with high-resolution colonoscopy using a magnifying colonoscope is another measure used to increase the detection rate of neoplastic lesions in patients with colitis [28, 29]. Many of these new methods may be promising but no technique has yet been convincing or has entered into routine clinical practice.

Last but not the least, it should be emphasised that, apart from a highly skilled endoscopist and histopathologist, for a program of surveillance to be efficient, it also has to rely on both the physician's and patient's compliance. There should be regular call back for all participating patients so that no patients are lost in follow-up.

Even then, cancer surveillance does not totally eliminate the risk of cancer. Despite many successful results, one must question as to whether colonoscopy surveillance, arguably efficacious for special clinic populations, is truly effective even in the community at large. In other words, will the results obtained from careful clinical trials – produced under ideal conditions – be reproducible when deployed in routine clinical practice? For example, it has been estimated, as a "best-case" scenario, that colonoscopic surveillance may decrease the incidence of cancer from 7–8% down to 0.5–1% and the author claims that no actual program is likely to enjoy such success. Therefore, "at risk" ulcerative colitis patients who are averse to take this cancer risk and who cannot accept the imperfect and in many respects inconvenient nature of colonoscopic surveillance, should be recommended for prophylactic colectomy.

Prophylactic Surgery: What Are the Options?

Panproctocolectomy and Ileostomy (PI)

For prevention of cancer development in patients with ulcerative proctocolitis, complete removal of all potential malignant colorectal mucosa has to be done. Before the advent of the surgical options of our days, panproctocolectomy with construction of a conventional ileostomy was the standard procedure for cancer prophylaxis in patients with longstanding ulcerative colitis. Such an operation eliminates further risks of colorectal cancer and no surveillance should be needed. Although cancer in the ileostomy in these patients has been demonstrated to occur many years after surgery, this is probably a different state of affairs [31]. Bowel metaplasia may occur where gut contents come into regular contact with the squamous epithelium of the skin, which is an important step in the development of these rare tumours, as is also true in some cases of adenocarcinoma of the oesophagus. Ileostomy cancer develops at the mucocutaneous junction of the ileostomy, and chronic irritation caused by trauma and/or chemical agents from stoma appliances or adhesives may be factors in its unclear etiology.

Colectomy and Ileorectal Anastomosis (IRA)

Conflicting results have been presented as regards the indications for colectomy with IRA for ulcerative colitis. Although many surgeons today are still reluctant to use the technique, emphasising not only the persistent cancer risk but also the poor function [32–34], others consider the operation a viable alternative when used selectively in patients without signs of mucosal dysplasia and whose rectum is not severely affected by inflammation or fibrosis [35–37]. The colectomy and IRA procedure for a condition that almost invariably involves an inflamed rectum certainly seems illogical. Apart from poor function, there is a significant risk of cancer development in the chronically inflamed mucosa. It is often argued that a substantial proportion of IRA patients – maybe even half of them – will have their rectum excised eventually due to persistent or relapsing proctitis [38]. However, in many cases, the proctitis often settles spontaneously or after local treatment or recurs periodically. Thus, the patient may enjoy reasonably good general health and bowel function. Therefore, even if 40–50% of the patients will ultimately require rectal excision, roughly half of the patients will continue to enjoy a satisfactory result and many of those who finally fail, have been able to postpone a major operation (IPAA) or an abdominal stoma for several years. Therefore, the time "bought" by IRA will get many young people through their formative years of education, allowing them to plan for a family and a professional career. However, the long-term risk of cancer in the rectal stump is the main strong argument that has been put forward against the use of this operation – a risk that increases with the duration of the disease and with the passage of time after the colectomy. The cumulative probability of cancer development approaches 5 and 15% after a 20 and 30-year observation, respectively [34, 39]. A very important predictive factor is the presence of severe dysplasia in the rectum or carcinoma of the colon at the time of surgery [40]. Bearing this in mind, the risk of rectal cancer should therefore be low in patients with a short antecedent disease history and in those without mucosal dysplasia in the colon/rectum. As regular well-designed colonoscopic surveillance is considered justified for the control of patients with longstanding panproctocolitis – in whom the cancer risk is 3–4 times higher – similar guidelines [19] should be quite appropriate and safe for surveillance of patients with an IRA. In other words, by using a meticulous follow-up system for patients with IRA, it should be possible to identify patients who are at a particular risk and urge them to undergo prophylactic rectal excision.

The controversy regarding colectomy and IRA and the place of this procedure in the treatment of UC has been characterised in the past by personal prejudices and overzealous condemnation of the technique by several of the more prominent experts on colorectal surgery [38]. Employed on a selective basis, IRA should a safe procedure with low mortality and morbidity and good prospects for success as a prophylactic procedure in many patients with longstanding ulcerative colitis. However, before surgery, the patients must be fully informed of any inconveniences and risks associated with the procedure, and, most importantly, they must be prepared to submit to lifelong endoscopy surveillance.

Restorative Proctocolectomy: Ileo Pouch-Anal Anastomosis (IPAA)

The interest in IRA may well have declined with the advent of proctocolectomy and the ileo pouch-anal anastomosis (IPAA). IPAA or restorative proctocolectomy, i.e. construction of a reservoir of distal ileum and an ileo pouch-anal anastomosis is the current most popular option for surgical treatment of ulcerative proctocolitis. There is no stoma or need for an external bag and the normal route of defecation is preserved, i.e. a normal body image. It has become the first choice operation to be recommended around the world. In the conventional technique, colectomy is combined with endoanal mucous proctectomy and the ileal pouch is hand-sewn to the pectinate line. In the currently most popular technique the abdominal dissection is carried out down to the levator muscle, the rectum is severed at this level and the ileal pouch is connected to the rectal stump by a stapling device. In analogy to the traditional total proctocolectomy procedure, it has been considered a curative and cancer-prophylactic procedure since all diseased mucosae are completely removed. At first sight, restorative proctocolectomy therefore seems to be an unmistakable opportunity; however, recent results imply that the IPAA procedure may not be the panacea it was thought to be. It is a demanding operation with a high potential for complications even in an experienced surgeon's hands and the functional results are sometimes far from perfect [41]; even its place as a cancer-prophylactic procedure may in fact be in question. An increasing number of cancers have been reported in these patients and the incidence is expected to rise as the length of follow-up increases [42].

Chronic inflammation in the ileal mucosa (pouchitis) is a frequent complication in continent ileostomy and has proved subsequently to be so even in the pelvic pouch (IPAA)[43]. A case of adenocarcinoma in the continent ileostomy [44] and sporadic reports of dysplasia in the ileal pouch mucosa, have currently appeared in the literature, suggesting that the morphological transformation of the ileal pouch mucosa might eventually result in cellular dysplasia and eventually carcinoma [45, 46]. The atrophic colon-like mucosa in the ileal pouch is hypothetically considered a potentially premalignant condition with risk of subsequent development of advanced neoplastic transformation. It has been suggested that dysplasia and aneuploidy, as demonstrated by these authors, reflect a different pathway of an atrophic mucosa-dysplasia carcinoma sequence. However, the results from long-term studies, both on continent ileostomy patients and subsequently on IPAA patients, are reassuring [47, 48]. The overall incidence of mucosal dysplasia in the ileal pouch mucosa proved to be low and no case of high-grade dysplasia or carcinoma was observed. Considering an observation time of an average of 30 years in these studies, and the comparatively large series of patients, these results imply that dysplastic and neoplastic transformation within the ileal pouch mucosa is extremely rare regardless of the type of adaptation and the risk for epithelial dysplasia in the ileal pouch mucosa to progress into cancer seems to be very low.

The published reports on cancer that develops in the IPAA patients operated on for ulcerative colitis, reflect a quite different issue, however [42, 48]. Irrespective of the technique used, IPAA leaves residual rectal mucosa behind and dysplasia in these rectal mucosal remnants with subsequent cancer development has proved to be a procedural risk, reflecting the continuous risk of malignant transformation in the chronically inflamed rectal mucosa. Thus, it has been demonstrated that even after a careful macroscopically complete mucosectomy, islands of remnants of rectal mucosa are left behind in about 20% of the cases [49], and in the alternative technique where the ileal pouch is stapled to the top of the anal canal, varying amounts of rectal mucosa as well as the anal transitional zone mucosa remain preserved. The rectal stump may even include part of the lower rectum in technically demanding cases. Thus, there is a potential risk for malignant development in the islands of mucosa remaining between the muscular cuff and ileal mucosa or in the retained mucosa in the anal transitional zone, the so-called residual epithelial cuff after the stapled technique. Moreover, it is convincingly demonstrated that this risk is impending in patients with a long history of antecedent ulcerative colitis, and with the diagnosis of dysplasia or cancer in the operative specimen at the time of colectomy [42, 48]). Therefore, although there are reports suggesting that an IPAA is a successful surgical approach for ulcerative colitis patients with coexisting colorectal cancer [50], it is doubtful if such an approach should be recommended.

Although some colorectal surgeons may question the need for routine surveillance for cancer in the IPAA patients [51], these observations imply that despite the fact that the cancer risk after IPAA may well be less than after the IRA procedure, a similar endoscopy surveillance is still justified. A close follow-up in all IPAA patients should be emphasised, with special attention focussed on those with a long antecedent disease history and those with dysplasia or cancer in the original specimen. In this context, it should be emphasised that the dysplasia or early cancer that arises from the residual rectal tissue in the muscular cuff after mucosectomy may not be easily detectable and endoscopy surveillance with deep random biopsies of the anal canal mucosa should be recommended.

References

1. Devroede GJ, Taylor WF, Sauer WG, Jackman RJ and Stickler GB (1971) Cancer risk and life expectancy of children with ulcerative colitis. N Engl J Med 285 1:17–21
2. Devroede G, Taylor WF (1976) On calculating cancer risk and survival of ulcerative colitis patients with the life table method. Gastroenterology 71(3):505–509

3. Eaden JA, Abrams KR and Mayberry JF (2001) The risk of colorectal cancer in ulcerative colitis: a meta-analysis. Gut 48(4):526–535
4. Macdougall IP (1964) The cancer risk in ulcerative colitis. Lancet 19:655–658
5. De Dombal FT, Watts JM, Watkinson G et al (1966) Local complications of ulcerative colitis: stricture, pseudopolyposis and carcinoma of colon and rectum. BMJ 1:1442
6. Hulten L, Kewenter J, Ahren C (1972) Precancer and carcinoma in chronic ulcerative colitis: a histopathological and clinical investigation. Scand J Gastroenterol 7(7):663–669
7. Shetty K, Rybicki L, Brzezinski A et al (1999) The risk for cancer or dysplasia in ulcerative colitis patients with primary sclerosing cholangitis. Am J Gastroenterol 94(6):1643–1649
8. Gyde SN, Prior P, Allan RN et al (1988) Colorectal cancer in ulcerative colitis: a cohort study of primary referrals from three centres. Gut 29(2):206–217
9. Edwards FC, Truelove SC (1964) The course and prognosis of ulcerative colitis. III. Complications. Gut 32:1–22
10. Edling NP, Eklof O (1961) Distribution of malignancy in ulcerative colitis. Gastroenterology 41:465–466
11. Hulten L, Kewenter J, Kock NG (1971) The long-term results of partial resection of the large bowel for intestinal carcinomas complicating ulcerative colitis. Scand J Gastroenterol 6(7):601–604
12. Slaney G, Brooke BN (1959) Cancer in ulcerative colitis. Lancet 2:694–698
13. Texter EC Jr (1957) The natural history of ulcerative colitis. J Chronic Dis 5(3):347–369
14. Carleson RFB, Philipsson J (1962) Ulcerative colitis: a follow-up investigation of a 20-year primary material. Acta Med Scand Dec 172:647–656
15. Dennis C KK (1961) Cancer risk in ulcerative colitis: formidability per patient year of late disease. Surgery 50:568–574
16. Itzkowitz SH, Harpaz N (2004) Diagnosis and management of dysplasia in patients with inflammatory bowel diseases. Gastroenterology 126(6):1634–1648
17. Chambers WM, Warren BF, Jewell DP et al (2005) Cancer surveillance in ulcerative colitis. Br J Surg 92(8):928–936
18. Mpofu C, Watson AJ, Rhodes JM (2004) Strategies for detecting colon cancer and/or dysplasia in patients with inflammatory bowel disease. Cochrane Database Syst Rev 2:CD000279
19. Eaden JA, Mayberry JF (2002) Guidelines for screening and surveillance of asymptomatic colorectal cancer in patients with inflammatory bowel disease. Gut 51(Suppl 5):10–12
20. Fireman Z, Wagner G, Weissman J et al (2001) Prevalence of short-segment Barrett's epithelium. Dig Liver Dis 33(4):322–325
21. Ullman T, Croog V, Harpaz N, Sachar D and Itzkowitz S (2003) Progression of flat low-grade dysplasia to advanced neoplasia in patients with ulcerative colitis. Gastroenterology 125(5):1311–1319
22. Lim CH, Axon AT (2003) Low-grade dysplasia: nonsurgical treatment. Inflamm Bowel Dis 9(4):270–272
23. Eaden J, Abrams K, McKay H et al (2001) Inter-observer variation between general and specialist gastrointestinal pathologists when grading dysplasia in ulcerative colitis. J Pathol 194(2):152–157
24. Karlen P, Kornfeld D, Brostrom O et al (1998) Is colonoscopic surveillance reducing colorectal cancer mortality in ulcerative colitis? A population based case control study. Gut 42(5):711–724
25. Lynch DA, Lobo AJ, Sobala GM et al (1993) Failure of colonoscopic surveillance in ulcerative colitis. Gut 34(8):1075–1080
26. Winawer S, Fletcher R, Rex D et al (2003) Colorectal cancer screening and surveillance: clinical guidelines and rationale-update based on new evidence. Gastroenterology 124(2):544–560
27. Taylor BA, Pemberton JH, Carpenter HA et al (1992) Dysplasia in chronic ulcerative colitis: implications for colonoscopic surveillance. Dis Colon Rectum 35(10):950–956
28. Itzkowitz SH, Marshall A, Kornbluth A et al (1995) Sialosyl-Tn antigen: initial report of a new marker of malignant progression in long-standing ulcerative colitis. Gastroenterology 109(2):490–497
29. Kiesslich R, Jung M, DiSario JA et al (2004) Perspectives of chromo and magnifying endoscopy: How, how much, when, and whom should we stain? J Clin Gastroenterol 38(1):7–13
30. Kawamura YJ, Togashi K, Sasaki J, Konishi F (2005) Acetic acid spray in colonoscopy: an alternative to chromoendoscopy. Gut 54(2):313
31. Provenzale D, Kowdley KV, Arora S, Wong JB (1995) Prophylactic colectomy or surveillance for chronic ulcerative colitis? A decision analysis. Gastroenterology 109(4):1188–1196
32. Quah HM, Samad A, Maw A (2005) Ileostomy carcinomas a review: the latent risk after colectomy for ulcerative colitis and familial adenomatous polyposis. Colorectal Dis 7(6):538–544
33. Albrechtsen D, Bergan A, Gjone E et al (1981) Elective surgery for ulcerative colitis: colectomy in 158 patients. Scand J Gastroenterol 16(6):825–831
34. Parc R, Legrand M, Frileux P et al (1989) Comparative clinical results of ileal-pouch anal anastomosis and ileorectal anastomosis in ulcerative colitis. Hepatogastroenterology 36(4):235–239
35. Pastore RL, Wolff BG, Hodge D (1997) Total abdominal colectomy and ileorectal anastomosis for inflammatory bowel disease. Dis Colon Rectum 40(12):1455–1464
36. Khubchandani IT, Sandfort MR, Rosen L et al (1989) Current status of ileorectal anastomosis for inflammatory bowel disease. Dis Colon Rectum 32(5):400–403
37. Leijonmarck CE, Lofberg R, Ost A, Hellers G (1990) Long-term results of ileorectal anastomosis in ulcerative colitis in Stockholm County. Dis Colon Rectum 3:195–200
38. Tonelli FBG et al (1989) Continenza e modificazioni della pressione del canale anale e della distensibilita rettale dopo ileorettoanastomosi. Chirurgia 2:289–296
39. Goligher JC (1984) Surgery of the anus, rectum and colon. Bailiere, London
40. Baker WN, Glass RE, Ritchie JK, Aylett SO (1978) Cancer of the rectum following colectomy and ileorectal anastomosis for ulcerative colitis. Br J Surg 65(12):862–868
41. Morson BC, Pang LS (1967) Rectal biopsy as an aid to

cancer control in ulcerative colitis. Gut 8(5):423–434
42. Delaini GG, Colucci G, Hulten L (2005) The ileoanal pouch procedure in the long-term perspective: a critical review. Tech Coloproctol 9:187–192
43. Lee SW, Sonoda T, Milsom JW (2005) Three cases of adenocarcinoma following restorative proctocolectomy with hand-sewn anastomosis for ulcerative colitis: a review of reported cases in the literature. Colorectal Dis 7(6):591–597
44. Svaninger G, Nordgren S, Oresland T, Hulten L (1993) Incidence and characteristics of pouchitis in the Kock continent ileostomy and the pelvic pouch. Scand J Gastroenterol 28(8):695–700
45. Cox CL, Butts DR, Roberts MP et al (1997) Development of invasive adenocarcinoma in a long-standing Kock continent ileostomy: report of a case. Dis Colon Rectum 40(4):500–503
46. Setti-Carraro P, Ritchie JK, Wilkinson KH et al (1994) The first 10 years' experience of restorative proctocolectomy for ulcerative colitis. Gut 35(8):1070–1075
47. Gullberg K, Stahlberg D, Liljeqvist L et al (1997) Neoplastic transformation of the pelvic pouch mucosa in patients with ulcerative colitis. Gastroenterology 112(5):1487–1492
48. Hulten L, Willen R, Nilsson O et al (2002) Mucosal assessment for dysplasia and cancer in the ileal pouch mucosa in patients operated on for ulcerative colitis: a 30-year follow-up study. Dis Colon Rectum 45 4:448–452
49. Borjesson L, Willen R, Haboubi N et al (2004) The risk of dysplasia and cancer in the ileal pouch mucosa after restorative proctocolectomy for ulcerative proctocolitis is low: a long-term term follow-up study. Colorectal Dis 6(6):494–498
50. O'Connell PR, Pemberton JH, Weiland LH et al (1987) Does rectal mucosa regenerate after ileoanal anastomosis? Dis Colon Rectum 30(1):1–5
51. Remzi FH, Preen M (2003) Rectal cancer and ulcerative colitis: Does it change the therapeutic approach? Colorectal Dis 5(5):483–5
52. Herline AJ, Meisinger LL, Rusin LC et al (2003) Is routine pouch surveillance for dysplasia indicated for ileoanal pouches? Dis Colon Rectum 46(2):156–159

Salvage Surgery After Restorative Proctocolectomy

Francesco Selvaggi, Guido Sciaudone, Antonio Giuliani, Crescenzo Di Stazio, Ilaria Guadagni

Introduction

The failure rate of restorative proctocolectomy (RP) varies from 5 to 15% of the cases [1, 2], but with the lengthening of follow-up, the rate exceeds 15% [3]. Failure of the RP refers to the necessity of fashioning a loop ileostomy with the pouch in site or the removal of the pouch with definitive ileostomy. The causes of failure include acute and chronic sepsis, bad functioning in regard to mechanical and functional causes and mucosal inflammatory processes. Procedures for avoiding loss of anal function come within the scope of salvage surgery.

Sepsis

Sepsis can be defined early or late. The incidence of such complications varies in 5–25% of cases after RPs [4, 5], and approximately half of these are responsible for the failure of the surgical operation. The majority of the cases depend on the anastomotic complications regarding the pouch anal or regarding the proximal ileum to the pouch. After modification via mucosectomy's technique, which is used preliminarily to remove all disease (prone mucosa), the sepsis rate is remarkably reduced. The experience of the surgeon in transanal surgery is the factor that can meaningfully influence any complications [3, 6, 7].

Early sepsis manifests itself as fever, tenesmus and loss of pus through the anus. In a certain number of cases, antibiotic therapy can resolve the infection. In others, however, TC-guided transanal or transabdominal drainage is necessary. In some cases, it is sufficient to open the pouch-anal anastomosis in order to guarantee adequate transanal drainage. In severe sepsis, laparotomic access is mandatory; it is in these cases that the removal of the pouch from its natural site is frequently carried out, whereas the closing of the ileostomy is done infrequently.

In the experience of Heuschen [8] with 131 patients with sepsis, approximately 16% of these could be treated conservatively. Failure was in relation to the procedure carried out. In fact, it occurred in 6% of the cases after minimal surgery and in 47% of the cases after major surgery. Consequently, it is obvious that premature sepsis represents an important risk factor regarding the success or failure of the procedure.

Late sepsis generally manifests itself with the appearance of abdominal or pelvic abscesses and/or with formation of fistulas. In the case of circumscribed sepsis, surgical or TC-guided drainage can resolve the inflammatory process, otherwise pouch salvage surgery, with the removal of the pouch from the pelvis and the positioning of it under the abdominal wall along with the creation of a mucosal fistula, can represent an adequate therapeutic choice. This procedure was successful in five patients of eight in the study of Keighley [9] and in two of four in the study of the Mayo Clinic Group [10].

In Fazio's study [11] of 35 patients with sepsis, of which 29 had leakage of the ileo-anal anastomosis, the patients were treated via abdominal surgery. The rescue of the pouch was achieved in 21 out of 22 patients with ulcerative colitis, preserving transanal evacuation to the detriment of the bowel function, which was characterised by an evacuative frequency of 9 motions within 24 h, (ranging between 4 and 35 motions). The quality of life (QoL) was good in 17 patients and bad in 13.

Cohen [12] performed salvage surgery on 24 patients and obtained acceptable results for 20. In 18 of these, the medium frequency of elimination was 5 evacuations/day and 1.5 nocturnally, with good continence in 13 of the patients. Galandiuk [13] operated for intra-abdominal sepsis on 29 patients and reported 17 failures, which emphasises that the possibility for failure increases with time.

Heuschen [8] reports 131 patients with sepsis on 706 PR. In the experience of the author, early sepsis involves a greater risk of failure that increases with time at a rate of 20% at 3 years and 40% at 10 years. The site of the fistula is proximal to the pouch in 13% of cases, at the level of the neorectal cuff in 31% and at the level of the ileo-anal anastomosis in 50% of cases. Treatment has been conservative in 18% of cases, with transanal surgery in 25% of cases and abdominal in 56% of cases. The difference in the failure is higher after major surgery (45%) than minor surgery (5%). The failure was also correlated to the dehiscence of the pouch-anal anastomosis and to the presence of a pouch-vaginal fistula. Experiences up to now demonstrate a great variability of results in relation to the severity of sepsis, the site regarding the pouch-anal anastomosis and to the duration of the follow-up.

Gorfine [14] of Mount Sinai in New York reports on 1 185 RPs: 51 patients with sepsis from leakage of the pouch-anal anastomosis in which 85 surgical procedures were carried out including 48 transanal surgeries in patients without ileostomy, 37 transanal surgeries in patients with ileostomy and 4 abdominal and perineal operations in patients with ileostomy. In 40% of patients he obtained a good result at a medium follow-up of 65 months. Comparing patients with and without ileostomy who received a surgical transanal procedure, the author did not see any evidence of differences in results. Moreover, he reports on the failure in all patients who had abdominal surgery. The author concludes, that in order to obtain good results, more surgical procedures are necessary, so that there are no differences between patients with and without ileostomy, which emphasises the failure of abdominal procedures used in the attempt to rescue the pouch.

Dehni [15] reported on the experience acquired from 54 patients who underwent salvage surgery, of which 47 had sepsis. In 19 patients with cases of abscess, he utilised a transanal approach preceded by surgical or radiological transanastomotic or perineal drainage. In the remaining cases he preferred an abdominoperineal approach. Altogether, 27 of the 40 patients evaluated after abdominoperineal surgery and 13 of the 18 after transanal surgery, obtained satisfactory results. Of the patients operated on for sepsis, 44 at a medium follow-up of 30 months obtained good results. Crohn's disease was subsequently diagnosed in three patients out of four who had pouch failure after salvage surgery.

Pouch-Vaginal Fistula

The symptoms of pouch-vaginal fistula consist of leakage of secretion or gas from the mucosa and/or faecal leakage through the vagina or the perineum. Its incidence is equal to approximately 5–10% of patients operated on for RP. The treatment depends on the severity of the symptoms. In the case of minimal symptoms, the application of a seton tie could be sufficient, even if long-term data on it does not exist [16].

In the case of incontinence, a defunctioning ileostomy can be performed and a seton tie can be inserted for drainage. Once the sepsis has been resolved, recanalisation will be possible. The insertion of a seton tie is probably the technique of choice in the presence of a cryptoglandular fistula. Ileostomy alone, in fact, is not in a position to guarantee satisfactory results [17].

Surgical procedures can be divided into abdominal and local. The first is concerned with abdominal revision and the advancement of the ileo-anal anastomosis. Local procedures, on the other hand, such as advancement flap repair and endoanal or endovaginal repair, precede fistulectomy.

It is obvious that the site of anastomosis influences surgical choice. According to some authors, in the presence of anastomosis in the distal rectum, it is possible to make a reconstruction and to perform a more distal anastomosis with success in 21 out of 26 patients [12, 16, 17]. In the case of a fistula that is derived from ileo-anal anastomosis, a local treatment is recommended.

Advancement flap repair determines success in 50% of cases. Transvaginal repair allows a direct access to the fistula avoiding sphincter damage. In one study, five patients out of seven obtained good results at a mean follow-up of 26 months [13]. Others authors have reported good results in 11 patients out of 14 at a mean follow-up of 18 months [18].

In reviewing the various results obtained with a transvaginal approach, the closing of the fistula has been demonstrated in 25 patients out of 35. Surgery with an abdominal approach is in a position to achieve good results in 80% of cases; with the perineal approach the percentage falls to 50% of cases [13, 16, 19, 20].

A further condition that can lead to the removal of the ileal pouch is represented via malfunction. Such an event is responsible for 20–40% of failure of the pouch [9, 10]. Karoui [21] reports a removal rate of 35% for poor functioning (24 out of 58 removals) due to outlet obstruction in 10 patients and incontinence in 14 patients. The success rate after medical or surgical treatment is extremely variable in the literature, ranging between 33 and 100% of cases [9, 22]. Surgical treatment can consist of an exclusively transanal approach or a combined abdominoperineal approach, depending on the reason of dysfunction and technical feasibility [23]. The most frequent causes of malfunction are represented by mechanical obstruction, sphincter dysfunction, reduced capacity of the reservoir or by mucosal inflammation [24]. The majority of the patients with poor functioning have an evacuation frequency of 10 motions/24 h or more, often associated with emission of small volumes of faeces and the presence of urgency, incontinence and evacuation difficulties [24].

Outlet obstruction (OO), which alone is responsible for 18–48% of the malfunction of the ileal reservoir [9, 10], can be determined by various factors including stenosis of the pouch-anal anastomosis, a long efferent limb (LEL) in an S-shaped form or by the presence of a residual of rectal mucosa at the level of the pouch-anal anastomosis (retained rectal stump).

Stenosis of Pouch-Anal Anastomosis

Ogunbiyi's study [9] on 198 PRs reports nine cases of OO due to stenosis of the pouch-anal anastomosis in four, LEL in two, prolapse of the pouch in one and stenosis of the remaining ileum above the pouch in two cases. All patients with stenosis of the pouch-anal anastomosis underwent a reconstruction of the reservoir with success in three patients out of four. A pouchpexy was performed with success in the patient with prolapse of the pouch. In the two patients with LEL, the efferent limb was successfully removed. In the two cases of stenosis above the pouch, one patient showed no improvement of clinical conditions after the construction of a pouch-anal anastomosis L/L, while for the other patient who was diagnosed with Crohn's disease after the construction of the reservoir, the resulting strictureplasty was successful.

A stenosis of the pouch-anal anastomosis, requiring a single dilatation, is described in the literature in a variable percentage from 4–40% of cases [1, 13, 25–31]. This event is more frequent in patients with UC [13, 28, 29] compared to those with FAP and shows a double incidence regarding mechanical anastomosis compared to those made by hand [29]. Senapati [31] in a study of 266 patients who underwent PR, reported stenosis in 14.2 and 39% of the patients, depending on whether the procedure had been carried out via manual or mechanical anastomosis. The first therapeutic approach to stenosis of the pouch-anal anastomosis, is dilatation under anaesthesia. With this procedure Senapati [31] reports a success rate of 26%, while Galandiuk [13] at a 31-month follow-up (range 1–98) reports a relapse rate of 59% with failure in 16% of the cases. The same author reports satisfactory results after repeated dilatations in more than 50% of cases (23 patients out of 42). In particular, in the case of a short stenosis, a posterior strictureplasty can be indicated. Stenosis of 2 cm of length can be corrected by an exclusive transanal approach. In the case of a long stenotic segment, on the other hand, a combined abdominoperineal approach is recommended [32, 33].

According to Dehni's [23] study of 23 patients who underwent transanal surgery, 4 because of fibrous stricture, the combined abdominoperineal conversion is mandatory. The transanal approach with removal of the stenosis and distal advancement of the pouch is particularly indicated in cases with concomitant vaginal fistula [32].

The remaining therapeutic options consist of the removal of the pouch with definitive ileostomy, which was necessary in 2.5–15% of the cases, or by abdominal salvage surgery, with removal of the pouch, removal of the fibrotic ring and reconstruction of the pouch-anal anastomosis restoring the proximal portion of pouch [24].

Maclean [34] of the Mount Sinai Hospital of Toronto, comparing patients who underwent rescue of the pouch through an abdominal approach in cases of pelvic sepsis or OO, reported a minor incidence of complications (33.3 *vs.* 61.5%, p=0.047) in patients with OO. This emphasises, moreover, that there was a greater risk of malfunction in those cases where it was necessary to refashion a new pouch then where it was possible to modify the old reservoir, depending on whether there was insufficient compliance due to fibrosis and a reservoir lacking in volume with a subsequent increase of evacuation frequency.

Long Efferent Limb

Parks and Nicholls's S-pouch [35] or Fonkalsrud's H-pouch [22] can determine the formation of an efferent limb of the terminal ileum, which constitutes the proximal side of ileo-anal anastomosis. A long efferent limb (LEL), >8 cm of length, fashioned in the first "debut" cases of the S-reservoir, needed catheterisation of the pouch to achieve evacuation in more than 50% of the patients [36].

Fonkalsrud [22], in his study of 601 PRs, reports an OO rate of 27.3%, with a success rate after surgical review in 93% of cases. In this experience, however, 221 patients had an H-reservoir and 4 had an S-reservoir constructed in the early 1980s. Those made at that time were abandoned because of an elevated incidence of emptying with the necessity of catheterisation.

The removal of the LEL is possible through a transanal approach, but it is technically feasible in less than 30% of patients [22, 37]. The technique consists of mobilisation of the pouch and separation of the ileo-anal anastomosis. The efferent limb is removed and a new manual anastomosis is fashioned between the pouch and the anal canal.

Sagar [10], in a study of 1 770 ileal pouches, evidenced 9 LELs (5–11 cm), all of which were in patients with an S-pouch, and 3 blind handle torsions in patients with J-pouches. After surgical treatment of the nine patients with LEL, five demanded construction of a new reservoir, which was successful in seven cases (78%). In the three patients with blind handle torsions, he did not fashion a new reservoir and only one patient benefited from the surgical treatment. Of a total of 26 patients who underwent this treatment, failure of the surgical procedure was recorded in 5, while 18 showed improvement which included a change from needing catheterisation to spontaneous evacuation [9, 10, 37, 38].

Retained Rectal Stump

The use of stapling in the realisation of the pouch-anal anastomosis or the insufficient execution of mucosectomy are the main causes of retention of rectal mucosa. In fact, with the double stapling technique, a little stump of rectal mucosa of variable length from 1.5–3 cm, in which the disease persists, is left In Situ. A certain degree of inflammation is commonly found on the biopsies carried out on the residual cuff of the columnar epithelium. However, this only causes symptoms in 2–15% of patients [39–42].

According to the experience of Herbst [38] in a study of 16 PRs with OO, in half of the patients, the functional disturbance was associated with an LEL of the S-pouch, five were associated with a stenosis of the pouch-anal anastomosis, and one was associated with a stenosis associated to an LEL, while two were associated with a long rectal stump. None of the patients had the reservoir reconstructed during a subsequent operation and surgery was successful in 80% of cases. The author concludes that with the use of a mechanical pouch-anal anastomosis, the incidence of a long rectal stump increases because of OO [38].

Lavery of the Cleveland Clinic, in one study focussing on 227 patients with PR, reports the presence of inflammation of the cuff, histologically demonstrated, in 82% of cases. This condition generated a clinical symptomatology in only 14.7% of the patients. The more frequent disturbances during cuffitis are bleeding, burning and urgency; moreover, neoplastic transformation of the residual rectal mucosa is possible [39, 40, 43]. Local treatment with steroids can determine remission of symptoms, but often definitive resolution of clinical presentation is possible only with surgical therapy.

Five patients of the series of Dehni [23] received a salvage procedure of the pouch for complications due to a long rectal stump with the presence of severe cuffitis in two cases, difficulty of emptying in two others and development of carcinoma on the stump in one case. Four of these patients demanded a new anastomosis carried out via a transanal approach and one demanded a review via an abdominalperineal approach.

If the retained portion of mucosa is short, a transanal approach can be possible, but in the majority of the cases, a combined abdominoperineal approach, that includes removal of the residual rectum followed by manual mucosectomy and transanal refashioning of the pouch-anal anastomosis is necessary.

Curran [42] reports three cases where there was a necessity to carry out a transanal mucosectomy for resolution of the symptomatology. In one of these cases the removal of the pouch was necessary. Fazio obtained good results associating the advance of the reservoir to a transanal [44].

Small Volume Reservoir

The first type of reconstruction after total proctocolectomy was the straight ileo-anal anastomosis. The unsatisfactory results of such a procedure together with the studies of Nicholls [45], which demonstrated the presence of an inverse relation between evacuation frequency and reservoir capacity, determined the spread of the pelvic pouches. However, constructing a pouch so as to have satisfactory functional results is not sufficient, because an adequate volume of the reservoir is necessary for the functioning of the neo-rectum with a reduction of evacuation frequency. In fact, insufficient volume of the reservoir can be responsible for the elevated number of evacuations and urgency. The demonstration of the importance of an adequate volume is represented in the differences in the results that can be observed between the J and the W-pouch [46].

The pouch enema and above all the mano-volumetry along with the determination of the threshold volume (TV) and the maximum tolerated volume (MTV) can define the capacity and compliance of the reservoir exactly. Medical therapy (loperamide, codeine and mass-forming drugs), often is not able to improve the evacuation frequency, so therefore, an abdominal operation becomes necessary in order to enlarge the pouch. Herbst demonstrated a meaningful reduction of evacuation frequency using this method [38] and Fazio [11] used this method in 7 of 35 patients reoperated on for sepsis.

Klas [47] reported that in five cases of insufficient volume of the reservoir for which he carried out a conversion from a J to a W pouch, daily evacuation frequency had been reduced, with much satisfaction on behalf of the patients, from 13–8 to 5–8 and the nocturnal episodes from 3–0 to 0–3. However, such an increase of the pouch, which certainly represents a more conservative method than *ex novo* construction of the reservoir, is not always feasible. This technique consists of the addition of a small intestinal loop to the proximal part of the pouch without removing it from its site, or as an alternative, mobilisation of the reservoir, modification of the J-pouch in order to construct a W-reservoir and finally a reconstruction of the pouch-anal anastomosis. In the case of a J-pouch with a long blind stump, its integration with an L/L suture is sufficient for increasing the volume of the pouch.

References

1. Marcello PW, Roberts PL, Schoetz DJ Jr et al (1993) Long-term results of the ileoanal pouch procedure. Arch Surg 128:500–503
2. Fiandra JFV (1993) The ileal pouch: indications for its use and results in clinical practice. Curr Pract Gastroenterol 4:22–28
3. Meagher AP, Farouk R, Dozois RR et al (1998) J ileal pouch-anal anastomosis for chronic ulcerative colitis: complications and long-term outcome in 1310 patients. Br J Surg 85:800–803
4. Pemberton JH, Kelly KA, Beart RW Jr et al (1987) Ideala pouch-anal anastomosis for chronic ulcerative colitis: long-term results. Ann Surg 206:504–513
5. Mc Mullen K, Hicks TC, Ray JE et al (1991) Complications associated with ileal pouch-anal anastomosis. World J Surg 15:763–766
6. Scott NA, Dozois RR, Beart RW Jr et al (1988) Postoperative intra-abdominal and pelvic sepsis complicating ileal pouch-anal anastomosis. Int J Colorectal Dis 3:149–152
7. Keighley MR, Grobler S, Bain I (1993) An audit of restorative proctocolectomy. Gut 34:680–684
8. Heuschen UA, Allemeyer EH, Hintz U (2002) Outcome after septic complications in J pouch procedures. Br J Surg 89:194–200
9. Ogunbiyi OA, Korsgen S, Keighley MR et al (1997) Pouch salvage long-term outcome. Dis Colon Rectum 40:548–552
10. Sagar PM, Dozois RR, Wolff BG, Kelly KA (1996) Disconnection, pouch revision and reconnection of the ileal pouch-anal anastomosis. Br J Surg 83:1401–1405
11. Fazio VW, Wu JS, Lavery IC (1998) Repeat ileal pouch-anal anastomosis to salvage septic complications of pelvic pouches: clinical outcome and quality of life assessment. Ann Surg 228:588–597
12. Cohen Z, Smith D, McLeod R (1998) Reconstructive surgery for pelvic pouches. World J Surg 22:342–346
13. Galandiuk S, Scott NA, Dozois RR et al (1990) Ileal pouch anal anastomosis: reoperation for pouch related complications. Ann Surg 212:446–452; Discussion 452–454
14. Gorfine SR, Fichiera A, Harris MT, Bauer JJ (2003) Long-term results of salvage surgery for septic complications after restorative proctocolectomy: does fecal diversion improbe outcome? Dis Colon Rectum 10(46):1339–1344
15. Dehni N, Cunningham C, Parc R (1998) Use of jejunal pouch with ileal interposition in salvage surgery after restorative proctocolectomy. Dis Colon Rectum 12(41):1587–1589
16. Keighley MR, Grobler SP (1993) Fistula complicating restorative proctocolectomy. Br J Surg 80:1065–1067
17. Paye F, Penna C, Chiche L et al (1996) Pouch-related fistula following restorative proctocolectomy. Br J Surg 83:1574–1577
18. Burke D, van Laarhoven CJ, Herbst F, Nicholls RJ (2001) Transvaginal repair of pouch-vaginal fistula. Br J Surg 88:241–245
19. Groom JS, Nicholls RJ, Hawley PR, Phillips RK (1993) Pouch-vaginal fistula. Br J Surg 80:936–940
20. Wexner SD, Rothenberger DA, Jensen L et al (1989) Ileal pouch vaginal fistulas: incidence, etiology, and management. Dis Colon Rectum 32:460–465
21. Karoui M, Cohen R, Nicholls J (2004) Results of surgical removal of the pouch after failed restorative proctocolectomy. Dis Colon Rectum 47:869–875
22. Fonkalsrud EW, Bustorff-Silva J (1999) Reconstruction for chronic dysfunction of ileo-anal pouches. Ann Surg 229:197–204
23. Dehni N, Remacle G, Dozois RR et al (2005) Salvage reoperation for complications after ileal pouch anal anastomosis. Br J Surg 92:748–753
24. Tulchinsky H, Cohen CRG, Nicholls RJ (2003) Salvage surgery after restorative proctocolectomy. Br J Surg 90:909–921
25. Metcalf AM, Dozois RR, Kelly KA et al (1985) Ileal "J" pouch-anal anastomosis: clinical outcome. Ann Surg 202:735–739
26. Fleshmann JW, Cohen Z, McLeod RS et al (1988) The ileal reservoir and ileo-anal anastomosis procedure: factors affecting technical and functional outcome. Dis Colon Rectum 31:10–16
27. Breen EM, Schoetz DJ Jr, Marcello PW et al (1998) Functional results after perineal complications of ileal pouch anal anastomosis. Dis Colon Rectum 41:691–695
28. Schoetz DJ Jr, Coller JA, Veidenheimer MC (1988) Can the pouch be saved? Dis Colon Rectum 31:671–675
29. Lewis WJ, Kuzu A, Sagar PM (1994) Stricture at the pouch-anal anstomosis after restorative proctocolectomy. Dis Colon Rectum 37:120–125
30. Beart RW Jr (1986) Proctocolectomy and ileo-anal anastomosis with a J-pouch. Aust N Z J Surg 56:467–469
31. Senapati A, Tibbs CJ, Ritchie JK (1996) Stenosis of the pouch-anal anastomosis following restorative proctocolectomy. In J Colorect Dis 11:57–59
32. Fazio VW, Tjandra JJ (1992) Pouch advancement and neoileal anastomosis for anastomotic stricture and anovaginal fistula complicating restorative proctocolectomy. Br J Surg 79:694–696
33. Prudhomme M, Dozois RR, Goldlewinski G et al (2003) Anal canal strictures after ileal pouch-anal anastomosis. Dis Colon Rectum 46:20–23
34. MacLean AR, O'Connor B, Parkes R, et al (2002) Reconstructive surgery for failed ileal pouch-anal anastomosis: a viable surgical option with acceptable results. Dis Colon Rectum 45(7):880–886
35. Parks AG, Nicholls RJ (1978) Proctocolectomy without ileostomy for ulcerative colitis. BMJ 2:85–88
36. Pescatori M, Manhire A, Bartram CI (1983) Evacuation

pouchography in the evaluation of ileo-anal reservoir function. Dis Colon Rectum 26:365–368

37. Nicholls RJ, Gilbert JM (1990) Surgical correction of the efferent ileal limb for disordered defaecation following restorative proctocolectomy with the S-ileal reservoir. Br J Surg 77:152–154
38. Herbst F, Sielezeneff I, Nicholls RJ (1996) Salvage surgery for ileal pouch outlet obstruction. Br J Surg 83:368–371
39. Lavery IC, Sirimarco MT, Ziv Y, Fazio VW (1995) Anal canal inflammation after ileal pouch-anal anastomosis: the need for treatment. Dis Colon Rectum 38:803–806
40. Thompson-Fawcett MW, Mortensen NJ, Warren BF (1999) 'Cuffitis' and inflammatory changes in the columnar cuff, anal transitional zone, and ileal reservoir after stapled pouch-anal anastomosis. Dis Colon Rectum 42:348–355
41. Schmitt SL, Wexner SD, Lucas FV et al (1992) Retained mucosa after double-stapled ileal reservoir and ileoanal anastomosis. Dis Colon Rectum 35:1051–1056
42. Curran FT, Hill GL (1992) Symptomatic colitis in the anal after restorative proctocolectomy. Aus N Z J Surg 62:941–943
43. Rotholtz NA, Pikarsky AJ, Singh JJ, Wexner SD (2001) Adenocarcinoma arising from along the rectal stump afther double-stapled ileorectal J-pouch in a patient with ulcerative colitis: the need to perform a distal anastomosis. Report of a case. Dis Colon Rectum 44:1214–1217
44. Fazio VW, Tjandra JJ (1994) Transanal mucosectomy, ileal pouch advancement for anorectal dysplasia or inflammation after restorative proctocolectomy. Dis Colon Rectum 37:1008–1011
45. Nicholls RJ, Pezim ME (1985) Restorative proctocolectomy with ileal pouch reservoir for ulcerative colitis and familial adenomatous polyposis: a comparison of three reservoir designs. Br J Surg 72:470–474
46. Selvaggi F, Giuliani A, Gallo C et al (2000) A randomized controlled trial to compare the J and W pouch configurations for ulcerative colitis in the maturation period, Dis Colon Rectum 43:615–620
47. Klas J, Myers GA, Starling JR, Harms BA (1998) Physiologic evaluation and surgical management of failed ileoanal pouch. Dis Colon Rectum 41:854–861

Management of the Difficult Ileal Pouch-Anal Anastomosis and Temporary Ileostomy

Susan Galandiuk

Introduction

There are several clinical scenarios when the operation of ileal pouch-anal anastomosis does not go as smoothly as planned, specifically with respect to obtaining enough length to construct an anastomosis. Although the technique of stapled ileal pouch-anal anastomosis has greatly facilitated the ability to obtain additional length, there are still situations in which this is technically difficult. In addition, there are situations in which a hand-sewn anastomosis is required, for example, in the UC or FAP patient with a low-lying rectal cancer, or the patient who has had a very short Hartmann pouch where, due to distal scarring, a stapler technically cannot be used to create an anastomosis. The most common situations in which it will be difficult to gain enough length to perform an "easy, tension-free anastomosis" are: [1] those patients who are obese, [2] those in whom reoperative surgery is performed and who have foreshortening of the mesentery due to scar tissue, [3] those patients who, based on their body habitus, have an unusually short small-bowel mesentery, [4] patients with an unusually long torso, [5] patients with familial adenomatous polyposis (FAP) who have mesenteric desmoid disease, as well as [6] patients who for a variety of reasons have undergone prior small-bowel resection. In these situations, particular attention to detail with respect to mobilization of the small-bowel mesentery and certain technical tips can be extremely helpful in facilitating the course of the operation. This chapter will be divided into two sections, the first dealing with maneuvers to help gain additional mesenteric length and allow the terminal ileum and J-pouch to reach the anal canal more easily and the second, with maneuvers to facilitate construction of a loop ileostomy in these individuals, which can itself be extremely difficult.

Maneuvers to Gain Additional Mesenteric Length

Mobilization of the Small-Bowel Mesentery

One of the key maneuvers in gaining length of the ileal J-pouch is complete mobilization of the small-bowel mesentery. The small-bowel mesentery adheres to the retroperitoneum in a diagonal fashion beginning in the lower right quadrant, extending upwards toward the left upper quadrant. The entire mesentery of the small bowel should be mobilized to the level of the second and third portions of the duodenum (Fig. 1). Division of the filmy adhesions between the small bowel mesentery and the duodenum permit additional stretch of the small bowel mesentery. In doing this maneuver, one must be careful not to do too much mobilization. Injudicious mobilization or use of electrocautery in the vicinity

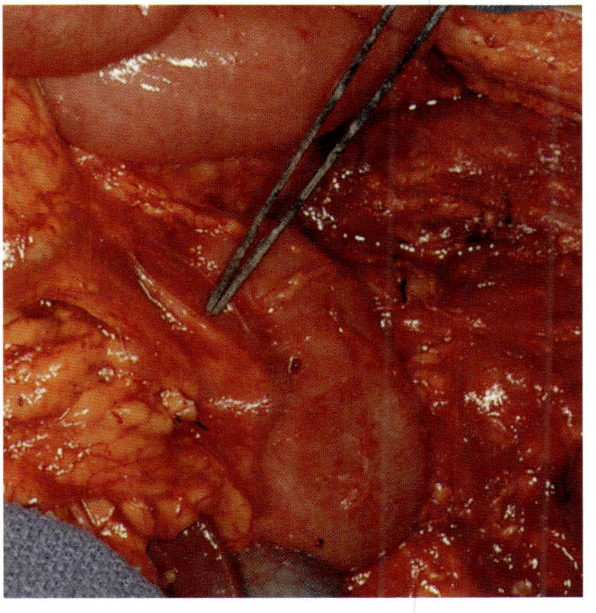

Fig. 1. Mobilization of the small-bowel mesentery up to the level of the third portion of the duodenum

of the pancreas can actually result in pancreatitis and should be avoided.

Peritoneal Windowing

The visceral peritoneum acts almost like a "sausage casing" in terms of holding in or confining the mesentery of the small bowel. If the visceral peritoneum covering the mesentery of the small bowel is sharply incised, the small-bowel mesentery stretches more easily. Because the blood supply to the ileal pouch is extremely important, much care needs to be taken when performing this maneuver. In order to do this, while avoiding injury to any of the underlying blood vessels, a very fine hemostat can be gently inserted underneath the peritoneum in order to lift it away from the underlying blood vessels and the electrocautery used to gently divide the peritoneum (Fig. 2a). This is done at 1 or 2-cm increments in a horizontal step-ladder-type fashion, while an assistant applies distal traction to the point of the terminal ileum that is chosen to be the apex of the J-pouch (Fig. 2b). As soon as the peritoneum is divided at each point, there is a gaping of the peritoneum in this area. When the anterior surface of the small-bowel mesentery's peritoneum is "windowed" in this manner, the small-bowel mesentery is then "flipped" or turned cranially so that it lies over the upper portion of the patient's abdomen and chest. Subsequently, the identical maneuver is then performed on the posterior aspect of the peritoneum covering the small-bowel mesentery beginning just above the level of the third portion of the duodenum and proceeding distally towards the mesenteric portion of the segment of terminal ileum chosen to be the apex of the J-pouch. One can usually gain approximately 2–3 cm or more of additional mesenteric length via this maneuver (Fig. 2c).

Division of Either the Ileocolic or Superior Mesenteric Blood Vessels

If the above maneuvers are still insufficient for providing adequate mesenteric length, some of the blood vessels supplying the terminal ileum can be divided. If the colectomy is performed at the same time as the ileal J-pouch anal anastomosis, it is important to pre-

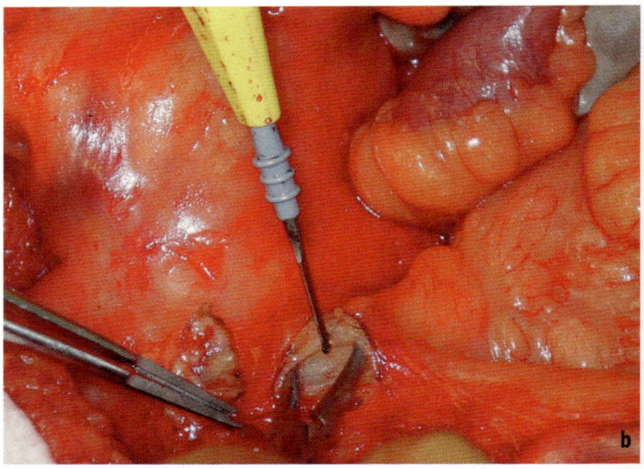

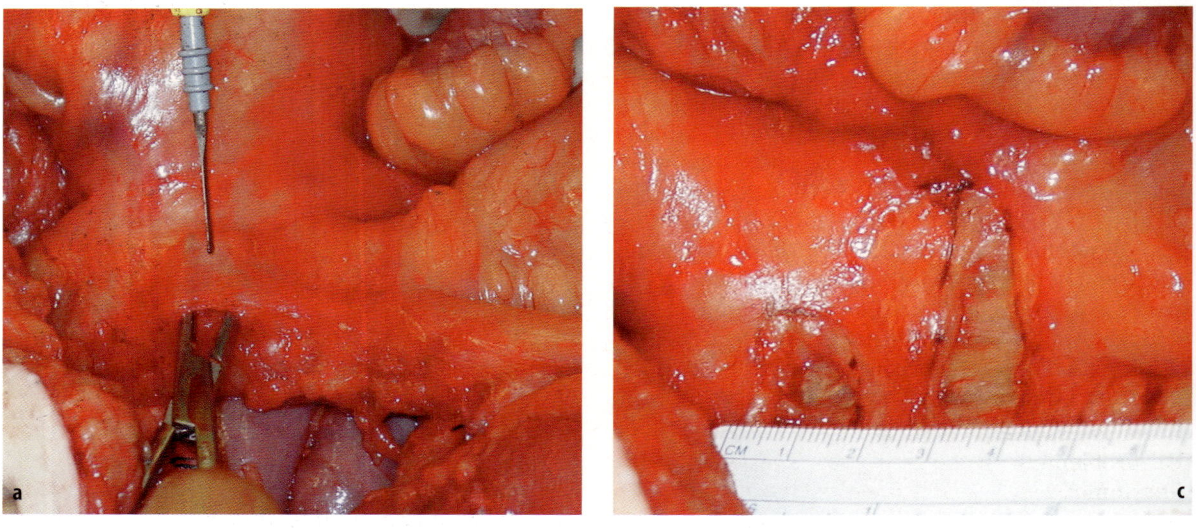

Fig. 2a-c. Peritoneal windowing to gain additional mesenteric length. **a** A hemostat is inserted underneath the peritoneum to lift it away from the underlying mesenteric blood vessels. **b** Electrocautery is then used to divide the peritoneum in a step-ladder-type fashion at regular intervals. **c** Several centimeters of additional mesenteric length can be gained using this maneuver serve the entire course of the ileocolic vessels. This is important so that, if additional mesenteric length is required, this vessel can be used as the main pouch blood supply. This is unfortunately not an alternative in patients who have already had a prior colectomy and present at a later stage for ileal J-pouch anastomosis. The terminal ileum is characterized by its arcade-like blood supply. Either the distal superior mesenteric or the ileocolic vessels can be divided, provided that the other blood vessels are intact and that good bowel perfusion can still be maintained via these arcades [1]. If there is inadequate mesenteric length, by placing distal traction on the J-pouch, one can easily ascertain by palpation alone whether the ileocolic vessels or the distal superior mesenteric vessels are under more tension. These vessels can be felt as tight cords or bands even in obese patients when the pulses of the vessels cannot easily be palpated. If one or the other of these vessels feels to be under more tension, these vessels can be clamped, divided and ligated and additional mesenteric length obtained. If there is a question as to what effect division of these vessels would have on pouch viability, vascular clamps can be used to occlude these vessels, and pouch viability ascertained before they are divided. With this technique, an additional 2–3 cm of mesenteric length can be attained.

Stapled Ileal Pouch-Anal Anastomosis

Performing stapled ileal J-pouch anal anastomosis is by far the easiest method with respect to mesenteric length, because in this situation, the transanally placed stapler pushes the perineum towards the abdomen and small-bowel mesentery, reducing the length needed by several centimeters compared to hand-sewn techniques. Purse string sutures are not reliable and frequently are placed incorrectly. Because of this, incomplete "doughnuts" are common. I prefer to use a triple-staple approach, in which no purse string suture is used [2]. The anvil of the stapler is placed through the enterotomy through which the GIA staplers that created the J-pouch are fired. This enterotomy is in turn then closed using a linear stapler and the shaft of the anvil pierced through the bowel just adjacent to this linear staple line. Since no purse string suture is required, the bowel is less likely to tear and there are fewer technical problems with the anastomosis, especially if an anastomosis is constructed under tension. In the very obese patient, the extra-large straight St. Marks retractor is invaluable. This is particularly useful in the patient who is well over 150 kg (Fig. 3), and particularly in obese male patients in whom the narrow pelvis further makes dissection difficult. The only

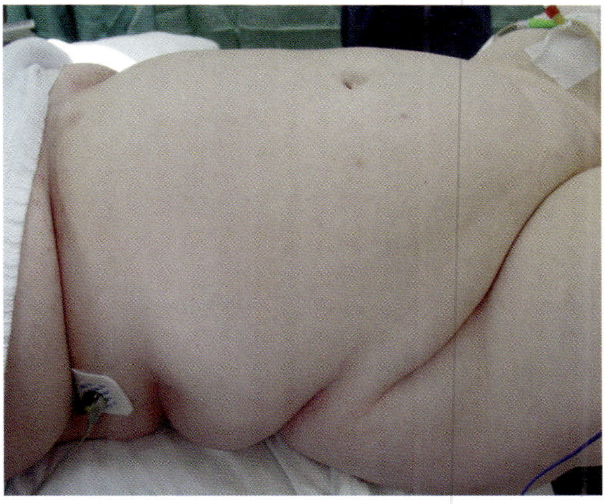

Fig. 3. Even in very large patients, ileal pouch-anal anastomosis can be performed. The extra-large straight St. Marks retractor is particularly helpful such as in this patient with a body mass index of 46.1

compromise one may have to accept with a stapled ileal J-pouch anal anastomosis is that, in a very large patient, one may have to accept an anastomosis that would be higher above the dentate line than in the ideal situation. In these cases, surveillance may need to be performed more frequently and one must be prepared to perform a mucosectomy should this become necessary. This clearly becomes a very serious issue in the case of familial adenomatous polyposis when one may also be dealing with patients who might not be compliant with follow-up surveillance. This must be discussed in great detail with patients preoperatively, particularly in the United States where many of these patients have a low rate of follow-up.

What to Do in Case of Extremely Difficult Hand-Sewn Anastomosis

Do not despair. Even in the most difficult circumstance, do not give up and excise the anal canal. I have frequently seen this done, and know from personal experience, that even in the most awful case when one thinks that all is lost, when one fears that there will be leaks and problems with healing, the anastomosis can still heal primarily and the patient obtain a satisfactory functional result. Even when the ileal J-pouch tears when it is brought down to the anal canal due to a large amount of tension on the anastomosis, it may still heal. One must, however, realize that the more tension there is on an anastomosis, the more likely the patient is to have a stricture postoperatively. It is therefore extremely important to check for this prior to loop ileostomy closure. If this is not treated with dilation prior to loop ileostomy closure, there is a much higher risk of dehiscence of the loop ileostomy closure site. There is also a higher rate of pouchitis and chronic pouchitis associated with untreated strictures. Such strictures may only require digital dilation or dilatation under anesthesia [3]. When performing a hand-sewn anastomosis, it is very useful to first place quadrant sutures to fix the pouch to the anal canal before making a pouch enterotomy at the apex of the pouch for the anastomosis. A hand-sewn anastomosis with a complete mucosectomy should be performed in cases in which there is a distal rectal cancer, for example a distal rectal cancer in ulcerative colitis or FAP which does not permit a stapler to be placed below it due to its very distal location.

Loop Ileostomy Formation

If one is constructing an ileal J-pouch anal anastomosis under tension, it is extremely important to always divert the patient no matter how difficult it appears that creation of the stoma will be. Imagine how miserable a situation it would be if the patient would have an anastomotic leak and required reoperation and diversion-it would be twice as difficult then. One must always optimize the conditions for successful anastomotic healing. If the anastomosis is created under tension, this includes diversion.

Preoperative Stoma Site Marking

It is extremely important to have the patient marked for a stoma site preoperatively [4]. This is most true in the obese patient and in the patient that has had previous open surgical incisions. If the patient should have a problem with the distal anastomosis and require diversion for longer than the normal 8 weeks postoperatively, it is imperative to have a stoma located in a location where the appliance will be able to adhere for at least 2–3 days. In patients in whom the ileal J-pouch anal anastomosis is constructed under tension, the superior mesenteric vessels and blood supply leading to the ileal J-pouch is tethered close along the patient's spine. This also tethers the vascular arcades along the anti-mesenteric border of the distal small bowel, so that it can be very difficult to mobilize a loop of bowel to create an end ileostomy. This will of course become easier as one proceeds proximally in the course of the small bowel. More proximal stoma placement will, however, be associated with higher volumes of ileostomy output. Unfortunately, in very heavy patients, the best external site for a loop ileostomy is often in the patient's right upper quadrant, requiring that the loop of bowel chosen for the stoma to be located much more proximally than one would wish.

Ileostomy Aperture

When creating the skin aperture, making the aperture too small makes it technically difficult to mature the stoma, while making it too large makes it harder to obtain stoma eversion. In most patients, making a skin aperture roughly the same size as the diameter of the bowel to be used to create the stoma or several millimeters larger will provide for a suitably sized skin aperture.

In most patients, a two-finger breadth opening in the abdominal wall is all that is required for a loop ileostomy. However, in patients in whom there is excessive tension or particularly in obese patients, where the small-bowel mesentery may be very large, it is important to create a large enough fascial defect in order to permit the bowel to pass easily through the abdominal wall. Since this is a temporary ileostomy, the larger fascial defect and the common parastomal hernia can easily be closed at the time of ileostomy closure.

Babcock or other types of clamps should be used for as brief a time as possible to grasp the bowel while it is brought through the abdominal wall. These clamps tend to rip through the bowel and cause an excessive amount of trauma even if they may be soft or "atraumatic". Once a clamp has been used to pass the bowel through the abdominal wall, it is quickly released and a dry gauze sponge or pad can be used to further manipulate the bowel, since this is much gentler to the bowel wall. If a significant amount of traction on the bowel is required, an umbilical tape passed immediately underneath the bowel, just at its mesenteric margin, will usually provide sufficient traction without disrupting the bowel wall, tearing it or interfering with or damaging its blood supply. One should always start with the small bowel just proximal to the ileal J-pouch and determine the most distal loop of small bowel that can reach and be adequately exteriorized through the ileostomy aperture. For an adequate loop ileostomy, 6–8 cm of bowel should be present above the skin surface depending upon the diameter of the small bowel.

Use of Stoma Rods

If there is excessive tension, a stoma rod may be used. I prefer short plastic ileostomy rods (Marlen). These have the advantage that they are relatively small, being only several centimeters in length, so that they do not interfere with the stoma appliance, as can larger rods that are meant for use with colostomies. Such rods should be left in place for 5 days after surgery in order to assure adherence of the bowel to the abdominal wall and subcutaneous tissue before removal. In a patient in whom a stoma is constructed under significant tension, these rods can easily cause a partial small-bowel obstruction when they are in place. It is not unusual that, due to this obstructed effect, the patient cannot be advanced beyond a liquid diet until the rod is removed. These rods also have the advantage of having an “eye” on both ends to permit them to be sutured to the skin so they cannot inadvertently “slip out” or be inadvertently removed. If there is difficulty in physically getting the bowel to reach to the skin, in very rare circumstances I have done a lipectomy of the area around the stoma site via the midline incision in order to “thin” the abdominal wall. This approach is used so as not to stretch the ileostomy skin aperture unduly. This is very rarely needed, since fat will almost always compress sufficiently and most obese patients have a fairly soft abdominal wall. One essential in dealing with such patients is, however, to have them seen postoperatively by a skilled enterostomal therapist. These patients will invariably require a convex stoma appliance, Eakin seals, and a stoma belt. There are many different stoma supply manufacturers. Some patients will even require very deep convexities or, appliances with special oval shapes. Without the use of such appliances, ileostomy retraction occurs. This is important, since, if retraction occurs, the stoma will no longer be diverting and the patient then passes a large amount of stool through their J-pouch. This not only causes anal excoriation, but may also impair healing of the distal ileal J-pouch anal anastomosis, the prime purpose of the ileostomy in the first place.

Conclusion

In performing ileal pouch-anal anastomosis in the technically challenging patient, due to anatomic or other reasons, the main key is patience and careful attention to detail. Even in the most difficult setting, satisfactory results can be achieved.

References

1. Dozois R (1990) Ulcerative colitis: surgical alternatives. In: Fazio V (ed) Current Therapy in Colon and Rectal Surgery. BC Decker, Toronto
2. Mahid SS, Christmas B, Tran D, Galandiuk S (2006) Triple staple technique for low rectal anastomoses eliminates the purse-string suture and facilitates stapled colorectal anastomosis. J Am Coll Surg 202:382-383
3. Galandiuk S, Scott NA, Dozois RR et al (1990) Ileal pouch-anal anastomosis: reoperation for pouch-related complications. Ann Surg 212(4):446-454
4. Keighley MRB (1996) Ostomy Management. In: Pemberton JH (ed) Shackelford's Surgery of the Alimentary Tract, volume IV: Colon. 5th edn. WB Saunders, Philadelphia

Open Questions in Restorative Proctocolectomy

Filippo Nifosì, Gianluca Colucci, Maurizio Mainente, Daniele Ortolani, Gian Gaetano Delaini

Introduction

Restorative proctocolectomy (RPC) has evolved as a procedure for the treatment of mucosal pathologies such as ulcerative colitis (UC) and familial adenomatous polyposis (FAP) while preserving intestinal continuity and anal continence [1]. The two key concepts on which it is based are ileoanal anastomosis [2] and construction of an ileal reservoir proposed, even if in different clinical situations, by Valiente and Bacon [3] and Kock [4] and subsequently integrated in the ileoanal anastomosis by Parks and Nicholls [5].

Since the period of the original description, the operation underwent many technical improvements which simplified the procedure, contained the morbility and improved the functional results [6, 7]. RPC with an ileal pouch-anal anastomosis (IPAA) is a complex and sophisticated operation; even if perioperative mortality is low (0–1%), specific surgical complications are about 25–40%, with the need to perform surgical revisions in 15–25% of cases [8]. Nevertheless, the functional results that may be obtained in terms of continence and acceptable intestinal function determine a high degree of satisfaction in relation to patient lifestyle [9]. Some controversies about some surgical aspects and patient selection criteria still exist even if issues about pouch duration and stability in the long run and its morphological and functional changes are actually considered much more important.

Open Questions Related to Technical Issues

Mucosectomy with Hand-Sewn Anastomosis or Double Stapling Technique

After performing mucosectomy and manual anastomosis, percentage of disorders pertaining fine tuning of continence is registered (such as spotting, daily and especially nightly soiling), which is definitely higher than the clinical situation after performing stapled anastomosis (30–50% vs about 10%) [10, 11]. Stapled anastomosis entails less handling of the anal canal, reduced sphincterial trauma, lower anastomotic tension and preservation of the transitional mucosa with a sensorial-discriminating function, which are all details to simplify the operation and improve functional results [12–14], as various retrospective and observational studies testify [6, 14, 15]. The different results appear to be less obvious if randomised studies only are taken into account [16–18]. Probably the heterogeneity of patients (including FAP cases), variability of the anastomosis level and methodological differences in the analysis of results may explain these discrepancies. Regardless, both from the Swedish [18] and Mayo Clinic [16] study, a trend showing a better night faecal continence emerges in patients with stapled anastomosis, which is a meaningful variable for patient overall well-being.

Manometric evaluations performed after IPAA show reduction in anal basal tone in comparison with preoperative values, but in all evaluations carried out, reduction of sphincterial tone is less obvious after a stapled suture [10, 12, 14–16,18]. Stapled anastomosis at the top of the anal canal preserves the anatomic functional integrity of the anal region whereas if performed at the dentated line, it causes damage to the internal sphincter and produces results similar to those of the manual technique [10, 11, 19]. Results of the stapled IPAA as a whole are functionally superior, as with the preservation of a suitable anal pressure gradient and transitional mucosa, which are important for the sampling [6, 10, 13, 14, 20]. Moreover, the stapled IPAA entails fewer septic complications and a lower risk of reservoir failure due to pelvic sepsis [6, 21, 22]. However, on these topics, unanimous agreement in the surgical community has not been reached [7, 8, 10, 13, 23, 25].

Pouch Configuration

Although the initial reservoir described by Parks and Nicholls [5] was triple limbs of the ileum shaped in

"S" configuration, surgeon creativity produced several designs – "J", "H", "K" and "W"– to overcome the difficulties of evacuation connected with the exit conduit of the S-shaped pouch and improve its functionality [8, 24]. The J-shaped configuration was adopted by most surgeons [6, 21, 23, 24] because of ease of construction using staplers and efficient evacuation even if its lower initial compliance may give rise to an increase in the defecation frequency at least in the initial period after the ileostomy take down [7]. Regardless, 1 year after surgery, the J-shaped pouch increases its ability by 300–400%, allowing suitable stabilisation of daily evacuations [25]. A comparative study into features of three different-shaped ileal reservoirs (S, J, K) showed that even if the S- and K-shaped reservoirs reach higher volumes 1 year after surgery (410 ml vs 305 ml), as a matter of fact, functional results do not differ much [24]. The W-shaped pouch has probably a small advantage in comparison with the J-shaped pouch in terms of evacuation frequency, at least in the first period after ileostomy closure, but this difference disappears with time [10], and 1 year after surgery, the two reservoirs give the same results [10, 26]. The choice among the various configurations is more a matter of personal taste, and as far as suitable ileal tract is concerned (at least 30-cm long), functional behaviour can be compared [24].

Omission of Diverting Loop Ileostomy

The complexity of IPAA and the seriousness of the functional consequences of pelvic sepsis from anastomotic dehiscence justify the almost routine adoption of the protective ileostomy [8]. Ileostomy does not completely eliminate the risk of pelvic sepsis, but it mitigates its negative consequences and facilitates its treatment [24, 25] even if at the price of a 10–30% of complications connected with its construction and closure [24, 27]. Even if several trials suggest the possibility of performing one-stage IPAA with overlapping pelvic complications, minor occlusive episodes and a shorter hospitalisation [28, 29], in other authors' experience [30–32], omission of the ileostomy is connected with an increase of anastomotic complications and pelvic sepsis. Despite an aggressive therapeutic attitude, the risk of reservoir failure in patients with septic complications is 31% after 5 years and 39% after 10 years since surgery [32]. In the light of these data, one-stage IPAA may be offered if the surgeon is an expert and in selected low-risk cases (patients with a suitable nutritional status, not undergoing immunosuppressive therapy, under treatment with a low steroid dosage) where the operation follows an ideal course without any technical incidents or problems of anastomotic tension [24, 30, 33]. However, it is noteworthy that the results of a recent experience investigating the reasons for long-term failure of RPC be taken into account, which demonstrate the omission of protective ileostomy as one major adverse prognostic factor [34].

Laparoscopic IPAA

Recently, we assisted to an increase of laparoscopic techniques in the field of gastrointestinal surgery, which also involved IPAA, whose laparoscopic practicability was shown with complications and overlapping results to the open approach [35, 36]. There are still some incontrovertible data missing about advantages of the mini-invasive approach in terms of surgical morbility, stress reduction and a faster healing process and more restricted intraabdominal adhesion formation, as data to compare open and laparoscopic surgery are presently unsuitable [8]. A recent randomised Dutch study [37] showed a comparable life-style between the two groups of patients, but the laparoscopic operation lasts longer, has higher costs and shows no clear advantages about the use of analgesics and duration of hospitalisation. The only real advantage that is presently well documented for the laparoscopic approach is the higher cosmetic effect [36]. Further prospective evaluations are necessary to define the role of laparoscopic IPAA.

Open Questions Related to Selection Criteria

Age

If at the beginning of the clinical experience with IPAA, given the complexity of the procedure, the higher age limit had been arbitrarily set at 55 years, this criterion does no longer represents an absolute bond [8]. Two recent studies showed that IPAA can be advised for patients older than 60 years in whom favourable results not considerably different from those in younger patients were reported [38, 39], as well as for 70-year-old, well-motivated patients with clinically acceptable results [40], even if those results were surely not ideal for younger patients.

Crohn's Disease

Crohn's disease (CD) is generally a contraindication to performing an IPAA [1, 25] because of the high risk of complications and illness relapse with a consequent destruction of the reservoir or its permanent loss of functionality in 30–45% of cases [41, 42]. The experience of Regimbeau et al. goes against the tide [43]; they performed the operation in a selected group of patients with known CD, with complications in 35% of patients, reservoir excision in 10% of cases and a functional result overlapping with the result of patients suffering from UC. Despite all the perplexities shown by some authors about the criteria used by the French surgeons to diagnose CD [34], their results compel us to reconsider the issue from a different perspective, as it is not properly suitable to compare the results of IPAA for CD with results for UC and FAP [44]. It must be emphasised that in case of Crohn's colitis, surgical relapses after 10 years since surgery are 25% after undergoing proctocolectomy and ileostomy and 50% after ileorectal anastomosis [45]. These values may well be compared with the percentages of the failure of IPAA for CD reported in the various series [42, 44, 45]. Delaini et al. [44] compared the results of two groups of patients suffering from Crohn's colitis at a distance; they underwent total proctocolectomy and continent ileostomy (Kock pouch) or conventional ileostomy. Reservoir excision was necessary due to a relapse of CD in 28% of patients with Kock pouch whereas in the group who underwent conventional ileostomy, 28% of patients underwent one or more ileal resections due to a relapse. Short-bowel syndrome occurred in 4% of patients in both groups. The results of this study show that loss of the small intestine due to pouch removal can be compared with those due to relapse after conventional ileostomy and does not inevitably lead to short-bowel syndrome. According to Delaini et al. [44], construction of a continent ileostomy and also of a pelvic reservoir in the case of selected CD (absence of ileal and anal-perineal illness) does not necessarily prognosticate a surgical catastrophe; this is a point of view that agrees with a recent study by the Cleveland Clinic [45] (12% reservoir excision, acceptable functional results, satisfactory quality of life).

Open Questions Related to Pouch Durability, Functional Stability and Pathophysiological Modifications of Ileal-Pouch Mucosa

Pouch Durability and Functional Stability in the Long Term

IPAA is an operation with a high potential for complications leading to reservoir failure in 10–15% of cases 10 years after surgery [43, 45]. Data present in the literature show that the risk of losing the reservoir progresses with time, that 75% of these events happen well after 1 year following surgery [34] and that the main causes are pelvic sepsis/fistulisation, reservoir disfunction and CD [23, 34, 46]. Risk of losing the reservoir is particularly high in patients developing postoperative septic complications, reaching values of 30% after 5 years and 40% after 10 years since surgery [32]. Fazio et al. [47] developed a predictive model to determine the risk of failure and allow patients an objective estimate of such an event in the light of an informed and well-thought-out choice among the various surgical options.

As for functional outcomes, despite the fact that short-term results are rather encouraging, there are concerns about continence stability in the long term, considering that the likely negative consequences of anastomotic complications adds to the physiological decline of the sphincterial function, which deteriorates with age [48]. If continence remains rather stable between 5 and 10 years since surgery [23], after 10–15 years since surgery, 18–32% of patients show a functional decay with an increase of incontinence episodes, usually intermittent and of a lower degree [49–51]. Noteworthy is the fact that the prevalence of incontinence in the long follow-up is no higher than that present before construction of the IPAA [49] and that patient quality of life remains excellent in all fields examined despite alteration of the intestinal function. This can also be contributed by patients' coping mechanisms to the new problems that arise [49, 51].

Long-Term Risk of Dysplasia/Cancer Development in Anal Transitional Zone/Columnar Mucosa After Stapled IPAA

The largest criticism about stapled IPAA is the risk of leaving in situ a 1- to 2-cm-long columnar cuff of mucosa above the anal transitional zone (ATZ) area, with symptomatic sequelae and the potential for neoplastic transformation over time [24, 52]. The risk of a dysplasia in the ATZ/columnar mucosa may be connected with the stage of illness, follow-up duration and UC or FAP diagnosis. Risk is 25% if the proctocolectomy specimen shows cancer, 10% if there is concomitant dysplasia. In patients with FAP, the risk of adenoma is 4–12% and of dysplasia 10–12% [53]. Considering that the risk of cancer onset after ileorectal anastomosis is 15–20% after 30 years since surgery [53], a theoretical risk of 2% after 30 years since surgery was calculated for the ATZ/columnar residual mucosa both in patients with UC and FAP. Neoplastic risk does not disappear after mucosectomy because in ileoanal pouches removed because of complications, residual islands of columnar mucosa between the reservoir serosa and the rectal muscular cuff were found in 20% of cases [54]; moreover, most carcinomas that occurred following IPAA were in patients who underwent mucosectomy [53, 54]. Recent investigations with a minimum follow-up of 10 years gave rather reassuring data, as development of dysplasia in the residual columnar mucosa was found in 0–4.5% of cases [53–55]. Evidence from examining doughnuts and mucosectomy specimens does not support the argument for routine mucosectomy, except for FAP patients with extensive rectal involvement and high-risk genotype and CU patients with associated dysplasia or cancer [53]. All other cases would be better served by sparing the anal canal mucosa due to functional improvement [11, 14], even if some controversy on this topic persists [7, 17, 25]. Regardless, it is advisable to perform an annual endoscopic biopsy follow-up [53, 55]. Endoscopic and histologic markers of an inflammation of the columnar mucosa were found in 35% and 50–75% of patients. Clinical symptoms affected only 15% of patients and did not compromise reservoir function [53].

Long-Term Risk of Cancer Development in the Pelvic Pouch

Adaptive alterations, both morphological and phlogistic, in the reservoir mucosa characterised by villous atrophy and crypt hyperplasia [56], and the report that some cases of dysplasia and cancer were found in ileal pouches [57, 58] caused concern that patients with IPAA might run the same risk in the long term as patients with long-lasting UC [46]. However, the supposed mucosal atrophy – dysplasia – cancer sequence [58] is not incontrovertibly corroborated, as the adaptation of the ileal mucosa is phenotypical and subject to regression after control of chronic inflammation [59]. It is a much-debated subject [60] whether carcinoma development is directly ascribable to the pouch mucosa or to the residual rectal mucosa whatever anastomotic technique is used, as pointed out in various studies [57, 61, 62].

Two recent studies [63, 64] one with a follow-up of 30 years [63], show that the development of dysplastic mucosal lesions of ileoanal reservoirs or Kock pouch is very low, ranging from 0 to 1.6% [63–65]. Further and more detailed data are necessary to confirm whether patients with serious villous atrophy and chronic pouchitis represent a subgroup with a particular risk of malignancy, as suggested by a Swedish study [58]. In the group of patients with FAP who underwent IPAA, the risk of developing adenomas in the reservoir is deemed 35% after 10 years and 75% after 15 years [66].

Pouchitis

Idiopathic and aspecific inflammation of the reservoir (pouchitis) is the most frequent and disturbing complication after IPAA [6, 7]. The cumulative risk of developing one or more episodes of pouchitis with rather serious symptoms requiring specific treatment is 50% after 5 years and in progressive relation with the length of follow-up [6, 67]. The rarity of this occurrence in patients suffering from FAP (3–14%) and the increased incidence in patients suffering from sclerosing cholangitis support the theory of pouchitis as a new form of intestinal inflammatory disease specific to the reservoir [68]. Usually pouchitis has a favourable course and quick response to antibiotics. Less than 10% of patients suffer from chronic disorders with difficult therapeutic control. Untreatable forms leading to reservoir excision are about 0.3–1.3% [67, 68]. Recent observations showed the effectiveness of probiotics in maintaining remission after antibiotic therapy and as a prophylaxis against pouchitis development in the first year after reservoir construction [69]. The effects of pouchitis on functional results have not been completely clarified even if some authors associate this complication with metabolic sequelae and significantly diminished quality of life [70].

Conclusions

If our expectancies about IPAA seem quite confirmed by functional outcomes and long-term results, we must not ignore that the probability of developing septic complications and pouchitis increases over time [46] and therefore the risk of pouch loss over the long term [34]. In relation to failed pouches, major revision surgery has a probability of being successful in 25–50% of cases, and, if objectively considered, functional outcomes after such major undertakings are often unsatisfactory [71, 72].

The most urgent issue in regard to IPAA in comparison with ileorectal anastomosis is, theoretically, rectal cancer risk that, even though substantially reduced, has not been completely eliminated [57, 58]; therefore, regular endoscopic follow-up is strongly recommended [46]. IPAA is a typical operation meant to improve quality of life and, despite various attempts to clarify this aspect, all studies conducted so far gave conflicting results [46].

If it is true that most patients are prompted to choose a procedure such as IPAA that preserves continence avoiding a stoma [73], it is also shown that a pelvic reservoir is advantageous in certain fields in comparison with a conventional ileostomy, but the differences seem less obvious in other respects [74], and reservoir malfunction may thwart the benefits of the preservation of body image [75].

Overall opinion regarding this operation is surely positive even if IPAA may not represent the ultimate panacea, as it was initially believed to be [46, 60]. If patients are suitably selected and the postoperative course is poor regarding complications, the result will generally be almost optimum with suitable preservation of continence and a good quality of life, as verified in most cases [46].

However, individual outcome after so complex an operation is sometimes unpredictable. Patients must be given detailed information about functional implications in the short and long term and the pros and cons of the different surgical options that, from time to time (conventional ileostomy in elderly patients and ileorectal anastomosis in young patients of child-bearing age as a bridge to a future IPAA) may represent reasonable alternatives [46, 67].

References

1. Onaitis MW, Mantyh C (2003) Ileal pouch-anal anastomosis for ulcerative colitis and familial adenomatous polyposis. Historical development and current status. Ann Surg 238:542-548
2. Ravitch MM, Sabiston DC (1947) Anal ileostomy with preservation of the sphincter: a proposed operation in patients requiring total colectomy for benign lesions. Surg Gyn Obst 84:1095-1099
3. Valiente MA, Bacon HE (1955) Construction of pouch using "pantaloon" technique for pull-through following total colectomy. Am J Surg 90:6621-6643
4. Kock NG (1969) Intra-abdominal "reservoir" in patients with permanent ileostomy; preliminary observations on a procedure resulting in fecal continence in five ileostomy patients. Arch Surg 99:223-231
5. Parks AG, Nicholls RJ (1978) Proctocolectomy without ileostomy for ulcerative colitis. Br Med J 2:85-88
6. Fazio VW, Ziv Y, Church JM et al (1995) Ileal pouch-anal anastomoses, complications and function in 1005 patients. Ann Surg 222(2):120-127
7. Radice E, Dozois RR (1999) Techniques of ileoanal anastomosis: historical evolution, refinements and current approaches. Tech Coloproctol 3:27-32
8. Lindsey I, MacMortensen N (2003) Surgical management of ulcerative colitis. In: Targan SR, Shanahan F, Karp LC (eds) Inflammatory bowel disease. From bench to bedside. Kluwer Academic Pub, pp 631-641
9. Seidel SA, Peach SE, Newman M, Sharp KW (1999) Ileoanal pouch procedures: clinical outcomes and quality-of-life assessment. Am Surg 65(1):40-46
10. Tonelli F, Monaci I, Garcea A, Batignani G (2000) What effect does ileoanal pouch anastomosis have on continence? In: Romano G (ed) Diagnosis and treatment of fecal incontinence. Idelson-Gnocchi, Napoli, pp 265-274
11. Rabau M (1999) Ileal pouch anal anastomosis: mucosectomy with hand-sewn anastomosis or double-stapling technique? Tech Coloproctol 3:265-274
12. Ascanelli S, Bartolo D (1999) Functional outcome after restorative proctocolectomy. Tech Coloproctol 3:145-151
13. Saigusa N, Kurahashi T, Nakamura T et al (2000) Functional outcome of stapled ileal pouch-anal canal anastomosis. Surg Today 30:575-581
14. Reissman PW, Piccirillo M, Ulrich A et al (1995) Functional results of the double stapled ileoanal reservoir. J Am Coll Surg 181:444-450
15. Mc Courtney JS, Finlay IG (1997) Totally stapled restorative proctocolectomy. Br J Surg 84(6):808-812
16. Reilly TW, Pemberton JH, Wolff BG et al (1997) Randomized prospective trial comparing ileal pouch-anal anastomosis performed by excising the anal mucosa to ileal pouch-anal anastomosis performed by preserving the anal mucosa. Ann Surg 225:666-677
17. Seow-Choen A, Tsunoda A, Nicholls RJ (1991) Prospective randomized trial comparing anal function after hand sewn ileoanal anastomosis with mucosectomy versus stapled ileoanal anastomosis without mucosectomy in restorative proctocolectomy. Br J Surg 78(4):430-434
18. Hallgren TA, Fasth SB, Oresland MO, Hulten L (1995) Ileal pouch-anal function after endoanal mucosectomy and handsewn ileoanal anastomosis compared with stapled anastomosis without mucosectomy. Eur J Surg 161:915-921
19. Deen KI, Williams JG, Grant EA et al (1995) Randomized trial to determine the optimum level of pouch-anal anastomosis in stapled restorative proctocolectomy. Dis Col Rectum 38:133-138
20. Michelassi F, Lee J, Rubin M et al (2003) Long-term functional results after ileal pouch anal restorative proctocolectomy for ulcerative colitis. A prospective observational study. Arch Surg 238:433-445
21. McLeod RS, Cohen Z (1998) Restorative proctocolectomy with stapled ileal pouch anastomosis. In: Rachmilewiz D (ed) 5th International Symposium of Inflammatory Bowel Disease. Kluwer Academic Publisher, pp 188-195
22. Ziv Y, Fazio VW, Church JM et al (1996) Stapled ileal pouch anastomosis in patients with ulcerative colitis. Am J Surg 171:320-323
23. Meagher AP, Farouk R, Dozois RR et al (1998) J ileal pouch-anal anastomosis for chronic ulcerative colitis: complications and long term outcome in 1310 patients. Br J Surg 85(6):800-803
24. Farouk R, Pemberton JH (1997) Surgical options in ulcerative colitis. Surg Cl N AM 77(1):85-94
25. Becker JM (1993) Surgical management of inflammatory bowel disease. Curr Op Gastroenterol 9:600-615
26. Keighley MRB, Yashioka K, Kmiot WA (1988) Prospective randomized trial to compare the stapled double lumen pouch and the sutured quadrupled pouch for restorative proctocolectomy. Br J Surg 75:1008-1011
27. Ganio E (1994) The arguments for and against a diverting ileostomy in pouch-anal anastomosis. In: Serio G, Delaini GG, Hulten L et al (eds) Inflammatory bowel disease. Graffham Press, Edinburg, pp 59-62
28. Sugerman HJ, Sugerman EL, Meador JG et al (2000) Ileal pouchanal anastomosis without ileal diversion. Ann Surg 232(4):530-541
29. Mowschenson PM, Cricthlow JF, Peppercorn MA (2000) Ileoanal pouch operation. Long term outcome with or without ileostomy. Arch Surg 135:463-466
30. Cohen Z, Mc Leod RS, Stephen W et al (1992) Contin-

uing evolution of the pelvic pouch procedure. Ann Surg 216:506-511
31. Williamson ME, Lewis WG, Sagar PM et al (1997) One-stage restorative proctocolectomy without temporary ileostomy for ulcerative colitis. Dis Colon Rectum 40:1019-1022
32. Heuschen UA, Allenmeyer EH, Hinz U et al (2002) Outcome after septic complications in J pouch surgery. Br J Surg 89:194-200
33. Heuschen UA, Hinz U, Allemeyer EH et al (2001) One- or two-stage procedure for restorative proctocolectomy: rational for a surgical strategy in ulcerative colitis. Ann Surg 234:788-794
34. Tulchinsky H, Hawley PH, Nicholls J (2003) Long-term failure after restorative proctocolectomy for ulcerative colitis. Ann Surg 238(2):224-234
35. Marcello PW, Milsom JW, Wong SK et al (2000) Laparoscopic restorative proctocolectomy. Case matched comparative study with open restorative proctocolectomy. Dis Colon Rectum 43:604-608
36. Dunker MS, Bemelman WA, Slors FM et al (2001) Functional outcome, quality of life, body image and cosmesis in patients after laparoscopic-assisted and conventional restorative proctocolectomy. A comparative study. Dis Colon Rectum 44:1800-1807
37. Maartense S, Dunker MS, Slors JF et al (2004) Hand-assisted laparoscopic versus open restorative proctocolectomy with ileal pouch anal anastomosis. A randomized trial. Ann Surg 240(6):984-992
38. Reismmanan P, Teon TA, Weiss EG et al (1996) Functional outcome of the double-stapled ileo-anal reservoir in patients more than 60 years of age. AM Surg 62:178-183
39. Tan HT, Vonnoly AB, Morton D et al (1997) Results of restorative proctocolectomy in the elderly. Colorectal Dis 12:319-322
40. Delaney CP, Daovand B, Remzi FH et al (2002) Functional outcome, quality of life and complication after ileal pouch-anal anastomosis in selected septuagenarians. Dis Colon Rectum 45:890-894
41. Sagar PM, Dezois RR, Wolff BG (1996) Long term results of ileo-pouch-anal anastomosis in patients with Crohn's disease. Dis Colon Rectum 39:893-898
42. Brown CJ, MacLean AR, Cohen Z et al (2005) Crohn's disease and indeterminate colitis and the ileal pouch-anal anastomosis: outcomes and pattern of failure. Dis Colon Rectum 48(8):1542-1549
43. Regimbeau JM, Panis Y, Pocaro M et al (2001) Long-term results of ileal pouch-anal anastomosis for colorectal Crohn's disease. Dis Colon Rectum 44:769-778
44. Delaini GG, Scaglia M, Lindholm E et al (2005) Is an ileal pouch an alternative for patients requiring surgery for Crohn's proctocolitis? Tech Coloproctol 9:222-224
45. Hartley JE, Fazio VW, Remzi FH et al (2004) Analysis of the outcome of ileal pouch-anal anastomosis in patients with Crohn's disease. Dis Colon Rectum 47(11):1809-1815
46. Delaini GG, Scaglia M, Colucci G, Hulten L (2005) The ileoanal pouch procedure in the long-term perspective: a critical review. Tech Coloproctol 9:187-192
47. Fazio VW, Tekkis PP, Renzi F, Laverty IC et al (2003) Quantification of risk for pouch failure after ileal pouch anal anastomosis surgery. Ann Surg 238:605-617
48. Laurberg S, Swash M (1989) Effect of aging on the anorectal sphincters and their innervation. Dis Colon Rectum 32:737-742
49. Fazio VW, O' Riordan MG, Lavery IC et al (1999) Long-term functional outcome and quality of life after stapled restorative proctocolectomy. Ann Surg 230(4):575-586
50. Bullard KM, Madoff RD, Gemlo BT (2002) Is ileoanal pouch function stable with time? Results of a prospective audit. Dis Colon Rectum 45:299-304
51. Hahnloser D, Pemberton JH, Wolff BG et al (2004) The effect of ageing on function and quality of life in ileal pouch patients. Ann Surg 240:615-623
52. Sequens R (1997) Cancer in the anal canal (transitional zone) after restorative proctocolectomy with stapled ileal pouch-anal anastomosis. Int J Colorectal Dis 12:254-255
53. Thompson-Fawcett MW, McMortensen NJ (1996) Anal transitional zone and columnar cuff in restorative proctocolectomy 83:1047-1055
54. Remzi FH, Fazio VW, Delaney CP et al (2003) Dysplasia of the anal transitional zone after ileal pouch-anastomosis. Results of prospective evaluation after a minimum of ten years. Dis Colon Rectum 46:6-13
55. Coull DB, Lee FD, Hendersone AP et al (2003) Risk of dysplasia in the columnar cuff after stapled restorative proctocolectomy. Br J Surg 90:72-75
56. Duff SE, O' Dwyer ST, Hulten et al (2002) Colorectal Dis 4(6):420-429
57. Hassan C, Zullo A, Speziale G et al (2003) Adenocarcinoma of the ileoanal pouch anastomosis: an emerging complication? Int J Colorectal Dis 18(3):276-278
58. Gullberg K, Lindoforss U, Zetterquisht H et al (2002) Cancer risk assessment in long-standing pouchitis. DNA aberrations are rare in transformed neoplastic pelvic pouch mucosa. Int J Colorectal Dis 17(2):92-97
59. Sylvester PA, Wong NA, Myerscough N et al (2002) Mucin expression in the ileoanal reservoir reflects incomplete mucosal adaptation. J Pathol 197(1):28-36
60. Borjesson L, Willen R, Haboubi N et al (2004) The risk of dysplasia and cancer in the ileal pouch mucosa after restorative proctocolectomy for ulcerative proctocolitis is low: a long-term followup study. Colorectal Dis 6:494-498
61. Stern H, Walfish S, Mullen B et al (1990) Cancer in an ileoanal reservoir: a new late complication. Gut 31:473-475
62. Hyman N (2002) Rectal cancer as a complication of stapled IPAA. Inflamma Bowel Dis 8:4345
63. Hulten L, Willen R, Nilsson O et al (2002) Mucosal assessment for dysplasia and cancer in the ileal pouch mocosa in patients operated for ulcerative colitis. A 30 year followup study. Dis Colon Rectum 45:448-452
64. Thompson-Fawcett MW, Marcus V, Redstone M et al (2001) Risk of dysplasia in long-term ileal pouches and pouches with chronic pouchitis. Gastroenterology 121(2):275-281
65. Herline AJ, Meisinger LL, Rusin LC et al (2003) Is routine pouch surveillance for dysplasia indicated for ileoanal pouches? Dis Colon Rectum 46:156-159
66. Parc YR, Olschwang S, Desaint B et al (2001) Familial

adenomatous polyposis: prevalence of adenomas in the ileal pouch after restorative proctocolectomy. Ann Surg 233:360-364

67. Hulten L (1998) Proctocolectomy and ileostomy to pouch surgery for ulcerative colitis. Word J Surg 22:335-341
68. Mahadevan U, Sandborn WJ (2003) Diagnosis and management of pouchitis. Gastroenterology 124(6):1636-1650
69. Gionchetti P, Amadini C, Rizzello F, Venturi A et al (2003) Diagnosis and treatment of pouchitis. Best Pract Res Clin Gastroenetrol 17(1):75-87
70. Keranen U, Luukkonen P, Jarvinen H (1997) Functional results after restorative proctocolectomy complicated by pouchitis. Dis Colon Rectum 40(7):764-769
71. Baixauli J, Delaney CP, Wu JS et al (2004) Functional outcome and quality of life after repeat ileal pouch-anal anastomosis for complications of ileoanal surgery. Dis Colon Retum 47(1):2-11
72. Tulchinsky H, Cohen CRG, Nicholls RJ (2003) Salvage surgery after restorative proctocolectomy. Br J Surg 90:909-921
73. McLeod RS, Baxten NN (1998) Quality of life of patients with inflammatory bowel disease after surgery. Word J Surg 22:375-381
74. Kohler LW, Pemberton JH, Zinsmeister AR, Kelly KA (1991) Quality of life after proctocolectomy. A comparison of Brooke ileostomy, Kock pouch, and ileal pouch-anal anastomosis. Gastroeneterology 101:679-684
75. O'Bichere A, Wilkinson K, Rumbues S et al (2000) Functional outcome after restorative proctocolectomy for ulcerative colitis decrease an otherwise enhancement quality of life. Br J Surg 89:802-807

Follow-Up of Restorative Proctocolectomy: Clinical Experience of a Specialised Pouch Clinic

Hagit Tulchinsky, Iris Dotan, Zamir Halpern, Micha Rabau

Introduction

Most patients with ulcerative colitis (UC) can be managed medically. However, about 20–30% will eventually require elective or emergency surgery. Restorative proctocolectomy with ileal pouch anal anastomosis (IPAA) has become firmly established as the operation preferred by most surgeons and patients because of the advantages of complete removal of the diseased colorectal mucosa, preservation of continence with relatively normal defecation and avoidance of a permanent ileostomy [1–5]. This chapter describes our experience with the follow-up of UC patients undergoing IPAA, focuses on potential short-term and long-term complications and presents our comprehensive, multidisciplinary approach.

Indications

Surgical treatment for UC patients is usually indicated due to one of three causes: (1) failure of medical therapy or dependence on therapy, mainly corticosteroids, with severe side effects; (2) prevention when dysplasia is diagnosed and treatment of colorectal cancer (CRC); and (3) a severe acute complication of UC, such as toxic megacolon or massive hemorrhage. The appropriate timing of elective surgery is determined by collaborative assessment of the gastroenterologist and the surgeon and should be tailored to each patient according to the specific clinical setup.

Ulcerative Colitis Refractory to Medical Therapy

Patients with chronically active UC and those with frequently recurrent disease, despite appropriate medical therapy, are candidates for elective surgery [6, 7]. These patients usually suffer from frequent bloody diarrhoea and abdominal cramps. They may also suffer from anaemia, mild-to-moderate chronic malnutrition and hypoproteinaemia. In addition to signs and symptoms, patients experience chronic disability and diminished physical, emotional and social quality of life [8]. In the pediatric population, growth impairment is an important indication for IPAA, often leading to significant growth acceleration [9]. Infrequently, surgery is also indicated for intractable and debilitating extraintestinal manifestations (EIM) of UC, such as peripheral arthritis, pyoderma gangrenosum, ocular, haematological and vascular manifestations [10]. Despite their well-known side effects, corticosteroids are still widely used for the treatment of UC. In contrast to their beneficial effect in remission induction of an acute flair [11], their use as maintenance is not effective and is associated with severe side effects, some of which are irreversible [12, 13]. Thus, prolonged treatment with systemic corticosteroids should be avoided [14]. Although it is widely agreed that steroid-dependent disease is a clear indication for surgery, there is no strict definition of steroid dependency or an agreed-upon time limit for this therapy. Thus, collaboration and mutual discussions between gastroenterologist, surgeon and patient are essential to determine the appropriate timing for surgery in these cases.

Cytotoxic agents, such as 6-mercaptopurine and azathioprine, are widely used as steroid-sparing agents to control chronic symptoms and maintain remission [15, 16]. Although severe side effects of these drugs are less frequent, they are not risk free; thus, side effects that preclude their use [17] or lack of response to immunosuppressive therapy may also be indications for surgery in UC patients [18].

Prevention and Treatment of Colorectal Cancer

Long-standing UC is a predisposing factor for development of CRC, as it is clear that cancer is more common in these patients compared to the age-matched general population [19, 20]. The actual prevalence varies in different series [21, 22], and the cumulative probability of developing CRC is 18% after 30 years of disease [23]. In addition to disease duration, disease extent also correlates with an increased risk of cancer, with the risk being most significant in patients with pancolitis [24]. Another two independent risk factors for CRC in UC patients are family history of CRC [25, 26] and primary sclerosing cholangitis (PSC) [27]. Common practice is to start an annual or biannual surveillance colonoscopy, as cancer risk increases over that of the background population. This would usually mean 8–12 years after disease onset for patients with pancolitis or upon diagnosis of concomitant PSC. Confirmed precancerous lesions, such as high-grade dysplasia or dysplasia-associated lesion or mass (DALM) would be an indication for proctocolectomy [28, 29]. In most inflammatory bowel disease (IBD) referral centres, confirmed low-grade dysplasia would also be an indication for surgery [30] although strict follow-up is an optional alternative suggested by others [31].

Diagnosis of already existing colorectal carcinoma is an obvious indication for surgery, and if curable intent is possible, surgery should include removal of the entire colon and rectum, as the presence of one proven cancer puts the patient in a significant risk of having a synchronous or developing a metachronous carcinoma [32]. In patients with good operative risk and adequate anal sphincter mechanism, IPAA is the most suitable procedure for cancer prophylaxis as well as preservation of reasonable quality of life.

Short- and Long-Term Complications of IPAA

While restoring the natural route of defecation, usually with improved quality of life and good long-term functional outcomes [33–35], IPAA may also be associated with various complications that, depending on duration of follow-up and diagnostic criteria, may occur in 10–60% of patients [36]. Complications may appear early or late and may be surgical or medical. Of note, clear distinction between purely medical or surgical complications seems to be artificial. Several complications are a combination of the two and thus require the surgeon's, as well as the gastroenterologist's, insight. Pouch dysfunction is the most frequent end result of a range of complications. Amongst the various complications reported that lead to pouch dysfunction are mechanical causes, functional disorders, pelvic sepsis and pouch inflammation. Systemic complications include new onset or persistent EIM as well as haematological, nutritional and electrolyte disturbances. The most dreaded condition, despite its rarity, is pouch and rectal-stump dysplasia or cancer [37]. However, the most common and frustrating long-term consequence is pouch inflammation [38]. A careful case selection is essential for a good outcome. Poor functional result or pouch failure are usually the end result of major unmanageable complications [39].

The Concept of a Comprehensive Pouch Clinic

At present, colorectal surgeons usually conduct the follow-up of patients after IPAA although this distinct patient population often requires medical as well as surgical follow-up, as shall be discussed in the following sections. With a primary goal of improving quality of patient care, we have established a multidisciplinary pouch clinic comprised of a colorectal surgeon and an IBD-oriented gastroenterologist. Patients are interviewed, examined and treated by both surgeon and gastroenterologist simultaneously at their outpatient clinic visit. Laboratory blood tests, pouch endoscopy and biopsies are done routinely 1 year post-IPAA or at the beginning of follow-up at the clinic and yearly thereafter or upon demand. Our experience, based on the follow-up of 125 UC patients after IPAA in such an approach, is integrated in the following sections.

Complications of IPAA that May End in Pouch Dysfunction

"Normal" or acceptable pouch function is hard to define since it varies from one person to another and from day to day in the same individual. Most patients with pouch dysfunction have an increased stool frequency, which is often associated with small amounts of stools. Incontinence may be the predominant symptom or may occur in association with frequency and urgency. The causes of pouch dysfunction can be divided into four categories: septic complications, mechanical or surgical complications, functional disorders and inflammation, mainly pouchitis and, to a lesser, extent cuffitis. Diagnosis is based on accurate history and physical examination combined with one or more auxiliary assessments, such as evaluation under anaesthesia, pouch endoscopy, anorectal physiology tests and various imaging techniques. The major conditions that may result in pouch dysfunction are described below.

Pelvic Sepsis

Pelvic abscess is usually the result of a leak or disruption of the ileoanal anastomosis, leak from the pouch suture line, or an infected haematoma. The prevalence of postoperative pelvic sepsis varies between 5% and 25% [40–42], this wide range being partially attributable to the lack of a standard definition. Symptoms and signs include fever, anal pain, tenesmus, purulent discharge, bleeding from the anus and leukocytosis. Diagnosis may be established by examination under anaesthesia alone or in combination with imaging studies such as contrast pouchography, computerised tomography (CT) and magnetic resonance imaging (MRI). Pelvic sepsis may be clinically evident in the immediate postoperative period, after ileostomy closure or after a long follow-up period. Late sepsis may be expressed as pouch dysfunction with frequency, urgency, incontinence or pouch-related fistula without systemic signs of sepsis. The treatment is modified according to the severity of sepsis. Some patients can be managed successfully with antibiotic treatment while others will need operative or CT-guided percutaneous drainage. It is clear that severe pelvic sepsis with extensive anastomotic breakdown results in a high failure rate despite salvage attempts [43].

Pouch Fistulae

Fistula originating from the ileoanal anastomosis or the pouch itself is a serious complication. The incidence varies between 5% and 17% and depends on the accuracy and duration of follow-up [44, 45]. It often requires further surgery and may alter ultimate functional outcome and lead to pouch excision. Fistulae may occur to the perineum, vagina, bladder or abdominal wall skin. Aetiologic factors include anastomotic dehiscence, pelvic sepsis, surgical experience, localised ischaemia, entrapment of the posterior vaginal wall in the stapling device and Crohn's disease. Pelvic sepsis is probably the major predisposing factor. Patients may be asymptomatic, some may have only minor symptoms whereas others may have disabling symptoms. Symptoms consist of purulent discharge and flatus or stool passing through the vagina, perineum or abdominal wall. Diagnosis is based on history and physical examination and may be confirmed by examination under anaesthesia. Other diagnostic modalities may be used to assess the tract, including endoanal ultrasound, pouchography, fistulography, CT and MRI. Initial management includes local procedures to drain the sepsis, and Crohn's disease must be excluded [46]. Most pouch-perineal fistulae originate from the ileoanal anastomosis. When superficial, these fistulae can be managed by fistulotomy. If the fistula is transsphincteric, it can be managed by staged fistulotomy using a seton or by a pouch advancement procedure. At our clinic, nine patients (7.6%) had a perineal fistula at a mean follow-up of 57 months. All were treated by staged fistulotomy. In none of these patients was the diagnosis changed to Crohn's disease.

Pouch-vaginal fistula (PVF) occurs in 6.3% (range 3–16%) of women who undergo IPAA [47]. Symptoms are discharge of flatus and faeces through the vagina. PVF are classified in relation to the ileoanal anastomosis (above, below or at the anastomosis), and management is challenging. Diversion may be considered in order to alleviate symptoms and control sepsis. Several surgical procedures have been described for the repair of PVF with variable success rates [48, 49]. Local procedures, such as transvaginal repair or endoanal ileal advancement flap, are appropriate for low fistulae whereas combined abdominoperineal procedures should be considered for high fistulae. Overall, more than 50% of patients maintain a functioning pouch without fistula recurrence, and about 20% require pouch excision [50]. Among the pouch clinic patients, four developed a PVF: two occurred early after a one-stage IPAA and were successfully treated by loop ileostomy. The other two patients had very mild symptoms and refused surgery.

Ileoanal Anastomotic Stricture

Stenosis of the ileoanal anastomosis is the most common perineal complication after IPAA. The precise definition is unclear and contributes to the wide range of incidence reported in the literature. Narrowing, which requires at least one dilatation under anaesthesia, has been reported in 4–40% of cases [51, 52]. The main causative factors are pelvic sepsis with subsequent fibrosis and tension on the anastomosis leading to ischaemia. Patients most frequently present with symptoms of straining, increased number of bowel movements per day, watery stool, urgency of defecation, a feeling of incomplete evacuation and abdominal or anal pain. Rectal examination and contrast pouchography if needed confirm the diagnosis. Anastomotic strictures can be noted before or after ileostomy closure. Most strictures, especially those found during an outpatient clinic visit before ileostomy closure, are annular and web like due to lateral adhesions across the anastomosis and can be treated successfully with a simple digital anal dilatation. Severe strictures usually require repeat dilatations. If a stricture persists in spite of repeated dilatations, surgery is required. Despite all salvage attempts, up to 15% of patients with severe anastomotic stricture will eventually come to pouch excision and permanent ileostomy [53].

Pouchitis

Pouchitis, defined as nonspecific inflammation of the ileal pouch, is the most common long-term complication of IPAA in UC patients [54]. Aetiology is poorly understood, and several mechanisms have been suggested, such as genetic susceptibility, immune alterations, faecal stasis resulting in bacterial overgrowth, lack of mucosal nutrients, ischaemia and missed diagnosis of Crohn's disease, none of which have been proved. Pouchitis may be a form of IBD that recurs in the pouch or a novel third form of IBD. It tends to occur in equal frequency irrespective of the pouch configuration. A number of factors have been studied as potential predictors for the development of pouchitis. A positive association was found between the presence of EIM and PSC and the risk of developing pouchitis [55, 56]. Smoking appears to protect from developing pouchitis [57]. Data regarding other predictive factors are more controversial and include previous course of extensive colonic disease, backwash ileitis and serum perinuclear antineutrophil cytoplasmic antibody (pANCA) staining pattern [58]. The true incidence of pouchitis in patients operated for UC is difficult to determine as it depends on diagnostic criteria used to define the syndrome, accuracy and intensity of evaluation as well as length and method of follow-up. Reported incidence varies between 5% and 59% [59–61]. Diagnosis should be based on clinical, endoscopic and histologic criteria [62]. To address this issue, a pouchitis disease activity index (PDAI) was developed taking into account clinical symptoms, endoscopic findings and histological changes, with pouchitis defined as a score greater than or equal to 7 points [63]. The use of clinical symptoms alone leads to overdiagnosis of pouchitis and unnecessary antibiotic use [62]. Pouchitis may appear late in the postoperative course, and its incidence increases with increased length of follow-up [64].

Clinically, patients present with a marked increase of stool frequency, usually watery but occasionally bloody, urgency and incontinence. Abdominal pain and pelvic discomfort, fever, fatigue, anorexia and malaise are often present. Pouchitis is a heterogeneous disease and can be classified depending on the activity (remission, mild to moderate or severe) and pattern (acute, acute relapsing and chronic persistent). It is usually well controlled with medical therapy and a variety of agents have been used. For the majority of patients, 10–14 days of antibiotic treatment will rapidly control symptoms [65]. Metronidazole is probably the most commonly used first-line agent and has been shown to be effective for active chronic pouchitis in a meta-analysis [66]. However, long-term use of metronidazole may be hazardous and cause peripheral neuropathy. Ciprofloxacin has been widely used as an alternative or in combination with metronidazole [67].

Relapse is common. About 60% of patients who experience one episode of acute pouchitis will develop recurrent attacks [68]. In patients with chronic pouchitis who respond to antibiotic treatment and are in remission, the use of probiotics seems to be effective in the prevention of further episodes. Gionchetti et al. [69] in a double blind, placebo-controlled trial found that oral administration of a mixture of probiotic bacterial strains (VSL3) was effective in secondary prevention of pouchitis. In total, about 4.5–21.5% of UC patients develop chronic pouchitis, which is defined as symptoms that persistent for more than 3 months or chronic antibiotic treatment [59, 70]. Chronic pouchitis may eventually lead to persistent use of anti-inflammatory agents, corticosteroids or immunosuppressive therapy [71]. A recent study found that patients who had suffered from chronic pouchitis had poorer functional results and general health perception when compared with patients with no or acute pouchitis [72]. About 1% of the patients develop chronic persistent pouchitis refractory to any medical treatment. In these patients, pouch excision is thus the only alternative since no other surgical approach has proved to alleviate symptoms and prevent recurrent pouchitis [60].

In our group of patients, the cumulative risk of developing at least one episode of pouchitis (that is, PDAI $\geqslant$7) was 50%. Of the patients who developed pouchitis, 28% had a single acute episode that responded to antibiotics, 45% had recurrent acute attacks and 27% had chronic pouchitis that required long-term maintenance antibiotic therapy. Patients with pouchitis were followed for a statistically significantly longer period of time compared with patients without pouchitis. This finding supports the observation that the incidence of pouchitis tends to increase with time. Thus, we recommend that patients be followed up on a regular basis after the operation.

Cuffitis

A stapled ileoanal anastomosis without mucosectomy is done routinely at the level of the anorectal junction; hence, a 1- to 2-cm strip of rectal columnar cuff is retained. Some degree of persistent inflammation of the rectal cuff is common. This may be severe enough to cause local symptoms of bleeding, burning and urgency in up to 15% of patients [73]. There may be disordered evacuation with frequency. Diagnosis, as with pouchitis, is based on clinical symptoms, endoscopy and histology taken from the rectal-cuff mucosa. In some patients, cuffitis coexists with pouchitis. Treatment consists of topical corticosteroids or 5-aminosalicylate. A few patients may need further systemic treatment or a salvage surgery [74]. In our group of patients, three (3%) were diagnosed with cuffitis. All were treated with corticosteroids or 5-aminosalicylate enemas with good response; no one needed a salvage operation.

Irritable Pouch Syndrome (IPS)

IPS is a functional disorder diagnosed in symptomatic patients who suffer mainly from increased bowel frequency, urgency and abdominal pain without endoscopic or histologic evidence of rectal cuff or pouch inflammation [75]. Clinical features overlap with those of pouchitis and resemble those of irritable bowel syndrome. The aetiology is unclear, and is probably multifactorial in nature. Brain–gut factors may play a role in the pathophysiology of IPS. It is currently a diagnosis of exclusion. A recent study by Shen et al. [76] reported that patients with IPS have significantly poorer quality-of-life scores than patients with normal pouches. Treatment is empiric and symptom oriented. Some authors had reported that dietary modifications, antidiarrhoeal medications (e.g. loperamide) or tricyclic antidepressants might be effective in treating these patients [75]. In our series, the incidence of IPS where patients had symptoms but pouch endoscopy and biopsies did not demonstrate a significant pathology (thus PDAI was <7) was 5.1%.

Small-Bowel Obstruction

Small-bowel obstruction is a common complication after major abdominal surgery. After IPAA, it may occur before ileostomy closure; however, it is more common after closure. The cumulative probability of developing small-bowel obstruction increases with longer duration of follow-up. The risk varies between 14% and 27% at 5 years after ileostomy closure whereas at 10 years, it increases to 31% [77]. While most patients may be treated conservatively, up to 17% of patients after IPAA require laparotomy with adhesiolysis or small-bowel resection due to this complication [78].

Nonsurgical Complications of IPAA

In contrast to IPAA complications that may result in pouch dysfunction or small-bowel obstruction, there are various complications that usually do not end in pouch dysfunction or excision. However, they may produce various signs and symptoms that interfere with the patients' health and quality of life and may require investigation, follow-up and treatment by both surgeon and gastroenterologist. Some of these conditions are related to the defunctionalised stage, i.e. the ileostomy, which are not discussed herein. Amongst the complications that may occur in the long-term follow-up of these patients, some merit specific attention.

Vitamin Deficiency

Patients after IPAA may develop vitamin B12 deficiency that often requires the exogenous addition of this vitamin; the mechanism is unknown [79]. A possible explanation for this complication is change in bacterial flora in the neoterminal ileum and pouch.

Iron-Deficiency Anaemia

Chronic pouchitis was reported as a risk factor for the development of iron-deficiency anaemia [79, 80]. Iron deficiency occurred in 10.4% of patients after IPAA. Massive, overt bleeding is a rare complication of patients after IPAA. Iron-deficiency anaemia was found in 22% of our patients. They were treated with oral or intravenous iron supplements. There was no correlation between pouch inflammation and iron-deficiency anemia. In the follow up of pouch patients, including those with a good pouch function, we recommend on periodic laboratory evaluation that should include a complete blood count, electrolytes and renal function tests, liver function tests and vitamin B12 and folic acid determinations.

New Onset or Persistent Extraintestinal Manifestations (EIM)

Cutaneous, peripheral articular, ocular, haematologic and vascular EIM are linked to exacerbation of UC, so by excision of the entire diseased colorectal mucosa, EIM amelioration is anticipated. Nevertheless, these manifestations may persist or be aggravated in some patients whereas others may even develop EIM for the first time after surgery, with or without pouchitis [81–83]. It was shown that 31% of colitic patients post-IPAA had joint symptoms. In two thirds, joint involvement was polyarticular and the symptoms were intermittent. Forty percent reported that their symptoms interfered with daily life. No relationship was found between pouchitis and the presence of joint symptoms [81]. Goudet et al. [82] assessed the clinical evolution of pre-IPAA EIM after surgery in a retrospective study. As expected, ocular manifestations and PSC were unaffected. Arthralgia, erythema nodosum and thromboembolic events benefited the most from IPAA and tended to improve or disappear.

Dysplasia

Dysplasia in the ileoanal pouch or the rectal cuff is a very rare complication after IPAA [84, 85]. Reported potential risk factors are cancer or dysplasia in the colectomy specimen, chronic pouchitis, and the time after IPAA [86]. The risk of developing dysplasia or cancer after IPAA had promoted us to perform annual surveillance by pouch endoscopy with random mucosal sampling from the pouch and the rectal cuff. Of note, in our pouch clinic, out of 105 patients screened of which 17% had diagnosed dysplasia or cancer in the colectomy specimen, none had cancer or dysplasia in the pouch or rectal cuff after a mean follow-up of 57 months (range 1–258) post IPAA.

Perspective

IBD patients after IPAA may well present with both medical and surgical complications. A comprehensive pouch clinic is a novel approach in their management. It seems to be more efficient and beneficial to patients as well as provide an ideal milieu for surgical and gastroenterological teamwork. We believe that it should be applied to all major centres treating pouch patients.

References

1. Wexner SD, Wong WD, Rothenberger DA et al (1990) The ileoanal reservoir. Am J Surg 159:178–183
2. Melville DM, Ritchie JK, Nicholls RJ et al (1994) Surgery for ulcerative colitis in the era of the pouch: the St Mark's Hospital experience. Gut 35:1076–1080
3. Kelly KA (1992) Anal sphincter-saving operations for chronic ulcerative colitis. Am J Surg 163:5–11
4. Dozois RR, Goldberg SM, Rothenberger DA et al (1986) Restorative proctocolectomy with ileal reservoir. Int J Colorectal Dis 1:2–19
5. Williams NS (1989) Restorative proctocolectomy is the first choice elective surgical treatment for ulcerative colitis. Br J Surg 76:1109–1110
6. Jowett SL, Seal CJ, Barton JR et al (2001) The short inflammatory bowel disease questionnaire is reliable and responsive to clinically important change in ulcerative colitis. Am J Gastroenterol 96:2921–2928
7. Blumberg D, Beck DE (2002) Surgery for ulcerative colitis. Gastroenterol Clin North Am 31:219–235
8. Bernklev T, Jahnsen J, Lygren I et al (2005) Health-related quality of life in patients with inflammatory bowel disease measured with the short form-36: psychometric assessments and a comparison with general population norms. Inflamm Bowel Dis 11:909–918
9. Sako M, Kimura H, Arai K et al (2006) Restorative proctocolectomy for pediatric patients with ulcerative colitis. Surg Today 36:162–165
10. Marion JF, Present DH (2004) Indications for surgery in inflammatory bowel disease from the gastroenterologist's point of view. In: Sartor RB, Sandborn WJ (eds) Kirsner's inflammatory bowel diseases, 6th edn. W.B. Saunders, Philadelphia, pp 585–596
11. Robertson DJ, Grimm IS (2001) Inflammatory bowel disease in the elderly. Gastroenterol Clin North Am 300:409–425
12. Sands BE (2000) Therapy of inflammatory bowel disease. Gastroenterelogy 118:568–562
13. Hanauer SB, Dossopoulos T (2001) Evolving treatment strategies for inflammatory bowel disease. Ann Rev Med 52:299–318
14. Sher ME, Weiss EG, Nogueras JJ et al (1996) Morbidity of medical therapy for ulcerative colitis: what are we really saving? Int J Colorectal Dis 11:287–293
15. Nielsen OH, Vainer B, Rask-Madsen J (2001) The treatment of inflammatory bowel disease with 6-mercaptopurine or azathioprine. Aliment Pharmacol Therapeut 15:1699–1708
16. Fraser AG, Orchard TR, Jewell DP (2002) The efficacy of azathioprine for the treatment of inflammatory bowel disease: a 30 year review. Gut 50:485–489
17. Present DH, Meltzer SJ, Krumholtz MP et al (1989) 6-Mercaptopurine in the management of inflammatory bowel disease: short and long term toxicity. Ann Intern 3:641–649
18. Hawthorne AB, Logan RF, Hawkey CJ et al (1992) Randomised controlled trial of azathioprine withdrawal in ulcerative colitis. BMJ 305:20–22
19. Ekbom A, Helmick C, Zack M et al (1990) Ulcerative colitis and colorectal cancer. N Eng J Med 323:1228–1233
20. Bernstein CN, Blanchard JF, Kliewer E et al (2001) Cancer risk in patients with inflammatory bowel disease: a population-based study. Cancer 91:854–862
21. Langholz E, Munkholm P, Davidsen M, et al (1992) Colorectal cancer risk and mortality in patients with ulcerative colitis. Gastroenterology 103:1444–1451
22. Lashner BA (1992) Recommendations for colorectal cancer screening in ulcerative colitis: a review of research from a single university-based surveillance program. Am J Gastroenterol 87:168–175
23. Eaden JA, Abrams KR, Mayberry JF (2001) The risk of colorectal cancer in ulcerative colitis: a meta-analysis. Gut 48:526–535
24. Eaden JA, Mayberry JF (2000) Colorectal cancer complicating ulcerative colitis: a review. Am J Gastroenterol 95:2710–2719
25. Askling J, Dickman PW, Karlen P et al (2001) Family history as a risk factor for colorectal cancer in inflammatory bowel disease. Gastroenterology 120:1356–1362
26. Nuako KW, Ahlquist DA, Mahoney DW et al (1998) Familial predisposition for colorectal cancer in chronic ulcerative colitis: a case-control study. Gastroenterology 115:1079–1083
27. Kornfeld D, Ekbom A, Ihre T (1997) Is there an excess risk for colorectal cancer in patients with ulcerative colitis and concomitant primary sclerosing cholangitis? A population based study. Gut 41:522–525
28. Bernstein CN, Shanahan F, Weinstein WM (1994) Are we telling patients the truth about surveillance colonoscopy in ulcerative colitis? Lancet 343:71–74
29. Blackstone MO, Riddell RH, Rogers BH et al (1981) Dysplasia-associated lesion or mass (DALM) detected

by colonoscopy in long-standing ulcerative colitis: an indication for colectomy. Gastroenterology 80:366–374
30. Ullman T, Croog V, Harpaz N et al (2003) Progression of flat low-grade dysplasia to advanced neoplasia in patients with ulcerative colitis. Gastroenterology 125:1311–1319
31. Rozen P, Baratz M, Fefer F et al (1995) Low incidence of significant dysplasia in a successful endoscopic surveillance program of patients with ulcerative colitis. Gastroenterology 108:1361–1370
32. Remzi FH, Preen M (2003) Rectal cancer and ulcerative colitis: does it change the therapeutic approach? Colorectal Dis 5:483–485
33. Michelassi F, Lee J, Rubin M et al (2003) Long-term functional results after ileal pouch anal restorative proctocolectomy for ulcerative colitis: a prospective observational study. Ann Surg 238:433–441
34. Wheeler JM, Banerjee A, Ahuja N et al (2005) Long-term function after restorative proctocolectomy. Dis Colon Rectum 48:946–951
35. Muir AJ, Edwards LJ, Sanders LL et al (2001) A prospective evaluation of health-related quality of life after ileal pouch anal anastomosis for ulcerative colitis. Am J Gastroenterol 96:1480–1485
36. Fazio VW, O'Riordain MG, Lavery IC et al (1999) Long-term functional outcome and quality of life after stapled restorative proctocolectomy. Ann Surg 230:575–584
37. Knupper N, Straub E, Terpe HJ et al (2005) Adenocarcinoma of the ileoanal pouch for ulcerative colitis – a complication of severe chronic atrophic pouchitis? Int J Colorectal Dis 20:1–5
38. Abdelrazeq AS, Lund JN, Leveson SH (2005) Implications of pouchitis on the functional results following stapled restorative proctocolectomy. Dis Colon Rectum 48:1700–1707
39. Tulchinsky H, Hawley PR, Nicholls J (2003) Long-term failure after restorative proctocolectomy for ulcerative colitis. Ann Surg 238:229–234
40. Dayton MT, Larsen KP (1997) Outcome of pouch-related complications after ileal pouch-anal anastomosis. Am J Surg 174:728–731
41. Heuschen UA, Hinz U, Allemeyer EH et al (2002) Risk factors for ileoanal J pouch-related septic complications in ulcerative colitis and familial adenomatous polyposis. Ann Surg 235:207–216
42. Fazio VW, Ziv Y, Church JM et al (1995) Ileal pouch-anal anastomoses complications and function in 1005 patients. Ann Surg 222:120–127
43. Gorfine SR, Fichera A, Harris MT et al (2003) Long-term results of salvage surgery for septic complications after restorative proctocolectomy: does fecal diversion improve outcome? Dis Colon Rectum 46:1339–1344
44. Paye F, Penna C, Chiche L et al (1996) Pouch-related fistula following restorative proctocolectomy. Br J Surg 83:1574–1577
45. Keighley MR, Grobler SP (1993) Fistula complicating restorative proctocolectomy. Br J Surg 80:1065–1067
46. Tekkis PP, Fazio VW, Remzi F et al (2005) Risk factors associated with ileal pouch-related fistula following restorative proctocolectomy. Br J Surg 92:1270–1276
47. Lolohea S, Lynch AC, Robertson GB et al (2005) Ileal pouch-anal anastomosis-vaginal fistula: a review. Dis Colon Rectum 48:1802–1810
48. Heriot AG, Tekkis PP, Smith JJ et al (2005) Management and outcome of pouch-vaginal fistulas following restorative proctocolectomy. Dis Colon Rectum 48:451–458
49. Shah NS, Remzi F, Massmann A et al (2003) Management and treatment outcome of pouch-vaginal fistulas following restorative proctocolectomy. Dis Colon Rectum 46:911–917
50. Johnson PM, O'Connor BI, Cohen Z et al (2005) Pouch-vaginal fistula after ileal pouch-anal anastomosis: treatment and outcomes. Dis Colon Rectum 48:1249–1253
51. Lewis WG, Kuzu A, Sagar PM et al (1994) Stricture at the pouch-anal anastomosis after restorative proctocolectomy. Dis Colon Rectum 37:120–125
52. Rossi HL, Brand MI, Saclarides TJ (2002) Anal complications after restorative proctocolectomy (J-pouch). Am Surg 68:628–630
53. Fazio VW, Tekkis PP, Remzi F et al (2003) Quantification of risk for pouch failure after ileal pouch anal anastomosis surgery. Ann Surg 238:605–614
54. Mahadevan U, Sandborn WJ (2003) Diagnosis and management of pouchitis. Gastroenterology 124:1636–1650
55. Penna C, Dozois R, Tremaine W et al (1996) Pouchitis after ileal pouch-anal anastomosis for ulcerative colitis occurs with increased frequency in patients with associated primary sclerosing cholangitis. Gut 38:234–239
56. Lohmuller JL, Pemberton JH, Dozois RR et al (1990) Pouchitis and extraintestinal manifestations of inflammatory bowel disease after ileal pouch-anal anastomosis. Ann Surg 211:622–627
57. Merrett MN, Mortensen N, Kettlewell M et al (1996) Smoking may prevent pouchitis in patients with restorative proctocolectomy for ulcerative colitis. Gut 38:362–364
58. Kuisma J, Jarvinen H, Kahri A et al (2004) Factors associated with disease activity of pouchitis after surgery for ulcerative colitis. Scand J Gastroenterol 39:544–548
59. Stahlberg D, Gullberg K, Liljeqvist L et al (1996) Pouchitis following pelvic pouch operation for ulcerative colitis. Incidence, cumulative risk, and risk factors. Dis Colon Rectum 39:1012–1018
60. Stocchi L, Pemberton JH (2001) Pouch and pouchitis. Gastroenterol Clin North Am 30:223–241
61. Meagher AP, Farouk R, Dozois RR et al (1998) J ileal pouch-anal anastomosis for chronic ulcerative colitis: complications and long-term outcome in 1310 patients. Br J Surg 85:800–803
62. Shen B, Achkar JP, Lashner BA et al (2001) Endoscopic and histologic evaluation together with symptom assessment are required to diagnose pouchitis. Gastroenterology 121:261–267
63. Sandborn WJ, Tremaine WJ, Batts KP et al (1994) Pouchitis after ileal pouch-anal anastomosis: a Pouchitis Disease Activity Index. Mayo Clin Proc 69:409–415
64. Cheifetz A, Itzkowitz S (2004) The diagnosis and treatment of pouchitis in inflammatory bowel disease. J Clin Gastroenterol 38:S44–S50
65. Sandborn WJ (2005) pouchitis and functional com-

plications of the pelvic pouch. In Fazio VW, Church JM, Delaney CP (eds) Current therapy in colon and rectal surgery, 2nd edn. Elsevier Mosby, Philadelphia, pp 229–232

66. Sandborn WJ, McLeod R, Jewell DP (1999) Medical therapy for induction and maintenance of remission in pouchitis: a systemic review. Inflamm Bowel Dis 5:33–39
67. Shen B, Achkar JP, Lashner BA et al (2001) A randomized clinical trial of ciprofloxacin and metronidazole to treat acute pouchitis. Inflamm Bowel Dis 7:301–305
68. Mahadevan U, Sandborn WJ (2003) Diagnosis and management of pouchitis. Gastroenterology 124:1636–1650
69. Gionchetti P, Rizzello F, Venturi A et al (2000) Oral bacteriotherapy as maintenance treatment in patients with chronic pouchitis: a double-blind placebo-controlled trial. Gastroenterology 119:305–309
70. Heuschen UA, Autschbach F, Allemeyer EH et al (2001) Long-term follow-up after ileoanal pouch procedure: algorithm for diagnosis, classification, and management of pouchitis. Dis Colon Rectum 44:487–499
71. Sandborn WJ, Pardi DS (2004) Clinical management of pouchitis. Gastroenterology 127:1809–1814
72. Abdelrazeq AS, Lund JN, Leveson SH (2005) Implications of pouchitis on the functional results following stapled restorative proctocolectomy. Dis Colon Rectum 48:1700–1707
73. Lavery IC, Sirimarco MT, Ziv Y et al (1995) Anal canal inflammation after ileal pouch-anal anastomosis. The need for treatment. Dis Colon Rectum 38:803–806
74. Tulchinsky H, McCourtney JS, Rao KV et al (2001) Salvage abdominal surgery in patients with a retained rectal stump after restorative proctocolectomy and stapled anastomosis. Br J Surg 88:1602–1606
75. Shen B, Achkar JP, Lashner BA et al (2002) Irritable pouch syndrome: a new category of diagnosis for symptomatic patients with ileal pouch-anal anastomosis. Am J Gastroenterol 97:972–977
76. Shen B, Fazio VW, Remzi FH et al (2005) Clinical approach to diseases of ileal pouch-anal anastomosis. Am J Gastroenterol 100:2796–2807
77. MacLean AR, Cohen Z, MacRae HM et al (2002) Risk of small bowel obstruction after the ileal pouch-anal anastomosis. Ann Surg 235:200–206
78. McMullen K, Hicks TC, Ray JE et al (1991) Complications associated with ileal pouch and anastomosis. World J Surg 15:763–767
79. M'koma AE (2006) Serum biochemical evaluation of patients with functional pouches ten to 20 years after restorative proctocolectomy. Int J Colorectal Dis 26:1–10
80. Tiainen J, Matikainen M (2000) Long-term clinical outcome and anemia after restorative proctocolectomy for ulcerative colitis. Scand J Gastroenterol 35:1170–1173
81. Thomas PD, Keat AC, Forbes A et al (1999) Extraintestinal manifestations of ulcerative colitis following restorative proctocolectomy. Eur J Gastroenterol Hepatol 11:1001–1005
82. Goudet P, Dozois RR, Kelly KA et al (2001) Characteristics and evolution of extraintestinal manifestations associated with ulcerative colitis after proctocolectomy. Dig Surg 18:51–55
83. Lohmuller JL, Pemberton JH, Dozois RR et al (1990) Pouchitis and extraintestinal manifestations of inflammatory bowel disease after ileal pouch-anal anastomosis. Ann Surg 211:622–627
84. Thompson-Fawcett MW, Marcus V, Redston M et al (2001) Risk of dysplasia in long-term ileal pouches and pouches with chronic pouchitis. Gastroenterology 121:275–281
85. Borjesson L, Willen R, Haboubi N et al (2004) The risk of dysplasia and cancer in the ileal pouch mucosa after restorative proctocolectomy for ulcerative proctocolitis is low: a long-term term follow-up study. Colorectal Dis 6:494–498
86. Veress B, Reinholt FP, Lindquist K et al (1995) Long-term histomorphological surveillance of the pelvic ileal pouch: dysplasia develops in a subgroup of patients. Gastroenterology 109:1090–1097

Management of Pouchitis

Paolo Gionchetti, Claudia Morselli, Fernando Rizzello, Rosy Tambasco, Gilberto Poggioli, Silvio Laureti, Federica Ugolini, Filippo Pierangeli, Massimo Campieri

Introduction

Total proctocolectomy with ileal pouch-anal anastomosis (IPAA) proposed for the first time by Parks in 1978 [1], represents nowadays the surgical treatment of choice for the management of patients with familial adenomatous polyposis (FAP) and ulcerative colitis (UC) [2, 3]. This procedure allows the removal of the whole diseased colorectal mucosal and has the great advantage of preserving the anal sphincter function. Most patients undergoing IPAA for severe colitis or for chronic continuous disease will achieve excellent functional results and physical well-being. In a prospective evaluation of health related quality of life (HRLQ) after IPAA, a significant improvement of HRQL has been shown, assessed with both generic and disease-specific measures, with many patients experiencing improvements as early as 1 month postoperatively [4]. However pouchitis, a non-specific (idiopathic) inflammation of the ileal reservoir, is the most common long-term complication after pouch surgery for UC [5].

Epidemiology, Risks Factors and Etiology

Frequency

The true incidence is still difficult to determine, depending on the diagnostic criteria used to define the syndrome, the accuracy of the evaluation and, particularly, on the duration of the follow-up. Reported incidence rates vary between 10 and 59%; most patients experience their first episode of acute pouchitis within 12 months after surgery, but some may suffer their first attack some years later [6]. Recently, Simchuk et al. performed a retrospective review of patients who underwent IPAA with a mean follow-up of 3 years: the incidence of pouchitis was 59%, but it increased with the duration of follow-up [7].

Risk Factors

The risk of developing pouchitis is much higher in patients with pre-operative extra-intestinal manifestations [8] and primary sclerosing cholangitis [9]. More controversial is the predictive role of anti-neutrophil cytoplasmic antibody with a perinuclear pattern (p-ANCA) [10-15] and of the pre-operative extent of UC [16-17]. Similarly to UC, smoking may be protective against the development of pouchitis (Table 1) [18]. The surgical technique (different type of reservoir) does not influence the frequency of pouchitis [19-20].

Etiology

The etiology is still unknown and is likely to be multifactorial; a variety of hypotheses have been suggested, including bacterial overgrowth due to faecal stasis, mucosal ischemia of the pouch, missed diagnosis of Crohn's disease, recurrence of UC and a novel form of IBD. Most likely pouchitis is the results of the interaction of a genetical and immunological susceptibility and an ileal mucosa that has adapted from its absorptive function to a new role of that of a reservoir with a colon-like morphology in response to faecal stasis [21].

Table 1. Pouchitis: predictive factors

Positive Association
Extra-intestinal manifestations
Primary sclerosing cholangitis
Antineutrophil cytoplasmic antibody with a perinuclear staining pattern (p-ANCA)
Extent of preoperative UC
Negative Association
Smoking

Diagnosis

The diagnosis of pouchitis should be based on clinical, endoscopic and histologic criteria; the key point is that endoscopic and histopathologic evaluation is required to make the diagnosis of pouchitis.

Clinical Diagnosis

The most frequent symptoms which characterise this syndrome include increased stool frequency and fluidity, rectal bleeding, abdominal cramping, urgency, malaise and tenesmus, and in most severe cases, incontinence and fever [21]. Patients with pouchitis may also have extra-intestinal manifestations such as arthritis, ankylosing spondylitis, pyoderma gangrenosum, erythema nodosum and uveitis [8]. These extra-intestinal manifestations may develop for the first time with pouchitis, but frequently patients have previously experienced these extra-intestinal manifestations before surgery.

Endoscopic Findings

A clinical diagnosis should be confirmed by endoscopy and histology. With endoscopy the mucosa of the neo-terminal ileum above the pouch should be normal. Inflammation of the pouch mucosa, with mucosal erythema, edema, friability, petechiae, granularity, loss of vascular pattern, mucosal haemorrhages, contact bleeding, mucus exudates, erosions and small superficial mucosal ulcerations can be present with varying degrees of severity [22-23]. Inflammation may be uniform or more severe to the distal part of the pouch.

Histologic Findings

Histologic examination shows acute inflammatory cell infiltrate with crypt abscesses and ulcerations on a background of chronic inflammatory changes with villous atrophy and crypt hyperplasia [24-25].

Disease Activity Score and Classification

Because of the great variability in the results of reports on the incidence of pouchitis and in the assessment of therapy due to the lack of standardised diagnostic criteria, Sandborn and colleagues developed a pouchitis disease activity index (PDAI). This 18-point index, calculated via three separate 6-point scales based on clinical symptoms, endoscopic appearance and histologic findings, represents an objective and reproducible scoring system for pouchitis [26]. Active pouchitis is defined by a total PDAI score ≥ 7 and remission is defined as a score <7. Once diagnosis is made, pouchitis can be further classified. The disease activity can be defined as remission, mild-moderate (increased stool frequency, urgency, infrequent incontinence) or severe (dehydration, frequent incontinence). Pouchitis can also be defined on the basis of the duration of disease: acute (≤ 4 weeks) or chronic (>4 weeks). Another way to classify this syndrome considers the following patterns: infrequent (a single or two acute episodes), relapsing (more than three acute episodes) in about two thirds of cases, continuous or chronic disease (a treatment responsive form requiring a maintenance therapy or a treatment-resistant form). About 15% of patients have a chronic disease and some of them require surgical excision or exclusion of the pouch because of impairment of reservoir function and poor quality of life.

The PDAI, nowadays, is the most frequently used scoring system in clinical studies to determine pouchitis disease activity. The validity of PDAI and the necessity of its application in epidemiological, pathophysiological or clinical studies, as well as in clinical practice in order to make a correct diagnosis of pouchitis, have been shown by Shen et al. [27] in a study evaluating the correlation between symptoms, endoscopy and histologic findings in patients with IPAA for UC. They found that symptoms alone do not reliably diagnose pouchitis, whereas an evaluation including symptoms, endoscopy and histology is the best way to make the diagnosis. In fact, 25% of patients with a high symptom score did not, in any of the cases, reach the PDAI diagnostic criteria and 36% of patients with minimal symptoms achieved a PDAI score $\geqslant 7$ because of significant endoscopic and histologic inflammation [27].

Differential Diagnosis

Before treatment is started, it is important to exclude other less frequent causes of pouch dysfunction or pouch inflammation, and this is particularly necessary in the case of a refractory patient. An anastomotic stricture, with consequent outlet obstruction and faecal stasis, is a common complication of IPAA; this increases stool frequency, makes the defecation painful with an incomplete evacuation predisposing to pouchitis. Diagnosis could be made by evacuation pouchography, while the stricture can usually be dilated with a finger or a rubber dilator.

Infectious etiology, caused by intestinal pathogens such as *Shigella, Escherichia coli, Salmonella, Clostridi-*

um difficile, should be ruled out by microbiology analysis and pouch biopsy. Multiple cases of cytomegalovirus infection have been reported showing the need for using monoclonal immunofluorescent staining for CMV for the examination of pouch biopsies when treatment with antibiotics has proven unsuccessful. In these patients the CMV infection must be excluded before starting immune modifier therapy [28-29].

Cuffitis is the inflammation of the retained rectal mucosa (columnar cuff) above the anal transitional zone (ATZ) after stapled anastomosis between the pouch and the top of the anal canal; this kind of inflammation, usually mild and not related to inflammation of the pouch, can cause anal discomfort, perianal irritation and pouch dysfunction. Clinically significant cuffitis should be defined using a triad of diagnostic criteria including clinical symptoms, endoscopic inflammation and acute histologic inflammation [30]. This syndrome rarely reaches dramatic proportions and clinical improvement can be obtained with topical corticosteroid, mesalazine suppositories and lidocaine gel applications. Scintigraphic pelvic pouch emptying scans can be used to evaluate patients who have inadequate pouch evacuation.

Fistulae and perianal abscesses should be suspected as being the expression of misdiagnosed Crohn's disease. Review of the proctocolectomy specimen and new biopsy samples are needed to make a correct diagnosis. If Crohn's disease is suspected, a small-bowel follow-through x-ray will rule out disease above the pouch. Approximately 5% of IPAA surgery is performed in patients whose primary diagnosis of UC is revised at some point after surgery to a definitive diagnosis of Crohn's disease. Other disorders that are able to mimic pouchitis symptoms are bile acid malabsorption, irritable pouch syndrome [31], and chronic pelvic sepsis.

Medical Treatment

Until now, few small placebo-controlled trials and small controlled comparisons of two active agents have been carried out and, as a consequence, the medical treatment of pouchitis is still widely empiric. The reason for this small amount of randomised double-blind controlled clinical trials may be found in the lack of a general agreement about the criteria for definition, diagnosis, classification and disease activity [32].

Antibiotics

The awareness of the crucial importance that faecal stasis and bacterial overgrowth may have in the pathogenesis of acute pouchitis has led clinicians to treat patients with antibiotics, which have become the mainstay of treatment, in absence of controlled trials. Usually metronidazole represents the most common first therapeutic approach, and most patients with acute pouchitis respond quickly to administration of 1–1.5 g/day [33-34]. A double-blind, randomised, placebo-controlled, crossover trial was carried out in 1993 by Madden et al. [22] to assess the efficacy of 400 mg three times a day of metronidazole *per os* in 13 patients (11 completed both arms of the study) with chronic, unremitting pouchitis, defined by the presence of recurrent or persistent symptoms with almost six bowel movements a day and typical endoscopic findings. Patients were treated for 2 weeks, with a 7-day wash-out period before the crossover to the second treatment. Metronidazole was significantly more effective than placebo in reducing the stool frequency (73 *vs.* 9%), even without improvement of endoscopic appearance and histologic grade of activity. Some patients (55%) experienced side effects from metronidazole including nausea, vomiting, abdominal discomfort, headache, skin rash and metallic taste [35]. Dysgeusia and peripheral neuropathy may limit long-term administration of metronidazole, while patients drinking alcohol may have a disulfiram-like reaction. Recently Shen and colleagues have compared the effectiveness and side effects of ciprofloxacin and metronidazole in a randomised clinical trial regarding the treatment of acute pouchitis. Seven patients received ciprofloxacin 1 g/day and nine patients metronidazole 20 mg/kg/day for a period of 2 weeks. The results of this study have shown that both ciprofloxacin and metronidazole are efficacious in the treatment of acute pouchitis; they reduced the total PDAI scores and led to a significant improvement of symptoms and endoscopic and histologic scores. However, ciprofloxacin led to a greater degree of reduction in the total PDAI score and to a greater improvement in symptoms and endoscopic scores; furthermore ciprofloxacin was better tolerated than metronidazole (33% of metronidazole-treated patients reported adverse effects; none were reported in the ciprofloxacin-treated group). The authors have suggested that ciprofloxacin should be considered the first-line therapy for acute pouchitis [36].

Other Agents

Anedoctal reports have suggested that oral or topical conventional corticosteroids may be of benefit to patients with pouchitis. Recently a double-blind, double-dummy, 6-week-controlled trial investigated the efficacy and tolerability of budesonide enema in the treatment of pouchitis compared with oral metronidazole. This study showed that budesonide enemas (2 mg/100 ml at bedtime) have a similar efficacy as oral metronidazole (0.5 g bid) in terms of disease activity, clinical and endoscopic findings (58 and 50% of patients, respectively, improved with a decrease in PDAI score ⩾3), but less side-effects (25 *vs.* 57%) and better tolerability, representing consequently a valid therapeutic alternative for active pouchitis [37].

While no data have been published on the efficacy of oral 5-ASA, uncontrolled studies have suggested the efficacy of topical 5-ASA either as suppositories or enemas in treatment of acute pouchitis [38]. As concerns immunosuppressive agents, cyclosporine enemas have been reported to be successful in chronic pouchitis in a pilot study [39] and other small studies have suggested that oral azathioprine may also be useful.

The observation reported in some studies [40], but not all [41], that the faecal concentration of SCFAs is lower in patients with pouchitis, led to the hypothesis that the topical administration of nutrients, such as SCFAs or butyrate or glutamine, may produce clinical benefit. Poor clinical results were obtained in uncontrolled trials using SCFAs enemas [42-43]. In a 3-week double-blind trial, glutamine and butyrate suppositories were compared in a group of 19 patients with chronic pouchitis with recurrent symptoms; the end-point was clinical remission. As the relapse rate was 40% for the glutamine group and 67% for the butyrate group and no placebo group was included, it was almost impossible to state if the two treatments were both ineffective and similarly effective [44]. In consideration of all these studies, nutritional therapy thus far should not be considered beneficial for pouchitis.

Bismuth, effective in UC and traveller's diarrhoea because of its anti-microbial and anti-diarrhoeal effects, was also investigated. One open-label long-term study evaluated the efficacy and safety of bismuth-citrate carbomer enemas in achieving and maintaining remission in a group of patients with chronic treatment-resistant pouchitis. After 45 days of nightly treatment, 83% of patients went into remission with a significant decrease of the mean total PDAI score from 12 to 6. Moreover, these patients entered a maintenance phase with enemas administered every third night for 12 months (60%) were able to maintain remission for 12 months [45]. On the other hand, a double-blind randomised trial in patients with active chronic pouchitis did not find a difference between bismuth enemas and placebo [46]. More recently, a 4-week treatment open trial showed patients benefited from bismuth subsalicylate tablets administered for chronic antibiotic-resistant pouchitis [47].

Allopurinol, a scavenger of oxygen-derived free radicals through inhibition of xanthine oxidase, was evaluated as post-operative prophylactic treatment (100 mg twice daily) against pouchitis in a randomised placebo-controlled double-blind study conducted at 12 centres in Sweden; however, it was not proven to be able to reduce the risk of a first attack of pouchitis [48].

Treatment of Chronic Pouchitis

Medical treatment of patients with chronic refractory pouchitis is particularly difficult and disappointing. The usual therapeutic strategy for these patients, who fail to respond to antibiotics or relapse once antibiotic therapy is stopped, includes: (1) a prolonged course of an antimicrobial agent, (2) a maintenance therapy with the most effective antibiotic at the lowest clinically effective dose, (3) cycles of multiple antibiotics at 1-week intervals. A possible therapeutic alternative for chronic refractory pouchitis is the use of a combined antibiotic treatment. We carried out a pilot trial to evaluate the efficacy of the association of two antibiotics in chronic active treatment-resistant pouchitis. Eighteen patients who were not responders to the standard therapy (metronidazole or ciprofloxacin or amoxycillin/clavulanic acid) for 4 weeks, were treated orally with rifaximin 2 g/day (non-absorbable, wide spectrum antibiotic) plus ciprofloxacin 1 g/day for 15 days; symptoms assessment, endoscopic and histologic evaluations were performed at screening and after 15 days using the PDAI. Sixteen out of 18 patients (88.8%) either improved (n=10) or went into remission (n=6); the median PDAI scores before and after therapy were 11 and 4 respectively (p<0.002) [49]. Unfortunately all patients relapsed within 2 months.

More recently, 44 patients with refractory pouchitis received metronidazole 800 mg – 1 g/day and ciprofloxacin 1 g/day for 28 days. Symptomatic, endoscopic and histological evaluations were undertaken before and after the antibiotic therapy, according to the PDAI score, and the related quality of life was assessed with the inflammatory bowel disease questionnaire (IBDQ). Thirty-six patients (82%) went into remission; the median PDAI scores before and after therapy were 12 and 3 respectively (p<0.0001). Patients' quality of life significantly improved with the treatment and median IBDQ strongly correlated with the disease activity and general satisfaction (from 96.5 to 175). Even in the eight patients who did not go into remission, the median PDAI score significantly improved from 14.5 to 9.5 as well as the median IBDQ score from 96 to 127 [50].

Oral-controlled release budesonide can be useful

for certain patients. In a small open trial, 16 patients with chronic pouchitis refractory to a 1-month antibiotic therapy (ciprofloxacin 1 g/day and metronidazole 1 g/day) were treated with budesonide CIR 9 mg/day for 8 weeks; the dose was gradually tapered (3 mg every month) and remission was defined as a clinical PDAI score ≤2 and an endoscopic PDAI ≤1. Twelve patients (72%) went into remission and the total PDAI score significantly decreased from 13 (range 8–16) to 3 (range 2-9) ($p<0.001$). Budesonide treatment increased the IBDQ score from 102 (range 77–176) to 182 (range 84–225) ($p<0.001$) [51].

In a subsequent study, 12 patients with active pouchitis refractory to ciprofloxacin and metronidazole for 1 month and oral budesonide for 8 weeks, were treated with three infusions of infliximab at a dosage of 5 mg/kg at week 0, 2 and 6. Ten patients (83.3%) achieved remission; the total PDAI score decreased from 13 (range 8–18) to 2 (range 0–9) ($p<0.001$). The IBDQ score strongly increased from 96 (range 74–184) to 196 (range 92–230; $p<0.001$) [52].

Probiotics

The term "probiotic" refers to "living organisms, which upon ingestion in certain numbers, exert health benefits beyond inherent basic nutrition" [53]. Recent observations have suggested a potential therapeutic role for probiotics in inflammatory bowel diseases (IBD), based on convincing evidence implicating intestinal bacteria in their pathogenesis [54].

On the basis of this information, we carried out a double-blind study comparing the efficacy of a highly concentrated probiotic preparation, VSL#3 (450 billion bacteria of eight different strains; VHS Pharma, USA) *vs.* placebo in maintenance treatment of chronic relapsing pouchitis. In our study, 40 patients who obtained clinical and endoscopic remission after one month of combined antibiotic treatment (rifaximin 2 g/day plus ciprofloxacin 1 g/day), were randomised to receive either VSL#3, 6 g/day (1 800 billion bacteria per day), or an identical-appearing placebo for 9 months. Relapse was defined as an increase of at least 2 points in the clinical portion of PDAI, which should be confirmed by endoscopy and histology. All the 20 patients who received the placebo relapsed; in contrast 17 of the 20 patients (85%) treated with VSL#3 were still in remission at the end of the study. All the 17 patients had a relapse within 4 months after suspension of the treatment. The results of this study suggested that oral administration of this highly concentrated probiotic preparation is effective in preventing relapse of chronic pouchitis, enhancing the concentration of protective bacteria and their metabolic activities in the ileal pouch [55].

These results have been recently confirmed by a study evaluating the efficacy of a single, daily dose of VSL#3 in maintaining antibiotic-induced remission (obtained after a 1 month treatment with metronidazole 800 mg/day plus ciprofloxacin 1 g/day) for 1 year in patients with refractory or recurrent pouchitis: 20 patients received VSL#3 at 1 800 billion bacteria once a day for 1 year and 16 patients received a placebo during the same period. Clinical, endoscopic and histological evaluations were made before 2 and 12 months after the randomisation. A parallel assessment of quality of life (QoL) was obtained with IBDQ. This study has substantially confirmed the observations made previously, with a maintenance remission rate of 85% at 1 year in the VSL#3 group and 6% in the placebo group. A high rating in the QoL score was obtained by the group treated with VSL#3 [56].

The same probiotic preparation was also more recently shown to be significantly superior to placebo in the prevention of pouchitis onset within the first year after surgery in a randomised double-blind placebo-controlled study. Forty consecutive patients who underwent IPAA for UC were randomised within a week after ileostomy closure, and received VSL#3 at a dosage of 3 g per day or an identical placebo for 12 months. They were assessed clinically, endoscopically, histologically at 1, 3, 6, 9 and 12 months, according to PDAI; QoL was also assessed at baseline at the end of the study. Patients treated with VSL#3 had a significantly lower incidence of acute pouchitis (10%) compared with those treated with placebo (40%) ($p<0.05$), and they experienced a significant improvement in quality of life, whereas this did not happen in the placebo group, indicating the effectiveness of a highly concentrated probiotic preparation in preventing pouchitis onset during the first year after surgery [57].

Preliminary data of a pilot study to evaluate the efficacy of high dosage of VSL#3 (6 g b.i.d. equivalent to 3 600 billion bacteria per day) administered for 1 month as treatment for mildly active pouchitis (PDAI score 7–12), have shown its potential usefulness in improving active pouch inflammation and health related quality of life [58].

Management

In a proposed algorithm for treatment of pouchitis, once diagnosis is confirmed by endoscopy and histology, and other causes of inflammation or pouch dysfunction have been excluded, the main treatment consists of metronidazole 250 mg three times/day or ciprofloxacin 500 mg b.i.d. for at least 2 weeks. In case of a subsequent prompt relapse, the patients can

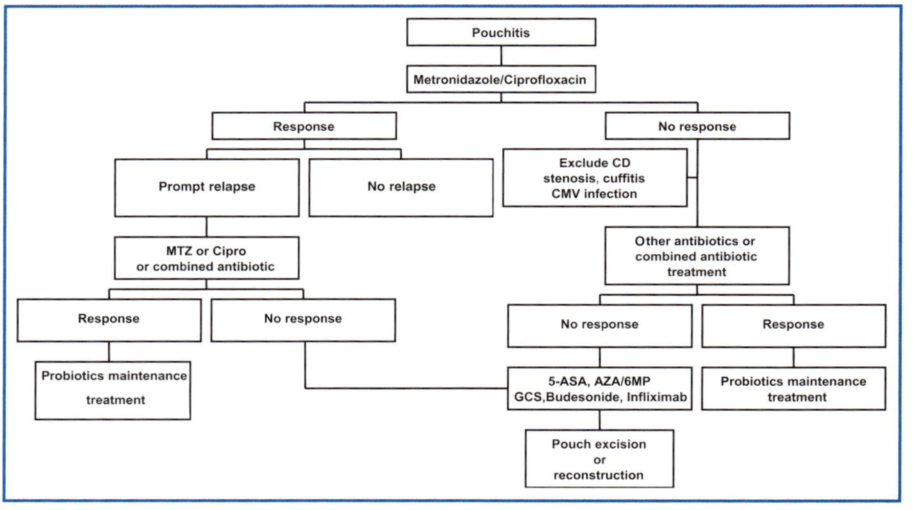

Fig. 1. Proposal for a treatment algorithm

be treated with a prolonged course of the same antibiotic or with a combined antibiotic treatment; in case of positive response we suggest starting maintenance treatment with highly concentrated probiotics. In refractory pouchitis, patients should be treated with other antibiotics or prolonged combined antibiotic treatment. Again, in case of response, maintenance probiotic treatment after the stopping of antimicrobial agents is suggested. When no positive response is obtained one should try other types of treatment such as topical corticosteroids, immunosuppressive agents, or topical bismuth. Patients who are refractory to all forms of medical treatment should be referred to a surgeon for a pouch reconstruction or pouch excision (Fig. 1).

References

1. Parks AG, Nicholls RJ (1978) Proctocolectomy without ileostomy for ulcerative colitis. BMJ 2:85–88
2. Pemberton JH, Kelly KA, Beart RW Jr et al (1987) Ileal pouch-anal anastomosis for chronic ulcerative colitis: long-term results. Ann Surg 206:504–513
3. Nicholls RJ, Moskowitz RL, Shepherd NA (1985) Restorative proctocolectomy with ileal reservoir. Br J Surg 72:S76–S79
4. Muir AJ, Edwards LJ, Sanders LL et al (2001) A prospective evaluation of health related quality of life after ileal pouch-anal anastomosis for ulcerative colitis. Am J Gastroenterol 96:1480–1485
5. Shepherd NA, Hulten L, Tytgat GNJ et al (1989) Workshop: pouchitis. Int J Colorectal Dis 4:205–229
6. Stahlberg D, Gullberg K, Liljeqvist L et al (1996) Pouchitis following pelvic pouch operation for ulcerative colitis: incidence, cumulative risk and risk factors. Dis Colon Rectum 39:1012–1018
7. Simchuk EJ, Thirlby RC (2000) Risk factors and true incidence of pouchitis in patients after ileal pouch-anal anastomosis. World J Surg 24:851–856
8. Lohmuller JL, Pemberton JH, Dozois RR et al (1990) Pouchitis and extraintestinal manifestations of inflammatory bowel disease after ileal pouch-anal anastomosis. Ann Surg 211:622
9. Zins BJ, Sandborn WJ, Penna CR et al (1995) Pouchitis disease course after orthotopic liver transplantation in patients with primary sclerosing cholangitis and an ileal pouch-anal anastomosis. Am J Gastroenterol 90:2177
10. Duerr RH, Targan SR, Landers CJ et al (1991) Antineutrophil cytoplasmic antibodies in ulcerative colitis: comparison with other colitides/diarrhea illness. Gastroenterology 110:1590
11. Reumaux D, Colombel JF, Duclos B et al (1993) Anti-neutrophil cytoplasmic auto-antibodies in sera from patients with ulcerative colitis after proctocolectomy with ileo-anal anastomosis. Adv Exp Med Biol 336:523
12. Vecchi M, Gionchetti P, Bianchi MB et al (1994) P-ANCA and development of pouchitis in ulcerative colitis patients after proctocolectomy and ileal pouch-anal anastomosis. Lancet 344:886
13. Sandborn WJ, Landers CJ, Tremaine WJ et al (1995) Antineutrophil cytoplasmic antibody correlates with chronic pouchitis after ileal pouch-anal anastomosis. Am J Gastroenterol 90:740
14. Patel RT, Stokes R, Birch D et al (1996) Influence of total colectomy on serum antineutrphil cytoplasmic antibody in pouchitis after proctocolectomy with ileal pouch -anal anastomosis for ulcerative colitis. Scand J Gastroenterol 31:594
15. Yang P, Oresland T, Jarnerot G et al (1996) Perinuclear antineutrophil cytoplasmic antibody in pouchitis after proctocolectomy with ileal pouch-anal anastomosis for ulcerative colitis. Scand J Gastroenterol 31:594
16. Samarasekera DN, Stebbing JF, Kettlewell MG et al (1996) Outcome of restorative proctocolectomy with ileal reservoir for ulcerative colitis: comparison of distal colitis with more proximal disease. Gut 38:574–577
17. Schmidt CM, Lazenby AJ, Hendrickson RJ et al (1998)

Pre-operatve terminal, ileal and colonic resection histopathology predicts risk of pouchitis in patients after ileo anal pull-through procedure. Ann Surg 227:654–662; Discussion 663–665
18. Merrett MN, Mortensen N, Kettlewell M et al (1996) Smoking may prevent pouchitis in patients with restorative proctocolectomy for ulcerative colitis. Gut 38:362
19. Oresland T, Fasth S, Nordgren S et al (1992) A prospective randomised comparison of two different pelvic pouch design. Scand J Gastroenterol 25:986–996
20. Sagar PM, Holdsworth PJ, Godwin PJ et al (1992) Comparison of triplicated (S) and quadruplicated (W) pelvic ileal reservoirs: studies on manovolumetry, fecal bacteriology, fecal volatile fatty acids, mucosal morphology, and functional results. Gastroenterology 102:520–528
21. Sandborn WJ (1994) Pouchitis following ileal pouch-anal anastomosis: definition, pathogenesis and treatment. Gastroenterology 107:1856–1860
22. Madden MV, Farthing MJ, Nicholls RJ (1990) Inflammation in the ileal reservoir: pouchitis. Gut 31:247–249
23. Di Febo G, Miglioli M, Lauri A et al (1990) Endoscopic assessment of acute inflammation of the reservoir after restorative proctocolectomy with ileoanal reservoir. Gastrointest Endosc 36:6–9
24. Moskowitz RL, Shepherd NA, Nicholls RJ (1986) An assessment of inflammation in the reservoir after restorative proctocolectomy with ileoanal ileal reservoir. Int J Colorectal Dis 1:167–174
25. Shepherd NA, Jass JR, Duval I et al (1987) Restorative proctoclolectomy with ileal reservoir: pathological and histochemical study of mucosal biopsy. J Clin Pathol 40:601–607
26. Sandborn WJ, Tremaine WJ, Batts KP et al (1994) Pouchitis after ileal pouch-anal anastomosis: a pouchitis disease activity index. Mayo Clinic Proc 69:409–415
27. *Shen B, Achkar JP, Lashner BA et al (2001) Edoscopic and histologic evaluation together with symptoms assessment are required to diagnose pouchitis. Gastroenterology 121:261–267
28. Moonka D, Furth EE, MacDermott RP, Lichtentein GR (1998) Pouchitis associated with primary cytomegalovirus infection. Am J Gastroenterol 93:264–266
29. Munoz-Juarez M, Pemberton JH, Sandborn WJ et al (1999) Misdiagnosis of specific cytomegalovirus infection of the ileoanal pouch as refractory idiopathic chronic pouchitis: report of two cases. Dis Colon Rectum 42:117–120
30. Thompson-Fawcett MW Mortensen NJ, Warren BF (1999) "Cuffitis" and inflammatory changes in the columnar cuff, anal transitional zone and ileal reservoir after stapled pouch-anal anastomosis. Dis Colon Rectum 42:348–355
31. Shen B, Achkar JP, Lashner BA et al (2002) Irritable pouch syndrome: a new category of diagnosis for symptomatic patients with ileal pouch-anal anastomosis. Am J Gastroenterol 97:972–977
32. Sandborn WJ, Mc Leod, Jewell DP (1999) Medical therapy for induction and maintenance of remission in pouchitis: a systematic review. Inflamm Bowel Dis 5:33–39
33. Hurst RD, Molinari M, Chung P et al (1996) Prospective study of the incidence, timing and treatment of pouchitis in 104 consecutive patients after restorative proctocolectomy. Arch Surg 131:497–502
34. Keighley MRB (1996) Review article: the management of pouchitis. Aliment Pharmacol Ther 10:449– 457
35. Madden M, McIntyre A, Nicholls RJ (1994) Double- blind cross-over trial of metronidazole versus placebo in chronic unremitting pouchitis. Dig Dis Sci 39:1193–1196
36. Shen B, Achkar JP, Lashner BA et al (2001) A randomized clinical trial of ciprofloxacin and metronidazole to treat acute pouchitis. Inflamm Bowel Dis 7:301–305
37. Sambuelli A, Boerr L, Negreira S et al (2002) Budesonide enema in pouchitis: a double-blind, double-dummy, controlled trial. Aliment Pharmacol Ther 16:27–34
38. Miglioli M, Barbara L, Di Febo G et al (1989) Topical administration of 5-aminosalicylic acid: a therapeutic proposal for the treatment of pouchitis. N Engl J Med 320:257
39. Winter TA, Dalton HR, Merrett MN et al (1993) Cyclosporine A retention enemas in refractory distal ulcerative colitis and pouchitis. Scand J Gastroenterol 28:701–704
40. Clausen MR, Tvede M, Mortensen PB (1992) Short chain fatty acids in pouch contents with and without pouchitis after ileal pouch-anal anastomosis. Gastroenterology 103:1144–1449
41. Sandborn WJ, Tremaine WJ, Batts KP et al (1995) Faecal bile acids, short-chain fatty acids and bacteria after ileal pouch-anal anastomosis do not differ in patients with pouchitis. Dig Dis Sci 40:1474–1483
42. De Silva HJ, Ireland A, Kettlewell M et al (1989) Short-chain fatty acids irrigation in severe pouchitis. N Engl J Med 321:416–417
43. Tremaine WJ, Sandborn WJ, Phillips SF et al (1999) Short-chain fatty acid (SCFA) enema therapy for treatment-resistant pouchitis following ileal pouch-anal anastomosis (IPAA) for ulcerative colitis. Gastroenterology 106:A784
44. Wischmeyer P, Pemberton JH, Phillips SF (1993) Chronic pouchitis after ileal pouch-anal anastomosis: responses to butyrate and glutamine suppositories in a pilot study. Mayo Clin Proc 68:978–981
45. Gionchetti P, Rizzello F, Venturi A et al (1997) Long-term efficacy of bismuth carbomer enemas in patients with treatment-resistant chronic pouchitis. Aliment Pharmacol Ther 11:673–678
46. Tremaine WJ, Sandborn WJ, Wolff BG et al (1997) Bismuth carbomer foam enemas for active chronic pouchitis: a randomised, double-blind, placebo-controlled trial. Aliment Pharmacol Ther 11:1041–1046
47. Tremaine WJ, Sandborn WJ, Kenan ML (1998) Bismuth subsalicylate tablets for chronic antibiotic-resistant pouchitis. Gastroenterology 114:A1101
48. Joelsson M, Andersson M, Bark T et al (2001) Allopurinol as prophylaxis against pouchitis following ileal pouch-anal anastomosis for ulcerative colitis: a randomised placebo-controlled double-blind study. Scand J Gastroenterol 36:1179–1184
49. Gionchetti P, Rizzello F, Venturi A et al (1999) Antibiotic combination therapy in patients with chronic, treatment-resistant pouchitis. Aliment Pharmacol Ther 13:713–718

50. Mimura T, Rizzello F, Helwig U et al (2002) Four week open-label trial of metronidazole and ciprofloxacin for the treatment of recurrent or refractory pouchitis. Aliment Pharmacol Ther 16:909–917
51. Gionchetti P, Rizzello F, Morselli C et al (2004) Eight-week open trial of oral budesonide for the treatment of refractory pouchitis. Gastroenterology 126:A123
52. Gionchetti P, Morselli C, Rizzello F et al (2005) Infliximab in the treatment of Refractory pouchitis. Gastroenterology 128:A578
53. Schaafsma G (1996) State of the art concerning probiotic strains in milk products. IDF Nutr Newsl 5:23–24
54. Campieri M, Gionchetti P (1999) Probiotics in inflammatory bowel disease:new insight to pathogenesis or a possible therapeutic alternative? Gastroenterology 116:1246–1249
55. Gionchetti P, Rizzello F, Venturi A et al (2000) Oral bacteriotherapy as maintenance treatment in patients with chronic pouchitis: a double-blind, placebo-controlled trial. Gastroenterology 119:305–309
56. Mimura T, Rizzello F, Schreiber S et al (2002) Once daily high dose probiotic therapy maintains remission and improves quality of life in patients with recurrent or refractory pouchitis: a randomised, placebo-controlled, double-blind trial. Gastroenterology 122:A81
57. Gionchetti P, Rizzello F, Helvig U et al (2003) Prophylaxis of pouchitis onset with probiotic therapy: a double-blind placebo controlled trial. Gastroenterology 124:1202–1209
58. Amadini C, Gionchetti P, Rizzello F et al (2002) High dose probiotics are effective in the treatment of mild pouchitis: a pilot study. Dig Liver Dis 34:A96

Bowel Transplantation for Inflammatory Bowel Disease

Raimund Margreiter

Introduction

Bowel transplantation has become a valuable option for patients with intestinal failure or short-bowel syndrome who do not tolerate total parenteral nutrition or have no vascular access for TPN. Up until March 31, 2005, a total of 1292 intestinal transplants (in altogether 1210 patients) have been reported to the international registry. Of these 1292 transplants, 570 of them were isolated small-bowel transplants, 490 combined small-bowel/liver transplants, and 232 were multivisceral transplants. Additionally, 772 transplants were performed in 721 pediatric recipients and 520 transplants in 489 adult patients [1].

It goes without saying that no bowel transplantation was done for inflammatory bowel diseases in the pediatric group, but 68 transplants were performed in adults for this indication. In total, we have experience with 16 isolated small-bowel transplants and ten multivisceral transplants, and four of the isolated intestinal transplants in three patients were performed for Crohn's disease.

Presently, appropriate indications, the timing of referral and the outcome of bowel transplantation are not well recognized among physicians caring for patients who may be candidates for this therapeutic option. Definitions of terms such as "intestinal failure" and "failure of parenteral nutrition" are not standardized and there is no accepted algorithm that integrates parenteral nutrition, intestinal rehabilitation and transplantation for patients with intestinal failure.

Herein, with special emphasis on inflammatory bowel diseases, we review the various aspects of bowel transplantation such as the indications for it, the current state of medical practice in intestinal transplantation, and its outcome.

History

Intestinal transplantation techniques were developed in animal models in 1959 and first attempted in humans in 1964 [2]. In those days, immunosuppression consisted of steroids and azathioprine after induction with an antilymphocyteglobulin. Under this type of rejection prophylaxis, altogether eight isolated intestinal transplants were performed. The first two transplants performed in Boston in 1964, however, have never been officially reported as files remain untraceable. The first well-documented case was reported from Minneapolis in 1967 [3]. Under unconventional immunosuppression, all but one graft failed within a few days. The last graft in this series was from a HLA identical sister and survived for 79 days. The recipient was able to be fed orally from day 23 until day 60 [4].

The first bowel transplant in the Cyclosporine era was performed in 1985 in Toronto [5]. Patient No. 8 in this series received 60 cm of jejunoileum from her sister in 1988 and became the first long-term survivor. It has to be said, however, that oral food intake was never sufficient and had to be supplemented by parenteral infusions. The patient experienced several episodes of rejection, developed end-stage renal disease and died a few years later [6].

On March 19, 1989, a 5-month old girl received 80 cm of jejunoileum from a neonate. This patient transplanted in Paris is still alive and well with a normally functioning graft [7]. Already in 1960, Starzl reported on a series of multivisceral transplants in dogs [8]. The same author performed the first human multivisceral transplant in 1983 in a 6-year-old girl in Pittsburgh. The girl, however, died only a few hours after surgery from exsanguination. The same happened to a 1-year-old male who underwent transplantation in 1986 in Chicago. In 1987, Starzl performed another transplantation in a 3.5-year-old girl and Williams in Chicago did the same in the following year in a 0.7-year-old neonate. Both children died 192 and 109 days, respectively, after transplantation from lymphoma. The type of IS consisted of OKT3 induction followed by cyclosporin and steroids. Both children were never discharged from the hospital [9, 10]. On December 26, 1989, a multivisceral transplant was carried out for the first time in an adult recipient

48 years of age in Innsbruck. This patient lived on oral food intake for 9 months when he died from tumor recurrence [11].

On November 13, 1988, Grant performed the first combined small-bowel/liver transplantation in London/Ontario in a 41-year-old woman with short-gut syndrome with a hypercoagulable state associated with low antithrombin III levels. The patient survived for several years [12].

Indications

It is now generally accepted that small-bowel transplantation is indicated in patients suffering from irreversible small-intestinal failure coexisting with failure of parenteral nutrition. The main causes of parenteral nutrition failure are recurrent line related sepsis, loss of venous access due to thrombosis and PN-related liver disease. Medicare and Medicaid Services in the US have established indications that include impending or overt liver failure due to TPN-induced liver injury, thrombosis of two or more central veins, the development of two or more episodes of systemic sepsis secondary to line infection per year that require hospitalization, a single episode of line-related fungemia, septic shock and/or acute respiratory distress, and frequent episodes of severe dehydration despite intravenous fluid supplementation in addition to TPN [13].

These criteria should help to avoid late referrals. A timely referral for pretransplant assessment is essential for allowing the optimization of physical and psychological factors and should be at a stage when the central venous access is adequate for surgery and management of postoperative complications which may include renal replacement therapy. Unfortunately, it is our experience, that most patients are not referred, but rather come on their own initiative.

Diseases Causing Intestinal Failure

Diseases leading to intestinal failure include loss of bowel length, loss of bowel function, or conventionally unresectable tumors involving the bowel or its feeding vessels. Short-bowel syndrome, the loss of intestinal length and absorptive surface areas due to surgical resection, are the most common cause of intestinal failure leading to bowel transplantation. The loss of mucosal absorptive surface area is associated with malabsorption and rapid transit through the jejunoileum leading to malnutrition, recurrent dehydration, and electrolyte abnormalities. Short-bowel syndrome can be caused by a variety of conditions and diseases in adults such as thrombosis or embolism to the superior mesenteric vessels, inflammatory bowel disease, volvulus, radiation enteritis, trauma or other causes of infarction.

In pediatric patients, most frequent causes of short-bowel syndrome are malrotation, volvulus, necrotizing enterocolitis, jejunoileal artresias, gastroschisis, and omphalocele among other congenital disorders. Transplant candidacy has to be considered in the context of alternatives to transplantation including the potential for rehabilitation or successful lifelong parenteral nutrition. In a large series, about 20% of adult patients with less than 100 cm of residual intestine could be weaned from TPN. In children, less than 30 cm of jejunoileum, lack of enterocolonic continuity, and lack of feeding tolerance early after birth correlate to failure of weaning from parenteral nutrition [14].

Functional Disorders

Functional disorders of the small bowel that may lead to intestinal failure include disorders of motility and disorders of enterocyte function. The most common motility disorders are chronic pseudo-obstruction, visceral myopathy, visceral neuropathy, total intestinal aganglionosis, and some forms of mitochondrial respiratory chain disorders that affect gastrointestinal motor function.

Epithelial disorders causing intractable secretory diarrhea or failure of absorption are more common in children and include microvillus inclusion disease, tufting enteropathy and autoimmune enteritis.

Tumors

Tumors involving the root of the mesentery are often benign but locally invasive and therefore lethal. The most common of these lesions are desmoid tumors in patients with familial adenomatous polyposis. Only complete resection of the tumor and sacrifice of the intestines can provide a cure. The most common of these lesions are desmoid tumors in patients with Gardeners' syndrome. This tumor often involves the mesenteric vessels and requires exenteration of the small bowel for complete resection. Since these tumors may involve other foregut organs such as the pancreas, stomach, duodenum or spleen, a multivisceral transplant is required in these patients. Patients with Gardeners' syndrome usually do not have intestinal failure and are therefore not dependent on parenteral nutrition prior to transplantation.

Types of Transplants

Intestinal transplantation may be performed as an isolated bowel transplant together with the liver as a combined small-bowel–intestinal transplant or as a multivisceral transplant procedure. The common element of these procedures is transplantation of the jejunoileum, with or without other organs. Soon after transplantation, most surgeons create an ileostomy to allow easy endoscopic surveillance of the graft for abnormalities. We prefer a technique where the distal end of the graft is brought out as a stoma wherever it is best situated; the ileum, however, is anastomosed with the remaining colon some 10–20 cm before its entrance into the abdominal wall. Gastrointestinal continuity is restored simply by stapling and transecting this chimney just distally to the anastomosis, which can then be used as a sentinel grafted tissue. We call this the "Innsbruck stoma."

Isolated Bowel Transplantation

Isolated intestinal transplantation may be performed with portal or systemic drainage. If the venous outflow is drained into the portal system via the superior mesenteric vein or directly into the portal vein, the transplant is called orthotopic. If, for technical reasons, portal drainage cannot be achieved, the superior mesenteric vein of the graft is anastomosed to the inferior vena cava; therefore, this type of transplant called heterotopic.

The graft artery is virtually in all cases anastomosed to the infrarenal aorta. In case of a segmental jejunoileum graft from a live donor, recipient iliac vessels are preferentially used for revascularization. The proximal end of the gut is attached to the first loop of native jejunum or to the third portion of duodenum. Isolated bowel transplant is carried out in patients with intestinal failure but no damage to the liver or other organs.

Combined Liver–Bowel Transplantation

Presently, most centers would transplant a liver and bowel that has an intact mesenteric–portal circulatory system en bloc. Therefore, the entire duodenum with a rim of pancreas is left with the graft. Because all the other upper abdominal organs such as the stomach, pancreas, spleen and duodenum are left in place, a portocaval shunt has to be created in order to provide venous drainage for these organs. This technique makes reconstruction of the biliary system unnecessary. Both grafts, however, can be transplanted simultaneously but not as a composite graft. Combined liver-intestinal transplantation is performed in patients with intestinal failure together with liver damage (considered irreversible), usually due to parenteral nutrition. Severe fibrosis on histology with bilirubin of more than 10 mg/dl may indicate a point of no recovery for liver function.

Multivisceral Transplantation

Multivisceral transplantation refers to en-bloc transplantation of the liver, stomach, pancreaticoduodenal complex as well as the small bowel, sometimes also including a kidney. Some authors, however, call it a multivisceral transplant if the stomach, pancreas and intestine are transplanted together without the liver. Exenteration of all native viscera which must precede the multivisceral transplants can be technically demanding in patients with portal hypertension due to diffuse splanchnic thrombosis or with severe adhesions after multiple laparotomies. Multivisceral transplantation is performed in patients with either diffuse thrombosis of all splanchnic veins usually associated with coagulation abnormalities, desmoid tumors involving the vascular supply of the liver, pancreas and intestines, or severe motility disorders.

Postoperative Management

Immunosuppression

The enormous amount of lymphatic tissue transplanted together with the bowel, be it in the form of mesenteric lymph nodes or mucosa-associated lymphatic tissue, is responsible for the heightened immunogenicity of an intestinal graft over other solid organs. This is the reason why recipients of a bowel transplant require more immunosuppression as compared to recipients of a kidney or heart transplant.

Following induction with lymphocyte depleting antibodies such as antithymocite globulin, Campath 1H (Genzyme, MA, USA), OKT3 (Ortho Biotech, NJ, USA) or with monoclonal anti-interleukin 2 (IL-2) receptor antibodies. Maintenance immunosuppression is usually based on the calcineurin inhibitor tacrolimus together with other anti-proliferative agents such as mycophenolate mofetil and steroids. There is a trend to minimize the use of the latter. The combination of tacrolimus and sirolimus seems not to have additional benefit over tacrolimus alone. Antibody preconditioning seems to allow less potent subsequent maintenance immunosuppression. Antibodies, however, are occasionally associated with severe adverse reactions caused by cytokine release [14, 15].

Infection Prophylaxis

Decontamination of bacterial and fungal organisms of the intestinal allograft is attempted before procurement by administering enteric antibiotics to the donor. Mechanical cleansing has turned out to be impractical in deceased donors. Since the graft is certainly not sterile, broad-spectrum antibiotics together with antifungal agents are given to the recipient during transplantation. Because of the powerful immunosuppression, patients are particularly at high risk for developing viral infections. The matching of allografts for cytomegalovirus is difficult to put into routine practice. Patients are given an antiviral agent (usually ganciclovir) prophylactically. Some centers add to this therapy CMV specific hyperimmunoglobulin in recipients of CMV positive grafts. Early diagnosis of CMV infection by a variety of means permits pre-emptive treatment of asymptomatic viremia [14].

Lymphoproliferative disorders related to Epstein-Barr virus mediated B-cell proliferation still represent a major problem after intestinal transplantation. In recent years, it occurs less frequently after a general reduction of immunosuppression, but it still occurs more often than after most solid organ transplantations. This complication is more common in the pediatric population with *de novo* EBV infection. Quantification of the viral load using quantitative polymerase chain reaction allow for the early implementation of therapeutic strategies including changes in the immunosuppression and medication of antiviral therapy. The use of rituximab, a humanized monoclonal antibody, directed against the CD20 molecule expressed on most B-cell lines and most PTLD clones, has led to a significant improvement in outcome [14].

Graft Monitoring

The enormous antigen load makes an intestinal transplant more prone to rejection than other solid organs. In addition, rejection may impair the absorptive capacity of the graft leading to further underimmunosuppression and aggravation of the rejection process. Therefore, timely diagnosis of any pathology of the graft is essential. For graft monitoring, routine endoscopies and biopsies are performed frequently in the early phase after transplantation. Starting at three times a week immediately following surgery, the frequency is continuously reduced over the following weeks. After restoration of the gastrointestinal continuity, biopsies can be obtained from above with the help of an endoscope and from below via a colonoscopic approach. It has to be emphasized, however, that these patients require lifelong monitoring and attention. Therefore, a close relationship between the physician following the patient, the patient himself and the transplant center is essential. Although most rejection episodes are observed during the first year, they may occur any time after transplantation. Rejection is clinically recognized by the development of diarrhea, but other gastrointestinal symptoms such as ileus, emesis, or general malaise may also occur. These symptoms should always prompt endoscopic evaluation of the graft which usually looks grossly normal unless rejection is severe. Therefore, multiple random biopsies should be taken and evaluated by a pathologist experienced with intestinal transplants. It should be recognized that no serum marker accurately diagnoses bowel rejection at present. Even concomitantly transplanted organs such as the liver or a pancreas are not reliable indicators for rejection of the intestinal component of the graft.

Results

Up until March 31, 2005, a total of 1292 intestinal transplants in 1210 patients have been reported at 65 centers to the International Intestinal Registry: 570 were isolated small-bowel transplants, 490 combined liver–small-bowel transplants and 232 were multivisceral transplants. Of the 1292, 772 intestinal transplants were performed in 721 pediatric recipients. For transplants carried out between 2003 and 2005, graft survival at 1 year was calculated to be around 80% with a patient survival percentage that was somewhat higher. Center experience, patient status prior to transplantation and induction therapy and the type of calcineurin inhibitor had a significant impact on outcome. Sepsis was the leading cause of death. Most survivors have full graft function with no requirement for parenteral nutrition (Figs. 1–4; Table 1) [1].

We have performed altogether 4 small bowel transplants in three patients suffering from end stage Crohn's disease. Patient characteristics are summarized in Table 1.

Patient #1 was a 35-year-old male who had a completely uneventful postoperative course and is alive and well with good graft function 64 months after transplantation.

Patient #2 was a 37-year-old female who lost the first graft 2 years after transplantation for chronic rejection and underwent re-transplantation in June

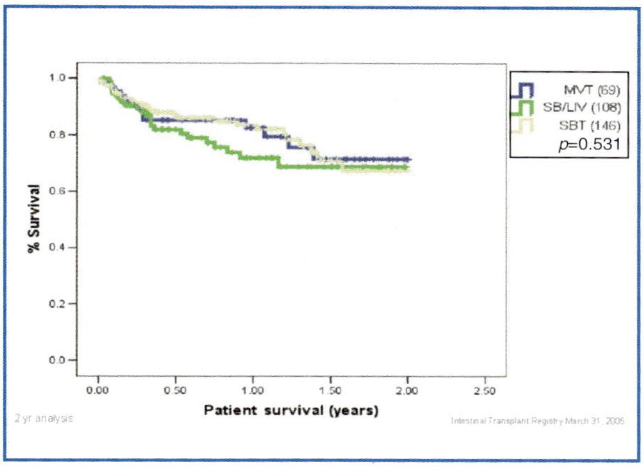

Fig. 1. 2003–2005 patient survival according to transplant type. *MVT*, multivisceral transplantation; *SB/Liver* combined small bowel-liver transplantation; *SBT*, small bowel transplantation alone

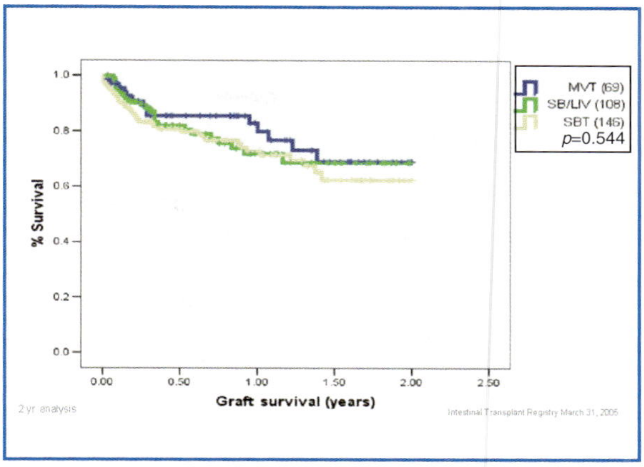

Fig. 2. 2003–2005 graft survival according to D-transplant type. *MVT*, multivisceral transplantation; *SB/Liver*, combined small bowel-liver transplantation; *SBT*, small bowel transplantation alone

2002. 42 months later she has a well function bowel allograft, but requires intermittent hemodialysis for chronic renal failure.

Patient #3 was a 60-year-old female suffering from endstage intestinal and renal failure due to chronic pyelonephritis und underwent combined small bowel-kidney transplantation on July 7, 2003. She developed early after transplantation a T-cell lymphoma of the intestinal graft requiring resection of the graft. 29 months later she is alive with good renal allograft function.

Recurrence of Crohn's Disease

Crohn's disease is considered to be an autoimmune disorder. Therefore, the possibility of recurrence within the graft is an important issue. So far, only two well-documented cases of recurrent disease have been reported. The first case was a 33-year-old female, who underwent small-bowel transplantation in December 1994. After induction with donor bone marrow infusion and with OKT3, immunosuppression consisted of tacrolimus and methylprednisolone. Only 7 months post-transplant did the

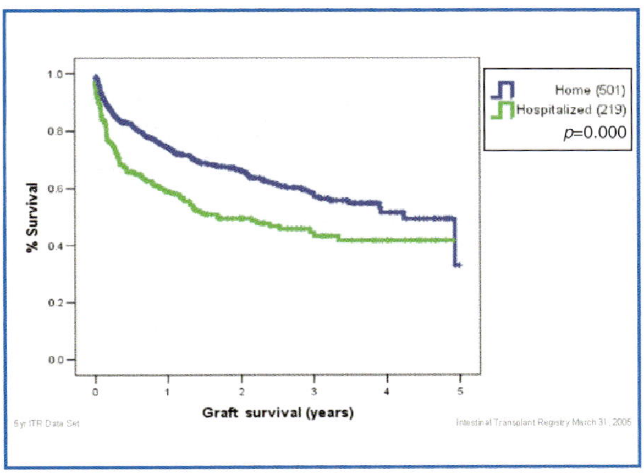

Fig. 3. Graft survival according to pretransplantation status of the recipients. *Home*, patients awaiting transplantations at home; *hospitalized*, patients awaiting transplantation at the hospital

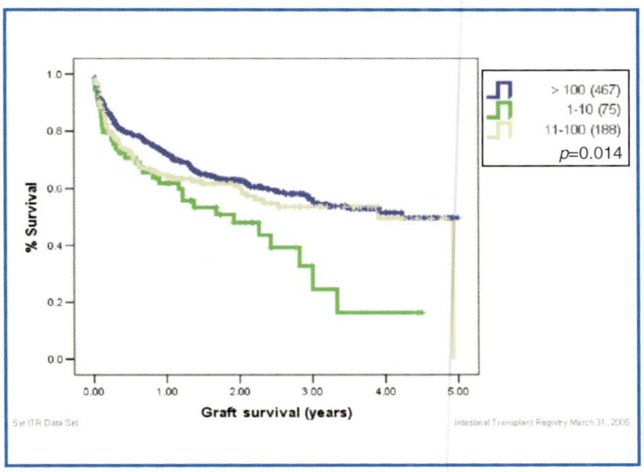

Fig. 4. Graft survival according to centre size: *>100*, number of transplants more than hundred; *11–100*, number of transplants between 11 and 100; *1–10*, transplants per centre

Table 1. Intestinal transplants for Crohn's disease (Innsbruck experience)

No.	Initials	Age	Gender	Underlying disease	Date	Immuno-suppression	Complication	Outcome
1	T.M.	35	M	Crohn's disease, short-bowel syndrome (after two resections)	14.08.98	ATG TAC Aza P	0	Well 64 months Good intestinal graft function
2	H.S.	37	F	Crohn's disease, short-bowel syndrome, impaired renal function	10.04.00	Zenapax TAC Aza P	Bleeding from anastomosis rejection	Graft loss (22.04.04)
3	H.S.	37	F	Loss of 1st intestinal graft	05.06.02	ATG TAC Aza P	Recurrent line sepsis two acute rejections	Well Good intestinal graft function 42 months on dialysis
4	S.H.	6	F	Crohn's disease, short-bowel syndrome, renal failure (pyelonephritis)	07.07.03 + kidney[a]	ATG TAC Aza P	T-cell lymphoma intestinal graft	Intestinal graft removed 29 months Good kidney function

[a] The kidney was transplanted separate from the small bowel
ATG, anti-thymocyte globulin; *TAC*, tacrolimus; *Aza*, azathioprine; *P*, prednisone

patient develop epithelial granulomas, which is characteristic of Crohn's disease. Resection of a bowel segment became necessary and the graft was eventually removed 17 months after transplantation. Histology revealed recurrent Crohn's disease and no signs of chronic or acute rejection [16].

The second case was a 19-year-old male who had an isolated small-bowel transplant in 1994. Maintenance immunosuppression included tacrolimus, azathioprine, and prednisolone. At 8 years post-transplantation, recurrent Crohn's disease was diagnosed that responded to prednisolone [17].

At another center, two patients transplanted for Crohn's disease were reported to have a significant incidence of granulomas in the graft. Both patients remained asymptomatic for as long as 40 months after transplantation [14]. Even if there are only few reports on disease recurrence, it has to be recognized that Crohn's disease can recur despite high-level immunosuppression.

Summary

Improved survival after intestinal transplantation mainly due to both patient condition at the time of transplantation and greater center experience, made small-bowel transplantation an attractive prospect for patients with complications on TPN and eventually became an alternative to conservative treatment of intestinal failure. Patient selection and lifelong surveillance are crucial to the long-term results.

References

1. The International Intestinal Transplant Registry (2005) www.intestinaltransplant.org
2. Lillehei RC, Goot B, Miller FA (1959) The physiological response of the small bowel of the dog to ischemia including prolonged in vitro preservation of the bowel with successful replacement and survival. Ann Surg 150:543–560
3. Lillehei RC, Idezuki Y, Feemster JA et al (1967) Transplantation of stomach, intestine and pancreas: experimental and clinical observation. Surgery 62:721–741
4. Fortner JG, Sichuk G, Litwin SD et al (1972) Immunological responses to an intestinal allograft with HLA identical donor-recipient. Transplantation 14:531–535
5. Cohen Z, Silverman RE, Wassef R et al (1986) Small intestinal transplantation using cyclosporine: report of a case. Transplantation 42:613–621
6. Deltz E, Schroeder P, Gebhardt H et al (1989) Successful clinical small bowel transplantation: report of a case. Clin Transplantation 3:89–91
7. Goulet O, Revillon Y, Canioni D et al (1992) Two and one-half-year follow-up after isolated cadaveric small bowel transplantation in an infant. Transplant Proc 24:1224–1225
8. Starzl TE, Kaupp HA Jr (1960) Mass homotransplantations of abdominal organs in dogs. Surg Forum 11:28–29
9. Starzl TE, Rowe MI, Todo S et al (1989) Transplanta-

tion of Multiple Abdominal Viscera. JAMA 261(10):1449–1457
10. Williams JW, Sankary HN, Foster PF et al (1989) Splanchnic Transplantation. JAMA 261(10):1458–1462
11. Margreiter R, Königsrainer A, Schmid TH et al (1992) Successful multivisceral transplantation. Transplant Proc 24:1226–1227
12. Grant D, Wall W, Mimeault R et al (1990) Successful small-bowel liver transplantation. Lancet 335:181–184
13. Buchman AL, Scolapio J, Fryer J AGA (2003) Technical review on short bowel syndrome and intestinal transplantation. Gastroenterology 124:1111–1134
14. Fishbein TM, Gondolesi GE, Kaufman SS (2003) Intestinal transplantation for gut failure. Gastroenterology 124:1615–1628
15. Middleton SJ, Jamieson NV (2005) The current status of small bowel transplantation in the UK and internationally. Gut 54:1650–1657
16. Sustento-Reodica N, Ruiz P, Rogers A et al (1997) Recurrent Crohn's disease in transplanted bowel. Lancet 349:688–691
17. Kaila B, Grant D, Pettigrew N et al (2003) Crohn's disease recurrence in a small bowel transplant. Am J Gastroenterol 99(1):158–162

Liver Transplantation for Primary Sclerosing Cholangitis and Inflammatory Bowel Disease

Ingmar Königsrainer, Ruth Ladurner, Claudia Schulz, Wolfgang Steurer, Alfred Königsrainer

Introduction

Primary sclerosing cholangitis (PSC) is a chronic cholestatic syndrome characterised by diffuse inflammation and fibrosis of both intra- and extrahepatic bile ducts [1]. Although PSC is most likely a multifactorial disease with genetic predisposition, its exact aetiology remains unknown. In 75% of cases, there is comorbidity with inflammatory bowel disease (IBD) such as ulcerative colitis (UC) and Crohn's disease. This underscores the role of immunological alterations in the pathophysiology of the disease. Mean age at diagnosis is 40 years, and men are affected about twice as often as women [2]. PSC lacks a definitive medical therapy. Promising regimens are high doses of ursodeoxycholic acid alone or in combination with immunosuppression. Endoscopic treatment of biliary strictures is frequently needed in the late course of PSC disease. Repeated stenting may be an option in treating dominant strictures [3]. Occasionally, surgical treatment of severe extrahepatic strictures is necessary. In general, however, most hepatobiliary surgeons are reluctant to perform such procedures, as they may complicate a future liver transplantation (Ltx) and reduce the chance of long-term survival following Ltx [4]. PSC runs an unpredictable clinical course leading to liver cirrhosis and terminal liver disease in the majority of affected individuals.

Primary Sclerosing Cholangitis and Liver Transplantation

At present, PSC is the fifth most important indication for liver transplantation in the United States [5]. There are two major difficulties associated with predicting the course of the disease in each individual case as well as the increased risk for hepatobiliary malignancies, primarily cholangiocellular carcinoma (CCC). The risk for CCC is highest during the first year of diagnosis and is not linked to the stage of disease [6, 7]. A PSC patient with cirrhosis and a liver tumour should also be evaluated for possible hepatocellular carcinoma (HCC) and in this case considered for Ltx if no extrahepatic metastases are detected and the tumour is within accepted criteria. Liver resection for HCC is rarely indicated in a PSC patient with advanced liver disease, as previous hepatobiliary surgery is a negative prognostic factor for transplant candidates [4].

The problem of identifying PSC patients with a high risk for developing CCC has not been resolved so far. No specific tumour markers exist. This has a great impact because CCC has traditionally been considered a contraindication to Ltx. Experience with CCC in patients undergoing Ltx is limited, and treatment guidelines are still lacking. The value of routine brush cytology obtained during endoscopic retrograde cholangiography remains unclear. Patients with severe dysplasia in cytologic smears should be considered as running a very high risk for CCC development and therefore evaluated to exclude possible systemic malignant disease. No consensus exists as to what imaging modality should be preferred in the management of these patients. Positron emission tomography (PET) is promising but its exact role remains unclear [8].

Studies indicate that Ltx results in highly selected patients with CCC are satisfactory if the patients undergo multidisciplinary treatment including chemotherapy and local radiation therapy prior to Ltx [9, 10]. Due to the fact that the diagnosis of CCC can be extremely difficult to establish, PSC patients are usually evaluated for Ltx even when CCC is suspected and the final decision to perform transplantation is taken during laparotomy. If a limited tumour without extrahepatic tumour growth is found, the procedure should be continued and transplantation performed. Positive lymph nodes contraindicate transplantation, and the patient is given palliative therapy. Brandsaeter et al. reported that clinical suspicion of cancer, recent diagnosis of PSC and previous colon cancer are predictors of malignancy, which was found in 20% of more than 500 patients [11]. Ideally, a PSC patient should be listed for Ltx at the time when survival with Ltx supersedes survival without Ltx. Prognostic models such as the Child-Pugh score or the model for end-stage liver disease (MELD) score have been demonstrated to be superior to PSC-specific prognostic models in predicting posttransplantation survival in PSC patients [12]. Short duration of PSC, a high bilirubin and an elevated MELD score are associated with poor outcome [13]. When assessing a PSC patient for Ltx a colonoscopy is mandatory. Patients with severe ulcerative colitis or mucosal dysplasia are candidates for colectomy before listing them for transplantation. Particular care is necessary to avoid life-threatening liver decompensation [14].

When reconstructing the biliary tract during transplantation two options are available. As experience with end-to-end biliary anastomosis is limited, most surgeons prefer a hepaticoenterostomy with a Roux-en-Y-loop in patients undergoing Ltx for PSC. There are a few reports that a duct-to-duct anastomosis is associated with a higher recurrence rate. From the pathophysiological point of view, neither alternative is logical since a possible source for malignancy remains untouched in situ. Whether an obligatory resection of the whole bile duct, meaning a pancreas head resection, is justified, has not yet been determined. Heightened attention is needed for the possibility of growth of malignant tissue infiltrating the choledochus duct. In this case, a simultaneous pancreatic head resection is generally accepted [15].

From the recipient's point of view and considering the development in waiting time in recent years, living related liver transplantation is the best option for PSC, not only in order to reduce waiting time but also to prevent patients from dropping off the list due to tumour formation [16]. Patients with PSC in general have good physical status with low Child-Pugh score and therefore face a long waiting time. The risk of developing CCC correlates directly with the length of time the disease remains untreated.

Outcome after Liver Grafting

Survival rates are comparable with those achieved in patients with other autoimmune liver diseases, such as primary biliary cirrhosis and autoimmune hepatitis, with 1-year patient survival exceeding 90 % in recently published series [14]. PSC patients are reported to have a slightly higher retransplantation rate without impact on long-term patient survival [4]. Again, this increased retransplantation rate has been ascribed to PSC-specific long-term complications, in particular, biliary strictures [17]. However, patient survival following Ltx has been shown to be clearly improved compared with the natural course of the disease predicted by prognostic models [18].

A number of pretransplantation factors have been shown to predict poorer posttransplantation survival, such previous hepatobiliary surgery, elevated creatinine levels, reduced nutritional status and the occurrence of hepatobiliary malignancy [4, 18]. Presence of IBD has also been claimed to affect survival following Ltx [18]. Other studies failed to identify IBD as a risk factor [4]. The greatest impact on long-term outcome is from CCC, which has been considered poor even in patients with occult tumours [19, 20].

Considering the lack of alternatives and the significant benefit in patients with small tumours, strict exclusion from transplantation is not justified. Moreover, improved patient survival has been reported in smaller series with strictly selected patients [21]. HCC is not observed frequently and has less impact on patient survival following Ltx in PSC patients [22].

Postoperative Complications

Hepatic artery thrombosis (HAT) with an incidence of 1–5% following adult Ltx is a feared complication frequently leading to graft loss and retransplantation. The reason for the increased incidence of hepatic artery thrombosis in PSC patients is unclear [17]. New immunosuppressive regimens have significantly reduced rejection episodes in liver allograft recipients. Patients with PSC, PBC or autoimmune hepatitis seem to experience more acute rejections compared with patients with alcoholic cirrhosis or chronic viral hepatitis who are thus on a higher level of immunosuppression [23]. On the other hand, some centres have also reported fully satisfactory results after early steroid withdrawal in patients with PSC [24]. With regard to postoperative infection episodes, positive bacterial cultures are found in bile samples from a large portion of PSC patients at the time of Ltx [25].

Another major concern is recurrent disease. Strictures can be single or multiple, anastomotic or nonanastomotic, and they can develop early within the first 3 months or later [26]. Differentiation of PSC-associated or nonrelated complications can be a challenge in follow-up. An increased rate of biliary problems in PSC liver allograft recipients, especially after duct-to-duct reconstruction of the biliary system, was identified by Sheng et al. more than 10 years ago [27].

Diagnostic criteria, prevalence and prognosis of PSC recurrence are not established. Cholangiography has been complicated because it is usually impossible to perform an endoscopic retrograde cholangiography in patients in whom a hepaticoenterostomy has been constructed. However, magnetic resonance cholangiography (MRC) now permits noninvasive cholangiography to be performed in these patients.

Even in a graft biopsy, PSC recurrence can be difficult to identify. In some cases, typical fibrous cholangitis and/or fibro-obliterative lesions are seen, supporting the diagnosis of recurrent PSC. About 20–40% of PSC patients will experience recurrent disease. The Mayo Clinic has defined PSC recurrence as either cholangiographic changes occurring more than 90 days after Ltx or characteristic liver biopsy findings, such as fibrous cholangitis and/or fibro-obliterative lesions with or without ductopenic biliary fibrosis or cirrhosis, namely in a PSC patient without HAT or stenosis, ABO incompatibility, chronic ductopenic rejection, early biliary complications or biliary strictures [28]. Therefore, the diagnosis of recurrent PSC should be made only in patients with typical cholangiographic findings and/or positive histology as well as patent arterial circulation. The improving quality of MRC will probably enable us to diagnose and characterise PSC recurrence more precisely in the near future. Pretransplantation colectomy has been claimed to be associated with a lower rate of recurrence [29]. The impact of different immunosuppression regimens has not yet been resolved. Cytomegalovirus (CMV) and donor–recipient gender mismatch have also been proposed as risk factors for recurrence [30].

The prognosis of PSC recurrence was originally thought to be favourable, with no cases progressing to graft failure [20], but more recent reports question this [28]. To date, no one can propose strategies for retransplantation.

Management of Inflammatory Bowel Disease

In spite of immunosuppressive medication, a significant number of patients undergoing Ltx due to PSC will experience an exacerbation of IBD following transplantation, in some cases necessitating colectomy. Patients without IBD prior to Ltx have also been diagnosed with de novo IBD in the posttransplantation period [31]. Dvorchik et al. described a high incidence of progression of IBD following Ltx [31]. Haagsma et al. found that tacrolimus is more frequently associated with posttransplantation exacerbation of IBD and that patients on triple immunosuppression (cyclosporine, azathioprine, prednisolone) have less active bowel disease in follow-up [32]. Discontinuation of steroids has also been reported to increase the risk of IBD exacerbation [33]. Colorectal cancer in patients with IBD and PSC undergoing Ltx has been reported in several series [28].

Conclusive evidence that immunosuppression administered following Ltx may further increase the risk of colorectal cancer compared with the risk in the nontransplanted PSC patient with IBD is still lacking [34, 35]. PSC patients with a diagnosis of IBD and in whom a colectomy has not been performed should undergo colonoscopy on a yearly basis. If dysplasia is detected, colectomy should be considered.

If severe colitis or dysplasia is found during the waiting period, colectomy can also be performed during laparotomy for the transplantation provided the patient's general condition permits. Indeed, the ideal time to perform colectomy is not yet known. So far, it is a matter of local preference and the condition of the individual patient.

Follow-Up

Due to the risk of PSC-specific complications, it is advisable that these patients be subjected to further detailed follow-up controls routinely, including a cholangiogram. The risk of developing de novo hepatobiliary malignancy is especially given in those patients with severe pretransplantation dysplasia. Surveillance of the remnant biliary duct should not be forgotten, and endoscopic ultrasound examination, including brush cytology, might be advisable.

Summary

PSC runs an unpredictable clinical course leading to liver cirrhosis and terminal liver disease in the majority of affected individuals. The ideal time to perform colectomy in colitis ulcerosa patients is still unclear; so far, it is a matter of local preference and patient condition. The problem of identifying PSC patients with a particular risk for developing CCC is multifactorial. Diagnostic features are still lacking. Living related donor liver transplantation for PSC could reduce waiting time and thus secondary complications as well as drop-out probability due to malignancy [16]. Major surgery with simultaneous pancreatic head resection may be necessary in cases with extrahepatic duct infiltration in order to achieve no residual tumour (R0) status [15].

References

1. Sherlock S, Dooley J (2002) Diseases of the liver and biliary system. Blackwell Science, Oxford
2. Olsson R, Danielsson A, Jarnerot G et al (1991) Prevalence of PSC in patients with ulcerative colitis. Gas-

troenterology 100:1319-1323
3. Stiehl A, Rudolph G, Kloters-Plachky P et al (2002) Development of dominant bile duct stenoses in patients with PSC treated with ursodeoxycholic acid: outcome of endoscopic treatment. J Hepatol 36:151-156
4. Brandsaeter B, Friman S, Broome U et al (2003) Outcome following liver transplantation for PSC in the Nordic countries. Scand J Gastroenterol 38:1776-1783
5. Levy C, Lindor KD (2006) Primary sclerosing cholangitis: epidemiology, natural history, and prognosis. Semin Liver Dis 26:22-30
6. Bergquist A, Ekbom A, Olsson R et al (2002) Hepatic and extrahepatic malignancies in primary sclerosing cholangitis. J Hepatol 36:321-327
7. Chalasani L, Baluyut A, Ismail A et al (2000) CCC in patients with primary sclerosing cholangitis: a multicenter case-control study. Hepatology 31:7-11
8. Keiding S, Hansen SB, Rasmussen HH et al (1998) Detection of cholangiocarcinoma in primary sclerosing cholangitis by positron emission tomography. Hepatology 28:700-706
9. Sudan D, De Roover A, Chinnakotla S et al (2002) Radiochemotherapy and transplantation allow long term survival for non respectable hilar carcinoma. Am J Transplant 2:774-779
10. Devroede J, Steeres JL, Burch PA et al (2000) Prolonged disease free survival after orthotopic liver transplantation plus adjuvant chemoirradiation for CCC. Liver Transpl 6:309-316
11. Brandsaeter B, Isoniemi H, Broome U et al (2004) Liver transplantation for primary sclerosing cholangitis; predictors and consequences of hepatobiliary malignancy. J Hepatol 40:815-822
12. Talwalkar JA, Seabe E, Kim W, Wiesener RH (2000) Predicting clinical and economic outcomes after liver transplantation using the Mayo primary sclerosing cholangitis model and Child-Pugh score. Liver Transpl 6:753-758
13. Brandsaeter B, Broome U, Isoniemi H et al (2000) Liver transplantation for primary sclerosing cholangitis in the Nordic countries: outcome after acceptance on the waiting list. Liver Transpl 9:961-969
14. Adam R, Mc Master P, O'Grady JG et al (2003) Evolution of liver transplantation in Europe: Report of the European Liver Transplant Registry. Liver Transpl 9:1231-1243
15. Varotti G, Gondolesi GE, Roayaie S (2003) Combined adult-to-adult living donor right lobe liver transplantation and pancreatoduodenectomy for distal bile duct adenocarcinoma in a patient with primary sclerosing cholangitis. J Am Coll Surg. 197:765-769
16. Oya H, Sato Y, Yamamoto S (2004) Living related donor liver transplantation for primary sclerosing cholangitis with hepatocellular carcinoma and Crohn's disease: a case report. Transplant Proc 36:2297-2298
17. Wiesner RH (2001) Liver transplantation for primary sclerosing cholangitis: timing, outcome, impact of inflammatory bowel disease and recurrence of disease. Best Pract Res Clin Gastro 15:667-680
18. Neuberger J, Gunson B, Kmolmitt P et al (1999) Pretransplant prediction of prognosis after liver transplantation in primary sclerosing cholangitis using a Cox regression model. Hepatology 29:1375-1379
19. Meyer CG, Penn I, James L (2000) Liver transplantation for cholangiocarcinoma: results in 207 patients. Transplantation 69:1633-1637
20. Goss J, Shackleton CR, Farmer DG et al (1997) Orthotopic liver transplantation for primary sclerosing cholangitis: a 12-year single center experience. Ann Surg 225:472-481
21. Hassoun Z, Gores GJ, Rosen CB (2002) Preliminary experience with liver transplantation in selected patients with unresectable cholangiocarcinoma. Surg Oncol Clin N Am 11:909-921
22. van de Fries W, de Man R, van Buuren HR (2003) Inflammatory bowel disease and liver transplantation for primary sclerosing cholangitis. Eur J Gastro Hepatol 15:657-663
23. Neuberger J (1999) Incidence, timing and risk factors for acute and chronic rejection Liver Transpl Surg 5:30-36
24. Kugelmas M, Spiegelman P, Osgood MJ et al (2003) Different immunosuppressive regimens and recurrence of PSC after liver transplantation. Liver Transpl 9:727-732
25. Olsson R, Bjornsson E, Backman L et al (1998) Bile duct bacterial isolates in primary sclerosing cholangitis: a study of explanted livers. J Hepatol 28:426-432
26. Feller RB, Waugh RC, Selby WS et al (1996) Biliary strictures after liver transplantation: clinical picture, correlates and outcomes. J Gastroenterol Hepatol 11:21-25
27. Sheng R, Zajko AB, Campbell WL, Abu-Elmagd K (1993) Biliary strictures in hepatic transplants: prevalence and type in patients with PSC vs those with other liver diseases. Am J Roentgenol 161:297-300
28. Graziadei JW, Wiesner RH, Marotta PJ et al (1999) Long-term results of patients undergoing liver transplantation for primary sclerosing cholangitis. Hepatology 30:1121-1127
29. Vera A, Moledina S, Gunson B et al (2002) Risk factors for recurrence of primary sclerosing cholangitis of liver allograft. Lancet 360:1943-1944
30. Jeyarajah DR, Netto GJ, Lee SP et al (1998) Recurrent PSC after orthotopic liver transplantation: is chronic rejection part of the disease process? Transplantation 66:1300-1306
31. Dvorchik I, Subotin M, Demetris AJ et al (2002) Effect of liver transplantation on inflammatory bowel disease in patients with primary sclerosing cholangitis. Hepatology 35:380-384
32. Haagsma H, Van den Berg AP, Kleibeuker JH et al (2003) Inflammatory bowel disease after liver transplantation: the effect of different immunosuppressive regimens. Aliment Pharm Ther 18:33-34
33. Papatheodoridis GV, Hamilton M, Mistry PK (1998) Ulcerative colitis has an aggressive course after liver transplantation for primary sclerosing cholangitis. Gut 43:639-644
34. Higashi H, Yanaga K, Marsh JW et al (1990) Development of colon cancer after liver transplantation of primary sclerosing cholangitis associated with ulcerative colitis. Hepatology 11:477-480
35. Loftus EV, Aguiar HI, Sandborn WJ et al (1998). Risk of colorectal neoplasia in patients with primary sclerosing cholangitis and ulcerative colitis following orthotopic liver transplantation. Hepatology 27:685-690

SECTION III

Familial Adenomatous Polyposis

Emergent Issues and Future Trends in Familial Adenomatous Polyposis

Gian Gaetano Delaini, Marco Scaglia, Gianluca Colucci, Tom Öresland

Introduction

Although this book is addressed to medical doctors, in this chapter, we have tried to look at the scientific literature with the eyes of someone who has an FAP or has a family member with this disease, in order to understand, for those who so urgently seek it, what lies just "around the corner" in terms of breaking news.

The Disease

Familial adenomatous polyposis (FAP) is a syndrome affecting 1:10 000 people and accounts for approximately 1% of colorectal cancer. It is an autosomal dominant syndrome caused by a germline mutation of the adenomatous polyposis coli gene (APC) located at chromosome 5q21. The disorder is characterised by the development of hundreds of colorectal adenomas during adolescence. Colorectal cancer will develop in nearly all affected persons by the sixth decade of life if prophylactic colectomy is not performed. Most cases begin as benign adenomatous colonic polyps.

One widely held opinion is that cancer is a genetic disease that arises from an accumulation of mutations that leads to the selection of cells with increasingly aggressive behaviour. These mutations may lead either to a gain of function by oncogenes or to a loss of function by tumour suppressor genes. Most mutations in cancer are somatic and are found only in the cancer cells. Most of our information on human cancer genes has been gained from hereditary cancers. In the case of hereditary cancers, the individual carries a particular germline mutation in every cell. In the past decade, more than 30 genes for autosomal dominant hereditary cancers have been identified.

Emergent Issues and Trends in Research

The ideal gold standard would be a gene technique that would allow the removal of the diseased gene and implant a disease-free gene. At present this is still pure speculation. Most of the research deals with systems for screening the germline mutations in the adenomatous polyposis coli (APC) gene that predisposes the disease susceptibility in familial adenomatous polyposis. Nowadays, there are technical systems that detect the mutations in APC gene. They might be useful in the molecular diagnosis of presymptomatic cases in FAP family. The clinical features of FAP patients may be related to the genotypes of their APC gene. However, there are other interesting ways of approaching the problem of a presymptomatic carrier risk assessment in familial adenomatous polyposis such as the combined use of molecular- and biomarkers. Predictive carrier testing for the inherited disorder of familial adenomatous polyposis can be conducted using DNA markers linked to the FAP locus. The presence of characteristic hypertrophic retinal lesions has been advocated as useful biomarkers for FAP. Bapat et al. [1] have compared molecular linkage and retinal screening techniques by evaluating the presymptomatic carrier risk of 40 at-risk individuals from 15 FAP families. Linkage analysis was informative in all the cases as was retinal lesion analysis in 25 cases. For identification of the at-risk population, predictive diagnosis by both techniques was completely concordant and identified 15 members at "high" and 10 at "low" risk of inheriting FAP. Another relevant matter regarding future trends in FAP research are the biomarkers for carcinogenesis and the use of drugs to prevent the evolution to the final stage of cancer.

Progression Markers during the Intestinal Carcinogenesis: Intermediate Biomarkers

Colon carcinogenesis is a multistep process in which an accumulation of genetic events within a single cell line leads to a progressively dysplastic cellular appearance, deregulated cell growth, and, finally, carcinoma. The "adenoma-carcinoma sequence" occurs through a series of mutations in cancer-causing genes and usually takes about 11 years. These genes (oncogenes, tumour suppressor genes, DNA mismatch repair genes) encode proteins that control vital cell functions such as growth and survival. Development of intermediate markers for chemoprevention trials is important. Premalignant lesions are a potential source of intermediate markers. Monitoring intermediate markers that correlate with a reduction in cancer incidence would allow a more expeditious evaluation of potentially active chemopreventive agents. If a disappearance of these lesions can be correlated with a reduction in cancer incidence, then markers of premalignancy may serve as intermediate endpoints for chemoprevention trials.

Intermediate biomarkers of abnormal cell growth and development have recently been used in chemoprevention trials in attempts to identify the efficacy of chemopreventive agents in human subjects. Measurements carried out include those related to cell proliferation, differentiation, and gene structure and expression in the colon. Among the modified patterns of cell proliferation identified by microautoradiographic or immunoperoxidase assays, a characteristic expansion in the size of the proliferative compartment has been observed in normal-appearing colorectal mucosa of human subjects with disease increasing cancer risk; the same patterns have been induced by chemical carcinogens in rodents. Moreover, this intermediate biomarker has been modulated by chemopreventive agents in both rodents and humans. Newer intermediate biomarkers being studied for application to human chemopreventive programs include normal and abnormal patterns of expression of mucins, intermediate filaments and cytoskeletal proteins, and the structure and expression of a variety of genes associated with normal and abnormal cell development. The application of these various intermediate biomarkers to chemoprevention studies is increasing the ability of investigators to analyse the effects of novel chemopreventive agents in the colon and in other organs.

How to Prevent the Carcinogenic Progression by Chemical Agents: the Chemoprevention

Cancer chemoprevention, as first defined by Sporn in 1976 [2], uses natural, synthetic, or biological chemical agents to reverse, suppress, or prevent carcinogenic progression. It is based on the concepts of multifocal field carcinogenesis and multistep carcinogenesis. In field carcinogenesis, diffuse epithelial injury in tissues such as the aerodigestive tract, results from generalised carcinogen exposure throughout the field and clonal proliferation of mutated cells. Genetic changes exist throughout the field and increase the likelihood that one or more premalignant and malignant lesions may develop within that field. Multistep carcinogenesis describes a stepwise accumulation of alterations, both genotypic and phenotypic. Arresting one or several of the steps may impede or delay the development of cancer. This has been described particularly well in studies involving precancerous and cancerous lesions of the head and neck, which focus on oral premalignant lesions (leukoplakia and erythroplakia) and their associated increased risk of progression to cancer. In addition to histologic assessment, intermediate markers of response are needed to assess the validity of these therapies in a timely and cost-efficient manner.

Non-steroidal Anti-Inflammatory Agents for Colon Cancer Prevention

Colon cancer prevention has now focused on novel targeted therapies, such as non-steroidal anti-inflammatory agents (NSAIDs). Aspirin, an inhibitor of COX-1 and -2, has been studied in several large randomised studies, but the effect on colorectal cancer prevention is unclear. The US Physician's Health Study, which enrolled 22 071 physicians as participants, reported that aspirin had no effect on the incidence of polyps or colon cancer [3]. However, Baron et al. conducted the Aspirin/Folate Polyp Prevention Study, a randomised, double-blind, placebo-controlled trial of daily aspirin (325 mg and 8 mg) and daily folate (1 mg) in 1121 patients with a recent history of colon adenomas [4]. This trial demonstrated that the 81-mg dose of aspirin prevented recurrence of colorectal adenomas (47% placebo *vs.* 38% aspirin 81 mg *vs.* 45% aspirin 325 mg; p=0.04). This translated into a relative-risk reduction of 19% in the 81-mg aspirin group and a non-significant reduction of 4% in the 325-mg aspirin group. This study also reported a relative-risk reduction of 40% in the 81-mg aspirin group for advanced lesions. In addition, Sandler et al. [5] reported on the Colorectal Adenoma Prevention Study, which randomised 635 patients with prior colorectal cancer to 325-mg aspirin or placebo. Twenty percent of the placebo group developed recurrent adenomas compared with 17% in the aspirin arm (p=0.0004), for an adjusted relative risk of 0.65. Aspirin intervention delayed the development of recurrent adenoma and also decreased the number of recurrent adenomas.

Although the role of aspirin remains debated, the

benefit of NSAIDs in chemoprevention has clearly been defined in certain high-risk subgroups [6]. In clinical trials of patients with FAP, sulindac (150 mg twice a day for 9 months) was shown to decrease the number of polyps by 44% and decrease the diameter of the polyps by 35% (p=0.014 and p<0.001, respectively) [7]. In a study, 77 patients with FAP (more than 5 polyps 2 mm in size) were randomised to receive placebo, 100 mg, or 400 mg of celecoxib twice daily [8]. Celecoxib is a selective COX-2 inhibitor. Response to treatment was reported as the mean percent change from baseline. After 6 months, the 30 patients assigned to 400 mg of celecoxib had a 28% reduction in the mean number of colorectal polyps (p=0.003) and a 30.7% reduction in the polyp burden (p=0.001) compared with 4.5 and 4.9% in the placebo group, respectively. This positive result led to the FDAs approval of celecoxib in the treatment of patients with FAP.

Other Agents under Trial

Other agents under investigation in colorectal chemoprevention include difluoromethylornithine (DFMO), which irreversibly inhibits ornithine decarboxylase and blocks cell proliferation. Ursodeoxycholic acid reduces the concentration of the secondary bile acid deoxycholic acid in the colon and affects arachidonic acid metabolism [9–11]. 3-hydroxy-3-methylglutaryl Coenzyme A reductase inhibitors are usually used in the setting of lowering cholesterol but also have antioxidant anti-inflammatory properties and inhibit cell proliferation [12]. Preclinical work in mutant APC murine models have shown that sulindac in combination with EGFR inhibitor EKI-785 can decrease intestinal polyps [13]. Almost one-half the mice treated with the combination agents did not develop polyps. With the recent success of bevacizumab, an antibody to the VEGF-receptor in metastatic colorectal cancer, and cetuximab, an antibody to EGFR, further strategies will be applied to prevention.

The continued study of immunology, tumour biology and natural history through controlled trials focusing not only on efficacy endpoints but also on biological markers in tissue and serum will help develop detailed risk models. Chemopreventive agents appear thus far to have efficacy in several tumour types, and we hope to define their future role in treating and preventing other cancers in high-risk individuals.

Advances in delaying the development of colorectal carcinoma have been shown in patients with FAP with celecoxib treatment. Current and future trials using celecoxib alone or in combination with chemotherapy and other biological therapies are targeting several cohorts including children with APC mutations, patients with FAP, HNPCC, prior colorectal adenoma, or prior history of sporadic adenomas [14]. The use of celecoxib in the prevention of polyps has resulted in continued efforts to define a high-risk population and to implement a chemopreventive agent in the treatment of cancer. With regard to aspirin use in the prevention of colon adenomas, two large randomised, placebo-controlled trials showed benefit. However, although the Aspirin/Folate Polyp Prevention Study and the Colorectal Adenoma Prevention Study reported positive results, a certain percentage of patients receiving aspirin intervention still developed colon adenomas. This suggests that aspirin use cannot be a substitute for colon surveillance and that further studies are necessary for effective colon cancer chemoprevention.

Surgical Prevention of Colorectal Cancer in FAP

Familial adenomatous polyposis coli (FAP) may not be considered a single disease entity with standardised guidelines for operative treatment. However, prophylactic colectomy after the manifestation of polyps but prior to the development of colorectal cancer remains the most effective prevention of colorectal cancer in FAP. The optimal timing of prophylactic surgery remains a clinical decision taken independently of mutation analysis. In the case of the classic FAP phenotype, restorative proctocolectomy and ileal pouch-anal anastomosis might be the procedure of choice. The development of reliable guidelines for attenuated FAP variants requires further evidence from clinical studies on surgical strategy and the advantages of prophylactic surgery over regular endoscopic screening with removal of polyps. A study by Winde et al. [15] has shown that low-dose rectal sulindac maintenance therapy is highly effective in achieving complete adenoma reversion without relapse in 87% of patients after 33 months. Rectal FAP phenotype should be crucial in the surgical decision. Colectomy with ileo-rectal anastomosis and regular chemoprevention might proceed to be a promising alternative to pouch procedures. Chemoprevention with lower incidence of FAP-related tumours via dysplasia reversion might be possible in the future.

The Aftermath of Prophylactic Colectomy

A patient after a proctocolectomy is cleared from colorectal cancer, but he is not entirely free from troubles. Duodenal adenomas might be the next problem, moreover desmoids are also a recognised entity in FAP. The lifetime risk of developing duodenal cancer in familial adenomatous polyposis (FAP) is about 5%. When and to what extent surgical intervention should be undertaken to prevent death from invasive carcinoma is controversial [16]. Of 48 proctocolectomies with a mean follow-up of 74 months (range, 3–288 months), Tulchinsky et al. [17] reported the development of extra-colonic manifestations including desmoid tumours (in 12), duodenal adenomas (in 9), pouch adenomas (in 5), and rectal stump adenomas (in 3), in 38 patients. Two patients died (4%) because of desmoid tumour and malignant fibrous histiocytoma.

Aiming to prevent duodenal polyps, enteral adenomatous polyposis coli gene replacement therapy in mice has awakened interest [18]. Preclinical studies of gene transfer for the treatment of desmoid disease in familial adenomatous polyposis [19] is under study and seems an attractive alternative for the treatment of desmoids, but it is too early to understand if this will develop into a clinical application.

Conservative surgical treatments such as pancreas-preserving total duodenectomy in familial adenomatous polyposis have been advocated, but surgery cannot be considered a future trend for a genetic disease.

New Screening Methods

Virtual colonoscopy, which is an electronic reconstruction of the colon from high-resolution abdominal computed tomographic (CT) scans or magnetic resonance imaging (MRI) studies, holds promise as a colon-screening tool. Current technology has already resulted in reliable identification of colonic lesions as small as a few millimetres. Complete colon preparation is still required, and the cost is not yet known. Research is under way to assess the potential of doing virtual colon studies without any preparation. If this succeeds, screening may well become both cost-effective and convenient. The utility of capsule endoscopy small-bowel surveillance in patients with polyposis [20] might find an indication in selected cases of more advanced duodenal adenoma that can be related to the presence of small-bowel polyps.

References

1. Bapat BV, Parker JA, Berk T et al (1994) Combined use of molecular and biomarkers for presymptomatic carrier risk assessment in familial adenomatous polyposis: implications for screening guidelines. Dis Colon Rectum 37(2):165–171
2. Sporn MB (1976) Approaches to prevention of epithelial cancer during the preneoplastic period. Cancer Res 36:2699–2702
3. Gann PH, Manson JE, Glynn RJ et al (1993) Low-dose aspirin and incidence of colorectal tumors in a randomized trial. J Natl Cancer Inst 85:1220–1224
4. Baron JA, Cole BF, Sandler RS et al (2003) A randomized trial of aspirin to prevent colorectal adenomas. N Engl J Med 348:891–899
5. Sandler RS, Halabi S, Baron JA et al (2003) A randomized trial of aspirin to prevent colorectal adenomas in patients with previous colorectal cancer. N Engl J Med 348:883–890
6. Ruschoff J, Wallinger S, Dietmaier W et al (1998) Aspirin suppresses the mutator phenotype associated with hereditary nonpolyposis colorectal cancer by genetic selection. Proc Natl Acad Sci USA 95:11301–11306
7. Giardiello FM, Hamilton SR, Krush AJ et al (1993) Treatment of colonic and rectal adenomas with sulindac in familial adenomatous polyposis. N Engl J Med 328:1313–1316
8. Steinbach G, Lynch PM, Phillips RKS et al (2000) The effect of celecoxib, a cyclooxygenase-2 inhibitor, in familial adenomatous polyposis. N Engl J Med 342:1946–1952
9. Narisawa T, Fukaura Y, Terada K, Sekiguchi H (1998) Prevention of N-methylnitrosourea-induced colon tumorigenesis by ursodeoxycholic acid in F344 rats. Jpn J Cancer Res 89:1009–1013
10. Rodrigues CM, Kren BT, Steer CJ, Setchell KD (1995) The site-specific delivery of ursodeoxycholic acid to the rat colon by sulfate conjugation. Gastroenterology 109:1835–1844
11. Ikegami T, Matsuzaki Y, Shoda J et al (1998) The chemopreventive role of ursodeoxycholic acid in azoxymethane-treated rats: suppressive effects on enhanced group II phospholipase A2 expression in colonic tissue. Cancer Lett 134:129–139
12. Davignon J, Laaksonen R (1999) Low-density lipoprotein-independent effects of statins. Curr Opin Lipidol 10:543–559
13. Torrance CJ, Jackson PE, Montgomery E et al (2000) Combinatorial chemoprevention of intestinal neoplasia. Nat Med 6:1024–1028
14. Clapper ML, Chang WC, Meropol NJ (2001) Chemoprevention of colorectal cancer. Curr Opin Oncol 13:307–313
15. Winde G, Schmid KW, Schlegel W, Fischer R, Osswald H, Bunte H (2005) Complete reversion and prevention of rectal adenomas in colectomized patients with familial adenomatous polyposis by rectal low-dose sulindac maintenance treatment: advantages of a low-dose nonsteroidal anti-inflammatory drug regimen in reversing adenomas exceeding 33 months. Am J Gastroenterol 100(7):1498-1502
16. de Vos tot Nederveen Cappel WH, Jarvinen HJ, Bjork J et al (2003) Worldwide survey among polyposis registries of surgical management of severe duodenal adenomatosis in familial adenomatous polyposis. Br J Surg 90(6):705–710
17. Tulchinsky H, Keidar A, Goldman G et al (2005) Surgical treatment and long-term outcome of patients with familial adenomatous polyposis: 16 years experience

at the Tel Aviv Sourasky Medical Center. Isr Med Assoc J 7(2):82–85
18. Lee J, Hargest R, Wasan H, Phillips RKS (2004) Liposome-mediated adenomatous polyposis coli gene therapy: a novel anti-adenoma strategy in multiple intestinal neoplasia mouse model. Dis Colon Rectum 47(12):2105–2113
19. Bright-Thomas RM, Agrawal A, Hargest R (2002) Preclinical studies of gene transfer for the treatment of desmoid disease in familial adenomatous polyposis. Br J Surg 89(12):1563–1569
20. Burke CA, Santisi J, Church J, Levinthal G (2005) The utility of capsule endoscopy small bowel surveillance in patients with polyposis. Am J Gastroenterol 100(7):1498–1502

Genetic Mutations in FAP and Conventional or Laparoscopic Surgical Approach

Ettore Contessini-Avesani, Fiorenzo Botti, Alberto Carrara, Chiara Rocha, Elisa Gilardoni, Barbara Oreggia

Introduction

Familial adenomatous polyposis (FAP) is a hereditary disease whose main characteristic is the great quantity of adenomatous polyps distributed throughout the colon and rectum and leading to their progressive degeneration. The complexity of the possible clinical presentations includes, in addition to severe or attenuated colorectal disorders, various extra-colonic manifestations such as gastric and duodenal polyposis and desmoid tumours that can require additional endoscopic or surgical treatment which complicates the therapeutic process and imposes continuative surveillance even when the colorectal disease is eradicated.

Analysis of the genetic pattern of the disease, as well as a better definition of the particular aspects of APC gene mutations on chromosome 5 and its relationship to the clinical aspects of the pathology, suggest a surgical therapeutic scheme based not only on clinical criteria but also on the genetic implications outlined [1].

Unfortunately, to date, a proven correlation between the variable characteristics of the genetic error and the clinical expressions of the pathology does not exist; nevertheless, on the basis of genetic analysis, which can precisely define attenuated and severe forms, it is possible to indicate a therapeutic option rather than another type of option. To understand whether the genetic traits could be useful in directing the therapy, we examined the literature existing on the subject and performed a retrospective analysis on patients operated on at our hospital without either the patients or ourselves knowing in advance the localisation of the genetic error.

The aim of our evaluation is to determine if the genetic disorder correlates with the clinical expressions, which would then lead to conservative surgery, or if the clinical criteria (for example the number and characteristics of the polyps in the rectum, presence of desmoids) should remain the only reliable factors playing a role in a correct technical choice [2].

Moreover, we analysed videolaparoscopic techniques to ascertain if they offer advantages over conventional open treatment, or if, in this specific case, the generic advantages of laparoscopy can be transferred to patients affected with FAP. In addition to the aesthetic benefits, appreciated mainly by younger patients, can laparoscopy reduce the risk of intestinal occlusions (reducing postoperative visceral adhesions) and the risk of the formation of desmoids (reducing the surgical scar, favoured site of these tumours)?

Some other problems that must be assessed: how to treat duodenal, periampullary and ampullary polyps and what kind of surveillance is advised in order to detect and treat the adenomas that can develop in ileoanal pouches, even many years after surgery.

Genetic Aspects in FAP

Familial adenomatous polyposis (FAP) is a hereditary disease characterised by the presence of adenomatous polyps in the colon and rectum, from a minimum of 100 (necessary number for diagnosis) up to more than 7 000, which are genetically determined by mutations of the APC (adenomatous polyposis coli) gene located on chromosome 5 [3]. Children have a 50% probability of being affected regardless of their sex. The onset is in the second and third decade of life, even if cases of early (13 months of age) or late onset (60 years) are reported. The incidence ranges from 1:8000 to 1:22000 and it is approximately estimated that one out of three patients with FAP does not have a familial history of the disease, as is therefore probably presenting a spontaneous mutation.

FAP is a generalised hyperproliferative disorder due to the constant activation of transcription and growth factors, as an ultimate result of the alterations of the protein codified by the APC gene. In addition to the typical colorectal disease, it presents various extra-colonic manifestations (gastroenteric and others) [4]. APC gene mutations responsible for FAP are of a germinal type, whereas the mutation of the somatic line is present in approximately 80% of the sporadic tumours of the colon-rectum.

From a clinical point of view, simple rectal exploration is often diagnostic: polyps in the ampulla may be evaluated with the exploring finger. Obviously, to observe the distribution, number and morphology of the polyps and to detect possible malignancies, only a complete endoscopic examination allows evaluation of the entire colon and rectum.

The main transcript of the APC gene is a 2843 amino acids protein, which is expressed in several adult tissues. This protein is implicated in signal transmission, negatively regulating the Wnt-1 path through its bind with a ß-catenin. The protein altered by the genetic mutation is not capable of binding the ß-catenin, which accumulates in the cytoplasm, determining constant activation of transcription and growth factors.

However, the main target of the germinal as well as the somatic mutations is exon 15, as it contains 75% of the codifying sequences of APC. In the majority of FAP patients, frameshift and nonsense germinal mutations were identified, with transcription of a truncated and hypofunctional protein. Germinal mutations are generally uniformly distributed between codons 200 and 1600, rarely above codon 1600. Moreover, they affect codons 1061 and 1309 more frequently. Together these account for one third of all these mutations.

It was demonstrated that the risk of developing specific FAP manifestations, as well as the disease severity on the large bowel, is related to the type of genetic mutation [5–7]. Severe forms of FAP are more frequently observed in mutations between codons 1250 and 1464. This implies an early onset, with symptoms (abdominal pain, diarrhoea, blood in the faeces) even before 20 years of age, a high number (carpet) of polyps in the colon and rectum and an early progression to malignancy.

On the other hand, the attenuated forms of FAP seem to be related to mutations of the 5' and 3' extremities of the gene, or the alternative splicing sites of codon 9. This form, called AFAP (attenuated familial adenomatous polyposis) [8], is characterised by a later onset of symptoms as well as the progression to cancer and by the presence of the so-called flat adenomas, which are mainly located in the right colon with a relative sparing of the rectum.

Mutations of codons 457 and 1444 are characteristic in patients who also present CHRPE, whereas desmoid tumours are limited to those who present mutations of codons 1403 and 1578. These, and other extra-colonic manifestations of FAP (osteomas, epidermal cysts, upper gastroenteric polyposis), can also often be observed in the presence of mutations between codons 1445 and 1578, or between 1395 and 1493.

We must mention that some clinically ascertained forms of FAP do not have a recognisable genetic mutation; that is to say, that these patients are negative for known mutations of the APC gene. These forms are characterised by a particular severity of the disease in the colon-rectum [9]. They present an early onset even with a low number of polyps which have a strong tendency to progress early to cancer, whereas extra-colonic manifestations are less frequent and severe. In these cases, screening of the call-up patients remains the domain of endoscopic examinations at a young age.

Molecular genetic techniques [10] allow individual analysis and, if a known mutation is found, allow certain diagnosis. In this way, the identification of sporadic cases is also possible. The identification of mutations of the codifying region of APC, due to the large size of the gene, is a long and expensive procedure so, in view of the fact that the majority of the mutations leads to the transcription of a truncate protein, it is faster and more convenient to evaluate mutations by means of protein analysis. More than 90% of mutations described to date result in a halt of the protein synthesis, with the expression of a truncate product. Blue White Assay and PTT (protein truncation test) are efficient and rapid methods for identifying truncate proteins.

Genetic Implication in Surgical Indication

Before the early 1980s, FAP and UC (Ulcerative Colitis) were treated with total colectomy and ileo-rectal anastomosis (IRA) or total proctocolectomy and permanent ileostomy (TP). As this radical option involved the sacrifice of the anal sphincter, both the surgeon and patient tended towards a less invaliding option even when the indication was not correct. As demonstrated by Church et al. [11], the risk of developing rectal cancer was higher before the early eighties before the introduction of restorative proctocolectomy with ileal pouch-anal anastomosis (IPAA) because the technical choice was not based only on clinical criteria, but was also conditioned by the desire to avoid a permanent ileostomy. However, the same author [12] outlined that, if the indication is correct, IRA is a good solution. In cases where there are few polyps in the colon and rectum, the risk of a subsequent proctectomy (because of the development of rectal cancer or of a high number of adenomas no longer endoscopically treatable) was very low.

IPAA made radical treatment possible, preserving the anal sphincter and reducing the risk of an inappropriate choice; therefore, this technique has become increasingly widespread. The rate of complications and the functional results are not particularly different to IRA, as described by various authors [13] and as emerging from our experience. Consequently, IPAA has become the primary choice for FAP treatment in centres specialising in major colorectal surgery. This attitude, justified also by the possibility of eradicating the colorectal disease and avoiding the risk of rectal cancer, should be re-evaluated as even ileo-anal pouches can present a progressive risk of developing adenomas which require endoscopic surveillance, just like the surveillance required for the rectum after IRA [14].

A total proctocolectomy, sacrificing the sphincter, is mandatory when a cancer is located near the dentate line, but the decision is more complex when the rectum can be spared. Clinical criteria appear to be non-univocal as regards the number (classically above or under 20) and characteristics of the polyps, the length of the rectum to spare (20 cm vs. 15 cm vs. 10 cm) [15] and the characteristics of the ileo-rectal anastomosis (hand-sewn or mechanical, side-to-end or end-to-end) that in the end can condition endoscopic removal of the polyps, functional results and any subsequent restorative proctectomy with IPAA (conversion of IRA to IPAA) respectively. In addition to the factors mentioned, the patient's desire to avoid an ileostomy (even if temporary) or the acknowledgement of sexual risks in men, or even the result of surgical treatment on relatives, appears to condition the choice of an IRA. If we also consider the possibility of performing the operation in a single laparoscopic time, avoiding temporary ileostomy with minimal aesthetic and abdominal wall damage in patients normally presenting few symptoms, IRA becomes a particularly appealing option. Thus, it has become important to encourage its renouncement in favour of a technique which is more complex and requires two surgical interventions with precise clinical indications and, if possible, supported by evidence of genetic error corresponding to a severe form of FAP destined to become a higher risk of cancer on the residual rectal stump.

Restorative proctocolectomy with IPAA, described by Parks and Nicholls in 1978 [16, 2], has a theoretical increased risk of complications compared to IRA, but this occurs only in a small percentage of cases, as opposed to IBD patients. This is probably due to the fact that hand-sewn ileo-anal anastomosis is performed on a healthy mucosa where there is no sign of inflammation.

The major risk in performing IPAA is the potential impossibility of mobilising the terminal ileum to reach the anal canal (usually due to the presence of intra-abdominal desmoids located in the mesentery, which shorten and retract the mesentery itself) in patients for whom the removal of the rectum is inevitable. In this case the only possible surgical solution is TP.

The criteria on which we base the indication of more radical surgery or less radical surgery have not changed in substance; we are always speaking of a maximum of 20 polyps in the residual rectum considering an average length of 15 cm, which is the maximum number acceptable for an IRA with subsequent endoscopic removal of polyps.

After the introduction of the IPAA, the cases of later reoperation to convert IRA also dropped; however, IPAA remains a possibility for those who undergo the less radical surgical treatment, since a tract of affected rectum remains in site and could escape endoscopic control and removal by developing an excessive number of polyps or presenting severe dysplasia or infiltrating carcinoma.

At present however, with refining genetic analysis techniques, the possibility of identifying the mutation carried by the patient (whether it is related to a severe phenotype or not) has taken on a fundamental role in the indication of the type of surgical treatment in terms of radicality.

In the presence of severe clinical features, the indication of radical surgery is clear regarding the entire removal of the affected part. Instead, in the presence of clinical features which are not particularly severe, before choosing a total colectomy with ileo-rectal anastomosis, it is necessary to consider the type of genetic mutation. In fact, it is now well known that mutations have been identified which involve a more indolent trait of the pathology and others which involve a marked severity of the disease irrespective of the clinical features at the moment of diagnosis. We must not forget those cases in this second group of patients for whom the choice of performing less radical surgery in the first place led to the necessity of reoperating at a later date because of the development of clinically more severe lesions in the tract of the residual rectum. In these cases, the surgeon had to convert IRA into a restorative proctectomy with IPAA, or into a TP with permanent ileostomy; the latter option being determined by technical reasons (short ileum vessels to reach the anal canal) or due to the disease (development of carcinoma in patients who did not go through follow-up).

Thus, the results of the genetic test can contribute to indicating the correct surgical treatment suited to the degree and severity of the disease, mainly to avoid patients undergoing a treatment which is under-estimated in terms of the real potential aggressiveness of the pathology. Endoscopic evaluation of clinical features remains without doubt an unavoidable datum, which, however, is subject to factors such as the subjectivity of the operator's judgment, which limit its adequacy and precision.

With the identification of mutations on the APC gene responsible for the disease , the introduction of genetic analysis methods [10] for the affected patients and, above all, the screening of their relatives, it is possible to determine the individuals at risk of developing the disease and the gravity with which it would present itself if it weren't treated. As concerns our case histories, we are not short of examples: we have treated two cousins with IPAA for a severe disease and the sister of one of them had also been operated on (in another surgical unit) for what the surgeon had defined as an IPAA, but which had preserved some centimetres of rectum. This woman came under our observation after annual endoscopic surveillance of the short residual rectum; the impossibility of continuing with endoscopic management led to surgery but at the time of the operation a carcinoma was already present, invading the transitional zone and making a Miles' operation necessary (Fig. 1).

Thus, it could be a matter of discussion whether to treat a patient with IRA who carries a mutation related to a potentially severe genotype that has a high tendency for developing rectal cancer, even if at the moment of surgery the rectum presented a not-so-high number of polyps still controllable via endoscopic removals. One could force the patient to undergo endoscopic management at ever-closer time intervals, with an increased risk of complications, thereby exposing him to the risk of being forced to undergo more radical surgery later.

Considering the fact that the two surgical solutions are very similar in terms of the quality of life as well as functional results [2] (except that restorative proctocolectomy is technically more complex to perform), the choice of the correct operation for FAP treatment seems less bound to the subjective judgment of surgeon; on the contrary it becomes more precise when supported by a prediction on genetic grounds. In order to compare claims made in literature against our case history findings, we highlighted a particular item of data concerning the ratio between the severity of the mutation, the type of operation performed and the need for a further operation (Figs. 2, 3).

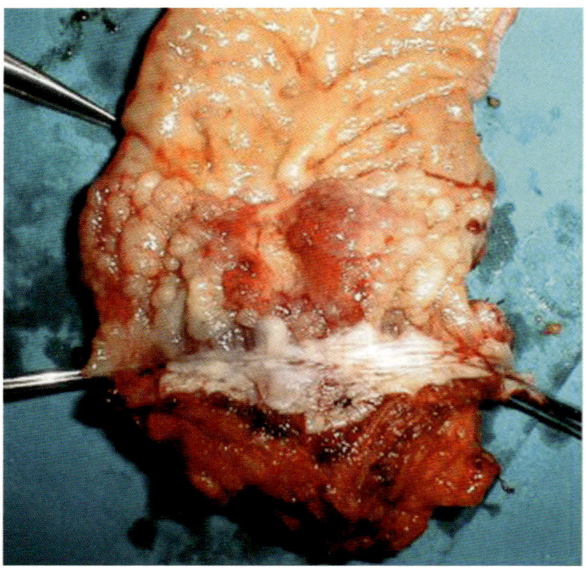

Fig. 1. Transitional zone invaded by carcinoma

When a slight mutation was present, IPAA was performed in seven cases and IRA in seven cases. None of the IRA operations performed so far, for a slight mutation, have required conversion to IPAA. Only endoscopic removal of rectal polyps has been necessary, but one patient who escaped follow-up died because of a hepatic metastasis probably due to rectal cancer. In patients with severe mutation, in one case we directly performed a Miles operation, sigmoid resection in one for palliative purposes, IPAA in ten cases and IRA in seven cases. Of the seven cases of IRA, five asked for conversion. In three of the five cases, a Miles operation was performed as cancer was detected in polyps that were so close to the anal canal that conversion to IPAA was not possible, while in two cases conversion was successfully performed to treat widespread polyps which could not be managed by endoscopic removal. However, the histological tests of one of these two patients indicated a stage B1 carcinoma that had not been detected in the preoperative stage. In three of these five cases, IRA had been performed at another hospital and decisions were not dictated by the clinical criteria in use at the time, but by the experience of the surgeon and the patient's wish to avoid a permanent ileostomy. In the two patients we previously operated on by performing IRA, one underwent a Miles operation as a carcinoma was detected on a polyp close to the dentate line which had not been noted during surveillance and endoscopic removal. IRA had been chosen for this patient due to the presence of a mesenteric desmoid, while in the other patient, genetic testing was not carried out in the preoperative stage, so the decision was dictated by a number of polyps bordering the rectum (around 20) and by the concurrent presence of jaundice, caused by duodenal adenomatous polyp. In this last case, despite the degenerated rectal polyp, conversion to IPAA was possible. To sum up, only two of the seven patients with severe mutation undergoing an IRA are still being treated for the routine removal of rectal polyps and at present have not requested conversion.

From an assessment of the literature and on the basis of our experience, it is clear that today the deci-

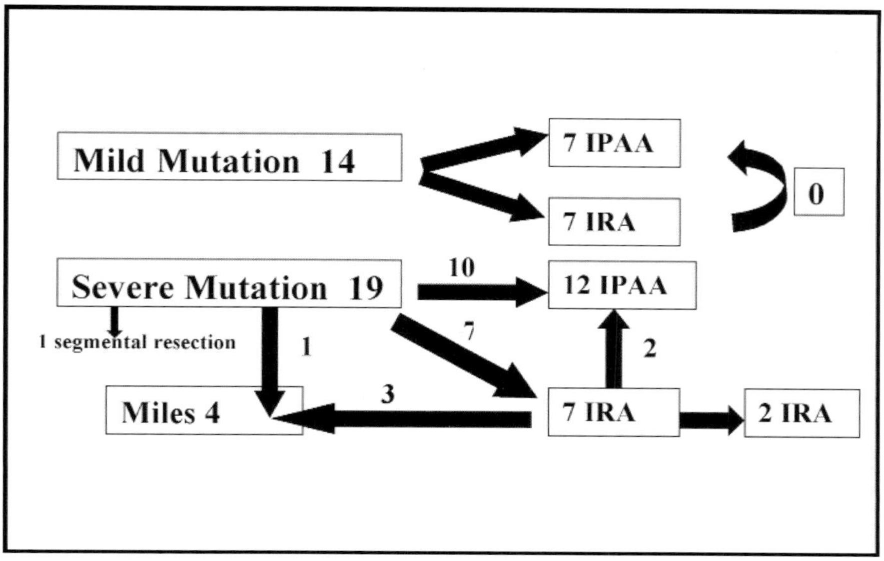

Fig. 2. IRA-genetic factors-IPAA. Retrospective aspects in our series of FAP patients. *Known mutation* = 33; *unknown* = 7; *total patients treated* = 40

Total proctocolectomy 5 of which 3 conversion due to cancer
Ileo-pouch-anal anastomosis 22 (4 conversion from IRA)
Ileorectal anastomosis (IRA) 19 (3 conversion to Miles)
Segmentary resection: 1
Desmoid tumors: 7
Colorectal cancer: 12 (10 patients)
Duodenotomy to remove an ampullary adenoma: 2
Palliative derivation for advanced ampullary cancer: 1
Total gastrectomy for gastric cancer
55% FAP patient with duodenal and gastric polyps
Dead (1 hepatic metastasis, 1 ampullary c., 1 C.C., 1 desmoid t)
Mean follow-up time 9.8 years - lost to follow-up: 1

Fig. 3. Case histories of 40 patients: surgical options and mutations. *Severe mutations* 19; *mild mutations* = 14; *unknown mutations* = 7

sion to leave the rectum must be prompted by the presence of sporadic rectal polyps and a slight genetic mutation, the absence of severe dysplasia or colon of the cancer and more rarely by the presence of intra-abdominal or mesenteric desmoids which advise against IPAA. As stated by several authors, it is difficult to perform endoscopic surveillance when there are many adjoining polyps; this increases the risk of progression to malignant transformation, even in patients who undergo regular follow-ups [17].

Thus, the risk of cancer of the rectum can easily be correlated to the above factors, as noted by Bertario's study [18] on patients in the Italian FAP registry, and particularly when cancer of the colon is present when IRA is performed in conjunction with a genetic error between codon 1250 and codon 1464.

Peculiar Aspects of Gastroenteric Extra-Colonic Manifestations of FAP

Among the possible extra-colonic manifestations are upper gastroenteric lesions, stomach polyps (25–60% of the patients) and duodenal polyps (24–73%) [19–21]. Hyperplastic polyps are commonly observed at a gastric level, whereas at a duodenal level and in the Vater's ampulla we mostly have real adenomas which are also subject to the rule of "adenoma-carcinoma" progression. Therefore, periodic endoscopic surveillance of the upper gastroenteric tract with possible removal of duodenal adenomas is essential.

An issue which is still open to discussion is the evaluation of the Vater's ampulla [22, 23]. It is known that FAP involves a higher risk of adenomas and carcinoma of the ampulla, in addition to duodenal polyposis (an estimated incidence around 60% *vs.* 3% of general population). The risk of developing adenomas and carcinoma of the Vater's ampulla is increased in patients affected with FAP with an incidence ranging from 50–86% considering adenomas, carcinoma In Situ and adenocarcinoma vs. the 2.9 cases per million people of the general population.

Nowadays the gold standard for diagnosis is represented by endoscopic retrograde cholangiopancreatography (ERCP) which allows evaluation of the morphology of the Vater's ampulla. When there is any doubt about the adenomatous localisations it is possible to perform biopsies of the mucosa after an endoscopic sphincterotomy. Alternatively, when sphincterotomy is contraindicated, a brushing cytologic exam could be indicated even if this method is not commonly used at present because of the high percentage of false negatives.

Magnetic resonance cholangiopancreatic (MRCP) could substitute for ERCP in diagnosing ampullary neoplasm, since it offers good imaging of the biliary tree and gives information on the dimension, extension and relationship to the nearby vascularisation of the possible tumour. Staging an ascertained papillary expansive lesion is left to endoscopic ultrasound (EUS). The possibility of performing internal sonographic scansions with different wavelengths (5 and 7.5 MHz) allows visualisation of the wall layers (determining dimension and grade of intramural invasion) as well as the nearby structures (with evaluation of the any lymph-node involvement and the presence of distant metastasis). Diagnostic use of EUS is now foreseen: it must be noted that this procedure has a medium level of invasiveness compared to MRCP (zero invasiveness) and ERCP (high invasiveness with risks of serious complications such as acute pancreatitis).

Bare local resection can be performed in benign adenomas. In this case it is possible to choose between an endoscopic approach and a surgical one. The former is indicated for adenomas with extra-ampullary growth (periampullary area) smaller than 1 cm and not carrying severe dysplasia, even if the risk of recurrence for incomplete removal is 20%. For adenomas larger than 1 cm and for ampullary ones, surgical polypectomy is indicated as well as resection of the papilla of Vater with reconstruction of the pancreatic and biliary duct by means of an eight shaped plastic.

Surgical removal treatment is possible for 75% of the patients with invasive adenocarcinoma and the primary technique is Whipple's pancreatoduodenectomy, with a mortality rate of less than 5%. In a subpopulation with increased probability of ampullary carcinoma, such as FAP patients, early diagnosis (in the preclinical phase or in the benign phase) should be promoted, since these patients represent a small group at high risk of pathology. In addition, precisely due to this exiguity of cases, promotion is not yet a reality, since there is no standard protocol in the literature for the follow-up, selection and timing of diagnostic exams.

To sum up, even though a higher incidence of ampullary neoplasm for FAP patients is well known, no procedure was identified as being sufficiently sensitive for a subgroup of patients more at risk of developing this manifestation. However, it is likely that, just like the correlation between genetics and severity of colorectal disease, the type of genetic alteration plays an important role also in the development of duodenal and ampullary lesions, again in terms of severity of the disease.

It is known that there are genetic mutations associated with an increased risk of superior gastroenteric polyposis, stomach and duodenum, such as mutations between codon 1445 and 1578, or between 1395 and 1493; but there are still no indications on the association between specific mutations and ampullary neoplasm. These genetic errors are part of the gene tract normally related to the severe form of FAP, as occurred in one of our patients who came under our observation for jaundice. While awaiting the ultimate genetic mapping, this patient underwent endoscopic removal of an ampullary polyp and contemporary total colectomy with IRA. Later, during short-term surveillance, a cancerised polyp was detected for which this patient was converted from IRA to IPAA; this evolution could have been expected according to the genetic finding of a severe mutation. However, in our series of patients there is an entire family of five female individuals with mild mutation presenting duodenal adenomas which are treated endoscopically; still, two of them had to undergo surgery. The mother presented an ampullary-pancreatic tumour that at the time of the operation allowed only palliative derivation, the daughter instead presented a progression of the duodenal polyps to severe dysplasia and the development of ampullary polyps diagnosed with RMN and EUS, which required surgical management by means of wide transduodenal ampullectomy. Considering the possibility that the duodenal lesions could be related to a genetically severe model of FAP as well as a non-severe one; and, as described in the literature, also in an AFAP, it is clear that endoscopic gastroduodenal surveillance is recommended to prevent the development of gastric and duodenal polyps for all patients regardless of the mutation [24]. At present the need for a follow-up protocol, based on the individual patient's characteristics and disease features, is increasingly pressing so that lesions can be identified in the preclinical phase, when radical treatment is still possible.

As already mentioned, even desmoid tumours are problematic in treating FAP [25, 26]. Intra-abdominal desmoid tumours may significantly affect the choice of surgical treatment or, if they develop during the postoperative stage, they are extremely difficult to treat and results are often unsatisfactory. Abdominal-wall desmoid tumours are less aggressive and easier to treat, and therefore can be entirely removed [27]. In our experience, parietal desmoid tumours appear in four out of five cases after surgery at the site of surgical scarring.

This aspect led us to think that long incisions and trauma on the muscles could support the subsequent development of abdominal-wall desmoids. Regarding this hypothesis, we are evaluating the impact that small scars such as the ones we have with the VDL approach, could have in determining desmoid development. Up to now only one of the patients operated on with the VDL approach has developed a desmoid tumour where the former protection ileostomy was.

Conventional and Videolaparoscopic Treatment

When IPAA is performed for UC some technical questions are still debated, especially about the type of ileoanal anastomosis (hand-sewn after mucosectomy or stapled without mucosectomy) and the number of surgical stages: one, two or three (total colectomy, restorative proctectomy with IPAA, removal of protection ileostomy). In patients affected with FAP, total colectomy and IRA are performed in a single operation without any protection ileostomy, whereas IPAA is usually a two-stage technique (with a loop ileostomy, to be removed about 2 months later); a single operation (avoiding the loop ileostomy) can be performed only with a stapled ileoanal anastomosis [28–30], but this could be regarded as a non-radical therapy because of the risk of adenomatous growth in the spared transitional mucosa. Both operations, IPAA and IRA, can be approached in a traditional or videolaparoscopic way.

The conventional approach involves a large central laparotomy through which total colectomy and total proctocolectomy are easily performed with a traditional technique familiar to all colorectal surgeons, even if details may differ according to the surgical school and points of view on the radicality of IPAA. Laparoscopic surgery has spread widely in the last 10 years thanks also to the continuous improvement of the instruments involved and to the enthusiasm of various surgical schools.

As regards colorectal surgery, the laparoscopic approach was initially used to treat benign diseases or in palliative operations because of the fear of neoplasm implantation on the scars of trocar accesses; however, despite its progressive diffusion and satisfactory employment in the oncology field, its use is still not completely accepted. The need to remove large and voluminous specimen from the abdomen has led to the use of videolaparoscopic-assisted techniques (VDLA), meaning short "service" incisions to carry out this part of the operation. Some problems still remain: a major technical complexity (difficult manoeuvres to be performed on delicate organs such as the colon, ileum and relative mesentery without the help of stereoscopic vision and tactile sensibility) and a long learning curve [31, 32], so that at present most major colorectal surgery is still performed using the traditional approach, whereas the laparoscopic technique is employed at specialised centres.

However, videolaparoscopy offers significant advantages for patients mainly of a young age who can appreciate the better cosmetic effect due to small scars or scars located in easily hidden sites (Pfannenstiel incision). In addition, postoperative pain is reduced, offering advantages in terms of hospitalisation, with an earlier recovery capacity and return to normal activity, which are in line with the literature [33, 34]. A more favourable immune response [35] and reduction or absence of visceral adhesions represents another reason for using the laparoscopic approach, thereby increasing its indications.

Videolaparoscopic Hand-Assisted Technique

Surgeons who support "pure" laparoscopic surgery use the service access essentially to remove the surgical specimen or for extra-body anastomosis, but the very need to perform this incision led to the development of instruments through which the surgeon could insert a hand into the patient's abdomen, while maintaining the pneumoperitoneum. These instruments (hand-ports) allow an incision a few centimetres long that can be located in the hypogastrium and therefore it is also aesthetically acceptable for the patient. They enhance both the efficacy of laparoscopy and the tactile sensitivity offered by the hand inserted in the abdomen.

This approach, which utilizes the hand-port, is called hand-assisted laparoscopy (HAL). With a sufficiently large protected access, it is possible to comfortably remove the specimen but most of all to insert a hand in the abdomen with the possibility of restoring tactile sense, of dislocating the intestine with a less traumatic traction than that of any laparoscopic instrument, thus obtaining better colon exposure. Even haemostasis in the case of a bleeding colic vessel can be easily conducted, reducing the blood loss and/or the need for conversion.

In comparing the conventional laparoscopic technique (VDLA) [32, 36] with HAL, results seem markedly superior in the latter case above all in terms of reduced operating time and consequently total costs, without reducing the known advantages of the laparoscopic approach compared to the traditional open approach [37]. Moreover, the learning curve for HAL appears to be shorter because technical gestures are more similar to the traditional ones. In FAP patients, contraindications are minimal and are generally related to the presence of desmoid tumours, mostly intra-abdominal ones, or to the presence of colic or rectal cancer, at least in our experience.

Hand-Assisted Technique with Personal Adjustments

When we began using HAL, the type of hand-port we chose was a Lap-Disc (Ethicon Endosurgery, USA;

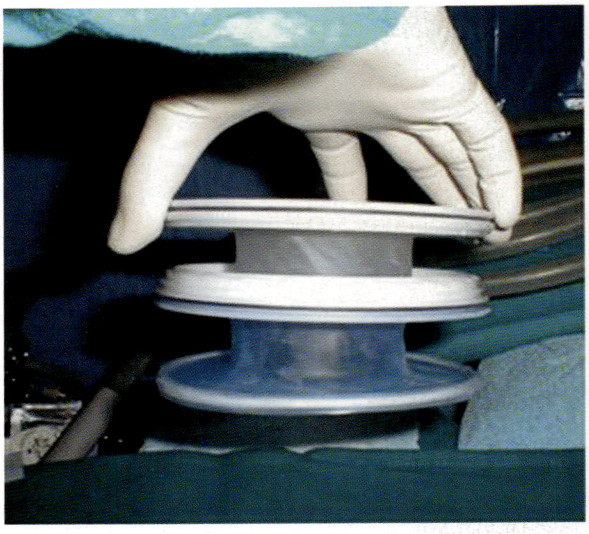

Fig. 4. Lap Disc

Fig. 4). This system is made of rubber rings and a double circle which allows its rotation and closure as a diaphragm around the hand, while at the bottom, the rubber ring models its form, which is generally opened in the hypogastrium site, on the abdominal wall (7-cm incision according to Pfannenstiel).

The patient is adjusted as for a cholecystectomy with parted legs and the operator in between, and the operation begins with a Pfannenstiel incision in the hypogastric region of exactly 7 cm. After opening the cutaneous tissue and subcutaneous tissue, we proceed by liberating the fascia vertically for 7 cm, opening it according to Kustner. We prepare a temporary suture between the peritoneum and fascia on the two sides of the incision to reduce the trauma caused by the divaricators in the first phase ("open") and by the hand in the second phase ("HAL"). Exposing the operative field in a traditional way, we proceed on the right to identify and lift the cecum and to mobilise it with its appendix and the last tract of ileum (Fig. 5).

We separate the ileum and cecum with a linear stapler (GIA60), taking care to spare as much ileum as possible. We identify the right ureter and gonadic vessels and complete the mobilisation of the cecum with the section of the terminal branches directed towards it, sparing the ileo-colic artery arch. We uncover the sigmoid-rectal junction and prepare the rectum and separate it from the sigma again with the linear stapler GIA60 already used. We proceed by further mobilising the sigma by tying and sectioning the sigmoidal vessels reached through the Pfannenstiel incision.

Inserting the first 10-mm trocar on the right side,

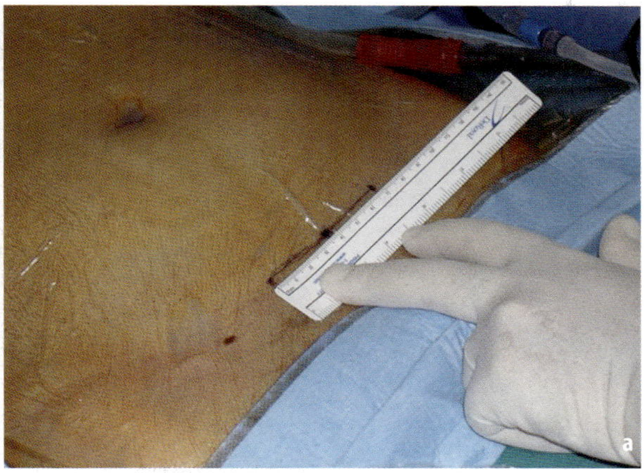

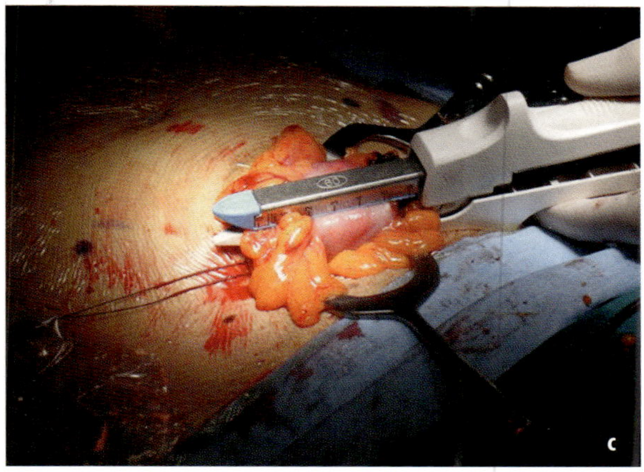

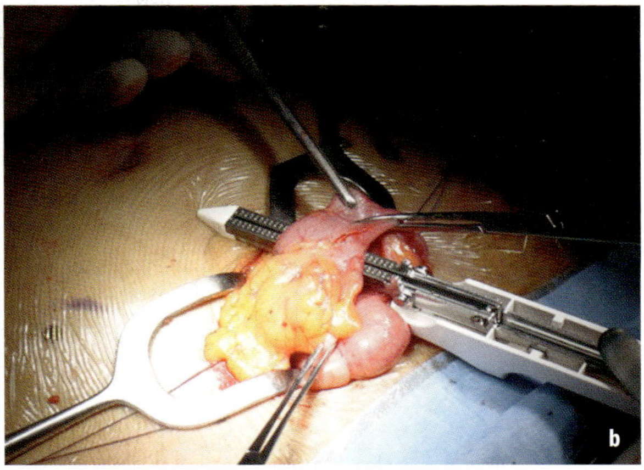

Fig. 5a Measurement of 7 cm before Pfannenstiel incision. **b** Separation of ileum from ciecum, with GIA. **c** Separation of sigma from rectum, with GIA

we place the Lap-Disc in the Pfannenstiel incision inducing pneumoperitoneum. We insert the second 10-mm trocar on the left symmetrically to the first. We introduce the video-camera which will remain on the right for the entire operation (the operation is possible with both the 0 and 30° optical camera, even if the second option offers a better view). We observe the visceral disposition and introduce the third and last trocar in the right hypochondrium near the rib arcade (Fig. 6).

Tractioning the sigmoid colon with the left hand and using a Babcock forceps through the upper trocar, we expose the colon mesentery starting the synthesis and section of the colic vessels with the instrument inserted in the left trocar. We generally use a radiofrequency instrument (Ligasure-Atlas™, Valleylab, CA, USA), particularly indicated for colic vessels; but also the last generation of ultrasound instruments (Ultracision®, Ethicon Endosurgery, OH, USA) can be used. These instruments allow a reduction in the instrument traffic which was responsible for the increased surgical time during the first years of experience with this surgery. Thus, it is possible to perform the entire operation with just one instrument.

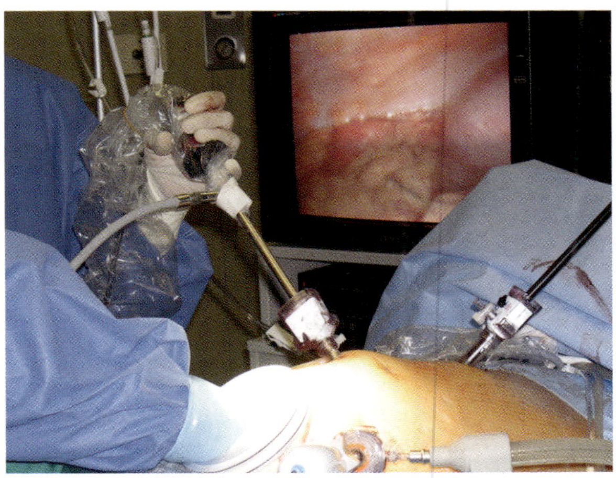

Fig. 6. Videolaparoscopic colectomy: right hand controlling Ligasure-Atlas and left hand in the patient's abdomen through Lap Disc

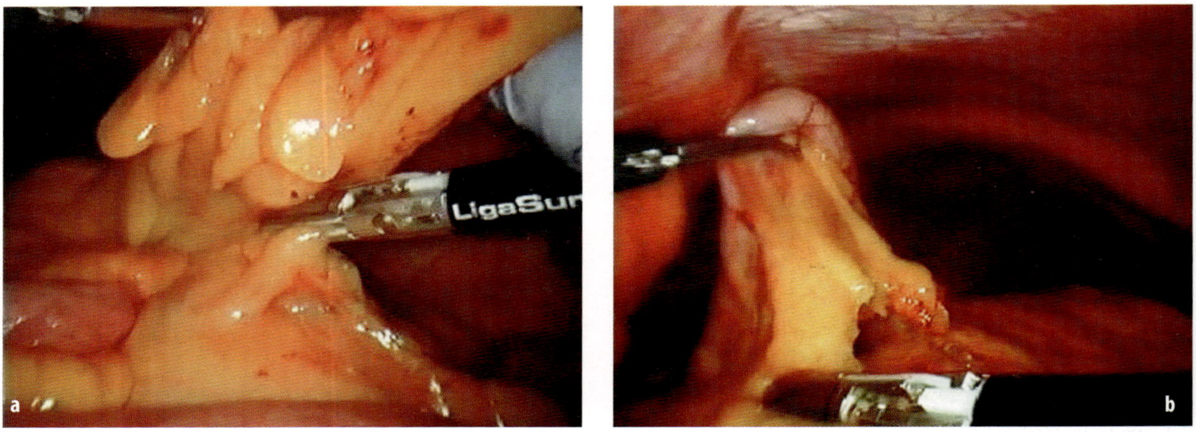

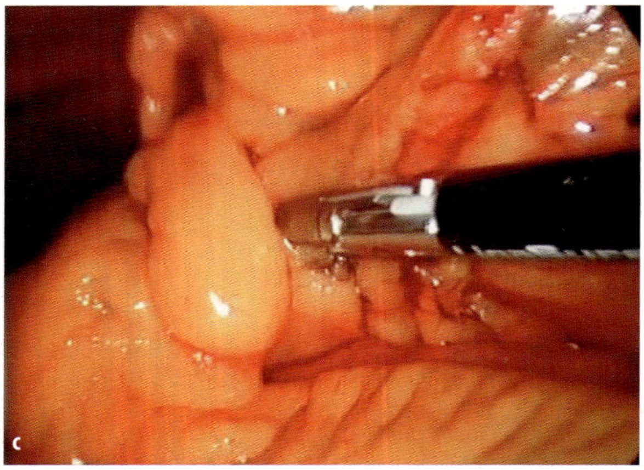

Fig. 7a Mobilisation of left colon. **b** Section of gastro-colic ligament. **c** Section of the middle colic artery

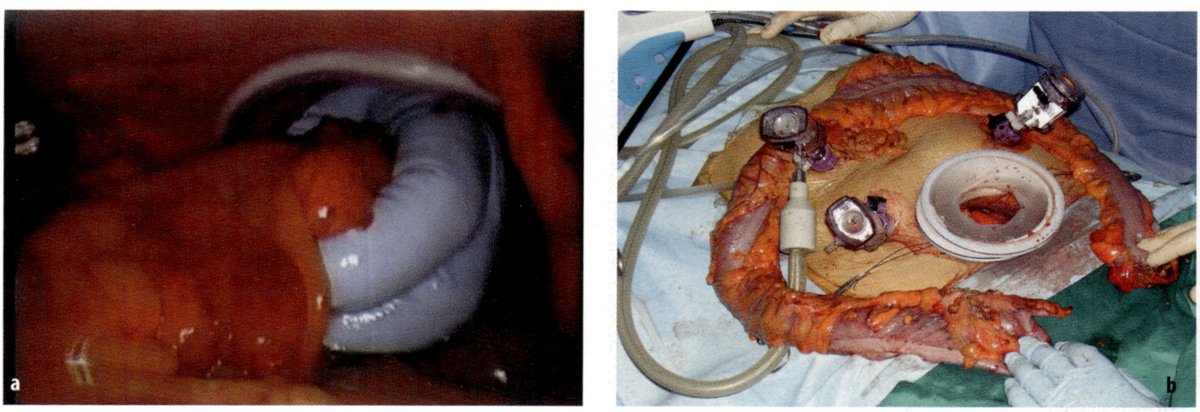

Fig. 8a, b. Extraction of specimen through Lap Disc

The curved end of the Ligasure-Atlas also allows a gentle dissection similar to that obtainable with fingers. Mobilisation of the left flexure (Fig. 7), like in open surgery, is a delicate phase of the operation that can be carried out after separating the omentum in the colic corner either continuing the liberation facing the spleen, or from above, after separating colon from the stomach, sectioning the gastrocolic ligament. In more complex cases either approach can be used. In order to facilitate gestures on the right colon and on the hepatic flexure, we rotate the patient to the left and begin mobilising the right colon, tractioning the cecum to the left with the hand. After recognising the duodenum we complete the section of the right colon mesentery and hepatic flexure until we obtain the complete liberation of the colon which can be easily removed through the Lap-Disc (Fig. 8).

The operation is carried out with a hand-sewn end-to-end anastomosis between the terminal ileum and the previously sectioned rectum (IRA). Preference for a hand-sewn anastomosis, which can be comfortably performed through the Pfannanstiel incision, is dictated by the need to preserve as much ileum length as possible to be able to perform an IPAA, when necessary, with maximum guarantee of success.

If a proctocolectomy is indicated, we proceed as already described for the colectomy, except for the fact that the rectum is not initially sectioned and that the pneumoperitoneum can be maintained by removing the colon through the Lap-Disc. This also allows a traction on the rectum so that pelvic dissection is facilitated (Fig. 9); once the pelvic floor is reached, the rectum is sectioned on the plane of the elevator muscle. Rectum removal, especially in men, is conducted following an intramesenteric plane in order to minimise the risk of neurological damage, unless a TME (total mesorectal excision) is indicated by the presence of cancer. After this first proctectomy, restorative surgery is carried out including mobilisation of the terminal ileum mesentery, preparation of the ileal pouch and of the ileo-anal anasto-

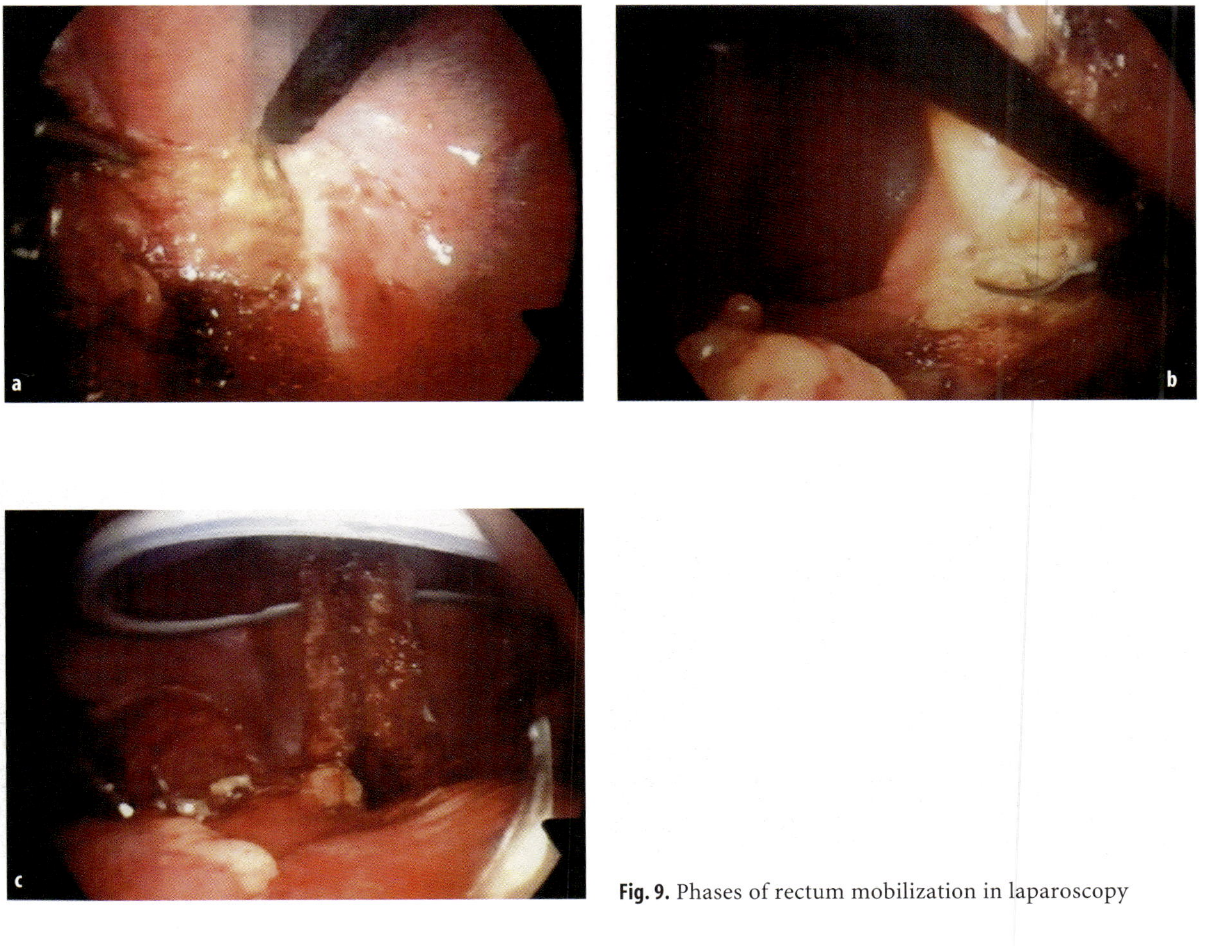

Fig. 9. Phases of rectum mobilization in laparoscopy

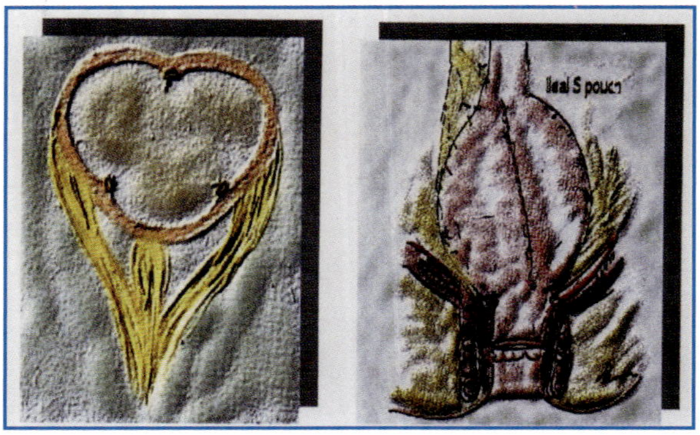

Fig. 10. S pouch (section design, position in the pelvis, operative view)

mosis, both protected by a loop-ileostomy. In our experience, this surgery is always performed using a traditional approach using the 7-cm Pfannenstiel incision, or enlarging it by a few centimetres, to mobilise the terminal ileum and prepare the "S" reservoir (three loop pouch) [38–40].

World literature documents the easier execution of the J pouch which can be entirely made with staplers, but in our opinion there are still good reasons to prefer a more handmade approach, with a hand-sewn S pouch that permits personal adjustments case by case, depending on the patient's characteristics. In our experience and in that of other authors [41], the terminal ileum sectioned on the ileo-cecal valve can reach a more distant site than the end of a J pouch. Even after mobilisation of the terminal ileum and section of the ileo-colic artery, which allows its maximum length, an S pouch does not modify the total length of the vascular arch. Moreover, the risk of needing to drop IPAA cannot be underestimated, even in expert hands, as it accounts for over 4% of the cases for different reasons [39] such as difficulties related to ileum vascularisation (Fig. 10).

Moreover, in our experience, as the mucosectomy has to be carried out from the dentate line, the "S" reservoir seems to be the most suitable. An aspect that is still being discussed, however, concerns the suitability of performing a mucosectomy and thus a hand-sewn, end-to-end, ileoanal anastomosis (for the S reservoir), removing the residual rectal mucosa (1.5–3 cm long) from the dentate line including the transitional epithelium between the anal and rectal mucosa. If a mucosectomy is not performed and stapling (often double stapling) is carried out, the entire transitional zone—at a minimum—is left: more centimetres of rectal mucosa may easily be left in relation to the thickness of the pelvic floor, the patient's sex and surgeon's skills.

The benefits of stapling include faster operating times, slightly better functional results and the possibility of avoiding a protective ileostomy. However, a 28% risk of adenomas forming in the transition zone and in the residual rectal mucosa exists, as demonstrated by Remzi et al. [43]. In our opinion, the risk

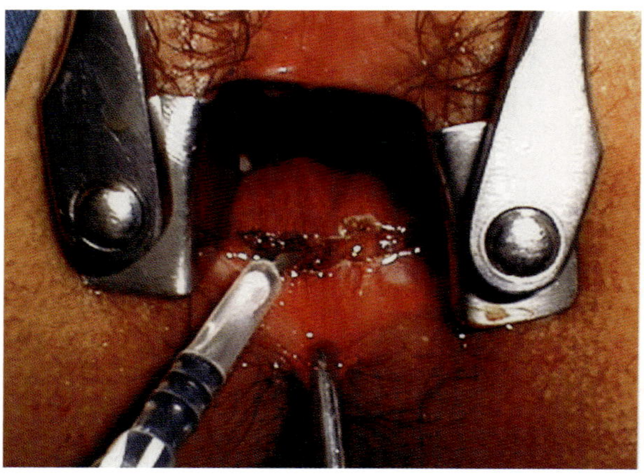

Fig. 11. Mucosectomy

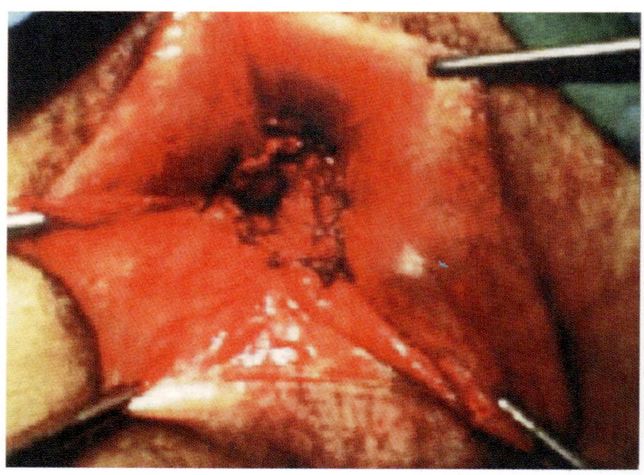

Fig. 12. Ileo-anal hand-sewn anastomosis

of cancer developing is relevant as it is not always easy to monitor and treat polyps close to the dentate line and malignant transformation can also occur during endoscopic follow-up [17].

Also Ooi et al. [44], in a recent work, points out the need for careful monitoring of the transitional zone left In Situ for cancer risks, and reconsiders the suitability of mucosectomy in patients with widespread polyps on the rectal mucosa. In our experience, we have always carried out mucosectomy from the dentate line and in the second case of FAP operated on in 1985, this decision was prompted by the discovery of a stage A Dukes carcinoma in the removed mucosa section. Once mucosectomy is carried out and the reservoir is located in the pelvic space, ileoanal hand-sewn anastomosis in one layer is executed (Figs. 11, 12).

From 1984 to 2005, we have operated on 40 cases of FAP with all the techniques in our possession, including the Kock pouch for a continent ileostomy in a patient who could not preserve the sphincters but wanted to reduce the problems related to definitive ileostomy. In 1996, we started treating FAP patients, when possible, with the videolaparoscopic techniques previously described. In this period, 9 out of 17 FAP patients were treated (2 with IRA, 7 with IPAA) with VDL or HALS, without any major complications when compared to the traditional open technique. Only two patients needed postoperative blood transfusion (one for each group) and no one in the laparoscopic group had an infection of the Pfannestiel incision. In our experience functional results such as continence, urgency, number of bowel movements and sexual functions do not differ significantly between IRA and IPAA and in patients operated with traditional or laparoscopic technique. With the HALS technique, the time needed to perform an IRA or IPAA is now quite similar to that needed in the traditional open technique; postoperative pain is normally lower and the patient can be discharged earlier. Moreover, the cost-effectiveness of laparoscopy increases with experience and patient satisfaction is greater. At the moment, the low number of patients operated on with this technique does not allow statistical evaluation of the risk of postoperative bowel occlusion and of desmoid tumour growth at the scar site. The laparoscopic experience obtained by treating IBD patients with HALS showed an absence of adherences in the second stage of the operation (proctectomy and IPAA) and this situation seems to reduce the risk of bowel occlusion. None of the nine patients treated with laparoscopy needed readmission, while 2 out of 31 patients treated traditionally were readmitted due to bowel occlusion and one needed surgery for adherences.

Conclusions

While the possibility of choosing the correct surgical option is certainly related to the surgeon's skills with all the technical solutions, the possibility of having genetical markers predicting the severity of the disease would make the surgeon's task easier in proposing different solutions for different presentations of the pathology. In fact we have experienced that extra-colonic manifestations of the disease also determine other aggravating factors and that eradication of the colorectal disease does not solve the problem.

We have been able to observe how in our case histories a non-radical choice such as IRA, when associated with a severe mutation, involved a high risk of conversion or demolition of the anal sphincters so in this case the choice of an IPAA seems justified. The more radical choice becomes more difficult in cases of severe mutation and clinical features compatible with IRA, when a patient requests the preservation of the rectum or when it is impossible to detect the genetic error. In these situations, it is advisable to evaluate the case without following a fixed scheme. By educating the patient on the need for constant follow-up, the risk of degeneration appears reduced; moreover, as outlined by our experience and in the literature, it is possible to convert IRA into IPAA in the majority of the cases especially when IRA was conducted preserving all the ileum. On the other hand, if we consider mucosal polyps growth at the pouch level (as recently highlighted in the literature [14, 45]) and their possible evolution to cancer, it is easy to see that the first surgical choice appears more important considering that even a radical solution such as IPAA could not completely solve the FAP problems at the colorectal level. The laparoscopic approach can achieve an almost complete absence of visceral adhesions. This has been assessed at further operations when total colectomy had been the first surgical step of an IPAA for Ulcerative Colitis (UC). This aspect, on one hand, involves a lower risk of occlusive complications and, on the other, makes conversion to IPAA more comfortable when necessary. It is clear that the videolaparoscopic approach is appealing particularly for young people due to the reduced aesthetic damage and IRA is appealing due to the possibility of performing a single operation without ileostomic protection.

References

1. Frield W, Caspari R, Sengteller M et al (2001) Can APC mutation analysis contribute to therapeutic decision in familial adenomatous polyposis? Experience from

680 FAP families. Gut 45:515–521
2. Contessini-Avesani E, Botti F, Negri C et al (2004) Familial adenomatous polyposis. Surgical treatment: when and how. Tech Coloproctol 8:S309–S314
3. Moisio AL, Jarvinen H, Peltomaki P (2002) Genetic and clinic characterization of familial adenomatous polyposis: a population based study. Gut 50:845–850
4. Crabtree D, Tomlinson IPM, Hodgson SV et al (2002) Explaining variation in familial adenomatous polyposis: relationship between genotype and phenotype and evidence for modifier genes. Gut 51:420–423
5. Scott RJ, Meldrum C, Crooks R et al (2001) Familial adenomatous polyposis: more evidence for disease diversity and genetic heterogeneity. Gut 48:508–514
6. Ponz de Leon M, Varesco L, Benatti P et al (2001) Phenotype-Genotype correlations in an extended family with adenomatosis coli and an unusual APC gene mutation. Dis Colon Rectum 44:1597–1604
7. Matsumoto T, Lida M, Kobori T et al (2002) Serrated adenoma in familial adenomatous polyposis: relation to germline APC gene mutation. Gut 50:402–404
8. Hernegger GS, Harvey MD, Moore G, Guillem JG (2002) Attenuated familial adenomatous polyposis: an evolving and poorly understood entity. Dis Colon Rectum 45:127–136
9. Bisgaard ML, Ripa R, Knudsen AL, Bulow SL (2004) Familial adenomatous polyposis patients without an identified APC germline mutation have a severe fenotype. Gut 53:266–270
10. Jarvinen HJ (2003) Genetic testing for polyposis: practical and ethical aspects. Gut 52(Suppl II):19–22
11. Church J, Burke C, McGannon E et al (2003) Risk of rectal cancer in patients after colectomy and ileorectal anastomosis for familial adenomatous polyposis: a function of available surgical options. Dis Colon Rectum 46:1175–1181
12. Church J, Burke C, McGannon E et al (2001) Predicting polyposis severity by proctoscopy: how reliable is it? Dis Colon Rectum 44:1249–1254
13. Bjork J, Akerbrant H, Iselius H et al (2001) Outcome of primary and secondary ileal pouch-anal anastomosis and ileorectal anastomosis in patients with familial adenomatous polyposis. Dis Colon Rectum 44:984–992
14. Contessini-Avesani E, Grossano L, Botti F et al (2001) Adenomas in the ileal pouch after restorative proctocolectomy in patients with familial adenomatous polyposis (FAP). Gut 49(Suppl III):A2275
15. Tonelli F, Valanzano R, Monaci I et al (1997) Restorative proctocolectomy or rectum-preserving surgery in patients with familial adenomatous polyposis: results of a prospective study. World J Surg 21:653–659
16. Parks AG, Nicholls RJ (1978) Proctocolectomy without ileostomy for ulcerative colitis. BMJ 2:85–88
17. Vasen HF, Van Duijvendjk P, Buskens E et al (2001) Decision analysis in the surgical treatment of patients with familial adenomatous polyposis: a Dutch-Scandinavian collaborative study including 659 patients. Gut 49:231–235
18. Bertario L, Russo A, Radice P et al (2000) Genotype and phenotype factors in patients with familia adenomatous polyposis. Ann of Surg 231(4):538–543
19. Kashiwagi, Spigelman AD (2000) Gastroduodenal lesion in familial adenomatous polyposis. Surgery Today 30:675–682
20. Bulow S, Bjork J, Christensen IJ et al (2004) Duodenal adenomatosis in familial adenomatous polyposis. Gut 53:381–386
21. Groves CG, Saunders BP, Spigelman AD, Phillips RKS (2002) Duodenal cancer in patients with familial adenomatous polyposis (FAP): results of a 10-year prospective study. Gut 50:636–641
22. Feldman M, Friedman L, Sleisengen M (eds) (2004) Sleisenger and Fordtran's gastrointestinal and liver disease. Saunders, Philadelphia, PA, USA
23. Chareton B, Caffic J, Landen S et al (1996) Diagnosis and therapy for ampullary tumors: 63 cases. World J Surg 20:707–712
24. Trimbath JD, Griffin C, Romans K, Giardiello FM (2003) Attenuated familial adenomatous polyposis presenting as ampullary adenocarcinoma. Gut 52:903–904
25. Sturt NJH, Gallagher MC, Bassett P et al (2004) Evidence for genetic predisposition to desmoid tumours in familial adenomatous polyposis independent of the germline APC mutation. Gut 53:1832–1836
26. Heiskanen I, Jarvinen HJ (1996) Occurrence of desmoid tumours in familial adenomatous polyposis and results of treatment. Colorectal Dis 11:157–162
27. Clarck SK, Neale KF, Landgrebe JC, Phillips RKS (1999) Desmoid tumors complicating familial adenomatous polyposis. Br J Surg 86:1185–1189
28. Heuschen UA, Allemeyer EH, Lucas M et al (2001) One- or two-stage procedure for restorative proctocolectomy. Ann Surg 234:788–794
29. Sugerman HJ, Sugerman EL, Meador JG et al (2000) Ileal pouch anal anastomosis without ileal diversion. Ann Surg 232:530–541
30. Gullberg K, Liljeqvist L (2001) Stapled ileoanal pouches without loop ileostomy: a prospective study in 86 patients. Int J Colorect Dis 16:221–227
31. Jakimowicz JJ (2000) Will advanced laparoscopic surgery go hand-assisted? Surg Endosc 14:881–882
32. Nakajima K, Lee SW, Cocilovo C et al (2004) Laparoscopic total colectomy.Hand-assisted vs. standard technique. Surg Endosc 18:582–586
33. Gurland BH, Steven D, Wexner (2002) Laparoscopic surgery for inflammatory bowel disease: results of the past decade. Inflamm Bowel Dis 8(1):46–54
34. Seow-Choen F, Eu KW, Leong AFPK, Ho YH (1999) A consecutive series of open compared to laparoscopic restorative proctocolectomy with ileo-pouch anastomosis for familial adenomatous polyposis. Tech Coloproctol 3:83–86
35. Novitsky YW, Litwin DEM, Callery MP (2004) The net immunologic advantage of laparoscopic surgery. Surg Endosc 18(10):1411–1419
36. Targarona EM, Gracia E, Garriga J et al (2002) Prospective randomized trial comparing conventional laparoscopic colectomy with hand-assisted laparoscopic colectomy. Surg Endosc 16:234–239
37. Kang JC, Chung MH, Chao PC et al (2004) Hand-assisted laparoscopic colectomy vs. open colectomy: a prospective randomized study. Surg Endosc 18:577–581
38. Gullberg K, Lindquist K, Lijeqvist L (1995) Pelvic

pouch-anal anastomoses: pros and cons about omission of mucosectomy and loop ileostomy: a study of 60 patients. Ann Chir 49(6):527–533
39. Mularczyk A, Contessini Avesani E et al (1999) Local regulation of postprandial motor responses in ileal pouches. Gut 45(4):575–80
40. Bullard KM, Madoff RD, Gemlo BT (2002) Is ileoanal pouch function stable with time? Dis Colon Rectum 45(3):299–304
41. Philip TM, Vincent TT (1991) Pelvic pouch procedures. Butterworth, London
42. Browning SM, Nivatvongs S (1998) Intraoperative abandonment of ileal pouch to anal anastomosis. the Mayo Clinic experience. J Am Coll Surg 186(4):441–445
43. Remzi FH, Church JM, Bast J et al (2001) Mucosectomy vs. stapled ileal pouch-anal anastomosis in patients with familial adenomatous polyposis: functional outcome and neoplasia control. Dis Colon Rectum 44:1590–1596
44. Ooi BS, Remzi FH, Gramlich T et al (2003) Anal transitional zone cancer after restorative proctocolectomy and ileoanal anastomosis in familial adenomatous polyposis: report of two cases. Dis Colon Rectum 40:1019–1022
45. Church J (2005) Ileoanal pouch neoplasia in familial adenomatous polyposis: an underestimated threat. Dis Colon Rectum 48:1708–1713

Clinical Significance of Extra-Colonic Manifestations of Familial Adenomatous Polyposis

Yehuda Kariv, Hagit Tulchinsky, Micha Rabau

Introduction

Familial adenomatous polyposis (FAP) is an inherited autosomal dominant disorder. It is characterized by the development of hundreds to thousands of adenomatous polyps in the colon and rectum, usually beginning at puberty, with a tendency to undergo malignant transformation by the fifth decade [1].Therefore, surveillance and management protocols have always focused primarily on early detection and prophylactic colectomy in affected persons. These measures have substantially reduced the risk of colorectal adenocarcinoma which was once the main cause of mortality, hence changing significantly the natural history of this disease manifestation. However, genotypic aberrations of the fundamental genetic defect that causes the syndrome, a germ-line mutation in the APC gene, may lead to additional phenotypic expressions in which extra-colonic organs develop neoplasms or other changes (Table 1). There is a large diversity in the expression and complexity of these extra-colonic manifestations (EM). Although some appear as clinically non-significant or are only cosmetically disturbing, others are potentially associated with high rates of morbidity and mortality. In contrary to the relatively straightforward management strategy of the colonic manifestation of the syndrome, some EM, like involvement of the upper GI tract and intra-abdominal desmoids, may be difficult to manage. This chapter describes the clinical significance of these manifestations and suggests management and surveillance strategies.

Table 1. Extra-colonic manifestations of familial polyposis

Upper gastrointestinal tract:
- Stomach: fundic gland polyps, adenomatous polyps, cancer
- Duodenum and small bowel: duodenal adenomas, periampullary cancer, small-bowel adenomas, cancer, lymphoid polyps of ileum
- Gallbladder, bile duct, pancreas: adenomas, cancer

Desmoid tumors: abdominal wall, mesentery, retroperitoneum, extremities

Bone and dental abnormalities: osteomas, unerupted teeth, supernumerary teeth, dentigerous cyst, odontomas

Cutaneous lesions: epidermoid cysts, sebaceous cysts, fibromas and lipomas

Ocular: pigmented ocular fundus lesions (POFLs)

Other neoplasia: adrenal adenomas, nasal angiofibromas, thyroid papillary adenocarcinoma, CNS tumors (glioblastoma multiforme, cerebellar medulloblastoma), hepatoblastoma

Upper Gastrointestinal Polyps and Cancer

Duodenal Neoplasia

After the colon and rectum, the duodenum is the second most commonly affected site of polyp development in FAP [2, 3]. Duodenal adenomas can be found in 30–70% of patients [2–4] and the lifetime risk of these lesions approaches 100% [4–6]. Duodenal/periampullary adenocarcinoma is a leading cause of cancer death in FAP patients following colectomy.

Duodenal cancer is rare in the general population, with an incidence of 0.01–0.04% [7]. Compared with the general population, FAP patients have a 100–330-fold higher risk of duodenal cancer [8, 9]. The estimated cumulative lifetime risk of developing duodenal cancer in FAP range from 4 to 10% [4, 10, 11]. The median age of duodenal cancer development is 52 years (range 26–58) [4]. Therefore, although most patients eventually develop duodenal polyps, these lesions occur at a later age and have lower potential for malignant change compared with colonic polyps.

Polyps can be found throughout the duodenum, but the second and third portion and the periampullary region are the most commonly affected sites. This pattern suggests a role for exposure of duodenal mucosa to bile acids in duodenal carcinogenesis [12, 13]. Data on the relationship between the severity of duodenal polyposis and specific mutations in the APC are inconsistent [14–16]. However, most reports indicate that mutations in exon 15 of the APC gene, particularly distal to codon 1400, give rise to a severe duodenal phenotype [11, 17, 18–20].

The adenoma-carcinoma sequence has been also observed in the setting of duodenal carcinogenesis in patients with both FAP and sporadic disease. Spigelman et al. showed that villous histology, moderate or severe dysplasia, and the presence of stage IV duodenal polyps were associated with malignant change [21].

The most useful system for rating the severity of duodenal polyposis was developed by Spigelman et al. This classification describes five (0–IV) stages. Points are accumulated for number, size, histology, and severity of dysplasia of polyps (Table 2). Approximately 70–80% of FAP patients have stage II or stage III duodenal disease, and 20–30% have stage I or stage IV disease [12, 22]. However, the estimated cumulative incidence of stage IV duodenal disease is 50% at age 70 years [4, 23]. The Spigelman classification correlates with risk of duodenal malignancy. Stages II, III, and IV disease are associated with a 2.3, 2.4, and 36% risk of duodenal cancer, respectively [22].

Duodenal polyposis slowly progresses in size, number, and histology, and eventually in Spigelman stage [24]. Heiskanen et al. reported worsening polyposis in 73% of 71 FAP patients followed for 11 years [5]. The median interval for progression by one stage was 4–11 years. The risk of developing stage III or IV disease exponentially increases after 40 years of age [25]. Endoscopic surveillance of the upper gastrointestinal tract for the development of neoplasia is recommended by most authorities. Screening for upper gastrointestinal disease should start at the time of FAP diagnosis [26]. The guidelines for continued endoscopic surveillance after baseline examination are according to the Spigelman stage (Table 3) [6, 22].

Table 2. Spigelman classification for duodenal polyposis in familial adenomatous polyposis

Points	1	2	3
Polyp number	1–4	5–20	>20
Polyp size (mm)	1–4	5–10	>10
Histology	Tubular	Tubulovillous	Villous
Dysplasia	Mild	Moderate	Severe

Stage 0, 0 points; stage I, 1–4 points; stage II, 5–6 points; stage III, 7–8 points; stage IV, 9–12 points

Table 3. Recommendations for management of duodenal polyposis in familial adenomatous polyposis adjusted to the Spigelman stage of duodenal polyposis [6]

Spigelman stage	Endoscopic frequency	Chemo-prevention	Surgery
0	4 years	No	No
I	2–3 years	No	No
II	2–3 years	Yes/no	No
III	6–12 months	Yes/no	Yes/no
IV	6–12 months	Yes/no	Yes

Treatment

Endoscopic treatment options for duodenal lesions include snare excision, thermal ablation, argon plasma coagulation, and photodynamic therapy (PDT). Most reports of endoscopic therapy use snare excision. However, endoscopic treatment is usually insufficient in guaranteeing a polyp-free duodenum and might cause complications. Recurrence rates of adenomatous tissue in the duodenum of FAP patients treated endoscopically range from 50 to 100% [26, 27–29]. Surgical procedures to treat duodenal polyposis include local excision (duodenotomy with polypectomy and/or ampullectomy), pancreas preserving duodenectomy, and pancreaticoduodenectomy. There are no randomized studies published to help guide surgical selection.

Local surgical treatment with duodenotomy has proven insufficient in guaranteeing a polyp-free duodenum, with most studies reporting high recurrence rates in patients with severe duodenal adenomatosis [5, 26–28, 30–33]. Farnell and colleagues found a lower recurrence rate of duodenal polyps of 32 and 43% at 5 and 10 years of follow up, respectively [34]. Nevertheless, duodenotomy may be indicated in patients with one or two dominant worrisome duodenal lesions in otherwise uninvolved or minimally involved intestine.

More radical surgery, in the form of pancreaticoduodenectomy, or pancreas preserving duodenectomy, has been indicated for patients with severe polyposis (stage III–IV), failed endoscopic or local surgical treatment, and carcinoma. [26–28, 31–39]. Low recurrence rates of polyposis have been reported with these procedures.

Pharmacological Treatment. Duodenal adenomas seem less responsive to chemoprevention with NSAIDs than colonic counterparts. The results of NSAID, COX 2 inhibitors and other compounds on regression or prevention of duodenal adenomas in FAP appear disappointing [40–42]. The response of earlier Spigelman stages might be better [43]. Suggested guidelines for chemoprevention are presented in Table 3.

Gastric Neoplasia

Gastric polyps occur in 23–100% of FAP patients [44–46]. Fundic gland polyps (FGP) are the most common gastric polyps in FAP. They usually appear in the gastric fundus and body, and have traditionally been regarded as non-neoplastic, possibly hamartomatous lesions. Similar polyps, although fewer in number, are sometimes observed in the general population and possibly associated with chronic use of proton pump inhibitors [47]. These polyps are considered to have little or no potential for malignant transformation; however, recent studies have reported that dysplasia and malignant transformation occur more frequently than previously believed (48, 49). Histologically, these polyps consist of simple hyperplasia of the fundic glands with microcytes. Endoscopically, these are multiple sessile lesions, 1–5 mm in diameter, that are the same color with the surrounding mucosa. They vary considerably in size and number. The polyps are sometimes numerous, and coalesce, forming an irregular matted surface mucosa. These polyps rarely cause symptoms and have been observed as early as 8 years of age.

Adenomatous polyps occur in the stomach of about 10% of patients with FAP. Most often, they are confined to the antrum but occasionally found in the body and fundus (44, 50]. The lifetime risk for gastric cancer in FAP is about 0.6%, believed in large part to arise from adenomatous polyps. Interestingly, Japanese and Korean FAP patients have a 3–4 times higher risk of gastric cancer compared with the general population [51, 52], whereas no increased risk has been found in Western countries [9].

Small-Bowel Neoplasia

Clinically significant small-bowel adenomas distal to the duodenum are uncommon in patients with FAP. Adenomas may occur throughout the small bowel but are concentrated for the most part in the proximal jejunum and the distal ileum. Studies using the capsule camera showed ileal polyps in 5% of FAP patients. Malignancy is unusual. In patients with FAP after restorative proctocolectomy, the incidence of neoplasia in the ileal pouch increases. The incidence of adenomas within the ileal pouch ranges between 20 and 62% and depends on duration of follow-up [53–56]. Parc et al. [57] found that the risk of developing adenomas at 5, 10, and 15 years was 7, 35, and 75%, respectively. The risk of cancer development in such adenomas has not been established, although three cases of pouch cancer have been reported [58]. Therefore, for all patients with FAP who have undergone restorative proctocolectomy, periodic endoscopic examination is indicated. Adenomas also occur in the terminal ileum of patients who have an ileostomy or Kock pouch after proctocolectomy without restoration. In addition, the risk of ileostomy carcinoma in these patients appears to be increased compared to the very low incidence of primary small-bowel carcinoma. By 2005, 11 ileostomy carcinomas were reported [59]. Other small bowel lesions include prominent lymphoid polyps that may occur in the terminal ileum of younger patients with FAP and should be differentiated from adenomas by biopsy [60].

Desmoid Tumors

Desmoid tumors (DTs) are benign fibrous growths which do not metastasize, but tend to invade locally. Although rare in the general population, DTs are not rare in FAP. They may arise in musculoaponeurotic structures throughout the body, but are most common in the abdomen. Desmoid tumors (DTs) affect between 4 and 20% of FAP patients. Within 10 years after colectomy, the cumulative risk of developing DTs is 16% [61], and the cumulative lifetime risk is 21% [62]. The peak incidence is between 28 and 31 years, although they may occur at any age [61, 63, 64].

Bertario et al. [65] described independent predictors of DTs in FAP patients: APC mutations beyond codon 1444, family history of desmoids, female gender, and the presence of osteomas. The female-to-male ratio of DTs in FAP is 1.4 [62, 63, 66]. In first-degree relatives of FAP patients with DTs, the relative risk of developing DTs is 2.5, when compared to FAP kindreds with no family history of DTs [61, 63]. Eleven to thirteen percent of patients are diagnosed with DTs before diagnosis of FAP, while 8–19% have a simultaneous diagnosis, and 68–82 % develop DTs after the diagnosis of FAP [63, 67].

Desmoid tumors (DTs) in FAP seem to occur on the basis of APC gene inactivation and accumulation of β-catenin in the cells. There is evidence to suggest that a mutation near or beyond codon 1444 may influence the process [68, 69].

A model of DT development has been suggested that is analogous to the adenoma-carcinoma sequence: mesenteric plaque-like precursor lesions progress to mesenteric fibromatosis that can give rise to desmoid tumors [70]. Desmoid tumors often develop in surgical scars, leading to the theory that surgical trauma is a potential initiating factor. Abdominal surgery precedes development of DTs in 68–83% of FAP patients, and in most cases a colectomy has been performed [63, 66, 71, 72]. There is no evidence to suggest that the extent or type of surgery influences DT development [62, 70, 73, 74]. Estrogen is considered to influence the development and growth of DTs [63]. Therefore, estrogen-blocking drugs are part of the usual treatment of these tumors.

Desmoid tumors are homogeneous, firm lesions that have no capsule. They vary in size from multiple small plaques to large tumors. Histological sections show highly differentiated fibroblasts and myofibroblasts, embedded in a matrix of collagen, with a normal number of mitoses and a lack of atypia. Desmoid tumors invade muscles and aponeuroses, attach to and erode bone and engulf rather than invade blood vessels, nerves, ureters and other hollow organs.

The histological diagnosis might be difficult. Occasional confusion with highly differentiated sarcoma may exist [75]. Transformation to sarcoma is extremely rare [76]. In FAP patients, 50% of DTs are intra-abdominal, 40% occur in the abdominal wall, and 10% on the extremities. Among the intra-abdominal DTs, 85–100% are located in the mesentery and 15% in the retroperitoneum [62, 67]. Desmoid tumors often present as a slow growing , non-tender, abdominal mass, although rapid growth has been reported [77] and they rarely regress spontaneously [66, 78]. Intra-abdominal DTs are often asymptomatic. The most common symptom is abdominal pain, which occurs in only about one third of patients. Discomfort, nausea, vomiting, diarrhea and hematochezia are less common. Desmoid tumors may cause small-bowel obstruction and hydronephrosis as a result of intestinal or ureteric compression [79]. Fistula between the tumor and the ureters or intestine [80, 81], abscess formation or intestinal perforation with peritonitis are infrequent complications [66]. Mesenteric vessels encasement may lead to ischaemia of the small bowel [82]. Development of DTs often impairs the outcome of patients with an ileal pouch-anal anastomosis, and it might become necessary to remove the pouch or create a permanent diverting stoma [74, 82]. A rapidly growing tumor might cause symptoms during pregnancy and interfere with normal maturation and delivery of the fetus prompting surgical resection [83]. The relation between FAP and mesenteric DTs is well established, and therefore it is recommended to perform a sigmoidoscopy whenever a mesenteric DT is diagnosed. [84–87]. Incidental intra-abdominal DTs were identified in 3% of FAP patients during the first laparotomy, and in 30% during a second laparotomy. Interestingly, an incidental finding of DTs influenced the intended procedure (e.g., ileal pouch anal anastomosis) in only 13 and 30% of the first and second laparotomy, respectively [88]. In addition, the incidental finding of desmoid reaction during laparotomy may have little bearing on the subsequent development of clinically significant intra-abdominal DTs [88].

Diagnosis

Desmoid tumors (DTs) in the abdominal wall are diagnosed by histological examination of a percutaneous biopsy; a CT scan is done to obtain accurate information on the extension of the abdominal tumor and to monitor the outcome of treatment [89]. Magnetic resonance imaging (MRI) has proved valuable in the diagnosis of DTs on the extremities [90]. When surgery is being considered, mesenteric angiography or MR angiography are useful in demonstrating the possible relationships to major mesenteric vessels [84].

Treatment

Medical treatment of DTs is still almost empirical as large prospective randomized studies are lacking. Sulindac, a COX inhibitor with prolonged effect is frequently used either alone or in combination with an anti-estrogen [66, 85, 91]. Desmoid tumors response rates to treatment with Sulindac alone or in combination with anti-estrogen or Warfarin were 33–50% in several studies [66, 84, 92, 93]; however, others have reported less encouraging results [72]. COX 2 inhibitors (Celecoxib) were also suggested, although clinical benefit has not yet been demonstrated [94, 95].

Anti-estrogens are frequently used in combination with a NSAID as first-line treatment in patients with non-complicated DTs [84, 85, 91, 96]. The choice is between tamoxifen or its analogues (toremifene, raloxifen). Several small studies demonstrate estrogen receptors in 33–75% of DTs [91, 97]. However, the effect of anti-estrogen therapy is not exclusively mediated through estrogen receptors, as some DT swithout estrogen receptors also responds to anti-estrogen [86, 97]. An overall response to this treatment is seen in about 50% of the patients [84, 86, 92]. Other reports were less optimistic [66, 93, 94].

Cytotoxic chemotherapy had proven valuable in the treatment of fibrosarcomas and, because of this, several studies have investigated its effect on DTs [72, 75, 98–101]. Some have demonstrated partial or complete response to a combination of doxorubicin and dacarbazine in 46–100% of patients [72, 98, 99]. Others could not reproduce similar results [100]. In addition, the morbidity and mortality related to cytotoxic chemotherapy is considerable [98–100]. Most authors therefore recommend that the use of cytotoxic chemotherapy should be limited to patients with large unresectable mesenteric or retroperitoneal DTs which do not respond to treatment with sulindac and anti-estrogen [75, 98–100, 102]. Other combinations of chemotherapeutic agents have been suggested for treating patients who had previously failed medical treatment or to those with inoperable aggressive fibromatosis [103, 104].

Radiotherapy is not recommended by most authors, since DTs are frequently located in the mesenterium, where irradiation might cause unacceptable complications [64–72]. In addition, its efficacy is questionable. Nevertheless, some do recommend radiotherapy for inoperable aggressive fibromatosis.

Other treatment modality has been reported

Small studies have reported remission with a combination of warfarin and sulindac. Others showed successful treatment with interferon, LHRH analogues, progesterons, ascorbic acid, prednisolone, testosterone, pirfenidone, imatinib mesylate and hyperthermia [92, 105–111]. Some patients with recurrent DTs of the extremities were successfully treated using isolated limb perfusion with tumor necrosis factor-alpha and melphalan [112].

Surgery for DTs of the abdominal wall or the extremities includes wide excision with tumor-free margins. Complications are few, but the reported recurrence rate is 10–68% [62, 78, 87, 113]. Mesenteric or retroperitoneal DTs usually exhibit expansive growth around parts of the small intestine and/or larger mesenteric vessels, and this often renders radical surgical excision impossible. Major complications such as abscess formation, fistulas or short-bowel syndrome were seen in up to 47% of patients after curative or palliative resection with postoperative mortality of 10–60% [64, 71, 72, 84]. Recurrence was seen at a mean interval of 5 years in 78% of the patients after presumed excision for cure [71]. On this basis, excision of a large DTs located in the mesentery or retroperitoneum should not be attempted in non-complicated cases, but only in patients with imminent or manifest bowel obstruction, intestinal ischaemia or hydronephrosis [64, 82, 102]. Surgery is usually targeted to relieve symptoms by performing intestinal bypass or segmental resection rather then tumor excision. Intestinal or multivisceral allograft or autograft transplantation has been proposed as a lifesaving procedure for otherwise untreatable patients with complicated DTs [114, 115].

A staging system that stratifies patients by disease severity of intra-abdominal DTs was recently suggested by the Collaborative Group of the Americas on Inherited Colorectal Cancer [116]. Size of tumor, presence of symptoms, and rate of growth mainly determine the staging and the treatment that is required. They recommend surgery for small symptomatic tumors that are not growing and can be resected with minimal sequela. Surgery should also be considered, when urgent treatment is required for large tumors, rapid growth or life threatening complications. Alternatives in these difficult situations are combination chemotherapy (adriamycin and dacarbazine) and radiation [116]. Intra-abdominal DTs may compromise ileoanal pouch function after restorative proctocolectomy, particularly if the pouch mesentery is involved. This may require a diverting stoma or pouch excision. Pouch salvage is possible in isolated cases with either surgical excision of the tumor or combination chemotherapy [117–119].

Prognosis

About 4–6% of DTs resolve spontaneously [66, 78]. In cases of unresectable mesenteric DTs, the mortality rate has been reported to be as high as 30% [120]. The overall survival rate after 10 years is 63% [84]. Death occurs 3–6 years after being diagnosed with DTs and at an age of 30–40 years [120]. Death due to colorectal cancer is still the most frequent cause of death in FAP patients, but among the EM, DTs are a frequent cause of death [120, 121]. In general, a tumor diameter >10 cm, multiple mesenteric DTs, bilateral hydronephrosis, and extensive mesenteric growth are considered to be bad prognostic signs. Low proliferation of Ki-67 in DTs is associated with RO resection, and has significant positive prognostic value [122].

Osteomas and Dental Abnormalities

Osteomas are the most common accompanying bone lesion seen in FAP, and the first extra-colonic lesion to be associated with FAP [123, 124]. Osteoma is a benign neoplasm of bone tissue that increases in size by slow continuous osseous growth and consists of well-differentiated compact or cancellous bone. It is a painless tumor and has no malignant potential. Since the mandible and skull are the most common locations, asymmetry of the maxillofacial region is typical. In children, it may precede the occurrence of colonic polyposis [125]. Subtle radiopaque jaw lesions are often evident at an early age via panoramic dental radiographs in patients with FAP with no other apparent extra-intestinal lesions [126, 127]. Long bone radiographs may demonstrate osteomas or hyperostosis.

Treatment for bone lesions of FAP depends on the symptomatic or cosmetic nature of the findings. They may require excision if they are severely deforming or interfere with function. In the past, the presence of osteomas was required to make the diagnosis of Gardner syndrome, a variant of FAP. However, with the discovery of the APC gene and the knowledge that FAP and Gardner syndromes arise from mutations of that gene, the term Gardner syndrome remains mainly of historical interest.

Various dental abnormalities have been described in FAP including unerupted teeth, supernumerary teeth, dentigerous cysts and odontomas [128]. These may precede the development of colonic polyposis, and the prevalence is estimated at 17%, compared with 1–2% in the general population.

Cutaneous Findings

The most common cutaneous findings in patients with FAP are epidermoid cysts [129, 130]. Epidermoid cysts of FAP syndrome occur around puberty in rather uncommon locations (e.g., face, scalp, extremities), and tend to be multiple [131]. Although cysts in FAP usually are asymptomatic, they may be pruritic and/or inflamed and may rupture. Pathological findings of the epidermoid cysts of FAP are similar to findings in non-FAP cysts; however, many have pilomatricoma-like changes [132].

Fibromas, ranging in size from millimeters to centimeters, are found most commonly on the cutaneous surface of the scalp, shoulders, arms, and back. Other skin lesions in FAP include lipomas, leiomyomas, neurofibromas, and pigmented skin lesions [129,130].

Treatment for the cutaneous manifestations FAP depends on the symptomatic or cosmetic nature of the findings. Therefore, no treatment is usually required. Specifically, treatment of cysts is similar to that used for ordinary cysts and involves excision or use of intralesional steroids if there is inflammation.

Ocular Manifestations

Pigmented ocular fundus lesions (POFLs) can be found in the majority of FAP patients [133]. They resemble congenital hypertrophy of the retinal pigment epithelium (CHRPE), an isolated patch that lacks an association with polyposis [134]. Since lesions in FAP are more variable in appearance, they have been termed POFL [133]. The POFLs in FAP are characterized as hamartomas of the retinal pigment epithelium based on histopathologic studies [135]. POFLs are multiple and bilateral, and may vary in size. The most common ophthalmoscopic features include small, flat, round, and hyperpigmented lesions that do not increase in number or size with age.

The presence of multiple POFLs is a specific and reliable clinical marker of FAP with extra-colonic manifestations [136]. POFLs are congenital, and can be detected using a simple dilated fundus examination, and as such they may be useful for the screening of affected families. Unfortunately, they are only present in approximately 70% of patients with FAP, making them a specific but relatively insensitive marker of the disease.

Phenotype-genotype correlation studies have demonstrated association of POFL-positive phenotype with mutation of the APC gene after exon 9, or deletion of the whole APC gene [137]. Uncommon ocular lesions in Gardner syndrome include orbital osteomas and soft tissue tumors of the brows or eyelids [133].

Thyroid Manifestations

Thyroid carcinoma occurs in 1–2% of FAP patients [138]. The relative risk of thyroid cancer has been estimated to be 7.6 (95% CL 2.5–17.7) in FAP [139] compared with the general population. FAP-associated thyroid cancer is typically characterized by female predominance, young age at tumor diagnosis (usually 30 years or below), papillary differentiation, and multifocal involvement [140]. Therefore, several authors have advocated periodic thyroid evaluation in young women with FAP [139,140]. An association between FAP and thyroiditis has also been reported [141].

Central Nervous System Tumors

Central nervous system (CNS) tumors appear in less than 1% of FAP patients. The association of colonic polyposis and CNS tumors is termed Turcot syndrome [142]. About two thirds of Turcot syndrome cases are associated with APC gene mutations and therefore are considered variants of FAP (Turcot type 2) [143]. They usually exhibit typical colonic polyposis and CNS tumors including medulloblastoma, anaplastic astrocytoma, and ependymomas. One third of patients with Turcot syndrome have a variant of HNPCC (Turcot type 1) [143]. A review of documented Turcot cases determined the average age at death to be 20.3 years. This raises the difficult question as to whether prophylactic colectomy, and specifically restorative proctocolectomy, should be performed [144].

Other Neoplasia

Several other malignancies are known to have an increased lifetime risk in FAP patients compared to the general population. These include pancreatic cancer, cholangiocarcinoma, hepatoblastoma, and possibly adrenal [145,146]. Both adenomatous changes and cancer have been reported in the gallbladder, bile duct and pancreas. The relative risk of pancreatic adenocarcinoma in the John's Hopkins FAP registry was 4.4 [139], whereas the absolute risk of pancreatic cancer is 2% or less.

Hepatoblastoma affects 0.75–1.6% of children with FAP, exhibits male predominance, and occurs mainly in the first 5 years of life and, therefore, may precede the development of FAP by many years [147, 148]. The risk in children with FAP is 800-fold higher than in the general population.

Adrenal adenomas have been shown to occur more frequently in FAP. Several cases of functioning adenomas and adrenal carcinomas have also been reported in FAP patients, but the association is uncertain [149, 150]. Most adrenal lesions are found incidentally on imaging studies done for other reasons and should be managed similarly to those in the general population.

References

1. Boardman LA (2002) Heritable colorectal cancer syndromes: recognition and preventive management. Gastroenterol Clin North Am 31:1107–1131
2. Tonelli F, Nardi F, Bechi P et al (1985) Extracolonic polyps in familial polyposis coli and Gardner's syndrome. Dis Colon Rectum 28:664–668
3. Sarre RG, Frost AG, Jagelman DG et al (1987) Gastric and duodenal polyps in familial adenomatous polyposis: a prospective study of the nature and prevalence of upper gastrointestinal polyps. Gut 28:306–314
4. Bulow S, Bjork J, Christensen IJ et al (2004) Duodenal adenomatosis in familial adenomatous polyposis. Gut 53:381–386
5. Heiskanen I, Kellokumpu I, Jarvinen H (1999) Management of duodenal adenomas in 98 patients with familial adenomatous polyposis. Endoscopy 31:412–416
6. Brosens LA, Keller JJ, Offerhaus GJ et al (2005) Prevention and management of duodenal polyps in familial polyposis. Gut 54:1034–1043
7. Lillemoe K, Imbembo AL (1980) Malignant neoplasms of the duodenum. Surg Gynecol Obstet 150:822–826
8. Pauli RM, Pauli ME, Hall JG (1980) Gardner syndrome and periampullary malignancy. Am J Med Genet 6:205–219
9. Offerhaus GJ, Giardiello FM, Krush AJ et al (1992) The risk of upper gastrointestinal cancer in familial adenomatous polyposis. Gastroenterology 102:1980–1982
10. Vasen HF, Bulow S, Myrhoj T et al (1997) Decision analysis in the management of duodenal adenomatosis in familial adenomatous polyposis. Gut 40:716–719
11. Bjork J, Akerbrant H, Iselius L et al (2001) Periampullary adenomas and adenocarcinomas in familial adenomatous polyposis: cumulative risks and APC gene mutations. Gastroenterology 121:1127–1135
12. Spigelman AD, Williams CB, Talbot IC et al (1989) Upper gastrointestinal cancer in patients with familial adenomatous polyposis. Lancet 2:783–785
13. Mahmoud NN, Dannenberg AJ, Bilinski RT et al (1999) Administration of an unconjugated bile acid increases duodenal tumors in a murine model of familial adenomatous polyposis. Carcinogenesis 20:299–303
14. Friedl W, Caspari R, Sengteller M et al (2001) Can APC mutation analysis contribute to therapeutic decisions in familial adenomatous polyposis? Experience from 680 FAP families. Gut 48:515–521
15. Soravia C, Berk T, Madlensky L et al (1998) Genotype-phenotype correlations in attenuated adenomatous polyposis coli. Am J Hum Genet 62:1290–1301
16. Saurin JC, Ligneau B, Ponchon T et al (2002) The influence of mutation site and age on the severity of duodenal polyposis in patients with familial adenomatous polyposis. Gastrointest Endosc 55:342–347
17. Bertario L, Russo A, Sala P et al (2003) Hereditary colorectal tumor registry: multiple approach to the exploration of genotype-phenotype correlations in familial adenomatous polyposis. J Clin Oncol 21:1698–1707
18. Groves C, Lamlum H, Crabtree M et al (2002) Mutation cluster region, association between germ-line and somatic mutations and genotype-phenotype correlation in upper gastrointestinal familial adenomatous polyposis. Am J Pathol 160:2055–2061
19. Matsumoto T, Iida M, Kobori Y et al (2002) Progressive duodenal adenomatosis in a familial adenomatous polyposis pedigree with APC mutation at codon 1556. Dis Colon Rectum 45:229–233
20. Leggett BA, Young JP, Biden K et al (1997) Severe upper gastrointestinal polyposis associated with sparse colonic polyposis in a familial adenomatous polyposis family with an APC mutation at codon 1520. Gut 41:518–521
21. Spigelman AD, Talbot IC, Penna C (1994) Evidence for adenoma-carcinoma sequence in the duodenum of patients with familial adenomatous polyposis: the Leeds Castle Polyposis Group (Upper Gastrointestinal Committee). J Clin Pathol 47:709–710
22. Groves CJ, Saunders BP, Spigelman AD et al (2002) Duodenal cancer in patients with familial adenomatous polyposis (FAP): results of a 10 year prospective study. Gut 50:636–641
23. Saurin JC, Gutknecht C, Napoleon B et al (2004) Surveillance of duodenal adenomas in familial adenomatous polyposis reveals high cumulative risk of

advanced disease. J Clin Oncol 22:493–498
24. Burke CA, Beck GJ, Church JM et al (1999) The natural history of untreated duodenal and ampullary adenomas in patients with familial adenomatous polyposis followed in an endoscopic surveillance program. Gastrointest Endosc 49:358–364
25. Moozar KL, Madlensky L, Berk T et al (2002). Slow progression of periampullary neoplasia in familial adenomatous polyposis. J Gastrointest Surg 6:831–837
26. Morpurgo E, Vitale GC, Galandiuk S et al (2004) Clinical characteristics of familial adenomatous polyposis and management of duodenal adenomas. J Gastrointest Surg 8:559–564
27. Alarcon FJ, Burke CA, Church JM et al (1999) Familial adenomatous polyposis: efficacy of endoscopic and surgical treatment for advanced duodenal adenomas. Dis Colon Rectum 42:1533–1536
28. Soravia C, Berk T,HaberG et al (1997) Management of advanced duodenal polyposis in familial adenomatous polyposis. J Gastrointest Surg 1:474–478
29. Bertoni G, Sassatelli R, Nigrisoli E et al (1997) Endoscopic snare papillectomy in patients with familial adenomatous polyposis and ampullary adenoma. Endoscopy 29:685–688
30. Penna C, Phillips RK, Tiret E et al (1993) Surgical polypectomy of duodenal adenomas in familial adenomatous polyposis: experience of two European centres. Br J Surg 80:1027–1029
31. Penna C, Bataille N, Balladur P et al (1998) Surgical treatment of severe duodenal polyposis in familial adenomatous polyposis. Br J Surg 85:665–668
32. de Vos tot Nederveen Cappel WH, Jarvinen HJ, Bjork J et al (2003) Worldwide survey among polyposis registries of surgical management of severe duodenal adenomatosis in familial adenomatous polyposis. Br J Surg 90:705–710
33. Ruo L, Coit DG, Brennan MF et al (2002) Long-term follow-up of patients with familial adenomatous polyposis undergoing pancreaticoduodenal surgery. J Gastrointest Surg 6:671–675
34. Farnell MB, Sakorafas GH, Sarr MG et al (2000) Villous tumors of the duodenum: reappraisal of local vs. extended resection. J Gastrointest Surg 4:13–21
35. Chung RS, Church JM, van Stolk R (1995) Pancreas-sparing duodenectomy: indications, surgical technique and results. Surgery 117:254–259
36. Kalady MF, Clary BM, Tyler DS et al (2002) Pancreas-preserving duodenectomy in the management of duodenal familial adenomatous polyposis. J Gastrointest Surg 6:82–87
37. Balladur P, Penna C, Tiret E et al (1993) Pancreaticoduodenectomy for cancer and precancer in familial adenomatous polyposis. Int J Colorectal Dis 8:151–153
38. Gallagher MC, Shankar A, Groves CJ et al (2004) Pylorus-preserving pancreaticoduodenectomy for advanced duodenal disease in familial adenomatous polyposis. Br J Surg 91:1157-1164
39. Mackey R, Walsh RM, Chung R et al (2005) Pancreas-sparing duodenectomy is effective management for familial adenomatous polyposis. J Gastrointest Surg 9:1088-1093
40. Nugent KP, Farmer KC, Spigelman AD et al (1993) Randomized controlled trial of the effect of sulindac on duodenal and rectal polyposis and cell proliferation in patients with familial adenomatous polyposis. Br J Surg 80:1618–1619
41. Debinski HS, Trojan J, Nugent KP et al (1995) Effect of sulindac on small polyps in familial adenomatous polyposis. Lancet 345:855–856
42. Phillips RK, Wallace MH, Lynch PM et al (2002) A randomised, double blind, placebo controlled study of celecoxib, a selective cyclooxygenase 2 inhibitor, on duodenal polyposis in familial adenomatous polyposis. Gut 50:857–860
43. Maclean AR, McLeod RS, Berk T et al (2001) A randomized trial comparing ursodeoxycholic acid and rofecoxib, a selective COX-2 inhibitor, in the treatment of advanced duodenal adenomas in patients with familial adenomatous polyposis. Abstract. Gastroenterology 120[Suppl 1]:A-254
44. Sawada T, Muto T (1997) Role of upper gastrointestinal surveillance in patients with familial adenomatous polyposis. Gastrointest Endosc Clin N Am 7:99–111
45. Offerhaus GJ, Entius MM, Giardiello FM (1999) Upper gastrointestinal polyps in familial adenomatous polyposis. Hepatogastroenterology 46:667–669
46. Kadmon M, Tandara A, Herfarth C (2001) Duodenal adenomatosis in familial adenomatous polyposis coli: a review of the literature and results from the Heidelberg Polyposis Register. Int J Colorectal Dis 16:63–75
47. Choudhry U, Boyce HW Jr, Coppola D (1998) Proton pump inhibitor-associated gastric polyps: a retrospective analysis of their frequency, and endoscopic, histologic, and ultrastructural characteristics. Am J Clin Pathol 110:615–621
48. Abraham SC, Nobukawa B, Giardiello FM et al (2000) Fundic gland polyps in familial adenomatous polyposis: neoplasms with frequent somatic adenomatous polyposis coli gene alterations. Am J Pathol 157:747–754
49. Sekine S, Shimoda T, Nimura S et al (2004) High-grade dysplasia associated with fundic gland polyposis in a familial adenomatous polyposis patient, with special reference to APC mutation profiles. Mod Pathol 17:1421–1426
50. Wallace MH, Phillips RK (1998) Upper gastrointestinal disease in patients with familial adenomatous polyposis. Br J Surg 85:742–750
51. Park JG, Park KJ, Ahn YO et al (1992) Risk of gastric cancer among Korean familial adenomatous polyposis patients: report of three cases. Dis Colon Rectum 35:996–998
52. Iwama T, Mishima Y, Utsunomiya J (1993) The impact of familial adenomatous polyposis on the tumorigenesis and mortality at the several organs: its rational treatment. Ann Surg 217:101–108
53. Polese L, Keighley MR (2003) Adenomas at resection margins do not influence the long-term development of pouch polyps after restorative proctocolectomy for familial adenomatous polyposis. Am J Surg 186:32–34
54. Parc Y, Piquard A, Dozois RR et al (2004) Long term outcome of familial adenomatosis polyposis patients after restorative coloproctectomy. Ann Surg 239:378–382
55. Thompson-Fawcett MW, Marcus VA, Redston M et al (2001) Adenomatous polyps develop commonly in the

ileal pouch of patients with familial adenomatous polyposis. Dis Colon Rectum 44:347–353
56. Groves CJ, Beveridge G, Swain DJ et al (2005) Prevalence and morphology of pouch and ileal adenomas in familial adenomatous polyposis. Dis Colon Rectum 48:816–23
57. Parc YR, Olschwang S, Desaint B et al (2001) Familial adenomatous polyposis: prevalence of adenomas in the ileal pouch after restorative proctocolectomy. Ann Surg 233:360–364
58. Church J (2005) Ileoanal pouch neoplasia in familial adenomatous polyposis: an underestimated threat. Dis Colon Rectum 48:1708–1713
59. Quah HM, Samad A, Maw A (2005) Ileostomy carcinomas a review: the latent risk after colectomy for ulcerative colitis and familial adenomatous polyposis. Colorectal Dis 7:538–544
60. Burt RW, Berenson MM, Lee RG et al (1984) Upper gastrointestinal polyps in Gardner's syndrome. Gastroenterology 86(2):295–301
61. Järvinen HJ (1997) Desmoid disease as a part of familial adenomatous polyposis coli. Acta Chir Scand 153:379–383
62. Heiskanen I, Järvinen HJ (1996) Occurrence of desmoid tumours in familial adenomatous polyposis and result of treatment. Int J Colorectal Dis 11: 157–162
63. Gurbuz AK, Giardiello FM, Petersen GM et al (1994) Desmoid tumors in familial adenomatous polyposis. Gut 35:377–381
64. Berk T, Cohen Z, McLeod RS et al (1992) Management of mesenteric desmoid tumors in familial adenomatous polyposis. Can J Surg 35:393–395
65. Bertario L, Russo A, Sala P et al (2001) Genotype and phenotype factors as determinants of desmoid tumors in patients with familial adenomatous polyposis. Int J Cancer 95:102–107
66. Clark SK, Neale KF, Landgrebe JC et al (1999) Desmoid tumours complicating familial adenomatous polyposis. Br J Surg 86:1185–1189
67. Knudsen AL, Bülow S (2001) Desmoid tumour in familial adenomatous polyposis: a review of literature. Fam Cancer 1:111–119
68. Lamlum H, Ilyas M, Rowan A et al (1999) The type of somatic mutation at APC in familial adenomatous polyposis is determined by the site of the germline mutation: a new facet to Knudson's 'two-hit' hypothesis. Nat Med 5:1071–1075
69. Palmirotta R, Curia MC, Esposito DL (1995) Novel mutations and inactivation of both alleles of the APC gene in desmoid tumours. Hum Mol Genet 4:1979–1981
70. Clark SK, Johnson Smith TGP, Katz DE et al (1998) Identification and progression of a desmoid precursor lesion in patients with familial adenomatous polyposis. Br Jr Surg 85:970–973
71. Rodriguez-Bigas MA, Mahoney MC, Karakousis CP et al (1994) Desmoid tumors in patients with familial adenomatous polyposis. Cancer 74:1270–1274
72. Soravia C, Berk T, McLeod RS et al (2000) Desmoid disease in patients with familial adenomatous polyposis. Dis Colon Rectum 43:363–369
73. Penna C, Tiret E, Parc R et al (1993) Operation and abdominal desmoid tumours in familial adenomatous polyposis. Surg Gynecol Obstet 177:263–268
74. Sagar PM, Möslein G, Dozois RR et al (1998) Management of desmoid tumours in patients after ileal pouch-anal anastomosis for familial adenomatous polyposis. Dis Colon Rectum 41:1350–1356
75. Lynch HT, Fitzgibbons R Jr, Chong S et al (1994) Use of doxorubicin and dacarbazine for the management of unresectable intraabdominal desmoid tumors in Gardner's syndrome. Dis Colon Rectum 37:260–267
76. Soule EH, Scanlon PW (1962) Fibrosarcoma arising in an extra-abdominal desmoid. Mayo Clin Proc 37:433-451
77. Häyry P, Reitamo JJ, Totterman S et al (1982) The desmoid tumour. 2. Analysis of factors possibly contributing to the etiology and growth behavior. Am J Clin Pathol 77:674–680
78. Reitamo JJ (1983) The desmoid tumour. 4. Choice of treatment, results and complications. Arch Surg 118:1318–1322
79. Porru D, Stancati S, Giliberto GL et al (2004) Bilateral ureteral compression by multiple abdominal desmoid tumors in Gardner syndrome: case report and literature review. Urology 64:1031
80. Maldjian C, Mitty H, Garten A et al (1995) Abscess formation in a desmoid tumor of Gardner's syndrome and percutaneous drainage: a report of three cases. Cardiovasc Intervent Radiol 18:168–171
81. Richard III HM, Thall EH, Mitty H et al (1997) Desmoid tumor-ureteral fistula in Gardner's syndrome. Urology 49:135–138
82. Church JM (1998) Mucosal ischaemia caused by desmoid tumors in patients with familial adenomatous polyposis. Dis Colon Rectum 41:661–663
83. Firoozmand E, Parger E (2001) Pelvic desmoid tumor: threat to mother and fetus. Am Surg 67:1213–1215
84. Clark SK, Phillip RK (1996) Desmoids in familial adenomatous polyposis. Br J Surg 83:1494–1504
85. Anthony T, Rodriguez-Bigas MA, Webwe TK et al (1996) Desmoid tumor. J Am Coll Surg 182:369–377
86. Serpell JW, Paddle-Ledinek JE, Johnson WR (1966) Modification of growth of desmoid tumours in tissue culture by antiestrogenic substances: a preliminary report. Aust N Z J Surg 66:457–463
87. Avisse C, Elbaz M, Pluot M et al (1997) Desmoid tumor of the abdominal wall: report of seven cases. Hernia 1:163–167
88. Hartley JE, Church JM, Gupta S et al (2004) Significance of incidental desmoids identified during surgery for familial adenomatous polyposis. Dis Colon Rectum 47:334–340
89. Brooks AP, Reznek RH, Nugent K et al (1994) CT appearances of desmoid tumors in familial adenomatous polyposis: further observations. Clin Radiol 49:601–607
90. Vandevenne JE, De Schepper AM, De Beuckeleer et al (1997) New concepts in understanding evolution of desmoid tumoures: MR imaging of 30 lesions. Eur Radiol 7:1013–1019
91. Tonelli F, Valanzano R, Brandi ML (1994) Pharmacologic treatment of desmoid tumours in familial adenomatous polyposis: results of an in vitro study. Surgery 115:473–479
92. Waddell WR, Kirsch WM (1991) Testolactone, sulin-

dac, warfarin and vitamin K1 for unresectable desmoid tumours. Am J Surg 161:416–421
93. Tsukada K, Church JM, Jagelman DG, et al (1992) Noncytotoxic drug therapy for intraabdominal desmoid tumor in patients with familial adenomatous polyposis. Dis Colon Rectum 35:29–33
94. Samuels BL (1999) Management of recurrent desmoid tumor after surgery and radiation: role of cytotoxic and non-cytotoxic therapies. Surg Oncol 8:191–196
95. Tulchinsky H, Keidar A, Strul H et al (2005) Extracolonic manifestations of familial adenomatous polyposis after proctocolectomy. Arch Surg 140:159–164
96. Klein WA, Miller HH, Anderson M et al (1987) The use of indomethacin, sulindac and tamoxifen for the treatment of desmoid tumors associated with familial polyposis. Cancer 60:2863–2868
97. Lim CL, Walker MJ, Mehta RR et al (1986) Estrogen and antiestrogen binding sites in desmoid tumors. Eur J Cancer Clin Oncol 22:583–587
98. Hamilton L, Blackstein M, Berk T et al (1996) Chemotherapy for desmoid tumors in association with familial adenomatous polyposis: a report of three cases. Can J Surg 39:247–252
99. Schnitzler M, Cohen Z, Blackstein M et al (1997) Chemotherapy for desmoid tumors in association with familial adenomatous polyposis. Dis Colon Rectum 40:798–801
100. Tsukada K, Church JM, Jagelman DG et al (1991) Systemic cytotoxic chemotherapy for desmoid in familial adenomatous polyposis. Dis Colon Rectum 34:1090–1092
101. Kitamura A, Kanagawa T, Yamada S et al (1991) Effective chemotherapy for abdominal desmoid tumour in a patient with Gardner's syndrome. Dis Colon Rectum 34:822–826
102. Middleton SB, Phillips RKS (2000) Surgery for large intra-abdominal desmoid tumours. Dis Colon Rectum 43:1759–1763
103. Okuno SH, Edmonson JH (2003) Combination chemotherapy for desmoid tumors. Cancer 97:1134–1135
104. Poritz LS, Blackstein M, Berk T et al (2001) Extended follow-up of patients treated with cytotoxic chemotherapy for intra-abdominal desmoid tumors. Dis Colon Rectum 44:1268–1273
105. Oohata Y, Mibu R, Uehara S et al (1997) Regression of an abdominal desmoid tumour in a patient with familial adenomatous polyposis by hyperthermoradiotherapy. Am J Gastroenterol 92:156–158
106. Nakada I, Ubukata H, Goto Y et al (1997) Prednisolone therapy for intraabdominal desmoid tumours in a patient with familial adenomatous polyposis. Gastroenterol 32:255–259
107. Geurs F, Kok TC (1993) Regression of a great abdominal desmoid tumor by interferon-alpha. J Clin Gastroenterol 16:264–265
108. Umemoto S, Makuuchi H, Amemiya T et al (1991) Intra-abdominal desmoid tumours in familial polyposis coli: a case report of tumour regression by prednisolone therapy. Dis Colon Rectum 34:89–93
109. Wilcken N, Tattersall MH (1991) Endocrine therapy for desmoid tumors. Cancer 68:1384–1388
110. Lindor NM, Dozois R, Nelson H et al (2003) Desmoid tumors in familial adenomatous polyposis: a pilot project evaluating efficacy of treatment with pirfenidone. Am J Gastroenterol 98:1868–1874
111. Mace J, Sybil Biermann J, Sondak V et al (2002) Response of extraabdominal desmoid tumors to therapy with imatinib mesylate. Cancer 95:2373–2379
112. Lev-Chelouche D, Abu-Abeid S, Nakache R et al (1999) Limb desmoid tumours: a possible role for isolated limb perfusion with tumour necrosis factor-alpha ang melphalan. Surgery 126:963–967
113. Rock MG, Pritchard DJ, Reiman HM et al (1984) Extra-abdominal desmoid tumors. J Bone Joint Surg Am 66:1369–1374
114. Chatzipetrou MA, Tzakis AG, Pinna AD et al (2001) Intestinal transplantation for the treatment of desmoid tumors associated with familial adenomatous polyposis. Surgery 129:277–281
115. Tryphonopoulos P, Weppler D, Levi DM et al (2005) Transplantation for the treatment of intra-abdominal fibromatosis. Transplant Proc 37:1379–1380
116. Church J, Berk T, Boman BM et al (2005) Collaborative Group of the Americas on Inherited Colorectal Cancer. Staging intra-abdominal desmoid tumors in familial adenomatous polyposis: a search for a uniform approach to a troubling disease. Dis Colon Rectum 48:1528–1534
117. Kono T, Tomita I, Chisato N et al (2004) Successful low-dose chemotherapy using vinblastine and methotrexate for the treatment of an ileoanal pouch mesenteric desmoid tumor: report of a case. Dis Colon Rectum 47:246–249
118. Sagar PM, Moslein G, Dozois RR (1998) Management of desmoid tumors in patients after ileal pouch-anal anastomosis for familial adenomatous polyposis. Dis Colon Rectum 41:1350–1356
119. Guy RJ, Mortensen NJ (2000) Successful resection of an ileoanal pouch mesenteric desmoid without pouch sacrifice: report of a case. Dis Colon Rectum 43:713–716
120. Bertario L, Presciuttini S, Sala P et al (1994) Causes of death and postsurgical survival in familial adenomatous polyposis: results from the Italian Registry of Familial Adenomatous Polyposis Writing Committee. Semin Surg Oncol 10:225–234
121. Belchetz LA, Berk T, Bapat BV et al (1996) Changing causes of mortality in patients with familial adenomatous polyposis. Dis Colon Rectum 39:384–387
122. Brueckl WM, Preuss JM, Wein A et al (2001) Ki-67 expression and residual tumour (R) classification are associated with disease-free survival in desmoid tumour patients. Anticancer Res 21:3615–3620
123. Gardner EJ, Plenk HP (1952) Hereditary pattern for multiple osteomas in a family group. Am J Hum Genet 4:31–36
124. Bilkay U, Edram O, Ozek C et al (2004) Benign osteoma with Gardner syndrome: review of the literature and report of a case. J Craniofac Surg 15:506–509
125. Takeuchi T, Takenoshita Y, Kubo K et al (1993) Natural course of jaw lesions in patients with familial adenomatosis coli (Gardner's syndrome). Int J Oral Maxillofac Surg 22:226–230
126. Giardiello FM, Offerhaus GJ, Tarboulsi EI et al (1991) Value of combined phenotypic markers in identifying inheritance of familial adenomatous polyposis. Gut

32:1170–1174
127. Offerhaus GJ, Levin LS, Giardiello FM et al (1987) Occult radiopaque jaw lesions in familial adenomatous polyposis coli and hereditary nonpolyposis colorectal cancer. Gastroenterology 93:490–497
128. Carl W, Herrera L (1987) Dental and bone abnormalities in patients with familial polyposis coli. Semin Surg Oncol 3:77–83
129. Ascari-Raccagni A, Baldari U, Righini MG (1999) Cutaneous symptoms of Gardner's syndrome. J Eur Acad Dermatol Venereol 12:80–81
130. Hood AB, Krush AJ (1983) Clinical and dermatologic aspects of the hereditary intestinal polyposes. Dis Colon Rectum 26:546–548
131. Marshall KA, Kuhlmann TP, Horowitz JH, et al (1985) Excision of multiple epidermal facial cysts in Gardner's syndrome. Am J Surg 150:615–616
132. Pujol RM, Casanova JM, Egido R, et al (1995) Multiple familial pilomatricomas: a cutaneous marker for Gardner syndrome? Pediatr Dermatol 12:331–335
133. Traboulsi EI (2005) Ocular manifestations of familial adenomatous polyposis (Gardner syndrome). Ophthalmol Clin North Am 18:163–166
134. Shields JA, Shields CL, Shah PG et al (1992) Lack of association among typical congenital hypertrophy of the retinal pigment epithelium, adenomatous polyposis, and Gardner syndrome. Ophthalmology 99:1709–1713
135. Kasner L, Traboulsi EI, Delacruz Z et al (1992) A histopathologic study of the pigmented fundus lesions in familial adenomatous polyposis. Retina 12:35–42
136. Traboulsi EI, Krush AJ, Gardner EJ et al (1987) Prevalence and importance of pigmented ocular fundus lesions in Gardner's syndrome. N Engl J Med 316:661–667
137. Olschwang S, Tiret A, Laurent-Puig P et al (1993) Restriction of ocular fundus lesions to a specific subgroup of APC mutations in adenomatous polyposis coli patients. Cell 75:959–968
138. Cetta F, Montalto G, Gori M et al (2000) Germline mutations of the APC gene in patients with familial adenomatous polyposis-associated thyroid carcinoma: results from a European cooperative study. J Clin Endocrinol Metab 85:286–292
139. Giardiello FM, Offerhaus GJ, Lee DH et al (1993) Increased risk of thyroid and pancreatic carcinoma in familial adenomatous polyposis. Gut 34:1394–1396
140. Plail RO, Bussey HJ, Glazer G et al (1987) Adenomatous polyposis: an association with carcinoma of the thyroid. Br J Surg 74:377–380
141. Herrera L, Carrel A, Rao U et al (1989) Familial adenomatous polyposis in association with thyroiditis: report of two cases. Dis Colon Rectum 32:893–896
142. Turcot J, Despres JP, St Pierre F (1959) Malignant tumors of the central nervous system associated with familial polyposis of the colon: report of two cases. Dis Colon Rectum 2:465–468
143. Paraf F, Jothy S, Van Meir EG (1997) Brain tumor-polyposis syndrome: two genetic diseases? J Clin Oncol 15:2744–2758
144. Gadish T, Tulchinsky H, Deutsch AA et al (2005) Pinealoblastoma in a patient with familial adenomatous polyposis: variant of Turcot syndrome type 2? Report of a case and review of the literature. Dis Colon Rectum 48:2343–2346
145. Jagelman DG, DeCosse JJ, Bussey HJ (1988) Upper gastrointestinal cancer in familial adenomatous polyposis. Lancet 1:1149–1151
146. Walsh N, Qizilbash A, Banerjee R et al (1987) Biliary neoplasia in Gardner's syndrome. Arch Pathol Lab Med 111:76–77
147. Bernstein IT, Bulow S, Mauritzen K (1992) Hepatoblastoma in two cousins in a family with adenomatous polyposis: report of two cases. Dis Colon Rectum 35(4):373–374
148. Hughes LJ, Michels VV (1992) Risk of hepatoblastoma in familial adenomatous polyposis. Am J Med Genet 43:1023–1025
149. Painter TA, Jagelman DG (1985) Adrenal adenomas and adrenal carcinomas in association with hereditary adenomatosis of the colon and rectum. Cancer 55:2001–2004
150. Marchesa P, Fazio VW, Church JM et al (1997) Adrenal masses in patients with familial adenomatous polyposis. Dis Colon Rectum 40(9):1023–1028

Desmoid Tumours in Familial Adenomatous Polyposis

Francesco Tonelli, Lucia Picariello, Gabriella Nesi, Alessandro Franchi, Rosa Valanzano, Corrado R. Asteria, Maria Luisa Brandi

Introduction

The term desmoid was first used by Muller [1] to describe the tendon-like aspect and the hard consistency of this type of proliferation (*desmos* in Greek means band). Desmoid tumours (DTs) are classified as extra- or intra-abdominal. The extra-abdominal DTs arise from fascial or musculoaponeurotic structures predominantly of the abdominal wall (Fig. 1a, b, c) and occasionally of the shoulder girdle, chest wall, inguinal region and extremities. They present as a firm, smooth, painless, progressively growing mass. Imaging investigations are useful in better defining the extent of the tumour which displays an iceberg growth with only a small proportion being clinically manifest. Interestingly, multiple extra-abdominal DTs are frequently discovered in very young patients under the age of 3 [2]. The intra-abdominal DTs develop in the folds of the mesentery or the mesocolon (Fig. 2a, b) even reaching the retroperitoneal tissue or they may grow exclusively in this region. These proliferations are usually single, round or oval in shape and up to 60 cm in size. Rather than a mass, a thickening of the mesentery that appears to be covered with hard white spots and causes retraction of the peritoneal folds is frequently reported in familial

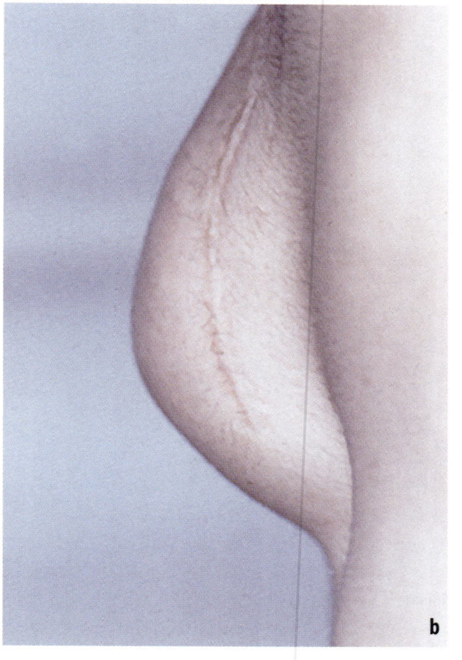

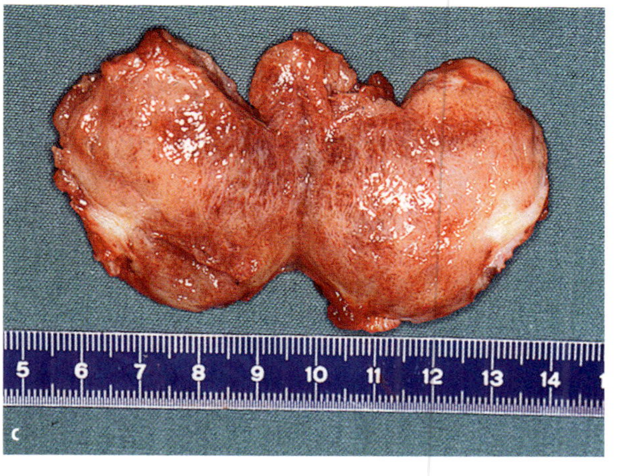

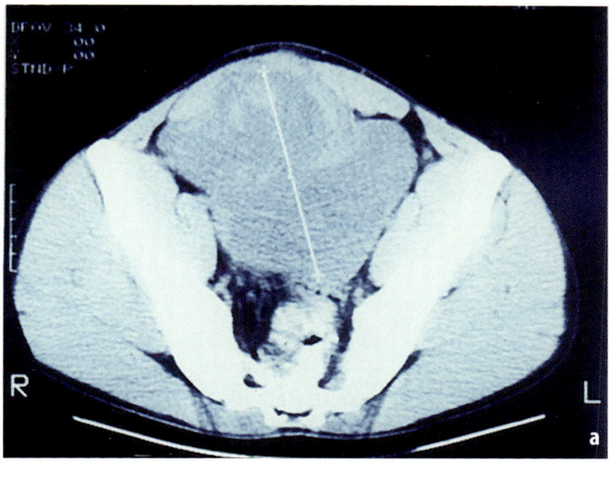

Fig. 1a. Tc scan revealing a large and invasive desmoid mass arising within the abdominal wall. **b** Lateral view of the abdomen showing a protruding desmoid mass along the scar of the previous prophylactic colectomy. **c** Desmoid mass specimen.

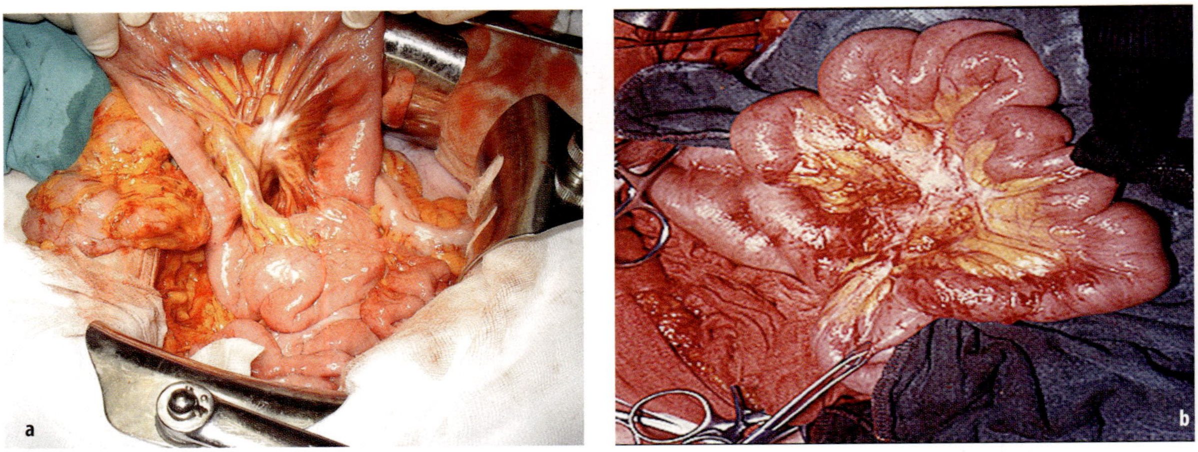

Fig. 2a. Intra-operative view shows a precursor desmoid lesion in the fold of the mesentery and **b** in the mesocolon

adenomatous polyps (FAP) patients. This process has been variously referred as mesenteric fibrosis or mesenteric fibromatosis [3-5]. However, whitish, thin plaque-like areas of the mesenteric folds have been frequently identified in FAP patients undergoing laparotomy (Fig . 3a, b). It has been suggested that these mesenteric abnormalities represent precursor lesions of mesenteric fibromatosis and mesenteric DT [6, 7]. A model of stepwise progression for DT development similar to the adenoma-carcinoma sequence observed for colorectal cancer has been proposed. A prospective study of 42 patients with FAP undergoing laparotomy was made performing a detailed examination of the small-bowel mesentery and biopsy of the lesions. Plaque-like areas of peritoneal thickening were observed in 30% of these patients and areas of diffuse mesenteric fibromatosis in 16%. Histology was similar to that of other desmoids [6]. The patients with mesenteric fibromatosis had undergone a significantly higher number of previous abdominal operations than those without [6].

Helical abdominopelvic CT scanning and MRI was employed to characterize and follow up these precursors. It has been suggested that rapidly growing DTs have high signal intensity on T2-weighted images [8]. Mesenteric fibromatosis were identified in 21% of asymptomatic patients. At the follow-up (median 27 months), patients with desmoid precursor lesions (DPLs) had a significantly greater degree of mesenteric fibromatosis and DT formation than the control group [7]. Furthermore, CT findings consistent with mesenteric fibromatosis were observed on reviewing the scans of patients subsequently developing DTs [9].

Intra-abdominal DTs can be associated with DTs arising in the abdominal wall. The similarity of intra-abdominal DTs to extra-abdominal DTs is evident in

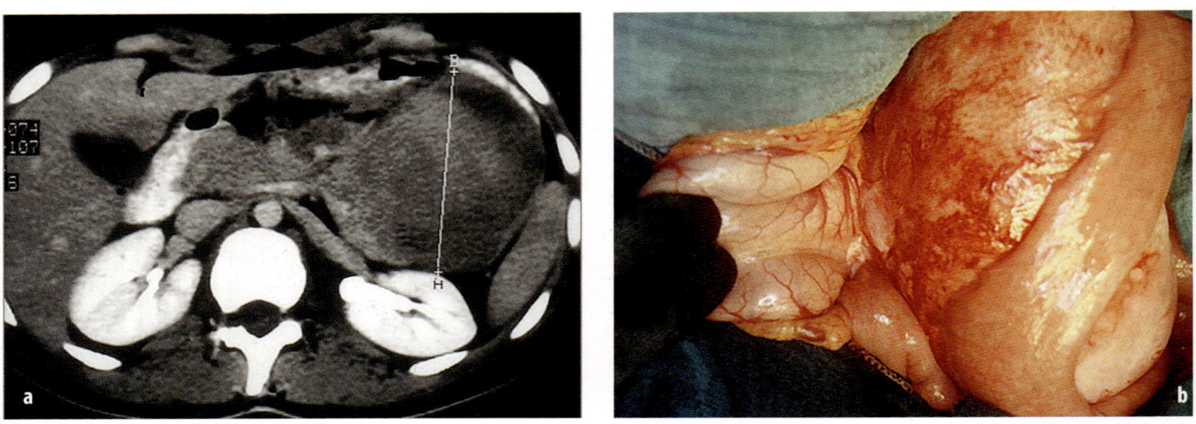

Fig. 3a. Tc scan shows a large desmoid mass arising within the mesentery. **b** Intra-operative view of desmoid mass

Table 1. Data of literature on operated desmoid tumours in familial adenomatous polyposis

Author (year)	Jones et al. [14] (1986)	Lofti et al. [15] (1989)	Penna et al. [13] (1993)	Gurbuz et al. [2] (1994)	Rodriguez-Bigas et al. [16] (1994)	Kadmon et al. [17] (1995)	Heiskanen et al. [18] (1997)	Soravia et al. [19] (2000)	Ho [20] (2002)
Patients ( )[a]	29 (8.9)	24 (13)	29 (12)	83 (10)	24 (38)	29 (17)	29 (14)	97 (12.4)	11 (1)
Male/female ratio	7/22	7/17	16/13	36/47	15/9	10/19	12/17	38/59	5/6
Family history	NA	3 (12.5)	NA	49 (59)	NA	3 (10.3)	4 (13.7)	41 (42.2)	NA
Pregnancy	NA	11 (65)	NA	22 (66)	NA	2 (10)	10 (59)	33 (60)	NA
Site	Mesentery 21 Abd. wall 5 Both sites 4	Mesentery 24	Mesentery 25 Abd. wall 4	Abd. 60, Extra-Abd. 11, Both sites 3 NA 9	Mesentery 8 Abd. wall 5, Both sites 11	Mesentery 19 Abd. wall 15 Extra-abd. 2	Mesentery 15 Abd. wall 10 Other sites 4	Mesentery 49 Abd. wall 10, Both sites 31, Extra-abd.	Mesentery 3 Abd. wall 4
Mean age at DT occurrence	29.8	34	32	31	28.5	34.5	28	29.9	33
DT development: mean tine from colectomy (years)	2	<4	4.9	NA	3.1	NA	3.2	4.6	2.0
Recurrence after surgery	25 (85)	24 (83)	20 (69)	43 (68)	20 (83)	22 (76)	20 (69)	77 (80)	4 (36)

[a]Rate of operated patients. *NA*, not available; *DT*, desmoid tumour; *Abd*, abdominal

the fact that these growths are histologically identical, they never metastasize and usually occur shortly after an abdominal operation. In the series from the polyposis registries of Denmark and Finland, DTs are located intra-abdominally in 50%, in the abdominal wall in 40% and on the extremities in 10% [10].While DTs are rare in the general population (two to four cases/million/year), they represent a major extra-intestinal manifestation of FAP. The risk for a FAP patient of developing a DT is one thousand times that of the general population [2]. The incidence increases steadily with age until the fifth decade of life [11]. Only a few patients manifest a DT before the diagnosis of colonic polyposis. The growth of DTs usually occurs after the colectomy and the mean age at diagnosis varies between 29 and 32 years in patients collected in the registries of the most important institutions [2]. The cumulative risk of DT developing 10 years after prophylactic colectomy is 16% and the cumulative lifetime risk is around 21% [12].

The true incidence of DTs in FAP is unknown. The incidence usually ranges between 7 and 12% when a retrospective review of surgical FAP series is considered [2, 12, 13]. In these studies, the diagnosis is generally made on clinical evidence of an abdominal mass. However, considering that several mesenteric DTs are asymptomatic or are discovered fortuitously on radiographic abdominal examination, the incidence is probably higher than usually reported. Furthermore, it is not clear whether mesenteric fibromatoses are always considered in these clinical series.

In our experience, DTs or their precursors such as mesenteric fibromatosis, retroperitoneal fibrosis or simply mesenteric fibrotic thickening have been found in 40 out of the 97 (41.2%) FAP operated patients. Twenty-seven patients (27.8%) developed abdominal wall or mesenteric DTs. The probable explanation of this relatively high frequency of desmoid reaction lies in a more accurate and prospective investigation. (Tables 1 and 2).

Table 2. Desmoids (D), fibromatosis (FB) and desmoid precursor lesions (DPL) in 40 out of 97 FAP patients (personal experience)

Abdominal wall D (M–F)	Mesenteric D (M–F)	Mesenteric FB (M–F)	Mesenteric DPL (M–F)	Retroperitoneal FB (M–F)
19 (9 /10)	8(1/7)	12(6/6)	7(4/3)	6(3/3)

Clinical Presentation

Desmoids can remain asymptomatic for a considerable length of time, all the while relentlessly enlarging and infiltrating adjacent structures. However, DTs may show a capricious, variable clinical behaviour, usually characterized by an indolent course, rarely by a spontaneous regression and sometimes by an aggressive and rapid growth and a tendency to invade surrounding structures. Desmoid tumours may cause abdominal pain, nausea, vomiting, diarrhoea and deterioration of the functional result in patients submitted to restorative surgery after total colectomy. The intra-abdominal tumour growth may induce small-bowel obstruction or other life-threatening complications such as intestinal perforation or intestinal infarct as the result of the compression of the blood vessels which may impair vascular supply and cause small-bowel ischaemia or mesenteric thrombosis [14, 16]. The consequences of mucosal ischaemia of the small bowel are bleeding or intestinal strictures [21]. Sudden enlargement of the DT can provoke deep vein thrombosis and fatal pulmonary embolism [22]. The tumoral mass may undergo colliquative necrosis and abscess formation which can determine an abdominal emergency or a spontaneous discharge into the intestinal lumen with fistula formation. Also mono- or bilateral hydronephrosis as a result of retroperitoneal invasion can be observed.

Desmoid tumours are the second most common cause of death in FAP patients after colorectal cancer. Intra-abdominal DTs can be responsible for death in up to 11% of FAP patients [23–25]. In the experience of the Johns Hopkins University, the survival rate from DTs evaluated by life-table analysis is 93% at 5 years and 79% at 20 years with a mean age of death in the affected patients of 40 years [2].

Patients who have had an ileal pouch-anal anastomosis (IPAA) and have developed a DT, show a worse functional result than IPAA patients not developing a DT [26, 27]. The occurrence of small-bowel obstruction or intestinal bleeding in IPAA patients with DTs usually requires the removal of the pouch [21, 26].

Histology

These lesions are typically poorly circumscribed with infiltration of the surrounding soft tissue structures. Histologically, DTs are composed of elongated, uniform, bland fibroblasts and myofibroblasts loosely arranged in sweeping bundles (Fig. 4a, b). Tumour cells are set within a collagenous to myxoid stroma

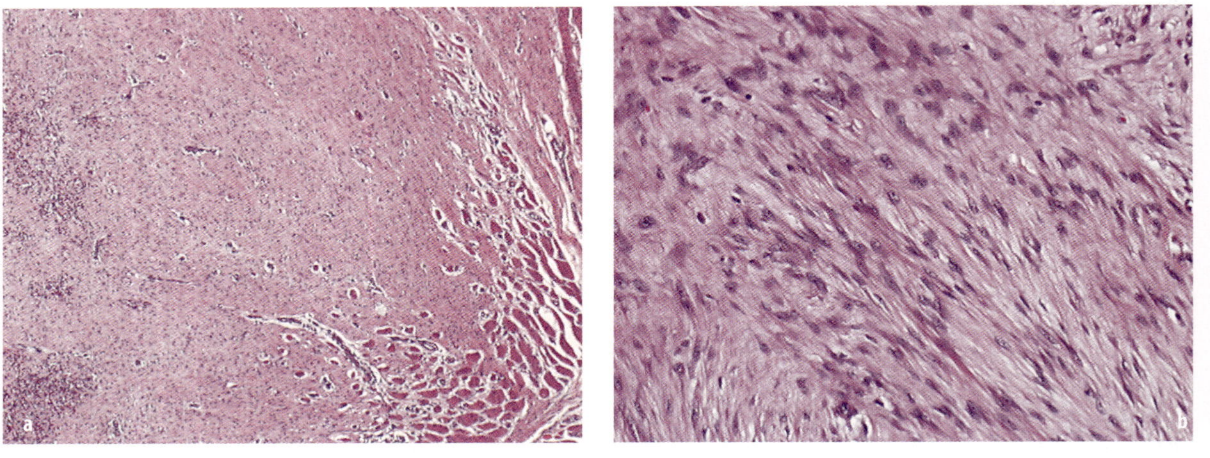

Fig. 4a. Desmoid tumour showing the typical infiltrative growth pattern of the skeletal muscle (original magnification, x50). [2] The lesion is composed of elongated, spindle-shaped cells with uniform cytological features (original magnification, x200).

causing the lesion to closely resemble normal cellular fibrous tissue or scar. Keloid-like collagen or extensive hyalinization may be present. One of the most characteristic features of DTs is its vascularity with numerous blood vessels showing thick walls and open lumina. Mitotic figures are virtually absent. In fact, the observation of even a few mitotic figures should raise the suspicion of a low-grade fibrosarcoma rather than DTs. On immunohistochemical analysis, tumour cells are generally positive for vimentin and actin. A few cells may also express desmin and S-100 protein. Ultrastructural studies further support the fibroblastic and myofibroblastic nature of DTs.

Aetiology and Risk Factors

The aetiology of DTs is unknown and their true nature is controversial. DTs are considered dysplastic lesions of connective tissue and classified as fibromatoses, which cover diseases such as Dupuytren's contracture, Peyronie's disease, plantar fibromatosis, idiopathic retroperitoneal fibrosis, etc. The absence of metastatic spread, the generally benign behaviour with slow growth or even regression, the histological features consisting of mature fibroblast without atypia or mitoses, and the absence of telomerase are consistent with a reactive or dysplastic lesion. However, their potentially rapid and aggressive growth and their tendency to recur after surgical removal have suggested a neoplastic origin. Favouring this view is also the fact that DTs will arise after inactivation of the *APC* tumour suppressor gene, occurring by point mutation or allelic deletion. Furthermore, it has been observed that the majority of the cells are represented by a clonal population [28]. It has also been shown that the proliferation of desmoid cell cultures is inhibited by the cellular transfection of wild-type *APC* [29]. The hypothesis has been proposed that the DPLs undergo a multi-step process analogous to the cascade suggested for the adenoma-carcinoma sequence developing firstly mesenteric fibromatosis and finally mesenteric DTs [6, 28]. The surgical trauma could favour somatic mutations of mesenteric fibroblasts, inducing their clonal expansion to produce a DT. This interpretation suggests the need of preventive measures in order to avoid the transformation of DPLs in true DTs, as well as for a rational oncological approach to aggressive DTs.

Gender and Pregnancy

The influence of the female gender regarding the development of DTs in FAP patients is controversial. In the past, several authors found no significant sex differences [2, 30] or a slight prevalence in the female sex, with a female/male ratio of 1.4 [31, 18]. More recently a clear preponderance of DTs among females clearly has been noted in studies concerning large series of FAP patients, and females have twice the odds of developing DTs compared with males [12, 32].

The effect of pregnancy on the behaviour of intra-abdominal DTs has been investigated in retrospective studies. Some authors have shown a tendency for DTs to develop soon after pregnancy [30, 33, 34], but others find that DTs present later, are smaller and significantly less aggressive in females who have been pregnant than in females who have not [35]. These authors suggest that hormones of pregnancy such as progesterone or prolactin, could have a beneficial effect and suggest that this type of hormonal treatment should be attempted. In their opinion, further prospective studies are needed to determine the consequences of pregnancy on DTs and the risk for a pregnant female of developing a DT, in order to advise women with a family history of DT against pregnancy [35].

Surgery

A surgical trauma is generally indicated as a precipitating factor for DT development (Table 3). In particular, in 68–83% of FAP patients, an abdominal operation precedes formation of DTs by a few months up to a few years. The mean time to DT development varies, but it is usually around 2 years [4, 11, 15, 30]. It appears that there is no correlation between the entity of the surgery and the occurrence of DTs. Desmoid tumours affect patients operated by subtotal colectomy and ileo-rectal anastomosis or by restorative proctocolectomy and IPAA in a similar percentage [13, 19, 31, 32], but even a minor abdominal surgical procedure such as appendectomy can induce DTs. Iterative surgery can increase the risk as Penna et al. [13] have shown, considering that 41% of DTs are discovered after at least two surgical interventions.

Early age at time of colectomy represents a risk factor. In the experience of Jarvinen [11], patients with postoperative DTs had undergo colectomy at a mean age of 26.1 years, significantly earlier than those not developing DTs (37.8 years, $p<0.01$).

Family History and Genetic Predisposition

The hereditary nature of DTs has become clearer when DTs and mesenteric fibromatosis were recog-

Table 3. Characteristics of desmoid lesions: personal experience in familial adenomatous polyposis

Type of D	Sex (M–F)	Age at diagnosis, mean (range)	Size: cm (range)	Time from colectomy, mean (range) years	Type of surgery IRA/IPAA
Abdominal wall D	9–10	29.3(11–61)	8.5(3–12)	4.9 (1–30)[a]	7/11[b]
Mesenteric D	1–7	35(25–61)	10 (3–17)	15.5(1–17)	6/2
Mesenteric FB	6–6	45(24–58)	4.8(4–9)	15(4–34)	11/1
DPL	4–3	35.8(14–57)	3.6(1–5)	3.4 (1–8)	2/2[c]
Retroperitoneal fibrosis	3–3	28.8 (11–36)	NA[d]	12 (1–17)	1/5
Extra-abdominal D	1	22	4	1	0/1

D, Desmoid; *FB*, Fibromatosis; *DPL*, Desmoid precursor lesion; *IRA*, Ileo-Rectal-Anastomosis; *IPAA*, Ileo pouch-anal anastomosis
[a]Diagnosis before colectomy: one case; at colectomy: one case; [b]One proctocolectomy and definitive ileostomy; [c]Diagnosis at colectomy in three patients; [d]Not applicable

nized as stigmata of FAP and a more accurate diagnosis of these complications was achieved. Desmoid tumours have been reported to be frequently associated with Gardner's syndrome [5]: a 32% incidence of desmoid reaction is found among affected members of the original Gardner's syndrome kindred 109. First-degree relatives of FAP patients with DTs have a greater risk of developing DTs than more distant relatives (25% for first degree vs. 11% for second degree and 8% for third degree) [2]. Bertario et al. [25] estimated the risk of developing DTs in 897 FAP patients scheduled on the Italian hereditary colorectal tumour registry and found that family history of DTs, osteomas and epidermoid cysts was significantly associated with the presence of the disease. Similarly, Sturt et al. [32] found that family history (especially if more than 50% of the members were affected with DTs) increased the odds ratio over sevenfold.

The *APC* gene responsible for the development of FAP has been investigated for specific mutations which may be related to DT development. Desmoid tumours will develop when both alleles of the *APC* gene are faulty, but one of the mutations encompasses the region 3' of codon 1444 [32, 36, 37]. Genotype-phenotype correlation within the location of *APC* mutation, the occurrence of DTs and the number of colonic polyps has been observed: *APC* mutations between codons 1444 to 1578 is associated with DTs and a severe form of polyposis, while mutations at the 3' region of *APC* are linked with DTs and an attenuated form of FAP [38, 39]. An aggressive growth pattern of DTs has been attributed to the presence of a germline *APC* mutation in codon 1445-1578 [38]. Mutations beyond codon 1309 or 1444 confer, respectively, a 17- and a 12-fold higher risk of DT development, compared with mutations located at or before codon 452 [12]. Therefore, families with a high incidence of DTs usually have the inherited germline mutation at 3' of codon 1444 and may have the environmentally induced somatic mutation in any point of the *APC* gene, whereas families with sporadic occurrence of DT have the germline mutation at 5' of codon 1444 and must have the somatic mutation at 3' of codon 1444. This fact explains the difference in the percentage of DTs among *APC* kindreds.

An uncommon mutation of the *APC* gene due to frameshift of codon 1924 is accompanied by a high incidence of DTs, a few or no colonic polyps and the rare occurrence of colorectal cancer. This syndrome is called hereditary desmoid disease [40].

Desmoid and Oestrogens

Mechanism of Action of Oestrogens

The oestrogenic bio-effects are mediated by specific receptor subtypes, ERα and ERβ, which exhibit a tissue-specific distribution. The unbound ERs exist as inactive intracellular receptors expressed in reproductive and not reproductive tissues. The mechanism of action is switched on after the interaction of the receptors with the ligand(s), which could be either the steroidal oestrogen, the polyphenolic phyto-oestrogens or the synthetic SERMs (selective estrogen receptor modulators). The latter exhibit either agonist or antagonist oestrogenic actions. The first generation of SERMs are represented by the triphenylethylenes tamoxifen and toremifene, which show agonist properties in the bone and uterus, but an antagonist action on the breast. The last generation of SERMs, represented by raloxifene and its analogues—LY-353381, EM-800 and CP-336156—are benzothiophene derivatives, showing anti-oestrogenic effects on the breast and uterus, but an oestrogen agonist effect on bone and cardiovascular systems.

The ER expression was shown by the authors both in DT tissues and in desmoid-derived cells in culture [41, 42]. Furthermore, we studied the gene expression of ERs in primary cultures obtained from desmoid tumoral tissue. The results showed that, in all the cultures, ERα and ERβ were variably expressed (Picariello et al., 2006, personal communication); in fact, in some patients the ERα expression was predominant in respect to ERβ. The extremely variable expression of the two ERs in these primary cell cultures underlines the individual differences among patients.

To evaluate if oestrogen could influence the DT derived cell growth, primary cell cultures obtained were cultured in presence or in absence of different concentrations of $17\beta E_2$, from 1 pM to 1 μM concentration for 1 week (Fig. 5) [41]. The results showed that 1 nM concentrations of $17\beta E_2$ stimulated cell proliferation in five of the seven cultures analyzed and the effect induced by oestrogen on cell proliferation was different from one cell culture to another. Any influence on cell proliferation by the oestrogen was observed in two of the seven cultures. These results confirmed that oestrogen induced a proliferative effect in the different cell cultures with a cell-specific potency. This could be due to the ER expression pattern and to the different $17\beta E_2$ potency in transactivating gene expression controlled by ERα and ERβ. In those cultures, where the increase of cell growth was great, there was a higher expression of ERαβ than ERβ, while in those cultures where the effect of oestrogens was slight or absent, a comparable expression of the two ERs was evident. Therefore, the characteristic pattern of ER expression in each culture could be responsible for the cell culture-specific proliferative potency of $17\beta E_2$ which displays a greater ERα selectivity with a higher potency in transactivating gene expression controlled by ERα rather than ERβ.

We also studied the effect of SERMs on the proliferation of desmoid cell cultures and the putative mechanism of action of SERMs. Firstly, we observed that tamoxifen inhibited the proliferative effect of $17\beta E_2$ [41]. Subsequently, we cultured desmoid cells in the presence of different concentrations of an analogue of raloxifene, LY117018 for one week (Fig. 6) [42]. LY117018 induced a dose-dependent inhibition of cell proliferation at the pharmacological dose of 5 μM concentration independently of a greater or lesser expression of each ER. This suggests that pharmacological concentration of raloxifene, as well as other SERM molecules (e.g. tamoxifen and toremifene), could directly inhibit the proliferation and function of DT cells acting through or independently of ERs. To investigate if the inhibition of cell proliferation by LY117018 was dependent on the apoptotic cell death process, the desmoid cells were stimulated with the drug and then the internucleosomal fragmentation of genomic DNA was evaluated. The results showed that DT derived cell cultures stimulated with 5 μM of raloxifene did not develop the typical nucleosomal ladder pattern of DNA degradation, clearly exhibited by the positive control (HL-60 cells stimulated for 4 h with 2.5 μg/ml camptothecin; personal observations). These data suggest

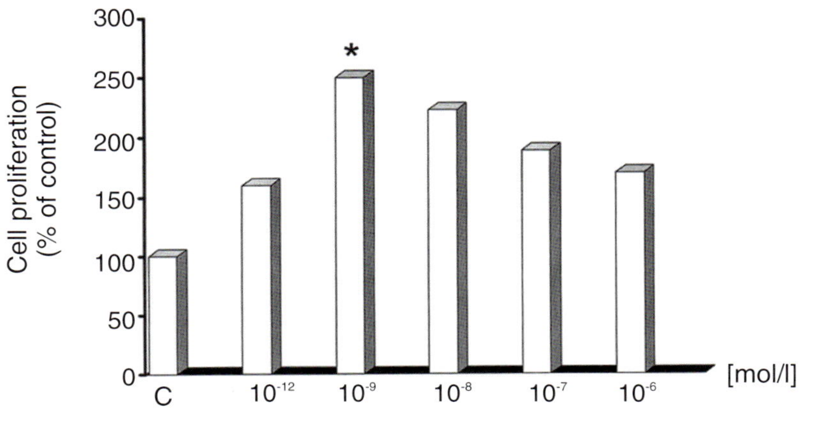

Fig. 5. Effects of $17ßE_2$ on cell growth of desmoid tumour cells. Cells were plated in phenol-red-free growth medium supplemented with 1% charcoal stripped foetal calf serum, containing different concentrations of $17ßE_2$. After 1 week cells were counted. Results were expressed as % of control values of three separate experiments. $*p<0.05$

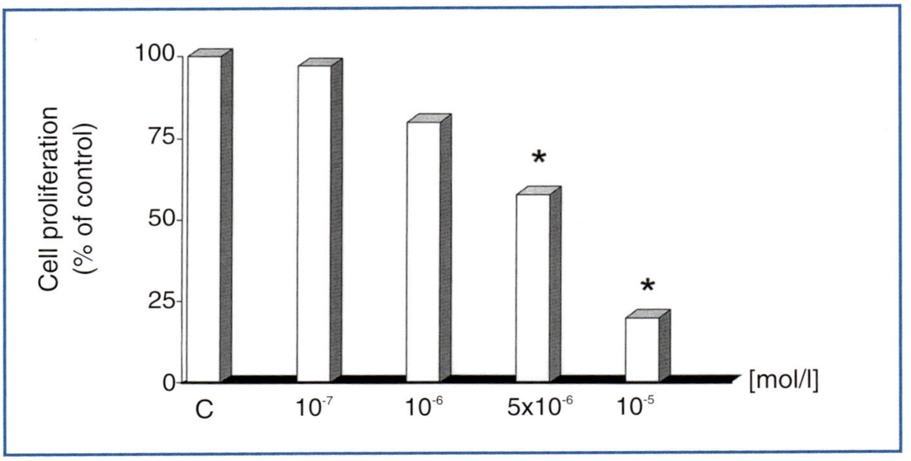

Fig. 6. Effects of LY117018, an analogue of raloxifene, on cell growth of desmoid cells. Cells were plated in growth medium containing different concentrations of LY117018. After 1 week cell number was evaluated. Results were expressed as % of control values of three separate experiments. *$p<0.05$

that the biological effect exerted by SERM molecules on DTs is mediated only in part by their binding to both ERα and ERβ, but is essentially due to a cytotoxic and cytostatic mechanism. The hypothesis to be evaluated is that raloxifene as well as triphenylethylenes reduce the synthesis of TGFβ1, a potent growth stimulator of mesenchymal cells. Recent studies have shown increased $17\beta E_1$ production, $17\beta E_1$ mRNA expression and $17\beta E_1$ receptor number in desmoid cells in culture compared with normal fibroblasts [43]. This growth factor enhances organic macromolecule accumulation in the extra-cellular matrix (ECM) via a reduction of matrix metalloproteinases (MMPs), a family of zinc-dependent neutral endopeptidases which are involved in the degradation of ECM, and an increase in the natural tissue inhibitors of MMPs. The growth of DTs is favoured by a decreased collagen degradation rather than by an increase of collagen synthesis. It has been shown that the presence of 1 μM toremifene in the cultural medium inhibited $17\beta E_1$ activity and consequently reduced collagen accumulation by increasing collagen degradation.

Treatment with SERMs

Anti-oestrogen therapy has been largely based on triphenylethylenes such as tamoxifen or its chlorinated derivate toremifene since its first use by Waddell in 1983 [44]. As for the use of NSAIDs, medical treatment with SERMs is empirical and controversial, being based largely on anecdotal reports and small, poorly controlled studies, most of which are retrospective [45]. The dose commonly used is 30 mg/day which is accompanied by a positive effect in about 50% of the cases. Other authors have employed higher doses of tamoxifen (120–200 mg/day) obtaining a cessation of growth in 63–77% of the patients [42, 47]. However, the best outcome was observed in the group of patients who received high-dose tamoxifen in combination with sulindac 300 mg. Development of ovarian cysts is a frequent side effect of tamoxifen treatment in the female patients. The response to tamoxifen is usually gradual and slow so that the achievement of a partial or complete regression lasts several months or years. If DTs are particularly aggressive with rapid growth, the effect of SERMs could be negative in the first months because the time period required for the action can be prolonged. It is not clear how long the treatment should be once a complete regression has been obtained. The likelihood of accelerated DT growth on the cessation of tamoxifen treatment should justify a prolonged or indefinite treatment [46]. However, the risk of endometrial cancer with 20 mg per day of tamoxifen has been recognized for many years [48, 49]. Conversely, lack of worrying endometrial stimulation seen with triphenylethylenes confers to raloxifene a more favourable profile, particularly in the long-term use of the drug. We studied the effect of 120 mg daily (a dosage double than recommended for prevention of osteoporotic fractures) of raloxifene on progression of DT and of mesenteric fibromatosis by evaluation of lesion size and symptoms in 13 FAP patients. The patients had a significant response to raloxifene therapy with complete remission in five cases and partial remission in five other cases [50]. None of the patients experienced major side-effects and no significant changes in biochemical parameters or endometrial thickness were observed. It is important to bear in mind that raloxifene was efficacious even if previous treatments with tamoxifen and sulindac had failed. Tables 4 and 5 focuses our personal experience respectively on chemoprophylaxis and on drug therapy.

Table 4. Chemoprophylaxis of desmoids: personal experience in familial adenomatous polyposis

Type of lesions	Patients	Drug	Duration, mean range (months)	Length of follow-up mean range (months)	Absence of progression	Regression	Recurrence
DPL	20	Tamoxifen/ raloxifen	65 (6–168)	79 (10–168)	18[b]	2[a]	
Abdominal wall D	15	Tamoxifen/ raloxifen	59 (2–120)	84 (2–154)	13[c]		2

D, Desmoid; *DPL*, Desmoid precursor lesion

[a]Intraoperative evaluation for second surgery; [b]No evidence at clinical examination or at CT scan; [c]No evidence of D at clinical examination or at US/CT scan

Table 5. Drug therapy of desmoids: personal experience in familial adenomatous polyposis

Type of desmoids	Patients	Drug	Duration months (range)	Lenght of follow-up months (range)	Progression	Regression	Stable
Mesentery D	8	Tamoxifen Raloxifen	65 (2–156)	57 (2–156)	2[a]	6	0
Retroperitoneal fibrosis	1 1	Tamoxifen Raloxifen	24 48	24 192	0	2	0
Abdominal wall D	2 1	Tamoxifen Raloxifen	14 44	14 60	2[a]	 1	

[a]Voluntary drop-out in one case

NSAIDs and Desmoid Tumours

Mechanism of Action of NSAIDs

Several reviews [51–53] have summarized the intriguing and accumulating evidence that non-steroidal anti-inflammatory drugs (NSAIDs) have potential as anti-cancer drugs. NSAIDs have been shown experimentally to stimulate apoptosis and to inhibit angiogenesis, two mechanisms that help to suppress malignant transformation and tumour growth.

The mechanism of action common to NSAIDs is the inhibition of cyclooxygenase (COX) enzymatic conversion of the polyunsaturated fatty acid arachidonic acid (produced by the hydrolysis of phospholipids catalyzed by phospholipase A) to prostaglandin G_2 (PGG_2) [56]. PGG_2 is converted to prostaglandin H_2 by the peroxidase activity of the COX enzyme, and then PGH_2 may be converted by tissue-specific isomerases to one of the five biologically active prostanoids: PGE_2, prostaglandin D_2, prostaglandin $F_{2\alpha}$, prostacyclin or thromboxane [57].

Two distinct isoforms of COX, designed COX-1 and COX-2 have been recognized [58, 59]. COX-1 is expressed constitutively in many tissues, and it plays a central role in platelet aggregation and gastric cytoprotection [58–59]. Although COX-2 is expressed constitutively in the human kidney and brain, its expression is induced in many tissues during inflammation, wound healing and neoplasia.

NSAIDs vary in their abilities to inhibit COX-1 or COX-2 at different concentrations and in different tissues [60, 61]. Aspirin is the only NSAID known to react covalently with COX-1 and COX-2 by selective acetylation of a specific serine residue at position 529 and 516, respectively [62, 63]. Aspirin acetylation of COX-1 results in a complete blockade of arachidonate oxidation to PGH_2, aspirin has thus been reported to be a more potent suppressor of PGH_2 formation by the activity of COX-1 than that formed by COX-2 [64]. The other NSAIDs such as ibuprofen and indomethacin, produce reversible or irreversible inhibition of both COX-1 and COX-2 by competing with the arachidonic acid for the active site of the enzyme [56].

Although NSAIDs are widely used and are effective, their long-term use is limited by gastrointestinal effects such as dyspepsia and abdominal pain, gastric and duodenal perforation or bleeding, and small bowel and colonic ulcerations. The discovery of COX-1 and COX-2 has led to the suggestion that the therapeutic effect of NSAIDs is primarily the result of inhibition of COX-2, whereas the toxicity of NSAIDs may primarily result from inhibition of COX-1 [65] In fact, NSAIDs toxicity in the gastrointestinal mucosa is the result of inhibition of COX-1 activity in platelets, which increases the tendency of bleeding, and in gastric mucosa, where prostanoids play an important role in protecting the stomach from erosion and ulceration [55]. While the conventional NSAIDs inhibit COX-1 and COX-2 to the same extent, the development of a new group of anti-inflammatory drugs, the coxibs, selective inhibitors of COX-2 (e.g. celecoxib, rofecoxib, valdecoxib, etoricoxib, lumiracoxib), represent a response to the unsatisfactory therapeutic profile of NSAIDs and it was hoped that coxibs would be better tolerated than non-selective NSAIDs and would be equally efficacious and that selective inhibition of COX-2 could be an effective strategy for preventing cancer.

Several prostaglandins such as PGE2, suppress immunosurveillance through down-regulation of lymphokines, T-cell and B-cell proliferation, cytotoxic activity of natural killer cells and secretion of TNFα and interleukin 10 [66]. It has been shown that there is a close relationship between PGE_2 and EGF-receptor signalling systems. PGE_2 induces the activation of metalloproteinases MMP2 and MMP9, increases expression of TGFα, transactivates EGF receptor, and triggers mitogenic signalling in gastric epithelial and colon cancer cells as well as in rat gastric mucosa in vivo. This mechanism may explain how PGE_2 exerts its trophic action on gastric and intestinal mucosa, resulting in hypertrophy and cancer. The inhibition of prostaglandin synthesis by NSAIDs can explain the anti-tumoral effect of these drugs.

Despite continuing uncertainty about the molecular pathways by which NSAIDs may inhibit neoplasia, there is mounting evidence that tumour inhibition, for example in colorectal cancer, may be mediated by at least two distinct cellular processes: the ability of NSAIDs to restore apoptosis in *APC*-deficient cells [67, 68] and their capacity, particularly in the case of coxibs, to inhibit angiogenesis. Apoptosis, or programmed cell death is needed to maintain homeostasis in continuously replicating tissues such as intestinal mucosa [69]. The suppression of apoptosis allows *APC*-deficient cells to accumulate and form adenomatous polyps. Further suppression of apoptosis occurs as these cells develop additional genetic mutations and phenotypic changes [70]. In Vitro, both non-selective NSAIDs and selective COX-2 inhibitors stimulate apoptosis in *APC*-deficient colonic cells that have not undergone malignant transformation [71]. Non-selective NSAIDs lose their ability to inhibit chemically induced tumours when polyps undergo malignant transformation. In contrast, selective COX-2 inhibitors stimulate apoptosis and suppress growth in many carcinomas, including cultured human cancers of the stomach, oesophagus, tongue, brain, lung and pancreas [72–77]. The precise mechanism by which NSAIDs restore apoptosis remains controversial [78], but treatment of colorectal carcinoma cells with NSAIDs or coxibs increases the concentration of arachidonic acid that, if unesterified, modulates mitochondrial permeability and causes release of cytochrome C, thus leading to apoptosis [79].

Other experimental models suggest that NSAIDs induce apoptosis by either COX dependent or COX independent mechanisms. In the latter case, the G0/G1 cell-cycle block caused by celecoxib in colon cancer cell lines and In Vivo models is related to a decreased expression of cyclins A and B1, and to the expression of cell-cycle inhibitory proteins p21WAF1 and p27KIP1 [80] as well as the coxib NS-398 enhanced apoptosis in cells which do not express COX-2 enzyme [78]. NSAIDs have also been reported to induce apoptosis through 15-lipoxygenase-1, independent of COX-2 [81]. However, many of these effects have been demonstrated only with high concentrations of NSAIDs In Vitro and are of uncertain clinical relevance.

Several studies have shown a relation between angiogenesis and COX-2 expression [82], so a second cellular process by which NSAIDs and in particular COX-2 inhibitors may inhibit tumour growth is through inhibition of angiogenesis and neovascularization [83]. COX-2 induces proangiogenic factors such as VEGF, inducible nitric oxide synthase, interleukins 6 and 8, and TIE_2 [83, 84], and it produces prostaglandins that have both autocrine and paracrine effects on proliferation and migration of endothelial cells In Vitro [82, 85]. COX-2 is overexpressed in "activated" tumour endothelial cells, whereas COX1 is expressed in normal endothelial cells [82]. COX-2 derived prostaglandins stimulate angiogenesis In Vivo, and COX-2 inhibition of endothelial cells slows down tumour growth. In particular, COX-2 modulates the production of angiogenic factors by tumour cells, whereas COX-1 regulates angiogenesis of endothelial cells in normal tissue [83]. Therefore the hypothesized mechanism by which NSAIDs block angiogenesis is the inhibition of COX-1 and COX-2 activity in endothelial cells. Other studies supported these data also in In Vivo models, focusing on the role of celecoxib in inhibiting of blood vessel formation, tumour growth and development of metastasis [86]. In contrast, toxic concentrations of aspirin or indomethacin are required to block vascular endothelial tube formation [83, 87]. These experiments suggest that COX-2 may be essential for tumour vascularization and growth.

Finally, Brueggemeier et al. [88] showed co-expression of the aromatase enzyme and COX-2 in human breast cancer, with a significant association with gene expression of both: Thus, COX-2 may be the cause of progression of oestrogen-dependent breast cancer by autocrine and paracrine mechanisms, by direct stimulation of tumour cell proliferation, or by indirect upregulation of aromatase activity [88].

Treatment with NSAIDs

The fact that both ß-catenin and mutated *APC* are implicated in colon cancer and DT development [89, 100] and that prostaglandins and cyclooxygenase have a role in colonic neoplasia and FAP progression [68, 91–93], has prompted the use of NSAIDs in the treatment of DTs. However, there are enough differences between desmoids and colonic neoplasms so that data, including blockade of angiogenesis, modulation of aromatase, and pro-apoptotic activity cannot be easily generalized from one tumour to another. We showed that there was a high expression of COX-1 and COX-2 in DT cells and tissues derived from different patients undergoing surgery (Picariello et al., 2006, personal communication). In particular, the amount of COX-2 protein was higher than that of COX-1, suggesting the role of COX-2 in the pathogenesis of this neoplasia. In addition, the expression of COXs was different in the different cultures, suggesting an extreme variability between individual tumours. Indomethacin or sulindac, an indomethacin analogue with prolonged effect, has been frequently used alone or in combination with anti-oestrogens. The mechanisms of action of the anti-COX drugs are complex: sulindac sulphide, the pharmacologically active metabolite of sulindac, induces a significant growth reduction in desmoid cells In Vitro [94], but the drug does not induce apoptosis at clinically significant concentrations in these cells. However, this NSAID molecule induces apoptosis in an endothelial cell line. The latter effect seems very important considering the role of the microvasculature in tumour growth and could explain the efficacy of sulindac sulphide in the treatment of DTs. Other recent studies have also shown that in DT cell cultures, the inhibition of COX-2 expression with a new coxib, DFU (5,5-dimethyl-3-(3-fluorophenyl)-4-(4-methylsulphonyl)phenyl-2(5H)-furon one), blocks the cellular growth, but does not promote apoptosis, suggesting that regulation of apoptosis does not play a major role in this neoplasm [95] and calling for other mechanisms to explain the effect of this drug.

Several small series of patients have been treated with a daily dosage of 200–400 mg of sulindac. The duration of treatment varied from a few months to several years. Overall, an objective response rate of about 50% was observed: in the majority of the patients a partial regression was shown and only in a few patients was a complete regression obtained [87, 96–97]. This treatment seems less efficacious in patients undergoing partial resection of their DT prior to medical therapy [19]. Most responses were observed after a few weeks of treatment.

More often, sulindac has been employed in combination with anti-oestrogen even if the effect is similar to that observed in patients treated with sulindac alone. Recently, 11 patients were treated with a combination of celecoxib, an anti-COX2, and tamoxifen, showing a complete regression in 1 patient, a partial regression in 3, a stable disease in 5 and no tumour recurrence in 2 patients in whom the drugs were used as adjuvant therapy after surgical excision [22]. As anti-cancer therapy, coxibs present important theoretical advantages: they are orally active, have moderate side effects, and have few medical contraindications. Their good toxicological profile allows long-term medical treatment. In conclusion, even if the small number of cases studied and appropriately referred to in the literature and the absence of prospective randomized trials makes estimation of the effect of NSAIDs difficult, they can be effective in controlling DT growth and should be used as a first-line treatment.

Other Drugs

A very small number or anecdotic cases are treated with other drugs sometimes in combination with NSAIDs or SERMs: warfarin and vitamin K [98], interferon-α-2b, progesterone, prednisolone, ascorbic acid, testosterone, analogues of LHRH, and pirfenidone [99–102]. Recently, imatinib mesylate has been shown to be active in two patients not affected by FAP with extra-abdominal DT refractory to other medical treatments. Interestingly, positivity for c-kit as well as PDGFR-α and PGDFR-β was found at immunohistochemical and qualitative RT-PCR analysis [103]. These data must be confirmed on DTs in association with FAP and on a larger series.

Prevention of Desmoid Tumours

Chemoprophylaxis against the onset of DTs has been suggested even if no data are reported in the literature. The ideal drug should be active in a large number of cases and have a favourable therapeutic index. Both NSAIDs and SERMs seem to have these characteristics, and raloxifen has no major side effects. All the FAP patients submitted to abdominal surgery who have a family history for DTs or a 3' *APC* mutation are candidates for a pharmacological prophylaxis. In our opinion, the patients in whom PDLs are found at surgery should also be submitted to chemoprophylaxis.

Our experience is detailed in Tables 4 and 5. The 20 patients with a DPL or a fibromatosis of the mesenteric fold were treated with tamoxifen or raloxifen and followed up for a mean time of 65 months and 79 months, respectively. No progression of the desmoid disease was observed in any patient and the lesions completely regressed in two patients after closure of the protective ileostomy.

Radiotheraphy

Radiotherapy is not indicated in the treatment of DTs, because these lesions are relatively insensitive to irradiation and, as a large area would have to be treated, actinic damage of the small bowel is inevitable.

Cytotoxic Chemotherapy

Systemic chemotherapy has been administered to patients with DTs continually growing despite treatment with NSAIDs or anti-oestrogens or rapidly increasing in size thus leading to life-threatening complications. However, chemotherapy is rarely employed because of its toxicity. The published reports regard single cases or small numbers of patients. All treated patients were affected with large tumours, had severe symptoms or major complications. The DTs continued to grow even if medically treated and were deemed unresectable. Various types of cytotoxic drugs were adopted [104–112]. The association with doxorubicin and dacarbazine have generally been chosen in recent years (Table 6). More than 50% of the treated patients achieved significant regression of the lesions and some patients were completely cured. The response to the therapy would appear to last a long time. It has been

Table 6. Results of chemotherapy for mesenteric desmoid

Authors	Type of chemotherapy	Desmoid numbers	Partial response >50%	Complete response
Tsukada et al. 1991 [102] [104]	Vincristine, cyclophosphamide, doxorubicin, 5-FU	8	3	2
Patel et al. 1992 [103] [105]	Doxorubicin, dacarbazine	4	2	2
Lynch et al. 1994 [106]	Doxorubicin, dacarbazine	2	–	1
Schnitzler et al. 1997 [107]	Doxorubicin, dacarbazine	5	3	–
Risum and Bulow [108] 2003	Doxorubicin	1	1	–
Okuno and Edmonson [109] 2003	Ifosfamide, etoposide, mitomycin, doxorubicin, Cis.	4	3	0
Kono et al. [110] 2004	Vinblastine, methotrexate	1	1	–

noted that this favourable response to chemotherapy of DTs defies the dogma in oncology that low-grade tumours without metastatic potential do not respond to chemotherapy [113].

Mesenteric Desmoid and Surgery

The presence of mesenteric DT can be incidentally discovered at the time of total colectomy and can preclude the scheduled procedure on account of technical reasons. In the experience of the Saint-Antoine Hospital of Paris, the presence of mesenteric DT ruled out construction of IPAA (three patients), conversion of an ileo-rectal anastomosis into an IPAA (three patients), removal of the rectum for carcinoma (two patients), construction of a continent ileostomy (two patients) and duodenal-pancreatic resection (two patients) [13]. According to Hartley et al. [113], this situation was discovered in 3% of the patients submitted to a first laparotomy and in 30% of those submitted to a second laparotomy, and also influenced the scheduled surgical procedure, generally IPAA. Similarly, Cohen observed significant mesenteric desmoid disease at the time of the attempted IPAA in seven patients and a definitive ileostomy was necessary [114].

The presence of a fibrous mesenteric mass or a mesenteric fibromatosis may preclude the construction of an IPAA for two reasons: (1) the shortness of the mesentery, (2) the impossibility of folding the ileal loops. In these cases we were able to perform a straight ileo-anal anastomosis since the terminal ileum must not be folded and can be carried down to the anal canal more easily than to the pouch, allowing the ileo-anal anastomosis to be performed without tension. However, the straight ileo-anal anastomosis has been abandoned on account of the unfavourable functional results. In our experience, multiple longitudinal myotomies of the last 15 cm of ileum provide a satisfactory functional result [115].

Surgical Treatment

For several authors, surgical intervention is the treatment of choice for DTs. A complete excision is recommended because partial excision may trigger a prompt recurrence. However, considering that DTs are basically benign, the advantage of surgery may be weighed with its consequences.

A different approach must be considered for abdominal wall or mesenteric DTs. Common opinion is that abdominal wall DTs can be removed, since the surgical procedure is relatively easy and the possibility of a radical removal is high even in presence of a huge mass. In order to obtain clear margins on histological examination excision in the muscular tissue is recommended, often with the sacrifice of most abdominal wall muscles. It is therefore important to treat DTs when they are small, otherwise a large musculoaponeurotic defect of the abdominal wall requires reconstruction with synthetic devices or myocutaneous flaps. However, some authors [16, 26, 114] maintain that surgery is not advisable even for DTs of the abdominal wall. In fact, the recurrence rate varies from 25 to 100% of cases, even when the DT has been radically resected [13, 15, 87] and the iterative operation can provoke the development of DT within the mesentery [18, 21–31]. Against imperative surgery, it must be considered that DTs can cease to grow [27] or even regress spontaneously [14, 33]. We are in favour of surgery for this type of DT, but believe it necessary to adopt a chemoprevention of the recurrence just after surgery. We treated 15 abdominal-wall DTs with radical surgery and employed SERMs as adjuvant therapy in the postoperative period. Recurrence was observed in two patients.

Conversely, mesenteric DTs can be removed only when small and relatively distant from the root of the small-bowel mesentery; since there is no plane of cleavage around the mass, enucleation is impossible and a concomitant resection of the surrounding intestinal tract is frequently needed. Otherwise, the risk is to remove a large part or the whole of the small bowel. Treatment of intra-abdominal DTs is usually reserved to cases in which complications occur such as small-bowel obstruction, bowel perforation, intestinal bleeding, hydronephrosis or deterioration of the functional results after IPAA. When surgery is chosen with curative intent, radical resection is achieved in about 20% of cases [14–16] with a mortality rate ranging from 2 to 10% [14, 19, 21]. In the other 80% of cases, partial resection or biopsy alone with or without intestinal bypass were performed. Severe complications are reported in up to 60% of cases [14]. Short-bowel syndrome, following wide or multiple bowel resections, is reported in 4.7–20% of cases [19, 21, 34]. Long-term parenteral nutrition and small-bowel transplantation can be necessary in some of these patients. The recurrence rate is around 70–80% (Table 3). The personal attitude was to avoid surgery and treat the lesions medically with SERMs or, in rare cases of refractory response, cytotoxic drugs. In the majority of cases we could arrest the growth of DTs and observe regression of symptoms and mass.

Conclusions

Abdominal wall and mesenteric DTs are a common manifestation in patients with FAP. The natural history is extremely variable and largely depends on the site of DT and its growth rate. Previous abdominal surgery, family history of DTs, *APC* germline mutation distal to codon 1444 and the female gender significantly increase the susceptibility of developing DTs. Prophylactic colectomy may be delayed in women with an attenuated FAP and in patients belonging to a family with evidence of DTs in more than 50% of the members. It seems probable that an attenuated form of mesenteric fibrosis represents the precursor of infiltrating fibromatosis and large mass. Even if the majority of DTs grow slowly and are asymptomatic, a minority of DTs may present a fast increase causing serious compression of intra-abdominal structures and life-threatening complications. In recent years, research has clarified the mechanism of actions of NSAIDs or SERMs and the rationale for their use in DTs. Considering the low toxicity of these drugs, they must be considered either as a first-line treatment when a DT or a mesenteric fibromatosis is diagnosed or as a preventive measure when DPLs are discovered at surgery. A close surveillance of the lesions by regular clinical and imaging assessment is mandatory. Progression of the tumour or occurrence of symptoms despite this treatment should promptly indicate cytotoxic chemotherapy. The medical treatment must be pursued for a long time, since shrinkage of DTs can be delayed by months or even years. However, regression can continue after discontinuation of the therapy. Surgical therapy is indicated when its consequences are not detrimental. Therefore, only extra-abdominal DTs or small mesenteric DTs that are located far from the mesenteric vessels and do not require a large intestinal resection, are susceptible of surgical resection. Postoperative therapy for prevention of recurrence is indicated.

References

1. Muller J (1838) Ueber den feinern Bau und die Formen der krankhaften Geschwulste. Reimer, Berlin
2. Gurbuz AK, Giardiello FM, Petersen GM et al (1994) Desmoid tumors in familial adenomatous polyposis. Gut 35:377–381
3. Tonelli F (1978) Abdominal desmoids and mesenteric fibromatosis in familial polyposis of the colon. Ital J Gastroenterol 10:27–36
4. Simpson RD, Harrison EG, Mayo CW (1964) Mesenteric fibromatosis in familial polyposis: a variant of Gardner's syndrome. Cancer 17:526–534
5. Richards RC, Rogers SW, Gardner EJ (1981) Spontaneous mesenteric fibromatosis in Gardner's syndrome. Cancer 47: 597–601
6. Clark SK, Johnson Smith TGP, Katz DE et al (1998) Identification and progression of a desmoid precursor lesion in patients with familial adenomatous polyposis. Br J Surg 85:970–975
7. Middleton SB, Clark SK, Matravers P et al (2003) Stepwise progression of familial adenomatous polyposis-associated desmoid precursor lesions demonstrated by a novel CT scoring system Dis Colon Rectum 46:481–485
8. Healey JC, Reznek RH, Clark SK et al (1997) MR appearances of desmoid tumours in familial adenomatous polyposis. Am J Roentgenol 169:465–472
9. Brooks AP, Reznek RH, Nugent K et al (1994) CT appearances of desmoid tumors in familial adenomatous polyposis: further observations. Clin Radiol 49:601–607
10. Knudsen AL, Bulow S (2001) Desmoid tumour in familial adenomatous polyposis: a review of literature. Famil Cancer 1:111–119
11. Jarvinen HJ (1997) Desmoid disease as a part of familial adenomatous polyposis coli. Acta Chir Scand 153:379–383
12. Bertario L, Russo A, Sala P et al (2001) Genotype and phenotype factors as determinants of desmoid tumors in patients with familial adenomatous polyposis. Int J Cancer 95:102–107
13. Penna C, Tiret E, Parc R et al (1993) Operation and abdominal desmoid tumors in familial adenomatous polyposis. Surg Gynecol Obstet 177:263–268
14. Jones IT, Fazio VW, Weakley FL et al (1986) Desmoid tumors in familial polyposis coli. Ann Surg 204:94–97 Lofti AM, Dozois RR, Gordon H et al (1989) Mesenteric fibromatosis complicating familial adenomatous polyposis: predisposing factors and results of treatment. Int J Colorectal Dis 4:30–36
15. Lofti AM, Dozois RR, Gordon H et al (1989) Mesenteric fibromatosis complicating familial adenomatous polyposis: predisposing factors and results of treatment. Int J Colorectal Dis 4:30–36
16. Rodriguez-Bigas MA, Mahoney MC, Karakousis CP et al (1994) Desmoid tumors in patients with familial adenomatous polyposis. Cancer 74:1270–1274
17. Kadmon M, Möslein G, Buhr H et al (1995) Desmoide bei Patienten mit familiärer adenomatöser Polyposis (FAP). Chirurg 66:997–1005
18. Heiskanen I, Jarvinen HJ (1997) Occurrence of desmoid tumours in familial adenomatous polyposis and results of treatment. Int J Colorectal Dis 11:157–162
19. Soravia C, Berk T, McLeod RS et al (2000) Desmoid disease in patients with familial adenomatous polyposis. Dis Colon Rectum 43:363–369
20. Ho JW, Chu KM, Tse CW, Yuen ST (2002) Phenotype and management of patients with familial adenomatous polyposis in Hong Kong: perspective of the Hereditary Gastrointestinal Cancer Registry. Hong Kong Med J 2002 Oct;8(5):342–347
21. Church JM (1998) Mucosal ischaemia caused by desmoid tumors in patients with familial adenomatous polyposis. Dis Colon Rectum 41: 661–663
22. Tulchinsky H, Keidar A, Strul H et al (2005) Extra-colonic manifestations of familial adenomatous polyposis after proctocolectomy Arch Surg 140:159–163
23. Arvanitis ML, Jagelman DG, Fazio VW et al (1990) Mortality in patients with familial adenomatous polyposis. Dis Colon Rectum 33:639–642

24. Iwama T, Myshima Y, Utsunomiya J (1993) The impact of familial adenomatous polyposis on the tumorigenesis and mortality at several organs: its rational treatment. Ann Surg 217:99–100
25. Bertario L, Presciuttini S, Sala P et al (1994) Causes of death and post-surgical survival in familial adenomatous polyposis: results from the Italian Registry of Familial Adenomatous Polyposis Writing Committee. Semin Surg Oncol 10:225–234
26. Sagar PM, Moslein G, Dozois RR (1998) Management of desmoid tumors in patients after ileal pouch-anal anastomosis for familial adenomatous polyposis. Dis Colon Rectum 41:1350–1356
27. Parc Y, Piquard A, Dozois RR et al (2004) Long-term outcome of familial adenomatous polyposis patients after restorative coloproctectomy. Ann Surg 239:378–382
28. Middleton SB, Frayling IF, Phillips RK (2000) Desmoids in familial adenomatous polyposis are monoclonal proliferations. Br J Cancer 82:828–832
29. Li C, Bapat B, Alman BA (1998) Adenomatous polyposis coli gene mutation alters proliferation through its beta-catenin regulatory function in aggressive fibromatosis (desmoid tumors). Am J Pathol 153:709–714
30. McAdam WA, Goligher IC (1970) The occurrence of desmoids in patients with familial polyposis coli. Br J Surg 57:618–631
31. Clark SK, Neale KF, Landgrebe JC et al (1999) Desmoid tumours complicating familial adenomatous polyposis. Br J Surg 86:1185–1189
32. Sturt NJH, Gallagher MC, Bassett P et al (2004) Evidence for genetic predisposition to desmoid tumours in familial adenomatous polyposis independent of the germline APC mutation. Gut 53:1832–1836
33. Caldwell EH (1976) Desmoid tumor: musculoaponeurotic fibrosis of the abdominal wall. Surgery 79:104–106
34. Eagel BA, Zentler-Munro P, Smith IE (1989) Mesenteric tumours in Gardner's syndrome: review of medical treatment. Postgrd Med J 65:497–501
35. Church JM, McGannon E (2000) Prior pregnancy ameliorates the course of intra-abdominal desmoid tumors in patients with familial adenomatous polyposis. Dis Colon Rectum 43:445–450
36. Miyaki M, Konishi M, Kikuchi-Yanoshita R et al (1993) Coexistence of somatic and germ-line mutations of APC gene in desmoid tumors from patients with familial adenomatous polyposis. Cancer Res 53:5079–5082
37. Palmirotta R, Curia MC, Esposito DL et al (1995) Novel mutations and inactivations of both alleles of the AP gene in desmoid tumors. Hum Mol Genet 4:1979–1981
38. Caspari R, Olschwang S, Friedl W et al (1995) Familial adenomatous polyposis: desmoid tumours and lack of ophthalmic lesions (CHRPE) associated with APC mutations beyond codon 1444. Hum Mol Genet 4:337–340
39. Couture J, Mitri A, Lagace R et al (2000) A germline mutation at the extreme 3' end of the APC gene results in a severe desmoid phenotype and is associated with overexpression of beta-catenin in the desmoid tumour. Clin Genet 57:205–212
40. Eccles DM, van der Lujit R, Breukel C (1996) Hereditary desmoid disease due to a frameshift mutation at codon 1924 of the gena APC. Am J Hum Mut 59:1193–1201
41. Tonelli F, Valanzano R, Brandi ML (1994) Pharmacologic treatment of desmoid tumors in familial adenomatous polyposis: results of an in vitro study. Surgery 115:473–479
42. Picariello L, Fiorelli G, Benvenuti S et al (1997) In vitro bioeffects of the antiestrogen LY117018 on desmoid tumor and colon cancer cells. Anticancer Res 17:2099–2104
43. Locci P, Bellocchio S, Lilli C et al (2001) Synthesis and secretion of transforming growth factor-ß1 by human desmoid fibroblast cell line and its modulation by toremifene. J Interferon and Cytokine Res 21:961–970
44. Waddell WR, Gerner RE, Reich MP (1983) Non steroidal anti-inflammatory drugs and tamoxifen for desmoid tumors and carcinoma of the stomach. J Surg Oncol 22:197–211
45. Kedar RP, Bourne TH, Powles TJ et al (1994) Effects of tamoxifen on uterus and ovaries of postmenopausal women in a randomised breast cancer prevention trial. Lancet 343:1318–1321
46. Fisher B, Costantino JP, Redmand CK et al(1994) Endometrial cancer in tamoxifen-treated breast cancer patients: findings from the National Surgical Adjuvant Breast and Bowel Project (NSABP) B-14. J Natl Cancer Inst 86:527–537
47. Clark SK, Phillips RKS (1996) Desmoids in familial adenomatous polyposis. Br J Surg 83:1494–1504
48. Brooks MD, Ebbs SR, Colletta AA et al (1992) Desmoid tumors treated with triphenylethylenes. Eur J Cancer 28:1014-1018
49. Hansmann A., Adolph C, Vogel T et al (2003) High-dose tamoxifen and sulindac as first-line treatment for desmoid tumors. Cancer 100:612–620
50. Tonelli F, Ficari F, Valanzano R et al (2003) Treatment of desmoids and mesenteric fibromatosis in familial adenomatous polyposis with raloxifene. Tumori 89:391–396
51. Taketo M (1998) Cyclooxigenase-2 inhibitors in tumorogenesis (part I). J Natl Cancer Inst 90:1529–1536
52. Taketo M (1998) Cyclooxigenase-2 inhibitors in tumorogenesis (part II). J Natl Cancer Inst 90:1609–1620
53. Janne PA, Mayer RJ (2000) Chemoprevention of colorectal cancer. N Engl J Med 342:1960–1968
54. Vane JR (1971) Inhibition of prostaglandin synthesis as a mechanism of action for aspirin-like drugs. Nature 231:232–235
55. Du Bois RN, Abramson SB, Crofford L et al (1998) Cyclooxygenase in biology and disease. FASEB J 12:1063–1073
56. Smith WL, Garavito RM, DeWitt (1996) Prostaglandin endo-peroxide H synthases (Cyclooxygenase)-1 and -2. J Biol Chem 271:33157–33160
57. Xie W, Robertson D, Simmons D (1992) Mitogen-inducible prostaglandin G/H synthase: a new target for nonsteroidal anti-inflammatory drugs. Drug Dev Res 25:249–265
58. Morrow JD, Roberts LJ (2001) Lipid-derived autacoids. In: Hardman JG, Limbird LE (eds) The pharmacological basis of therapeutics. McGraw-Hill, New York, pp 669–685

59. Roberts LJ, Morrow JD (2001) Analgesic-antipyretic and anti-inflammatory agents and drugs employed in the treatment of gout. In: Hardman JG, Limbird LE (eds) The pharmacological basis of therapeutics. McGraw-Hill, New York, pp 687–731
60. Patrignani P, Filabozzi P, Patrono C (1982) Selective cumulative inhibition of platelet thromboxane production by low-doses aspirin in healthy subjects. J Clin Invest 69:1366–1372
61. FitzGerald GA, Oates JA, Hawiger J et al (1983) Endogenous biosynthesis of prostacyclin and thromboxane and platelet function during chronic administration of aspirin in man. J Clin Invest 71:678–688
62. Roth GJ, Majerus P (1975) The mechanism of the effect of aspirin on human platelets: acetylation of a particulate protein fraction. J Clin Invest 56:624–632
63. Lecomte M, Laneuville O, Ji C et al (1994) Acetylation of human prostaglandin endo-peroxide synthase-2(cyclooxygenase-2) by aspirin. J Biol Chem 269:13207–13215
64. Cipollone F, Patrignani P, Greco A et al (1997) Differential suppression of thromboxane biosynthesis by indobufen and aspirin in patients with unstable angina. Circulatio 96:1109–1116
65. Vane JR (1994) Towards a better aspirin. Nature 367:215–216
66. Stolina M, Sharma S, Zhu L et al (2000) Lung cancer cyclooxygenase-2 dependent inhibition of dendritic cell maturation and function. Pro Am Assoc Cancer Res 41:619 (abstract 620)
67. Tsujii M, DuBois RN (1995) Alteration in cellular adhesion and apoptosis in epithelial cells overexpressing prostaglandin endo-peroxide synthase 2. Cell 83:493–501
68. He TC, Chan TA, Vogelstein B et al (1999) PPAR-delta is an APC-regulated target of nonsteroidal anti-inflammatory drugs. Cell 99:335–345
69. Afford S, Randhawa S (2000) Apoptosis. Mol Pathol 53:55–63
70. Bedi A, Pasricha PJ, Akhtar AJ et al (1995) Inhibition of apoptosis during development of colorectal cancer. Cancer Res 55:1811–1816
71. Pasricha PJ, Bedi A, O'Connor K et al (1995) The effects of sulindac on colorectal proliferation and apoptosis in familial adenomatous polyposis. Gastroenterology 109:994–998
72. Uefuji K, Ichikura T, Shinomiya N et al (2000) Induction of apoptosis by JTE-522, a specific cyclooxygenase-2 inhibitor in human gastric cancer cell lines. Anticancer Res 20:4279–4284
73. Souza RF, Shewmake K, Beer DG et al (2000) Selective inhibition of cyclooxygenase-2 suppresses growth and induces apoptosis in human oesophageal adenocarcinoma cells. Cancer Res 60:5767–5772
74. Sumitani K, Kamijo R, Toyoshima T et al (2001) Specific inhibition of cyclooxygenase-2 results in inhibition of proliferation of oral cancer cell lines via suppression of prostaglandin E2 production. J Oral Pathol Med 30:41–47
75. Joki T, Heese O, Nikas DC et al (2000) Expression of cyclooxygenase 2 (COX-2) in human glioma and in vitro inhibition by a specific COX-2 inhibitor, NS-398. Cancer Res 60:4926–4931
76. Tsubouchi Y, Mukai S, Kawaito Y et al (2000) Meloxicam inhibits the growth of non-small cell lung cancer. Anticancer Res 20:2867–2872
77. Molina MA, Sitja-Arnau M, Lemoine MG et al (1999) Increased cyclooxygenase-2 expression in human pancreatic carcinomas and cell lines: growth inhibition by nonsteroidal anti-inflammatory drugs. Cancer Res 59:4356–4362
78. Marx J (2001) Cancer research. Anti-inflammatories inhibit cancer growth, but how? Science 291:581–582
79. Scorrano L, Penzo D, Petronilli V et al (2001) Arachidonic acid causes cell death through the mitochondrial permeability transition: implications for tumor necrosis factor-alpha apoptotic signalling. J Biol Chem 276:12035–12040
80. Grosch S, Tegeder I, Niederberg E et al (2001) COX-2 independent induction of cell arrest and apoptosis in colon cancer cells by the selective COX-2 inhibitor celecoxib. FASEB J 15:2742–2744
81. Shureiqi I, Chen D, Lotan R et al (2000) 15-lipoxygenase-1 mediates nonsteroidal anti-inflammatory drug-induced apoptosis independently of cyclooxygenase-2 in colon cancer cells. Cancer Res 60:6846–6850
82. Leahy KM, Ornberg RL, Wang et al. (2002) Cyclooxygenase-2 inhibition by celecoxib reduces proliferation and induces apoptosis in angiogenic endothelial cells in vivo. Cancer Res 62:625–631
83. Tsujii M, Kawano S, Tsujii S et al (1998) Cyclooxygenase regulates angiogenesis induced by colon cancer cells. Cell 93:705–716
84. Dannenberg AJ, Altorki NK, Boyle JO et al (2001) Cyclo-oxygenase 2: a pharmacological target for prevention of cancer. Lancet Oncol 2:544–551
85. Araki Y, Okamura S, Hussain S et al (2003) Regulation of cyclooxygenase-2 expression by the Wnt and Ras pathways. Cancer Res 63:728–734
86. Masferrer JL, Leahy KM, Koki AT et al (2000) Antiangiogenic and anti-tumour activities of cyclooxygenase-2 inhibitors. Cancer Res 60:1306–1311
87. Jones MK, Wang H, Peskar BM et al (1999) Inhibition of angiogenesis by nonsteroidal anti-inflammatory drugs: insight into mechanisms and implications for cancer growth and ulcer healing. Nat Med 5:1418–1423
88. Brueggemeier RW, Quinn AL, Parrett ML et al (1999) Correlation of aromatase and cyclooxygenase gene expression in human breast cancer specimens. Cancer Lett 140:27–35
89. Tejpar S, Nollet F, Li C et al (1999) Predominance of -catenin mutations and -catenin dysregulation in sporadic aggressive fibromatosis (desmoid tumor). Oncogene 18:6615–6620
90. Sparks AB, Morin PJ, Vogelstain B et al (1998) Mutational analysis of the APC/-catenin/Tcf pathway in colorectal cancer. Cancer Res 58:1130–1134
91. Williams CS, Smalley W, DuBois RN (1997) Aspirin use and potential mechanisms for colorectal cancer prevention. J Clin Invest 100:1325–1359
92. Williams CS, Mann M, DuBois RN (1999) The role of cyclooxygenases in inflammation, cancer, and development. Oncogene 18:7908–7916
93. Oshima M, Dinchuk JE, Kargman SL et al (1996) Suppression of intestinal polyposis in Apc delta716 knockout mice by inhibition of cyclooxygenase 2

(COX-2). Cell 87:803–809
94. Picariello L, Brandi ML, Formigli L et al (1998) Apoptosis induced by sulindac sulfide in epithelial and mesenchymal cells from human abdominal neoplasms. Eur J Pharm 360:105–112
95. Poon R, Smits R, Catherine L et al (2001) Cyclooxygenase-two (COX-2) modulates proliferation in aggressive fibromatosis (desmoid tumor). Oncogene 20:451–460
96. Tsukada K, Church JM, Jagelman DG et al (1992) Noncytotoxic drug therapy for intra-abdominal desmoid tumors in patients with familial adenomatous polyposis. Dis Colon Rectum 35:29–33
97. Klein WA, Miller HH, Anderson M et al (1987) The use of indomethacin, sulindac and tamoxifen for the treatment of desmoid tumors associated with familial polyposis. Cancer 60:2863–2868
98. Waddell WR, Kirsch WM (1991) Testolactone, sulindac, warfarin, and vitamin K1 for unresectable desmoid tumors. Am J Surg 161:416-421
99. Geurs F, Kok TC (1993) Regression of a great abdominal desmoid tumor by interferon-alpha. J Clin Gastrenterol 16:264–265
100. Heidemann J, Ogawa H, Otterson MF et al (2004) Antiangiogenic treatment of mesenteric desmoid tumors with toremifene and interferon alfa-2b: report of two cases. Dis Colon Rectum 47:118–122
101. Nakada J, Ubukata H, Goto Y et al (1997) Prednisolone therapy for intra-abdominal desmoid tumours in a patient with familial adenomatous polyposis. Gastroenterol 32:255–259
102. Lindor NM, Dozois RR, Nelson H et al (2003) Desmoid tumors in familial adenomatous polyposis: a pilot project evaluating efficacy of treatment with pirfenidone. Am J Gastroenterol 98:1868–1874
103. Mace J, Biermann JS, Sondak V et al (2002) Response of extra-abdominal desmoid tumors to therapy with imatinib mesylate. Cancer 95:237–239
104. Tsukada K,Church JM, Jagelman DG et al (1991) Systemic cytotoxic chemotherapy and radiation therapy for desmoid in familial adenomatous polyposis. Dis Colon Rectum 34:1090–1092
105. Patel SR, Evans HL, Benjamin RS (1992) Combination chemotherapy in adult desmoid tumors. Cancer 72:3244–3247
106. Lynch HT, Fitzgibbons R Jr, Chong S et al (1994) Use of doxorubicin and dacarbazine for the management of unresectable intraabdominal desmoid tumors in Gardner's syndrome. Dis Colon Rectum 37:260–267
107. Schnitzler M, Cohen Z, Blackstein M et al (1997) Chemotherapy for desmoid tumors in association with familial adenomatous polyposis. Dis Colon Rectum 40:798–801
108. Risum S, Bulow S (2003) Doxorubicin treatment of an intra-abdominal desmoid tumour in a patient with familial adenomatous polyposis. Colorectal Dis 5:585–586
109. Okuno SH, Edmonson JH (2003) Combination chemotherapy for desmoid tumors. Cancer 97:1134–1135
110. Kono T, Tomita I, Chisato N et al (2004) Successful low-dose chemotherapy using vinblastine and methotrexate for the treatment of an ileoanal pouch mesenteric desmoid tumor: report of a case. Dis Colon Rectum 47:246–249
111. Gega M, Yanagi H, Yoshikawa R et al (2006) Successful chemotherapeutic modality of doxorubicin plus dacarbazine for the treatment of desmoid tumors in association with familial adenomatous polyposis. J Clin Oncol 24(1):102–105
112. Patel SR, Benjamin RS (2006) Desmoid tumors respond to chemotherapy: defying the dogma in oncology. J Clin Oncol 24:1–2
113. Hartley JE, Church JM, Gupta S et al (2004) Significance of incidental desmoids identified during surgery for familial adenomatous polyposis. Dis Colon Rectum 47:334–340
114. Cohen Z, Berg T (1998) Invited editorial. Dis Colon Rectum 41:1355–1356
115. Tonelli F, Batignani G, Ficari F et al (1997) Straight ileo-anal anastomosis with multiple ileal myotomies as an alternative to pelvic pouch. Int J Colorectal Dis 12:261–266

The Endoscopic Procedures in Familial Adenomatous Polyposis (FAP): a Critical Review

Walter Piubello, Fabrizio Bonfante, Morena Tebaldi

Introduction

To have a better understanding of the role of endoscopy in familial adenomatous polyposis, it is necessary to clarify some concepts in colon cancer development. Colon cancer (CRC) arises from a dysplastic precursor lesion called adenomatous polyp (or adenoma). Approximately 30–40% of people over 50 years of age will develop an adenoma, but not all adenomas will progress to CRC. In the general population some individuals tend to develop one or only a few adenomas and endoscopic polypectomy is often sufficient for removing them, thereby markedly reducing the subsequent development to CRC. Adenomas arise when both copies of the APC gene are lost. Indeed, the APC gene is considered the "gatekeeper" of the colon, protecting against the development of adenomas. The loss of APC gene function permits adenoma formation and sets the stage for subsequent molecular alterations of genes such as k-ras and p53, which promote further progression to CRC (Fig. 1). Some people develop multiple polyps of the colon at a younger age due to inheritance of a germline mutation of a gene that predisposes to CRC. Since these patients are at increased risk of CRC (and other types of cancer), it is important to recognize these syndromes earlier (Table 1). Therefore, endoscopic procedures play a crucial role in the diagnosis, staging and follow-up of these conditions.

Familial Adenomatous Polyposis

In these patients, the disease begins at the age of 8–10 years with a small number of colonic polyps, increasing progressively until the colon becomes studded with adenomas. Endoscopy mainly plays a diagnostic role (Fig. 2) since colorectal cancer should be considered an inevitable consequence in the natural history of FAP, appearing approximately 15 years after the onset of the polyps. For this reason prophylactic proctocolectomy is the procedure of choice for this condition. After the proctocolectomy, the ileal pouch could develop polyps even if the risk of pouch cancer in FAP is unclear. Therefore, long-term endoscopic surveillance (pouchoscopy) is recommended [1].

It is known that FAP patients frequently develop

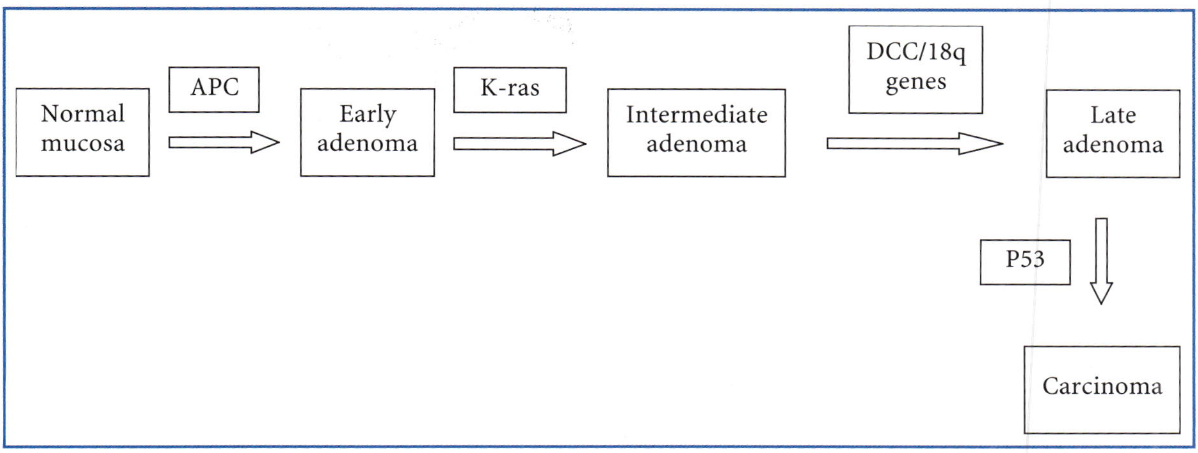

Fig. 1. Steps of colon carcinogenesis

Table 1. Features of adenomatous polyposis syndromes

Syndrome	Type of polyps	Location of polyps	Other manifestations	Germline gene mutation
FAP (autosomal dominant)	Adenomas (100s-1000s)	Colon, duodenum, jejunum, ileum, stomach, (fundic gland polyps)	Benign: desmoid tumours, osteomas, epidermoid cysts, CHRPE[a] Malignant: medulloblastoma, hepatoblastoma, thyroid cancer, adrenal cancer	APC
Attenuated FAP (autosomal dominant)	Adenomas (5–100)	Colon, duodenum, stomach	Osteomas (mandible)	APC (5' and 3') APC E1317Q
MYH polyposis (autosomal recessive)	Adenomas (5–100)	Colon, duodenum, stomach	Osteomas, CHRPE[a]	MYH[b]

[a]*CHRPE*, congenital hypertrophy of the retinal pigment epithelium; [b]*MYH*, is a gene that repairs DNA damage (if defecting, the resulting loss of APC function causes an increase in multiple adenomas)

tumours (either benign or malignant) in other organs besides the colon, mainly in the upper GI tract (stomach, small intestine). Gastric polyps occur in 30–100%, but adenomas are uncommon, occurring in approximately 5% of FAP patients usually in the gastric antrum (Fig. 3). The development of gastric carcinoma in FAP patients is only very high in Japan where the gastric cancer rate in the general population is higher. In other populations it occurs in less than 5% of the population. Proximal small-bowel cancer is one of the two leading causes of death in FAP patients with previous colectomy [2, 3]. It develops

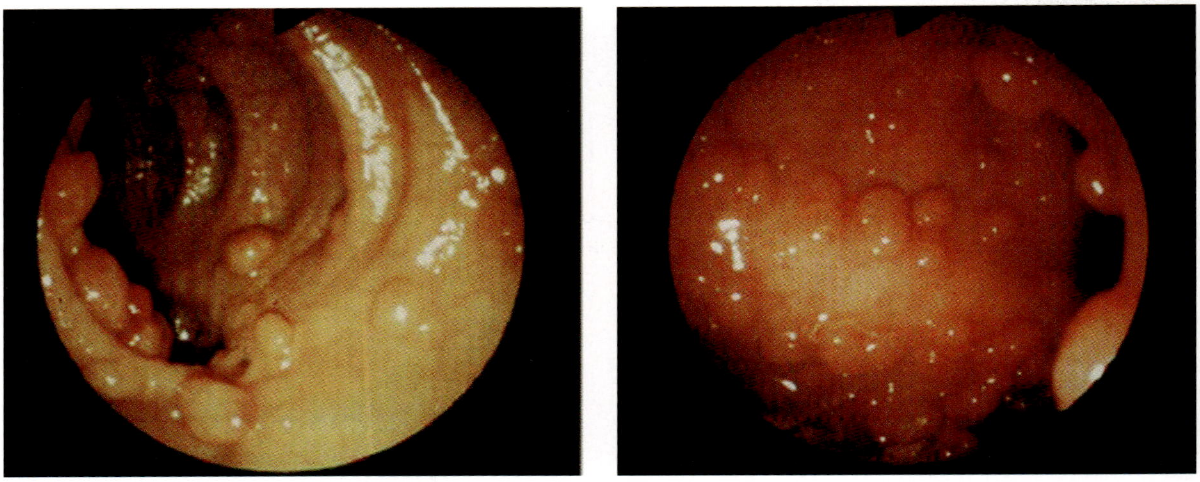

Fig. 2. Diffuse polyposis of the colon

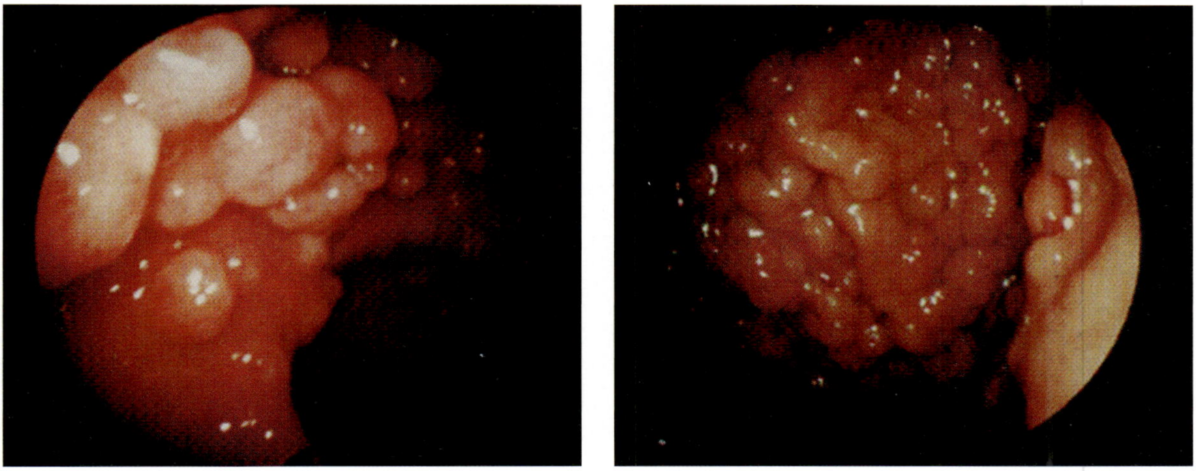

Fig. 3. Gastric polyps in FAP

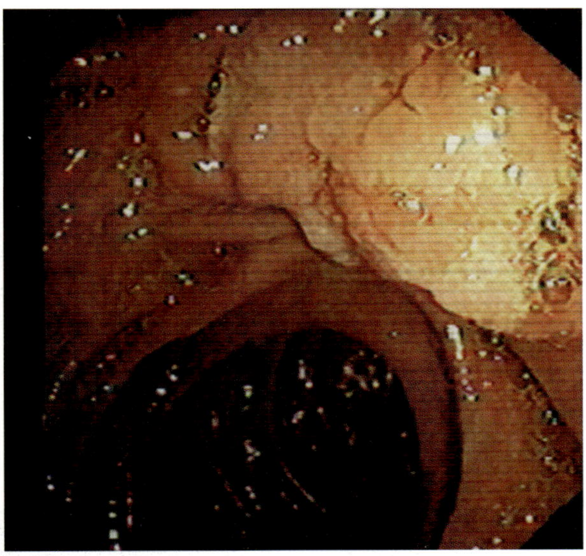

Fig. 4. Duodenal adenoma in FAP

from pre-existing adenomas which are present in approximately 100% of these patients in the duodenum (Fig. 4). Duodenal adenomas can be classified through macroscopic and histologic criteria in five stages (0–IV) following the Spigelman's classification (Table 2) [4, 5].

In all FAP patients submitted to proctocolectomy, screening and surveillance for duodenal and small-bowel polyps are mandatory. Duodenoscopy (side vision) should be performed, taking several biopsies from the duodenal papilla and from all the polyps,

Table 2. Spigelman's score and classification (modified)

Score	No. of duodenal polyps		Size (mm)	Histology	Dysplasia
1 point	1–4		1–4	Tubulous	Low grade
2 points	5–20		5–10	Tubulous-villous	–
3 points	> 20		>10	Villous	High grade
Classification	**Stage** 0	**Point** – (no polyps)			
	I	1–4			
	II	5–6			
	III	7–8			
	IV	9–12			

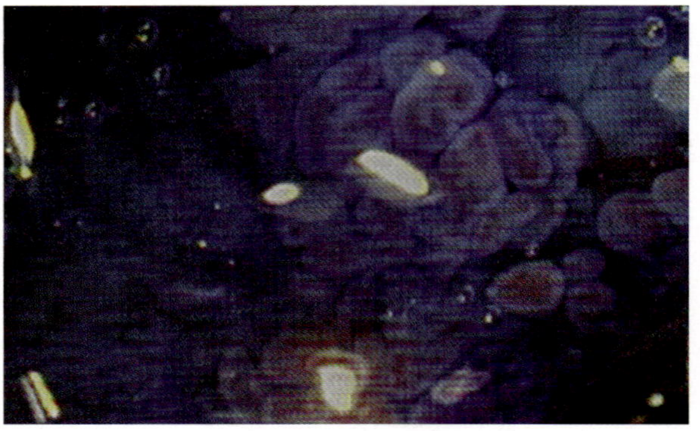

Fig. 5. Duodenal chromoendoscopy (methylene blue)

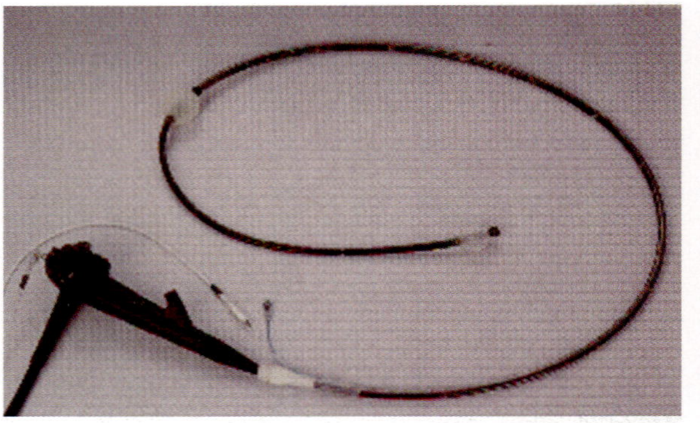

Fig. 6. Double balloon enteroscopy

also by means of chromoendoscopy (Fig. 5). At the first duodenoscopy, the prevalence of duodenal adenomatosis is 58–74% in the major series, and only about 10% of adenomas are diagnosed histologically.

The risk of duodenal carcinoma is related to the Spigelman stage (about 7% in stage IV, 0.7% in stage 0–III) [6]. In Spigelman stage III–IV, endoscopic ultrasonography is recommended to ensure that invasive growth has not occurred. The regular endoscopic surveillance of the duodenum should be offered to all FAP patients (Table 3) [7]. The first upper endoscopy should be carried out at the age of 30 years and include multiple random biopsies taken from the duodenal mucosa in patients without visible polyps. Endoscopic surveillance (included ultrasonography) is recommended at intervals of 3 months in patients who are not suitable for or refuse surgery.

Screening or surveillance for small-bowel polyps is difficult with current technologies. By means of traditional push enteroscopy (PE), up to only 30% of the small-bowel length can be visualized. A new promising endoscopic method for allowing complete visualisation, biopsies and treatment in the small bowel is the double balloon enteroscopy (DBE; push and pull; Fig. 6), but the use of this technique in FAP patients is not yet routine [8].

Table 3. Programme for surveillance and treatment of duodenal adenomatosis

Spigelman's stage	Frequency of endoscopy
0	5 years[a]
I	5 years[b]
II	3 years[b]
III	1–2 years[b]
IV	Endoscopic ultrasonography Consider pancreas sparing and pylorus sparing duodenectomy

[a]Including multiple random biopsies from the mucosal fold in patients without visible polyps; [b]Including multiple biopsies from polyps

Capsule endoscopy (CE) is another recent technology that allows a non-invasive endoscopic assessment of the entire small bowel (Fig. 7) [9]. Published clinical trials have shown that CE carries a high diagnostic yield in patients suffering from obscure gastrointestinal bleeding [10–13]. Beyond this role, the value of CE in other small bowel disorders has to be evaluated. CE may also be used to search for tumours or tumour-like lesions in patients that present with a known increased risk of small bowel carcinomas such as familial adenomatous polyposis, Peutz-Jeghers syndrome and familial juvenile polyposis. The comparison between CE and DBE in detecting small bowel tumours is shown in Table 4 [12–16].

In FAP patients, preliminary results [17] suggest that capsule endoscopy can only be used additionally to identify patients with significant distal jejunal polyposis. However, this is suggested to be a rather infrequent situation. The correlation between the findings of capsule endoscopy and conventional endoscopy is reported in Table 5. Active control of the capsule endoscopy, the precise assessment of polyps size and the opportunity to obtain biopsies are important long-term future requirements for extending the indication to FAP patients.

In the first study that compares the value of CE and DBE in the diagnosis of small intestinal polyposis [18], the diagnostic yield of DBE was superior in comparison to CE in almost the same area explored. Even Yamamoto et al. [19] have shown that with this method, total enteroscopy can be achieved by combining antegrade and retrograde examinations, however, DBE in comparison with CE is an inconvenient and invasive procedure that requires specialized equipment, sedation of the patients, fluoroscopy and

Table 4. Comparison between capsule endoscopy (CE) and push enteroscopy (PE) in detecting small-bowel tumours

Author	Year	No. of patients	No. of tumours (%)		
			Total	PE	CE
Cosentino et al. [14]	2003	33	4 (10.7)	4	2
Delvaux et al. [15]	2002	57	1 (1.8)	0	1
Ell et al. [12]	2002	32	2 (6.3)	2	2
Mylonaky et al. [16]	2002	38	2 (5.3)	2	2
Pennazio et al. [11]	2002	50	3 (6)	2	2

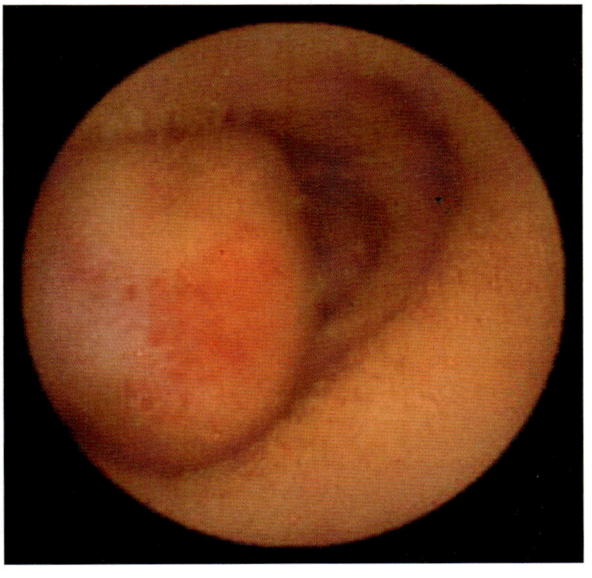

Fig. 7. Ileal polyp at capsule endoscopy

Table 5. Correlation of Spigelman's score (modified) measured by capsule endoscopy and conventional endoscopy

Capsule endoscopy (score)	Conventional endoscopy (score)			
	No. of patients			
	0	1–2	3–4	5–6
0	5	1	-	-
1–2	1	-	1	-
3–4	1	±	7	-
5–6	-	-	-	7

a prolonged examination time.

At the end of this report, the role of endoscopic procedures in FAP patients can be summarized as follows (Table 6):

- Conventional colonoscopy should be performed with multiple biopsies and polypectomy, starting at the age of 8–10, considering prophylactic proctocolectomy when the number of polyps are increasing and the risk of carcinoma is very high (10–15 years from the onset of polyps).
- Pouchoscopy, after proctocolectomy, should be performed because the ileal pouch could develop polyps even if the real risk of pouch cancer is unclear.
- Gastric endoscopy to show fundic gland polyps (frequent) and adenomas (rare).
- Duodenoscopy with side view to remove all the polyps, particularly near the papilla, and to perform several random biopsies by using chromoendoscopy with methylene blue.
- Endoscopic ultrasonography in patients with Spigelman stages III–IV.

Table 6. Endoscopic procedures in FAP

GI site	Endoscope	Findings	Time and follow-up
Stomach	Conventional	Fundic gland polyps (adenoma)	At first diagnosis
Duodenum	Side vision (±chromoendoscopy)	Adenomas	Spigelman stage (endoscope ultrasonography stages III–IV)
Small bowel	Capsule endoscopy, double balloon enteroscopy	Polyps	At first diagnosis? Surveillance?
Colon	Conventional	Adenomas (100s–1000s)	-
Ileal pouch	Conventional	Polyps	?

- Capsule endoscopy to better explore the small bowel.
- DBE to eventually remove the intestinal polyps found at CE examination.

References

1. Groves CJ, Beveridge G, Swain DJ et al (2005) Prevalence and morphology of pouch and ileal adenomas in familial adenomatous polyposis. Dis Colon Rectum 48:816–823
2. Arvanitis ML, Jagelman DG, Fazio VW et al (1990) Mortality in patients with familial adenomatous polyposis. Dis Colon Rectum 33:639–642
3. Nugent KP, Spigelman AD, Phillips RK (1993) Life expectancy after colectomy and ileorectal anastomosis for familial adenomatous polyposis. Dis Colon Rectum 36:1059–1062
4. Spigelman AD, Williams CB, Talbot IC (1989) Upper gastrointestinal cancer in patients with familial adenomatous polyposis. Lancet 2:783–785
5. Spigelman AD (2004) Extracolonic polyposis in familial adenomatous polyposis: so near and yet so far. Gut 53:322–327
6. Bülow S, Bjiörk J, Christensen IJ et al (2004) Duodenal adenomatosis in familial adenomatous polyposis. Gut 53:381–386
7. Saurin JC, Gutknecht C, Napoleon B et al (2004) Surveillance of duodenal adenomas in familial adenomatous polyposis reveals high cumulative risk of advance disease. J Clin Oncol 22:493–498
8. May A, Nachbar L, Ell C (2005) Double-balloon enteroscopy (push and pull enteroscopy) of the small bowel: feasibility and diagnostic and therapeutic yield in patients with suspected small bowel disease. Gastrointest Endosc 62:62–70
9. De Franchis R, Rondonotti E, Abbiati C et al (2004) Small bowel malignancy. Gastrointest Endosc Clin N Am 14:139–148
10. Lewis BS, Swain P (2002) Capsule endoscopy in the evaluation of patients with suspected small intestinal bleeding: results of a pilot study. Gastrointest Endosc 56:349–353
11. Pennazio M, Santucci R, Rondonotti E et al (2002) Capsule endoscopy: diagnostic yield and comparison with push enteroscopy in patients with obscure gastrointestinal bleeding: the Italian multicentre experience. Endoscopy 34 (suppl II):A91
12. Ell C, Remke S, May A et al (2002) The first prospective controlled trial comparing wireless capsule endoscopy with push enteroscopy in chronic gastrointestinal bleeding. Endoscopy 34:685–689
13. Piubello W, Bonfante F, Tebaldi M et al (2005) Pillcam videocapsule endoscopy and obscure gastrointestinal bleeding: our experience. Dig Liver Dis 37(suppl 1):160
14. Cosentino F, Morandi E, Rubis-Passoni G et al (2003) Wireless capsule endoscopy: limits and complications. Abstracts of the 2003 Meeting of the Italian Federation for Digestive Disease, Italian Federation for Digestive Disease, Florence, p 41
15. Delvaux M, Saurin JC, Gaudin JC et al (2002) Comparison of wireless endoscopic capsule and push-enteroscopy in patients with obscure occult/overt digestive bleeding: results of a prospective, blinded, multicentre trial. Gastrointest Endosc 55:AB88
16. Mylonaky M, Fritscher-Ravens A, Swain PC (2002) Clinical results of wireless capsule endoscopy. Gastrointest Endosc 55:AB146
17. Schulmann K, Schmiegel W (2004) Capsule endoscopy for small bowel surveillance in hereditary intestinal polyposis and non-polyposis syndromes. Gastrointest Endosc Clin N Am 14:149–158
18. Matsumoto T, Esaki M. Horiyama T et al (2005) Comparison of capsule endoscopy and enteroscopy with the double-balloon method in patients with obscure bleeding and polyposis. Endoscopy 37:827–832
19. Yamamoto H, Kita H, Sugano K et al (2004) Clinical outcomes of double-balloon endoscopy for the diagnosis and treatment of small intestinal diseases. Clin Gastroenterol Hepatol 2:1010–1016

FAP History Through a Patient's Story

Gian Gaetano Delaini, Gianluca Colucci, Filippo Nifosì

This is the story of Rosa Gallo, a young and bright student of medicine, who died of Gardner's syndrome at 21 years of age; this story allows us to more easily explain the history of the disease, the various aspects of which (aetiology, clinical history, diagnostic and therapeutical approach) are extensively covered in several chapters of this book.

Rosa Gallo was born on 6 August 1982, second born of the Gallo family, 4 years younger than the first born, Carmine. She was a happy child and soon stood out among her friends of the same age, for her lively wit. Fondly loved by mom and dad, the two children grew up happy and carefree. In 1990, Rosa's paternal aunt, who moved from Altavilla Salentina to Milan, underwent coloscopy due to lower gastrointestinal (GI) bleeding. The result of the examination would upset the life of the whole Gallo family: the diagnosis was familial adenomatous polyposis coli (FAP). All first degree relatives underwent coloscopy, and Rosa's father, Rosario, was found to be bearer of this disease. Now the high presence of rectal cancer in the Gallo family could be explained (Fig. 1).

FAP coli is a well-described autosomal syndrome characterised by diffused polyposis of the colon. The first description of intestinal polyposis dates back to 1721 with Menzelio [1]. In 1882, Cripps [2] described the inhered predisposition (brother and sister, both affected by FAP) while Smith [3] found the progress of the disease from an adenoma to a cancer that was then histologically described, in 1890 by Handford [4]. This disease is the most diffused heritable cause

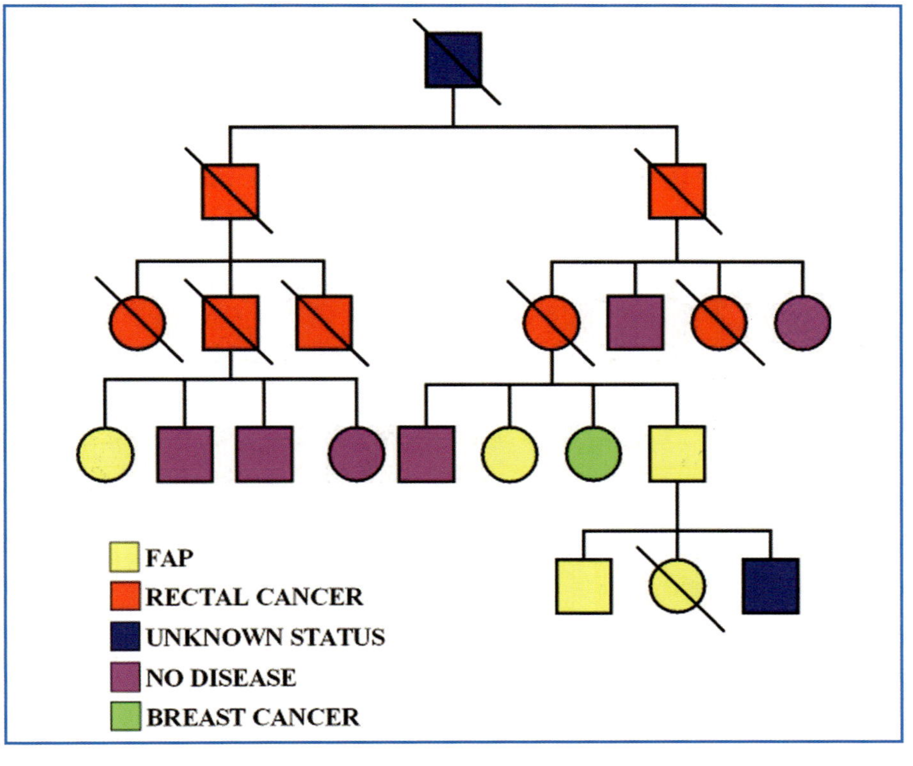

Fig. 1. Gallo family genetic tree

of colorectal cancer (CRC), second only to the Lynch syndrome. FAP stems from mutation of the APC gene localised on 5q21. The APC gene plays several important roles in cells, influencing cell adhesion, cytoskeleton and cell cycle [5, 6.] Since the first description in 1986 [7], much progress has been accomplished in determining the mutations causing this disease, thanks to the cloning technique, and over 1,000 mutations have been found [8], which have been inserted into an international reference database (http://perso.curie.fr/tsoussi). Now it seems certain that there is a correlation between genotype and phenotypic manifestation of the disease, as mutation in different areas of the APC leads to different manifestations of the disease [9]

Clinically, FAP is characterised by the presence of a high number (>100) of adenomatous polyps of the colon and rectum [10]. These polyps are characterised by a neoplastic degeneration, and these patients with them, if they do not undergo prophylactic colectomy, will develop colon cancer and will be doomed because of this neoplasty. Sometimes the disease has a slower course and a lower number of polyps, probably because of a milder form of the disease called attenuated adenomatous polyposis coli AAPC [11]. Usually in AAPC, polyps are right-sided and the rectum is spared. The disease develops over time. Bulow [12], in a now historic review, determined that the onset of polyps usually begins at 16 years of age (range: 5–38), at 29 years of age (range 12–73) the first symptoms begin (generally lower GI bleeding) and at 36 years of age (range: 17–63) rectal/colonic cancer appears.

Besides in the colon–rectum, the disease is characterised by the high incidence (from 28% to 68%) [13–15] of polyps in the stomach and duodenum. With the diffusion of the prophylactic colectomy, this associated pathology grew increasingly important, as extension of the average duration of life in these patients brought to light the risk of neoplastic degeneration. It also evidenced the need to perform a suitable follow-up with gastroscopy [16] and stratification of patients using Spigelman's classification [17] to determine which patients may be treated with endoscopic polypectomy only and which must undergo surgery, usually consisting of a pancreaticoduodenectomy.

Rosa's father and aunt were operated in London by Prof. Nicholls and underwent total colectomy with ileorectal anastomosis because preoperative examinations revealed the absence of polyps at rectum level.

The surgical therapy chosen to treat FAP was restorative proctocolectomy with ileal pouch anal anastomosis [18–20] due to the high risk of neoplastic degeneration in the residual rectal stump even though ileal rectal anastomosis might be a surgical option acceptable by patients with rectal sparing and a good compliance to follow-up [21, 22].

The years went by peacefully. Rosario's and his sister's follow-ups showed an absence of residual disease. The risk of this disease hung over Rosario's children, too. At 18 years of age, Carmine underwent the first colonoscopy and the diagnosis, for him, too, was FAP. He was then hospitalised at the Verona Surgery Clinic and underwent restorative proctocolectomy with ileal pouch anal anastomosis (RP-IPAA). The postoperative course went without complications, and after about 45 days, the loop ileostomy was closed.

Rosa, who by the time was a happy-go-lucky teenager, attended high school with very good results. She was always happy; she supported her family with her happiness and maturity during the

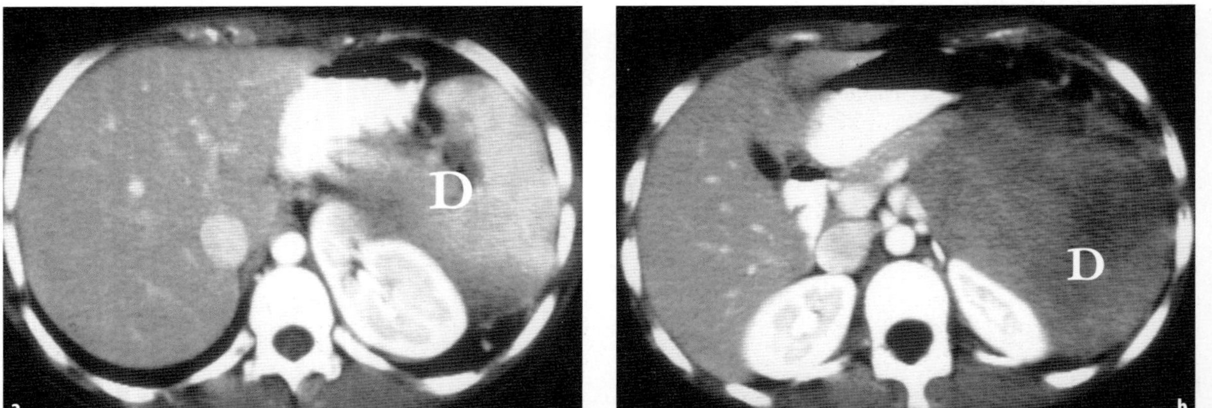

Fig. 2a, b. Preoperative computed tomography (CT) scan. *D*, desmoid tumour

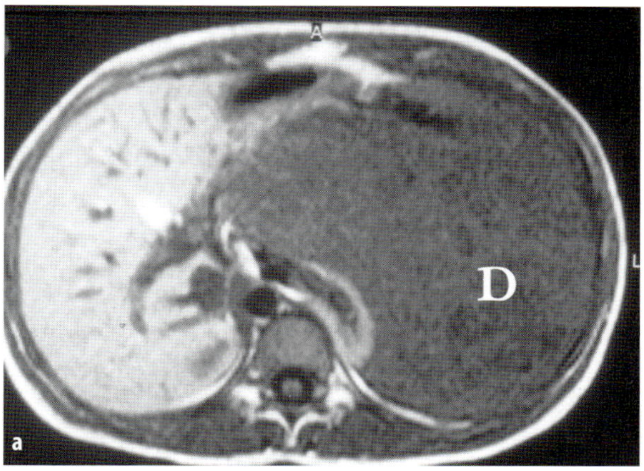

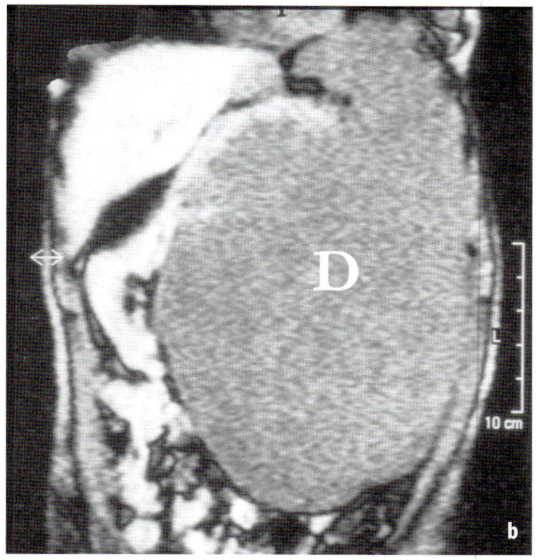

Fig. 3a, b. Preoperative magnetic resonance imaging (MRI) scan. *D*, desmoid tumour

hard times, well aware of the risk that she could suffer from the disease, too. In May 1998, when she was 17 years old, Rosa began to complain about a pain localised in the left side, which grew increasingly annoying. Her parents decided to subject the girl to a series of examinations. Rosa underwent colonoscopy, which revealed many polyps in the colon and rectum. Moreover, she underwent a computed tomography (CT) scan (Fig. 2) and magnetic resonance imaging (MRI) (Fig. 3), which revealed a voluminous mass filling the left hemiabdomen and infiltrating the spleen, pancreas, kidney and left ureter. The diagnostic procedure included, moreover, an ophthalmology exam, which revealed congenital hypertrophy of the retinal pigment epithelium. The cranial radiography did not reveal supernumerary teeth or osteomas. The diagnosis was then clear: Gardner's syndrome.

FAP may be associated with the presence of many extraintestinal manifestations characterising various syndromes, such as Gardner's syndrome [23] and Turcot's syndrome [24]. Table 1 summarises the main features of these syndromes.

The Voluminous Mass was a Desmoid Tumour

Desmoid (from the Greek desmos, which means tendon like) tumours are begnin tumours arising from the muscle-aponeurotic structures [25]. They are usually well differentiated but with an aggressive behaviour. Even if they have no metastatic potential, they can locally infiltrate the adjacent structures, leading to morbility/mortality because of the deformity resulting from the pressure or obstruction of vital structures/organs [26–28]. They represent 0.03% of all neoplasies [29] but this incidence increases up to 13% in patients with FAP [30], affecting mostly women (female:male ratio 2:1). Generally, desmoid tumours are localised in the abdominal wall or in the shoulder girdle, but in Gardner's syndrome, they mostly develop in the retroperitoneal space [31]. Many of these tumours are revealed after RP-IPAA [32, 33] or may be revealed, despite the preoperative staging, only during laparotomy and presenting small-sized masses, making deciding upon the kind of treatment difficult and controversial [34]. In order to determine approach to these tumours and assess their response to therapy, a method of staging intra-abdominal desmoid tumours was recently formulated [35].

In the effort to reduce the abdominal mass, before performing surgical resection, Rosa was treated with tamoxifen and sulindac, which she had to stop after 3 months due to the appearance of side effects (abdominal and limb cramps).

Despite anecdotes about the spontaneous reduction of the mass of desmoid tumours, the latter, as already stated above, tend to grow, sometimes fast, showing signs connected with infiltration of the surrounding structures or of space filling. As we will later see, the surgical approach proved to be at once subject to a high rate of relapses and to a high rate of complications [36], leading us to explore the possibility of using pharmacologic therapy as a primary choice.

Schematically, we can say that the drugs used may be divided into 5 groups: hormonal modulators, that is non-steroidal anti-inflammatory agents (NSAIDs); cAMP modulators, that is, cytotoxic

Table 1. Physical characteristics associated with Gardner's and Turcot's syndromes

Gardner syndrome		
Skin	Epidermal cyst Sebaceous cyst	
Craniofacial	Osteomas Dental abnormalities	Supernumerary teeth Missing teeth Root abnormalities
Gastrointestinal	Multiple gastric polyps Multiple duodenal polyps Multiple colonic polyps (FAP) Desmoid tumours (abdominal or/and thoracic wall; mesenteric)	
Endocrine	Cushing syndrome Multiple endocrine neoplasia	
Turcot syndrome		
Skin	Café au lait spots Multiple lipomas	
Gastrointestinal	Basal cell carcinoma of scalp Multiple colonic polyps (FAP) Hepatic nodular hyperplasia Gastric carcinoma	
Central nervous system	Glioma Glioblastoma multiforme Astrocytoma	

FAP, familial adenomatous polyposis coli

chemotherapeutic agents and other various agents (interferon gamma and, recently, imatinib mesylate). Cytotoxic drugs did not prove to be particularly effective in treating desmoid tumours, and their use was reserved to a few patients who did not respond to the other agents. Various therapeutic patterns were used, all including doxorubicin in association with other agents, also associated in some cases with radiotherapy [37–40] The action pattern of the NSAIDs is not yet clear, but it seems to be connected with a decreased prostaglandin synthesis due to cyclooxygenase reduction. The results obtained show a regression (either partial or complete) of the mass ranging from 0% [36] to 45% [41]. The side effects, though, are high, with a GI bleeding (in 29% of cases), gastric ulcer, nausea or vomiting [41].

The use of antiestrogens has its rationale in the proof, in many cases, of the presence of receptors for progesterone on desmoid tumour cells. By blocking these receptors, as in other neoplasties, activation of some genes is negatively inhibited (such as ornithine decarboxylase), influencing cell growth [42]. Moreover, there is an action pattern that is independent from the presence of receptors and is connected with stimulation of the secretion of the growth factor-b, which in turn inhibits the growth of abnormal fibroblast present in the desmoid tumour. Results in the literature are extremely various, with a success rate (either complete or partial response) ranging from 25% to 100% [41, 43, 44]. This treatment, though, due to the lower side effects, may be considered a first-line therapy and tried in most patients, even if it seems (the studies include a decreasing number of patients) to have better results if progesterone is expressed [43].

The introduction of imatinib mesylate (which proved extremely effective to treat another class of solid tumours, that is, GI stromal tumour), seems to offer some hope, considering the remarkable results described in a report [45], even if its usage seems to be limited to cases expressing the CD117 surface receptor.

A new abdomen CT showed growth of the abdominal mass, compelling us to choose surgery as an option.

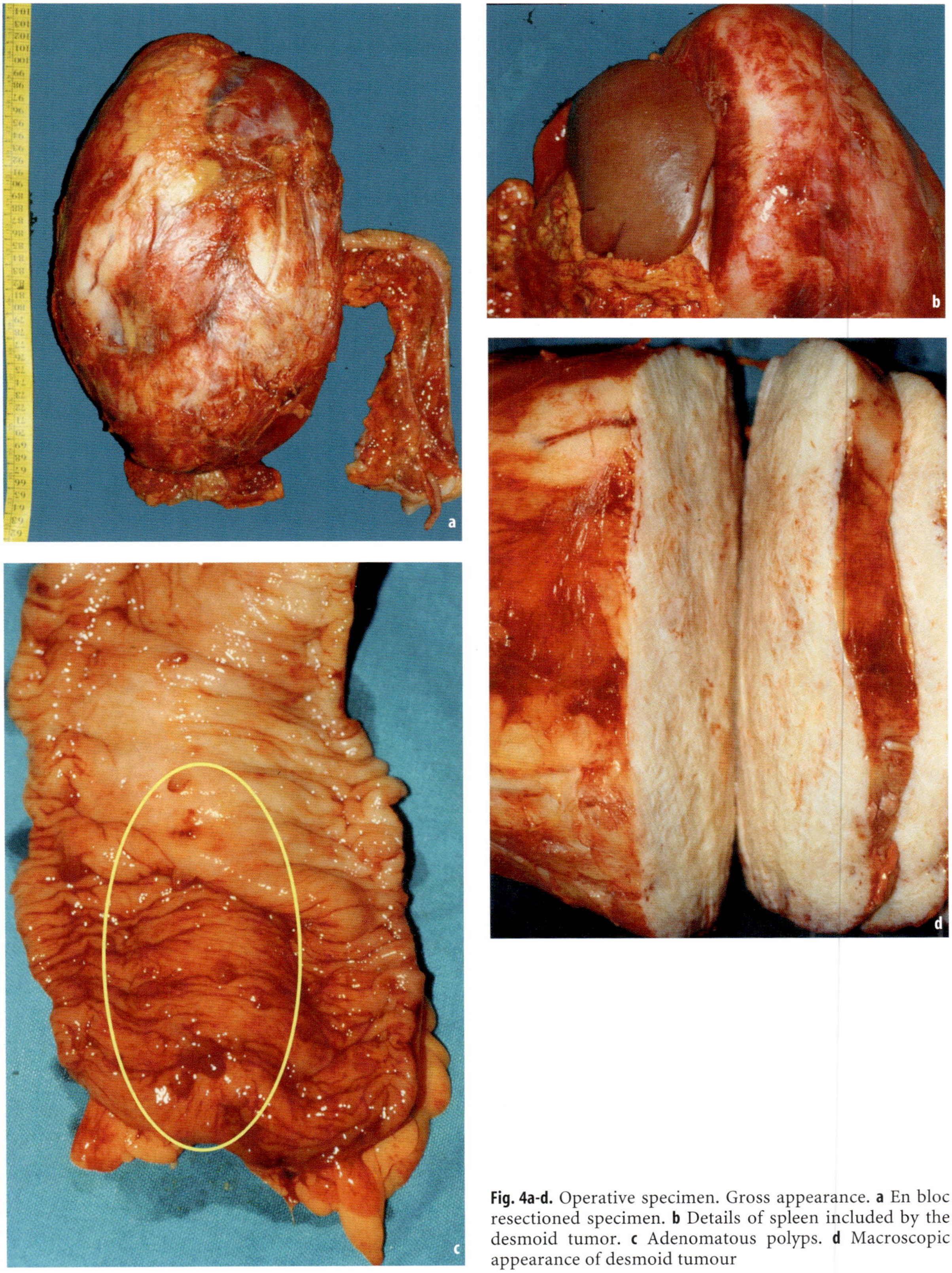

Fig. 4a-d. Operative specimen. Gross appearance. **a** En bloc resectioned specimen. **b** Details of spleen included by the desmoid tumor. **c** Adenomatous polyps. **d** Macroscopic appearance of desmoid tumour

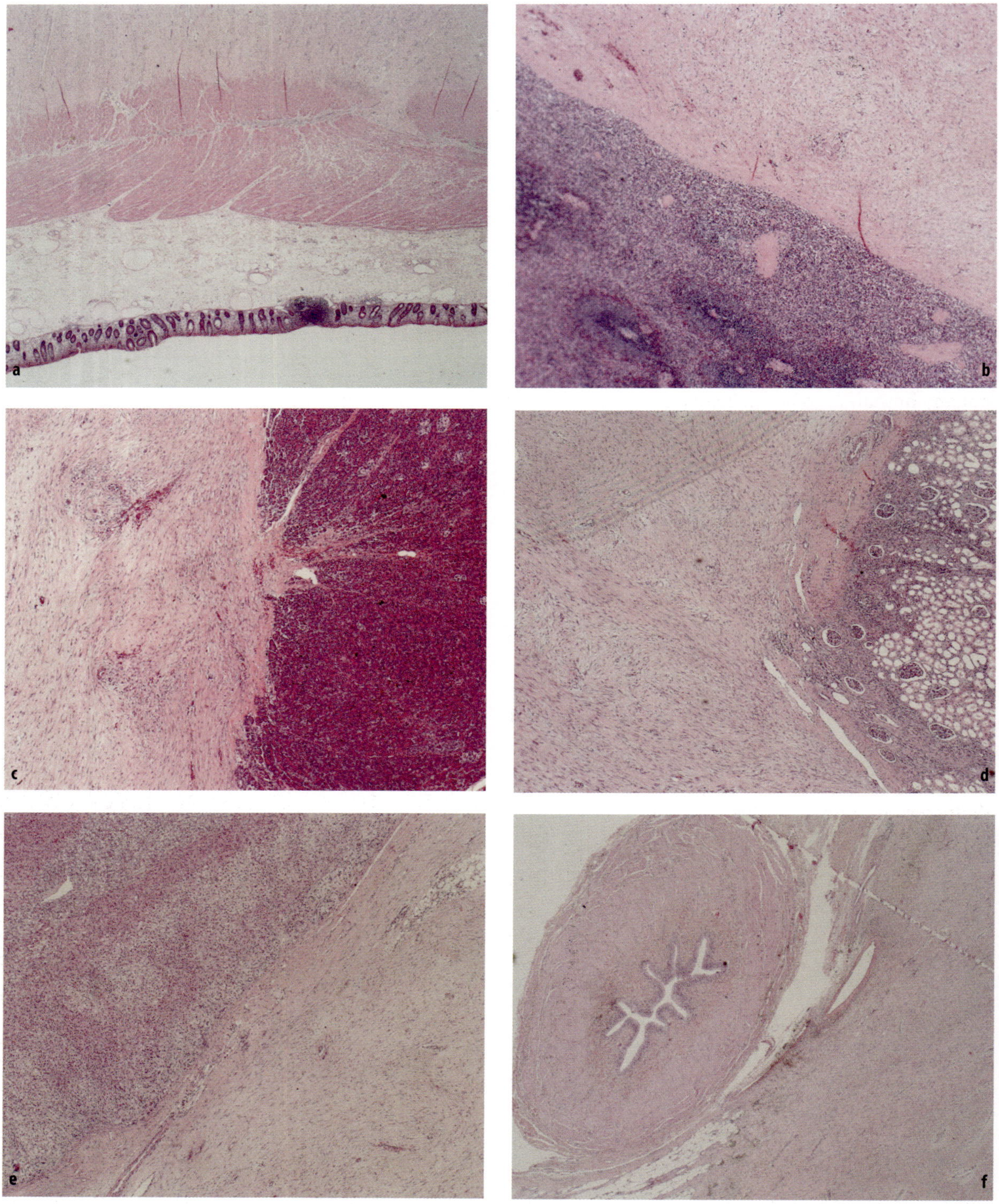

Fig. 5. Operative specimen: histologic involvement of colon (**a**); spleen (**b**); pancreas (**c**); kidney (**d**); surrenalic gland (**e**); ureter (**f**)

Resective therapy is considered the only alternative to pharmacological therapy if the latter fails, but it must be carefully considered due to the high rate of recurrence and the need to perform extended incisions to resect the tumours [46–48].

On 8 October 1998, Rosa underwent an en bloc resection of a large desmoid tumour (including pancreatic tail, spleen, left kidney, ureter and surrenal gland) (Figs. 4a–c and 5a–f), total colectomy with terminal ileostomy and closure of the rectal stump. The postoperative course was very good, and the MRI revealed complete resection of the tumorous mass (Fig. 6). Rosa was then dismissed. Rosa's recovery was unbelievable. She resumed school after a short while and managed to lead an ordinary life despite the stoma, which she managed autonomously without any limitation to her daily living.

In June 1999, at the end of school year, Rosa was hospitalised again to close the ileostomy. Preoperative exams, particularly the MRI did not reveal the presence of a desmoid tumour. On 25 June, Rosa was then subjected to surgery. At laparotomy, many nodules were revealed (likely recurrence of desmoid tumour) in the mesentery. Some nodules were resected, but it was not possible to remove them all without performing too wide a resection on the small bowel. The ileostomy was resected and, after mobilisation of the ileum, a side-to-end ileorectal anastomosis was made. Also in this case, there were no important complications during the postoperative course, and Rosa was dismissed after 2 weeks.

After just 8 months, during follow-up, an MRI revealed a new abdominal mass of about 10 cm in diameter. Moreover, a fast-growing mass in the abdominal–thoracic area was found. Rosa again underwent surgery. At laparotomy, a voluminous desmoid tumour was found (12–14 cm) growing from the mesentery and involving the origin of the mesenteric artery. Resection of such a mass was impossible without resecting over 80% of the small intestine. Some small desmoid tumours were then removed along the abdominal incision, and the abdominal–thoracic mass (a new desmoid tumour). Postoperative hospitalisation lasted 10 days only, and Rosa was dismissed. In the meantime, proving to be very brave, Rosa moved to Verona by herself and to attend the faculty of medicine at the university. The next 2 years went by rather peacefully. Rosa, always smiling and in a good mood, often walked down the hospital aisles, alternating her role of a bright student of medicine with the role of the patient undergoing periodical follow-ups. The big abdominal desmoid tumour seemed to have stopped growing, apparently responding well to the new therapy with raloxifene.

At the beginning of January 2003, Rosa began to report recurring abdominal pains, nausea and intestinal subocclusion. The situation slowly progressed; her appetite diminished and she consequently lost weight [actual body mass index (BMI): 17.5]. Considering the symptomatology, oral intake was stopped and was positioned at the central line. The abdominal radiograph showed a pattern of intestinal subocclusion. The MRI revealed persistence of the previously described mass and the appearance of new nodules in the abdomen and abdominal wall. After 2 days, the physicians decided, considering the persistence of the symptoms, to perform surgery again. Laparotomy revealed a situation of diffused adherences and two new desmoid masses. Some jejunal loops were dilated and strictly connected to the bigger desmoid tumour. A jejunal–ileal bypass was created. The postoperative course was difficult, with slow reactivation of intestinal movements.

Rosa, at this point, seeing there were no further alternatives, was sent to the surgical clinic in Innsbruck managed by Prof. Margreiter to be evaluated for an intestinal transplant. After careful clinical

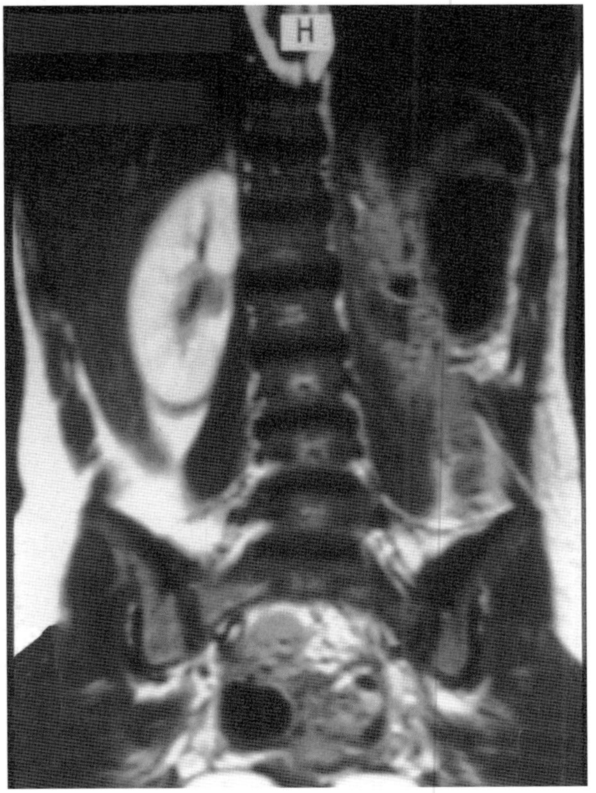

Fig. 6. Postoperative magnetic resonance imaging (MRI) scan

evaluation and a thorough explanation of the surgery to be performed (Fig. 7) and short- and long-term risks, Prof. Margreiter proposed that Rosa undergo intestinal or multiorgan transplant. With her usual bravery, Rosa accepted and was placed on the waiting list.

The multiorgan transplant is a very complicated procedure, especially due to postoperative management of rejection. Even if the experiences in major centres are limited, the multiorgan transplant, in the case of large desmoid tumours, is becoming a reality [49–53]. However, besides the risks connected with the procedure, there is the possibility of recurrence of the desmoid tumour, with the risk of having to perform new resective operations [54].

During the following months, Rosa resumed an ordinary life. Despite the fact that her parents wanted and encouraged her to go home, she returned to live in Verona with her mates and resumed studying, taking exams and getting the best grades. Follow-ups revealed a stationary situation, with a discreet nutritional status. In November 2003, things began to get worse. Rosa began to report the return of abdominal pains and fever. She was then treated at the outpatient clinic but on 25 November 25 2003 had to be hospitalised due to the reappearance of sepsis white blood cell count (WBC): 20,000, fever 40.5°C). A broad-spectrum antibiotic therapy was then started and a abdomen CT was performed. The latter revealed the presence of an abdominal purulent concentration. Rosa was then subjected to a new laparotomy and drainage of the purulent concentration, which was probably due to a fistula between a jejunal loop and the bigger desmoid tumour. Because of the abdominal situation, only drainage of this abdominal abscess was done. Her case was then declared urgent, and she was placed on the top of the transplant list.

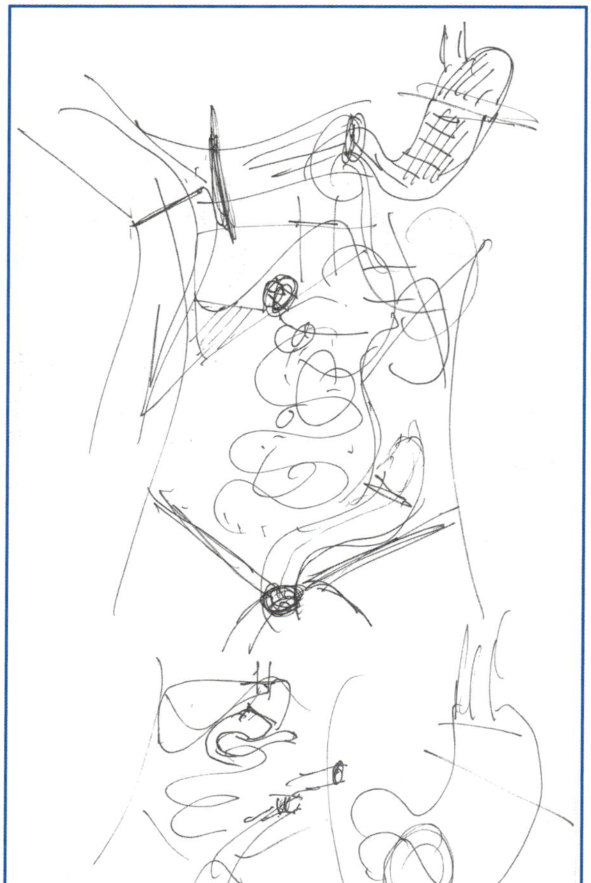

Fig. 7. Picture drawn by Prof. Margreiter during the informed consent process

The postoperative course was extremely difficult. After an initial period of relative well-being, bacterial and fungal infections occurred, becoming increasingly difficult to control with therapy. A new abdominal abscess close to the abdominal wall was drained percutaneously. After more than 2 months of hospitalisation, on 15 February 2004, Rosa received the long-awaited call: a donor was found. Rosa was moved to Innsbruck at once. While going into the operating theatre, she said goodbye to Prof. Delaini with a smile on her face; he had been following her since the beginning of the disease and saw her as far as Innsbruck: "Professor, these surgeons will try to kill me anyway. Please, oversee the operation", she said. Surgery was extremely complicated. In the demolitive stage, all desmoid abdominal tumours were abscessed, resecting the aorta vena cava. The desmoid tumours of the abdominal and thoracic wall were then abscessed, demolishing a large portion. Rosa was then subjected to a multivisceral transplant: liver, pancreas, stomach (with gastric anastomosis), duodenum, jejunum and ileum. A terminal ileostomy was made. The abdominal wall was reconstructed by a large abdominal Gore-Tex patch. The final stage of the operation was characterised by difficulty controlling bleeding and the need to perform an abdominal patching. After 4 days, the abdominal patches were removed. On 5 March, Rosa underwent a new surgery to drain an infected retrogastric haematoma [positive for methicillin-resistant ***Staphylococcus aureus*** (MRSA)]. The remaining operative course was without complications. Rosa began a by-mouth feeding even though prudentially a Port-a-Cath was inserted.

Antirejection therapy, after some initial adjustments and the need to undergo a unique dialysis session due to worsening of kidney function following a temporary high haematic concentration of FK-506, had a very good range and response. The duodenal biopsies through ileostomy did not reveal the appearance of any sign of acute or chronic rejection. Moreover, echo-colour Doppler revealed very good hepatic perfusion. On 13 May 2004, Rosa was dismissed, and follow-ups at the outpatient clinic were scheduled. The first 2 months went by satisfactorily despite the need to undergo 2 cycles of high-dosage corticosteroids to avoid rejection. During this period, Rosa could even leave her apartment near Innsbruck, where she lived with her parents, and travel to Altavilla Salentina.

On 11 July 2004, Rosa was hospitalised due to upper GI bleeding that, at gastroscopy, revealed two duodenal ulcers that only required the transfusion of 3 units of blood. This event, which apparently was not so serious, was the initial cause of a miserable course. Rosa began to have a series of bacterial infections, which required broad-spectrum antibiotic therapy and removal of the Port-a-Cath (16 July). Subsequently, a state of sepsis began to appear (on 27 July), with an increase of lactates and worsening of the cardiocirculatory condition. To support circulation, it was necessary to begin the administration of pressor amines. On 4 August a massive left pleuritic effusion was surgically drained, which on 6 August required a review due to bleeding with haematoma. Moreover, following the development of respiratory insufficiency, Rosa was intubated, and respiratory function was mechanically supported.

Following the bacterial infections came fungal infections and the development of coagulative deficiencies. On 20 August, a surgical tracheostomy was performed. After a few hours, Rosa's circulatory status worsened and despite all efforts, she died at 21.04 on 21 August 2004. The autopsy was performed 1 day later, but it only confirmed the damage caused by the septic shock.

Rosa Gallo was an extraordinary young woman who, despite her short life, deeply changed all who knew her. With her wonderful smile and her incredible stamina, she faced her disease and trouble serenely. This book is the first step towards the realisation of a dream that led her to attend the faculty of medicine: to help all people suffering with FAP. Thank you, Rosa.

References

1. Menzelio D (1721) De excrescentis verrucoso cristosis copiose in intestinis crassis dysenteriam passi observatis. Acta Medicorum Berolinensium IX:68–71
2. Cripps WH (1882) Two cases of disseminated polypus of the lower bowel occurring in one family. Trans Path Soc London 33:165–168
3. Smith T (1887) Three cases of multiple polypi of the lower bowel occurring in one family. St. Bartholomew's Hosp Rep 23:225–229
4. Handford H (1890) Disseminated polypi of the large intestine becoming malignant; strictures (malignant adenoma) of the rectum and of splenic flexure of the colon; secondary growths in the liver. Trans Path Soc London 133–137
5. Kita K, Wittmann T, Nathke IS, Waterman-Storer CM (2006) APC on microtubule plus ends in cell extensions can promote microtubule net growth with or without EB1. Mol Biol Cell [Epub ahead of print]
6. Gayther SA, Wells D, Sen-Gupta SB et al (1994) Regionally clustered APC mutations are associated with a severe phenotype and occur at a high frequency in new mutation cases of adenomatous polyposis coli. Hum Mol Genet 3:53–56
7. Herrera L, Kakati S, Gibas L et al (1986) Gardner syndrome in a man with an interstitial deletion of 5q. Am J Med Genet 25:473–476
8. Laurent-Puig P, Beroud C, Soussi T (1998) APC gene: database of germline and somatic mutations in human tumors and cell lines. Nucleic Acids Res 26:269–270
9. Fearnhead NS, Britton MP, Bodmer WF (2001) The ABC of APC. Hum Mol Genet 10:721–733
10. Bussey HJR (1975) Familial polyposis coli. John Hopkins University Press, Baltimore
11. Soravia C, Berk T, Madlensky L et al (1998) Genotype-phenotype correlations in attenuated adenomatous polyposis coli. Am J Hum Genet 62:1290–1301
12. Bulow S (1987) Familial polyposis coli. Dan Med Bull 34:1–15
13. Bulow S, Bjork J, Christensen IJ et al (2004) Duodenal adenomatosis in familial adenomatous polyposis. Gut 53:381–386
14. Church JM, McGannon E, Hull-Boiner S et al (1992) Gastroduodenal polyps in patients with familial adenomatous polyposis. Dis Colon Rectum 35:1170–1173
15. Bjork J, Akerbrant H, Iselius L et al (2001) Periampullary adenomas and adenocarcinomas in familial adenomatous polyposis: cumulative risks and APC gene mutations. Gastroenterology 121:1127–1135
16. Groves CJ, Saunders BP, Spigelman AD, Phillips RK (2002) Duodenal cancer in patients with familial adenomatous polyposis (FAP): results of a 10 year prospective study. Gut 50:636–641
17. Spigelman AD, Williams CB, Talbot IC et al (1989) Upper gastrointestinal cancer in patients with familial adenomatous polyposis. Lancet 2:783–785
18. Krausz MM, Duek SD (2005) Restorative proctocolectomy with ileal pouch-anal anastomosis for ulcerative colitis and familial adenomatous polyposis: twenty years follow-up in 174 patients. Isr Med Assoc J 7:23–27
19. Penna C, Tiret E, Kartheuser A et al (1993) Function of ileal J pouch-anal anastomosis in patients with familial adenomatous polyposis. Br J Surg 80:765–767
20. Ziv Y, Church JM, Oakley JR et al (1996) Results after restorative proctocolectomy and ileal pouch-anal anastomosis in patients with familial adenomatous polyposis and coexisting colorectal cancer. Br J Surg 83:1578–1580
21. Soravia C, Klein L, Berk T et al (1999) Comparison of ileal pouch-anal anastomosis and ileorectal anastomo-

sis in patients with familial adenomatous polyposis. Dis Colon Rectum 42:1028–1033
22. Van DP, Slors JF, Taat CW et al (1999) Functional outcome after colectomy and ileorectal anastomosis compared with proctocolectomy and ileal pouch-anal anastomosis in familial adenomatous polyposis. Ann Surg 230:648–654
23. Gardner EJ (1962) Follow-up study of a family group exhibiting dominant inheritance for a syndrome including intestinal polyps, osteomas, fibromas and epidermal cyst. Am J Hum Genet 14:390
24. Turcot J, Despres J, St. Pierre F (1959) Malignant tumors of the central nervous system associated with familial polyposis of the colon: report of two cases. Dis Colon Rectum 2:468
25. Clark SK, Phillips RK (1996) Desmoids in familial adenomatous polyposis. Br J Surg 83:1494–1504
26. Knudsen AL, Bulow S (2000) [Desmoid tumor in familial adenomatous polyposis] Ugeskr Laeger. 162:5628–5631
27. Gonzalez CF, Herranz AF, Duran MR et al (1994) [Obstructive uropathy in Gardner syndrome: a new case and an alternative therapeutic option]. Actas Urol Esp 18:128–132
28. Campos FG, Habr-Gama A, Kiss DR et al (2003) [Extracolonic manifestations of familial adenomatous polyposis: incidence and impact on the disease outcome] Arq Gastroenterol 40:92–98
29. Shields C J, Winter D C, Kirwan WO, Redmond HP (2001) Desmoid tumours. Eur J Surg Oncol 2:122–135
30. Klemmer S, Pascoe L, DeCosse J (1987) Occurrence of desmoids in patients with familial adenomatous polyposis of the colon. Am J Med Genet 28:385–392
31. Bessler W, Egloff B, Sulser H (1984) Case report 253. Gardner syndrome with aggressive fibromatosis. Skeletal Radiol 11:56–59
32. Araki Y, Isomoto H, Shirouzu K et al (1991) Occurrence of desmoid tumors following surgery for familial adenomatosis coli – report of two cases. Kurume Med J 38:9–14
33. Clark SK, Smith TG, Katz DE et al (1998) Identification and progression of a desmoid precursor lesion in patients with familial adenomatous polyposis. Br J Surg 85:970–973
34. Hartley JE, Church JM, Gupta S et al (2004) Significance of incidental desmoids identified during surgery for familial adenomatous polyposis. Dis Colon Rectum 47:334–338
35. Church J, Berk T, Boman BM et al (2005) Staging intra-abdominal desmoid tumors in familial adenomatous polyposis: a search for a uniform approach to a troubling disease. Dis Colon Rectum 48:1528–1534
36. Jones IT, Jagelman DG, Fazio VW et al (1986) Desmoid tumor in patients with familial polyposis coli. Ann Surg 204:94–97
37. Tsukada K, Church JM, Jagelman DG et al (1991) Systemic cytotoxic chemotherapy and radiation therapy for desmoid in familial adenomatous polyposis. Dis Colon Rectum 34:1090–1092
38. Poritz LS, Blackstein M, Berk T et al (2001) Extended follow-up of patients treated with cytotoxic chemotherapy for intra-abdominal desmoid tumors Dis Colon Rectum 44:1268–1273
39. Patel SR, Benjamin RS (2006) Desmoid tumors respond to chemotherapy: defying the dogma in oncology. J Clin Oncol 24:11–12
40. Lynch HT, Fitzgibbons R Jr, Chong S et al (1994) Use of doxorubicin and dacarbazine for the management of unresectable intra-abdominal desmoid tumors in Gardner's syndrome. Dis Colon Rectum 37:260–267
41. Tsukada K, Church JM, Jagelman DG et al (1992) Noncytotoxic drug therapy for intra-abdominal desmoid tumor in patients with familial adenomatous polyposis. Dis Colon Rectum 35:29–33
42. Kulaylat MN, Karakousis CP, Keaney CM et al (1999) Desmoid tumour: a pleomorphic lesion. Eur J Surg Oncol 25:487–497
43. Tonelli F, Ficari F, Valanzano R, Brandi ML (2003) Treatment of desmoids and mesenteric fibromatosis in familial adenomatous polyposis with raloxifene. Tumori 89:391–396
44. Bauernhofer T, Stoger H, Schmid M et al (1996) Sequential treatment of recurrent mesenteric desmoid tumor Cancer 77:1061–1065
45. Mace J, Sybil B , Sondak V et al (2002) Response of extraabdominal desmoid tumors to therapy with imatinib mesylate. Cancer 95:2373–2379
46. Berk T, Cohen Z, McLeod RS, Stern HS (1992) Management of mesenteric desmoid tumours in familial adenomatous polyposis. Can J Surg 35:393–395
47. Clark SK, Neale KF, Landgrebe JC, Phillips RK (1999) Desmoid tumours complicating familial adenomatous polyposis. Br J Surg 86:1185–1189
48. Kadmon M, Moslein G, Buhr HJ, Herfarth C (1995) [Desmoid tumors in patients with familial adenomatous polyposis (FAP) Clinical and therapeutic observations from the Heidelberg polyposis register]. Chirurg 66:997–1005
49. Chatzipetrou MA, Tzakis AG, Pinna AD et al (2001) Intestinal transplantation for the treatment of desmoid tumors associated with familial adenomatous polyposis. Surgery 129:277–281
50. Gajate ML, Elias ME, Martinez PA et al (2004) [Intestinal transplantation in adults: present situation and future prospects]. Rev Esp Anestesiol Reanim 51:537–548
51. Lattimer JK, Birkhoff J, Olsson CA (1987) The treatment of ureteral obstruction in Gardner's syndrome: renal autotransplantation. J Urol 138:133–135
52. Soon JL, Lau WK, Seow-Choen F, Cheng CW (2005) Unresectable desmoid tumours causing obstructive uropathy in familial adenomatous polyposis. Asian J Surg 28:233–237
53. Jovine E, Masetti M, Cautero N et al (2002) Modified multivisceral transplantation without a liver graft for Gardner/Desmoid syndrome and chronic intestinal pseudo-obstruction. Transplant Proc 34:911–912
54. Misiakos EP, Pinna A, Kato T et al (1999) Recurrence of desmoid tumor in a multivisceral transplant patient with Gardner's syndrome. Transplantation 67:1197–1199

Ileo-Rectal Anastomosis *vs.* Ileo-Anal Pouch as the Surgical Treatment for Familial Adenomatous Polyposis

Omer Aziz, Paris Tekkis

Introduction

Surgery for Familial Adenomatous Polyposis

The surgical treatment of familial adenomatous polyposis (FAP) is aimed at minimising the risk of colorectal cancer whilst leaving the patient with a good functional outcome and one that is socially acceptable to them [1]. The ideal operation for FAP should therefore be safe with regards to post-operative morbidity and mortality, preserve faecal continence, spare pelvic innervation to the sexual organs, and eliminate cancer risk [2]. Because patients with FAP are generally young and often asymptomatic at the time of presentation for surgery, the prospect of undergoing a "proctocolectomy and end ileostomy" is one they understandably find difficult to accept, making surgical options for FAP that remove the need for a permanent stoma attractive. The two most common options that offer this are the "colectomy and ileo-rectal anastomosis" (IRA) and "proctocolectomy with ileal pouch anal anastomosis" (IPAA), with no clear consensus on which of these two options is the best first-line treatment. This is because surgery that preserves intestinal continuity for FAP involves balancing certain risks and benefits, all of which must be taken into account individually before the final surgical option is decided. These are considered in turn below.

Rectal Cancer Risk

IRA carries a definite cancer risk in FAP due to the remaining rectal stump [3, 4], with a long-term rectal cancer risk reported to increase from 4% at 5 years to 25% at 20 years post-operatively [5]. More recently it has been suggested that absolute patient age is the determinant factor for cancer development rather than the length of post-operative follow-up [6]. This has led some to suggest that IRA should be converted to IPAA before the age of 50 [7]. Several factors are thought to increase the rectal cancer risk with IRA, namely colorectal polyp density, and presence of colorectal cancer at presentation, both of which are associated with higher proctectomy rates [8, 9]. Supporting this is the finding that having greater than 1000 adenomas in the colon is associated with double the risk of developing colorectal cancer [10]. Other factors thought to increase colorectal cancer risk in the retained rectum include length of rectal stump [11], age of patient at surgery [8], site of the APC mutation [8, 9] and adequacy of rectal surveillance [12]. Despite this, recent evidence does suggest a role for performing IRA in selected patients with FAP, namely those with relative rectal sparing (<10 adenomas), attenuated adenomatous polyposis coli or in adolescents and teenagers with mild polyposis coli [13, 14]. A study by Church et al. found IRA performed since 1983 (termed the "IPAA era") to carry a significantly lower rate of proctectomy for rectal cancer than those performed before 1983 (termed the "pre-IPAA era") [15]. The authors attributed this to a greater number of patients in the IPAA era having undergone the procedure despite severe polyposis in order to avoid a permanent ileostomy in an otherwise young and asymptomatic patient. Although they demonstrated that careful selection of patients for IRA can result in a successful outcome, a limitation of the study was the significantly shorter length of follow-up in the IPAA era group. With restorative proctocolectomy and IPAA, although the incidence of adenomatous polyps in the ileal reservoir and the risk of malignant transformation is reduced, this cannot be eliminated [7, 16]. This is particularly the case with IPAA using stapled anastomosis where mucosectomy (as in the case of hand-sewn anastomosis) is not possible, and results in retained rectal mucosa with a potential to undergo adenomatous change [17-19]. Although both IPAA and IRA reduce the risk of colorectal cancer in FAP, neither completely remove this risk, resulting in a requirement for endoscopic surveillance.

Functional Outcome

Bowel habit and other functional outcomes are thought by many to be better preserved and more physiological with IRA as compared to IPAA [20, 21]. Restorative proctocolectomy with mucosectomy and hand-sewn IPAA is thought to carry a relatively higher risk of postoperative functional impairment and incontinence due to increased manipulation of the anal canal [22]. Stapled IPAA, on the other hand, results in preservation of the anal transition zone mucosa 1–2 cm above the dentate line, which is thought to be important in the control of continence. This has been shown by many to result in better functional outcome and quality of life after IPAA [13, 19, 22]. In the case of IPAA, it has been suggested that functional outcome is poorer in patients with ulcerative colitis (UC) than those with FAP [23]. It has also been suggested that secondary IPAA, often performed following failed IRA (due to rectal cancer or poor functional outcome), is associated with poorer bowel function than a primary IPAA procedure [24].

Post-operative Morbidity

Although both IPAA and IRA procedures qualify as major abdominal operations, performing an IRA is perceived as being an easier and less complicated procedure, associated with less post-operative morbidity [15]. Factors that are thought to play a part in this include increased operative time, hospital stay and blood loss, all of which have been suggested as being greater with IPAA [13]. This procedure may also involve the formation of a temporary defunctioning ileostomy in order to minimise the risk of anastomotic leakage and pelvis sepsis [25]. There are however complications and disadvantages related to this additional procedure, which requires closure under general anaesthetic at a later date [26, 27]. This has led to several groups avoiding defunctioning ileostomy with IPAA altogether, with encouraging results [27, 28]. The question of whether IRA is suitable for young patients, who are more likely to require a later rectal excision due to polyp recurrence or rectal cancer, or whether these patients are better served with a one-stage restorative proctocolectomy, mucosectomy, and IPAA, particularly in those with severe FAP phenotype, has been considered and remains to be answered [13]. Secondary IPAA is a procedure in which technical difficulties are more common than primary IPAA for both UC and FAP [29, 30], with some suggesting significantly higher complication rates due to technical difficulties and increased age at presentation [31], and others suggesting that it can be performed safely [20].

Long-term Complications

Desmoid tumours are known to occur in 5–15% of patients with FAP and known to cluster in families [32]. The conversion of IRA to IPAA may not be possible due to the presence of low rectal cancer or an abdominal desmoid tumour [24]. The question of whether an IPAA or IRA affects the development of intra-abdominal desmoid tumour is also unclear [33, 34], with some suggesting that this may be greater in IPAA due to increased handling and mobilisation of the small bowel mesentery [14]. Other long-term adverse events include perianal irritation and anastomotic stricture formation [35].

Quality of Life

The risk of sexual dysfunction is also thought to be greater with IPAA as compared to IRA, mainly due to the increased handling of the pelvic floor and therefore risk of nerve damage [2]. Other factors that affect a patient's the quality life are restrictions to their social activities (including occupation), and changes to their diet in order to maintain manageable bowel function [35]. Scoring systems such as the "Short Form-36 Health Survey questionnaire" and "European Organisation for Research and Treatment of Cancer QoL questionnaire" have been used to compare IPAA and IRA for FAP, with inconclusive results [36], whilst other systems have suggested better results following IPAA for FAP [37].

Current Evidence

Whilst it is clear that the ideal surgical intervention for FAP would involve minimal colorectal malignancy risk, whilst obtaining a good functional outcome, quality of life, and low post-operative morbidity; it is unclear from the literature as to which of the IPAA and IRA techniques best offer this, and in which patients. This chapter aims to systematically review and present the existing comparative literature on IPAA as compared to IRA for the primary treatment of FAP, using meta-analytic techniques where appropriate. The specific questions that we aim to answer are:

- does one technique carry significantly less early post-operative morbidity (bowel obstruction, haemorrhage, intra-abdominal sepsis, anastomotic separation, wound infection and need for reoperation within 30 days) than the other?
- How does the functional outcome compare between the two techniques with regards to stool frequency, urgency, night defecation, inconti-

nence, pad requirement and need for anti-diarrhoeal medication?

- Is there a significant difference in the dietary restrictions and social dysfunction between IRA and IPAA techniques?
- How does male and female sexual dysfunction compare between the two techniques?
- What are differences between IPAA and IRA in the incidence of long-term complications (anastomotic stricture, perianal irritation, intra-abdominal desmoid formation and cancer in the pouch/rectum)?

Please note that where appropriate meta-analysis of these outcomes has been performed in line with recommendations from the Cochrane Collaboration and the Quality of Reporting of Meta-analyses (QUORUM) guidelines [38, 39]. Statistical analysis for categorical variables has been carried out using the odds ratio as the summary statistic. This ratio represents the odds of an adverse event occurring in the IPAA group compared with the IRA group. An odds ratio of less than one favours the IPAA group, and the point estimate of the odds ratio is considered statistically significant at the $p<0.05$ level if the 95% confidence interval does not include the value one. For continuous variables such as bowel frequency per 24-h period, statistical analysis has been carried out using the weighted mean difference (WMD) as the summary statistic [40]. For studies that presented continuous data as means and range values, the standard deviations (SD) have been calculated using statistical algorithms and checked using "bootstrap" resampling techniques. Thus all continuous data have been standardised for analysis.

Literature Review

Since 1991, seventeen studies comparing the results from primary IRA and primary IPAA for FAP [2, 13, 14, 20, 25, 29, 31, 35-37, 41-48] have been published in the peer-reviewed literature (including all languages). One of these studies reported on a mixed patient group of both FAP and UC patients [47], making it difficult to draw conclusions from its results. In addition to this, in four papers, the authors reported on overlapping patient groups (these patients had already been reported on in another paper) [25, 36, 45, 46]. In this case the most informative and highest quality paper was selected to represent this patient group. The results from the remaining twelve studies (containing 1002 subjects) published between 1991 and 2003 comparing primary IPAA to primary IRA for FAP and were therefore included in this review [2, 13, 14, 20, 29, 31, 35, 37, 41-44]. Table 1 shows the characteristics of these twelve studies with 535 (53.3%) patients undergoing IPAA

Table 1. Characteristics of studies included in the systematic review

Author	Institution	Year	Design	IPAA	IRA	Group	Male (%)	Follow-up (months)
Madden [35]	St. Marks	1991	R	24	62	IPAA	42	62
						IRA	53	78
Ambrose [2]	Mayo Clinic, Minnesota	1992	R	91	18	IPAA	55	48
						IRA	56	72
Rodriguez [42]	Santander, Spain	1992	R	11	8	IPAA	55	26
						IRA	25	3
Penna [29]	St. Antoine, Paris	1993	R	120	23	IPAA	N/A	N/A
						IRA		
Ziv [13]	Cleveland Clinic, Ohio	1995	R	7	17	IPAA	57	36
						RA	53	46
Rotondano [43]	Napoli, Italy	1997	R	15	25	IPAA	N/A	46
						IRA		54
Tonelli [14]	Florence, Italy	1997	Pr	24	14	IPAA	63	61
						IRA	57	82
Soravia [20, 24]	Mount Sinai, Toronto	1999	R	38	60	IPAA	48	72
						IRA	42	92.4
Van Duijvendijk [44]	Leiden, Netherlands	1999	R	118	161	IPAA	57	79
						IRA	49	144
Ko [41]	Lahey Clinic, Massatussets	2000	R	30	14	IPAA	N/A	120
						IRA		168
Bjork [31]	Multicentre, Sweden	2001	R	20	43	IPAA	40	84
						IRA	51	128
Gunther [37]	Erlangen, Germany	2003	R	37	22	IPAA	59	118
						IRA	50	180

R, retrospective patient identification, prospective data collection; *Pr*, prospective study and 467 (46.7%) undergoing IRA as the primary treatment for FAP. Please note that the mean/median length of follow-up for both IPAA and IRA groups was at least 36 months in all but one study.

Early Post-Operative Morbidity

Early post-operative complications such as bowel obstruction, haemorrhage, intra-abdominal sepsis, anastomotic separation, wound infection, and the need for 30-day re-operation were reported by the ten studies shown in Table 2. The results from meta-analysis of post-operative complications from these studies are shown in the Forrest plot in Fig. 1. Please note that squares indicate point estimates of treatment effect (odds ratio), with the size of the square representing the weight attributed to each study and 95% confidence intervals indicated by horizontal bars. The diamond represents the summary odds ratio from the pooled studies with 95% confidence intervals. There was no significant difference between IRA and IPAA groups in the incidence of bowel obstruction, post-operative haemorrhage, intra-abdominal sepsis, anastomotic separation, and post-operative wound infection. There was however a significantly reduced need for re-operation within 30 days of 11.6% with IRA *vs.* 23.4% with IPAA (OR 2.11, CI 1.21-3.70).

Long-Term Complications

Long-term adverse events such as perianal irritation, anastomotic stricture, desmoid formation, cancer in pouch/rectum, and need for further operation on the pouch (IPAA) or rectum (IRA) were reported by the ten studies shown in Table 3. It is important to note that further operation on the rectum after IRA involves excision of retained rectum and either proctectomy or secondary IPAA, whereas in the case of IPAA this involves either a redo IPAA or pouch excision and end ileostomy. The results from meta-analysis of post-operative complications from these studies are shown in the Forrest plot in Figure 2. Results significantly favouring IRA over IPAA included a reduced incidence of perianal irritation of 57.4% with IRA as compared to 62.7% with IPAA (OR=2.48, CI 1.36–4.55), and reduced incidence of anastomotic stricture formation of 2% with IRA *vs.* 8.1% following IPAA. Results significantly favouring IPAA over IRA included a reduced incidence of cancer in the pouch or retained rectum at 0% (0/187) following IPAA *vs.* 5.5% after IRA group (OR=0.13, CI 0.03–0.61), and a reduced need for further surgery to the pouch or rectum of 3.1% in the IPAA *vs.* 27.7% in the IRA group. There was no significant difference between IPAA and IRA groups in the incidence of intra-abdominal desmoids.

Dietary Restriction, Social and Sexual Dysfunction

The studies reporting on dietary restriction, social restriction, and sexual dysfunction are shown in Table 4. The results from meta-analysis of these outcomes are shown in the Forrest plot in Figs. 3 and 4. The incidence of social restrictions following 58 IPAA and 85 IRA procedures (33, 35), was found to be significantly lower at 3.5% following IRA as compared to 13.8% following IPAA (OR=6.04, CI 1.53–23.78). There was no significant difference between IPAA and IRA in terms of need for dietary restriction and male and female sexual dysfunction.

Table 2. Studies reporting early post-operative complications

Author	Early post-operative complications					
	Bowel obstruction	Haemorrhage	Abdominal sepsis	Anastomotic separation	Wound infection	30-day reoperation
Ambrose [2]	*		*			
Bjork [31]	*	*	*	*	*	*
Gunther [37]	*	*	*		*	*
Madden [35]	*	*	*	*	*	*
Penna [29]	*		*			
Rodriguez [42]	*		*	*	*	
Soravia [20, 24]	*		*	*	*	*
Tonelli [14]	*		*			*
Van Duijvendijk [44]	*			*		*
Ziv [13]	*				*	

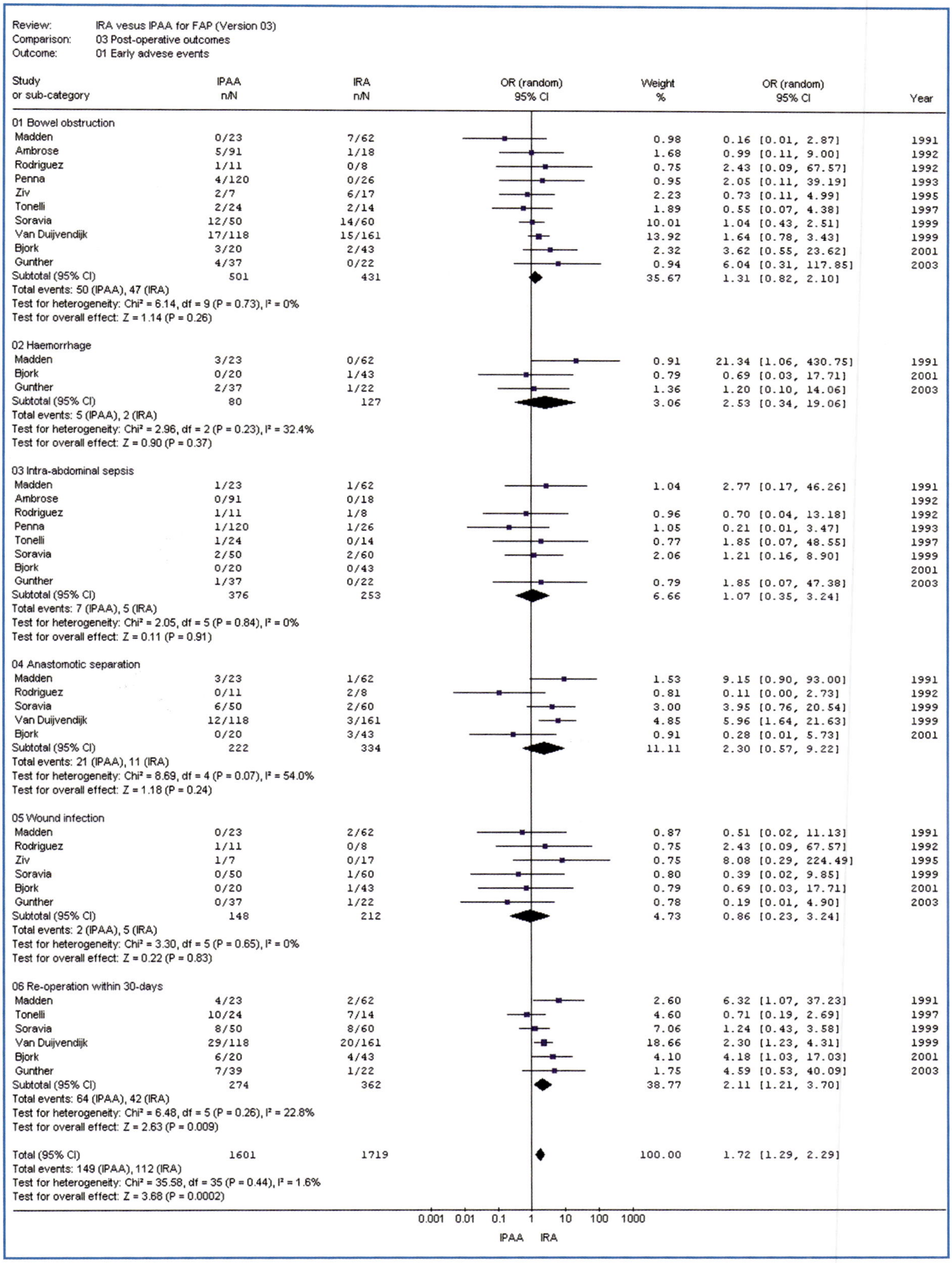

Fig. 1. Meta-analysis of post-operative complications

Table 3. Studies reporting long-term complications

Author	Long-term complications				
	Perianal irritation	Anastomotic stricture	Intra-abdominal desmoids	Cancer in pouch/rectum	Reoperation on rectum
Ambrose [2]	*		*	*	*
Bjork [31]	*	*		*	*
Ko [41]	*				
Madden [35]	*	*			
Penna [29]			*		
Rodriguez [42]				*	*
Soravia [20, 24]	*	*	*	*	*
Tonelli [14]	*		*		*
Van Duijvendijk [44]	*	*	*	*	*
Ziv [13]		*	*		

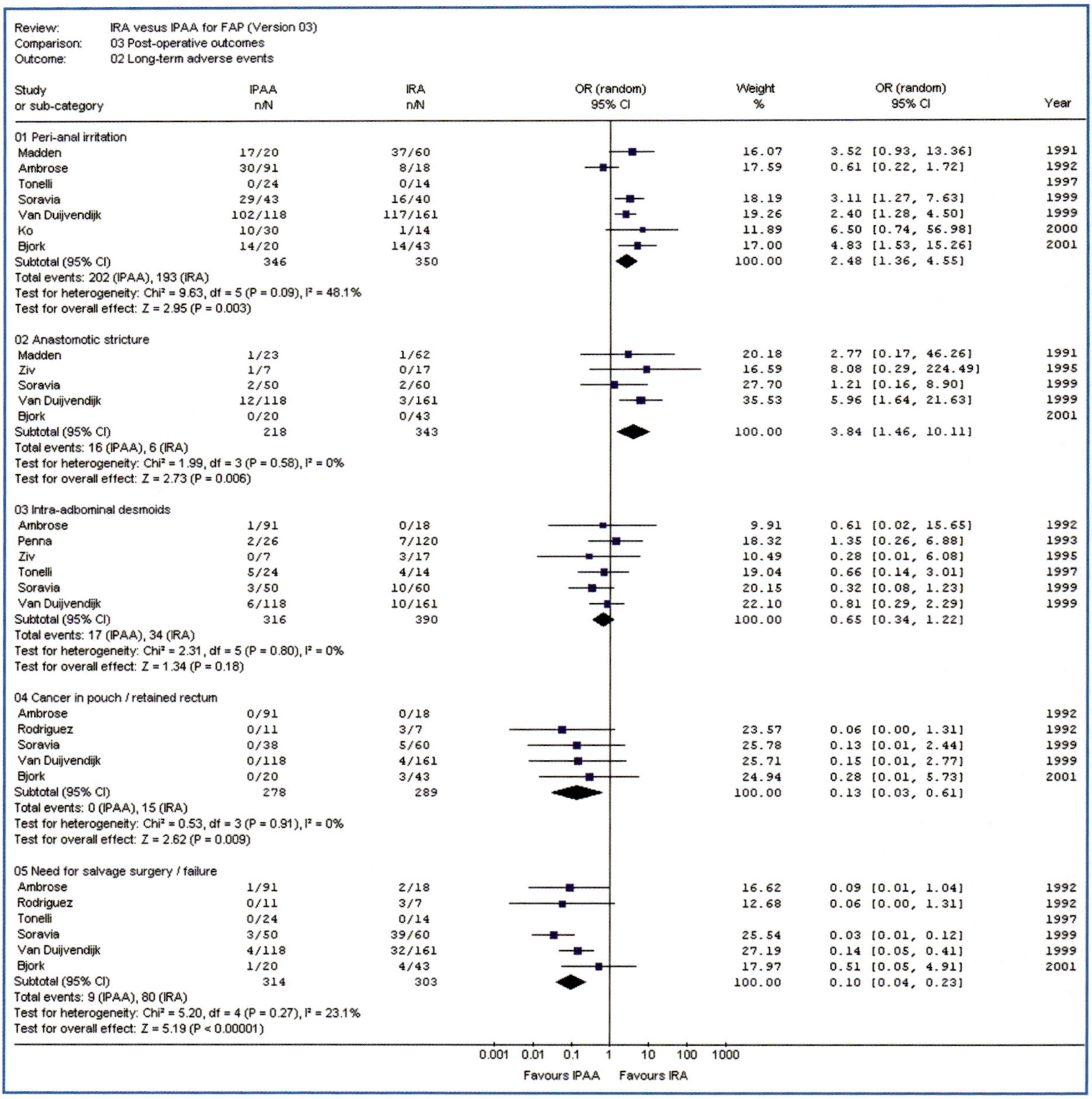

Fig. 2. Meta-analysis of long-term complications

Table 4. Studies reporting dietary restriction, social restriction and sexual dysfunction

Author	Quality of life			
	Dietary restrictions	Social restrictions	Male sexual dysfunction	Female sexual dysfunction
Ambrose [2]			*	*
Bjork [31]	*	*	*	*
Gunther [37]				
Ko [41]	*	*		
Madden [35]	*		*	
Penna [29]	*			
Rodriguez [42]			*	*
Rotondano [43]			*	*
Soravia [20, 24]	*			
Tonelli [14]			*	*
Van Duijvendijk [44]	*			

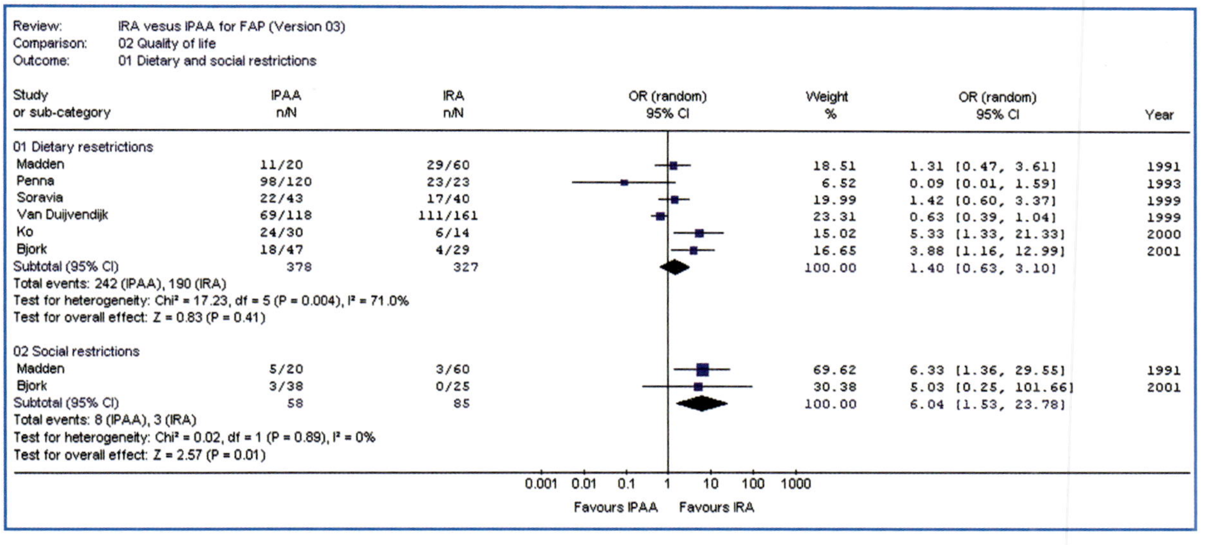

Fig. 3. Meta-analysis of dietary and social restrictions

Functional Outcome

The studies reporting on functional outcome including bowel frequency (number of motions during the day, night, or over a 24-h period), need for night defecation, incontinence (during day, night, or 24-h period), faecal urgency (inability to hold stool for more than 15 min), incontinence pad requirement, and the need for anti-diarrhoeal medication (Table 5). Figures 5 and 6 shows the results from meta-analysis of these outcomes and are depicted as a Forrest plot.

Results significantly favouring IRA over IPAA included: reduced bowel frequency of 2–6.1 per 24 h *vs.* 3.8–8 per 24 h (WMD=1.62, 95% CI 1.05–2.20), reduced need for night defecation of 8.2 *vs.* 44.1% (OR=6.64, CI 2.99–14.74), reduced incontinence during the night of 3.8 *vs.* 21% (OR=8.03, CI 4.22–15.25), reduced incontinence rate over a 24-h period 30 *vs.* 50.5% (OR=2.71, 95% CI 1.81–4.07), and reduced requirement for incontinence pad use during a 24-h period of 5.4 *vs.* 14.5% (OR=2.72, CI 1.02–7.23). The only functional outcome significantly favouring the IPAA group was faecal urgency, which was 39.2% with IRA *vs.* 14.2% following IPAA (OR=0.43, CI 0.23–0.80). There was no significant difference between IPAA and IRA groups in bowel frequency at night, daytime incontinence, and need for anti-diarrhoeal medication.

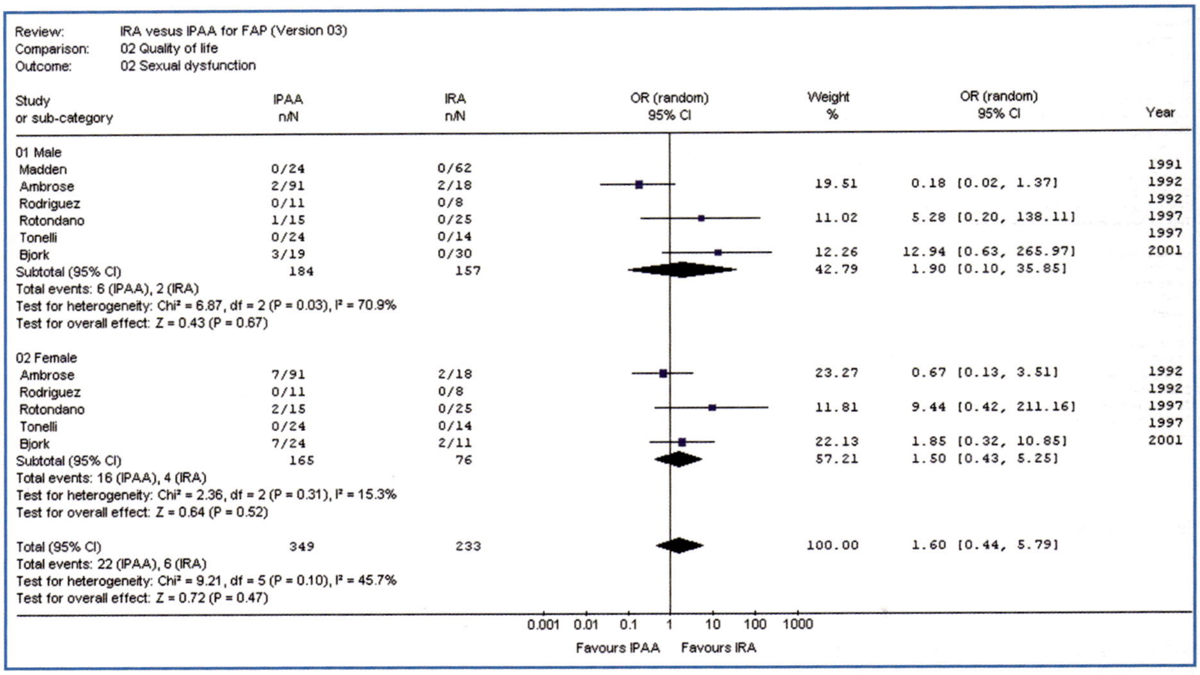

Fig. 4. Meta-analysis of sexual dysfunction

Table 5. Studies reporting functional outcome with IPAA *vs.* IRA

Author	Functional outcome								
	Bowel frequency		Night stools	Incontinence			Faecal urgency	Pad use	Anti-diarrhoeal medication
	Night	24h		Day	Night	24h			
Ambrose [2]	*	*		*	*				*
Bjork [31]			*	*	*		*		*
Gunther [37]									
Ko [41]								*	
Madden [35]		*	*			*	*	*	*
Penna [35]		*	*	*	*		*		*
Rodriguez [42]		*	*			*			
Rotondano [43]		*				*			
Soravia [20, 24]				*	*		*	*	*
Tonelli [14]	*			*	*	*	*	*	*
Van Duijvendijk [44]	*	*		*	*	*			*
Ziv [13]		*							*

Discussion

This systematic review has highlighted some very important differences in outcome between restorative proctocolectomy and IRA for the patient with FAP. The results on functional outcome suggest a favourable outcome towards the IRA procedure with regards to stool frequency over a 24-h period, need for defecation at night, incontinence (both over a 24-h period and at night) and pad usage. These finding are perhaps expected in a patient with a retained, functioning rectum. Interestingly, IPAA was not significantly different to IRA in stool frequency at night, day incontinence, and need for anti-diarrhoeal medication, all of which are outcomes that may make it acceptable for many young patients. Another inter-

Review: IRA vesus IPAA for FAP (Version 02)
Comparison: 16 Functional outcomes Figure
Outcome: 01 Bowel frequency

Study or sub-category	N	IPAA Mean (SD)	N	IRA Mean (SD)	WMD (random) 95% CI	Weight %	WMD (random) 95% CI	Year
02 At night								
Ambrose	91	1.00(1.00)	18	1.00(1.00)		32.91	0.00 [-0.51, 0.51]	1992
Tonelli	24	0.50(0.70)	14	0.90(0.60)		33.76	-0.40 [-0.82, 0.02]	1997
Van Duijvendijk	118	2.00(2.00)	161	1.40(1.90)		33.33	0.60 [0.13, 1.07]	1999
Subtotal (95% CI)	233		193			100.00	0.06 [-0.53, 0.65]	
Test for heterogeneity: Chi² = 9.79, df = 2 (P = 0.007), I² = 79.6%								
Test for overall effect: Z = 0.20 (P = 0.84)								
03 Per 24 hours								
Madden	24	5.10(3.25)	62	3.00(2.50)		10.30	2.10 [0.66, 3.54]	1991
Ambrose	91	5.00(2.00)	18	4.00(2.00)		13.10	1.00 [-0.01, 2.01]	1992
Rodriguez	11	6.10(1.80)	8	3.10(1.10)		11.12	3.00 [1.69, 4.31]	1992
Penna	120	4.00(1.00)	23	3.00(0.75)		17.05	1.00 [0.65, 1.35]	1993
Ziv	7	4.00(3.50)	17	2.00(0.75)		5.23	2.00 [-0.62, 4.62]	1995
Rotondano	15	5.30(1.20)	25	3.00(0.50)		15.58	2.30 [1.66, 2.94]	1997
Tonelli	24	3.80(1.30)	14	3.00(0.70)		15.59	0.80 [0.16, 1.44]	1997
Van Duijvendijk	118	8.00(3.00)	30	6.10(2.90)		12.03	1.90 [0.73, 3.07]	1999
Subtotal (95% CI)	410		197			100.00	1.62 [1.05, 2.20]	
Test for heterogeneity: Chi² = 23.79, df = 7 (P = 0.001), I² = 70.6%								
Test for overall effect: Z = 5.57 (P < 0.00001)								

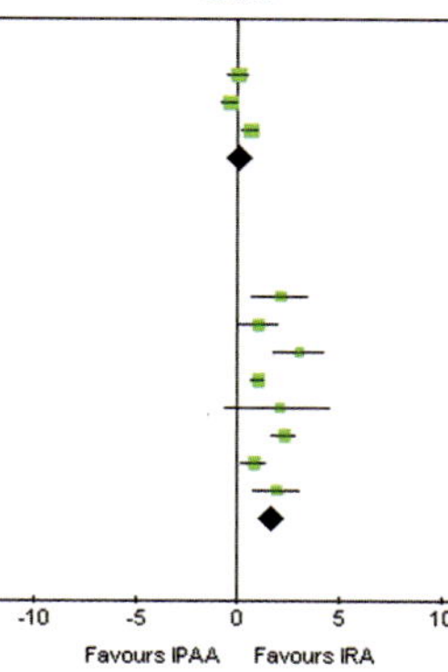

Fig. 5. Meta-analysis of bowel frequency

esting finding was that faecal urgency (the ability to defer defecation for at least 15 min) was significantly better in the IPAA group. This finding is important, as urgency can be a very detrimental outcome, particularly with regards to patient embarrassment, social behaviour, and ultimately patient satisfaction with the IRA procedure. A patient may therefore prefer the IPAA and increased frequency of stools, or even pad usage, for this outcome. Whether hand-sewn or stapled IPAA offers the best functional option for the patient undergoing surgery for FAP remains to be seen.

There was no significant difference between IPAA and IRA in the quality of life outcomes of dietary restriction and male and female sexual dysfunction. This is an important finding, particularly with regards to sexual dysfunction, as the patient facing FAP surgery is often young and likely to want to conceive at a later point in their lives. Normal sexual function is also an important outcome with regards to patient satisfaction with the procedure. One outcome that was significantly different between IPAA and IRA groups, was social restriction as a result of the procedure, which significantly favoured the IRA group. These results should, however, be treated with caution as there were only two studies reporting this outcome, containing at total of 58 patients in the IPAA and 85 patients in the IRA groups respectively.

As previously mentioned, restorative proctocolectomy with IPAA is perceived to be a more complicated procedure than IRA because of the increased pelvic dissection and potential for damage to the internal anal sphincter. The result of this meta-analysis showed that the incidence of all post-operative complications was significantly higher with IPAA (10%), as compared to IRA (6.8%). This was also reflected in an increased rate of 30-day re-operation with IPAA (23.4%) *vs.* IRA (11.6%). With regards to the individual post-operative outcomes, there was no significant difference between IPAA and IRA for bowel obstruction, haemorrhage, intra-abdominal sepsis, anastomotic separation and wound infection. The findings of this paper support this, although the magnitude of this overall increase (3.2%) is probably smaller than expected. The use of temporary defunctioning ileostomy adds another procedure to the primary IPAA where it is used, and although our study did not mention the morbidity associated with its reversal, there was little on this documented in the papers included in our meta-analysis.

With regards to long-term adverse events, IRA was associated with significantly less perianal irritation than IPAA (57.4 *vs.* 62.7%) as well as anastomotic stricture formation (2 *vs.* 8.1%). There was, however, no significant difference between the groups for the incidence of intra-abdominal desmoids, and no evidence that this is higher for primary IPAA as compared to IRA (5.4% with IPAA *vs.* 8.7% with IRA).

Although the choice of whether to perform IRA or IPAA as the primary operation for young patients with FAP relies on several factors as illustrated by our paper, the risk of cancer recurrence plays a significant part in this decision. Cancer recurrence was 5.5% following IRA as compared to 0% following IPAA, which is not surprising as the retained rectum (following IRA) has a higher chance of undergoing polyposis than the stapled IPAA with 1–2 cm of retained rectal mucosa, and the hand-sewn IPAA

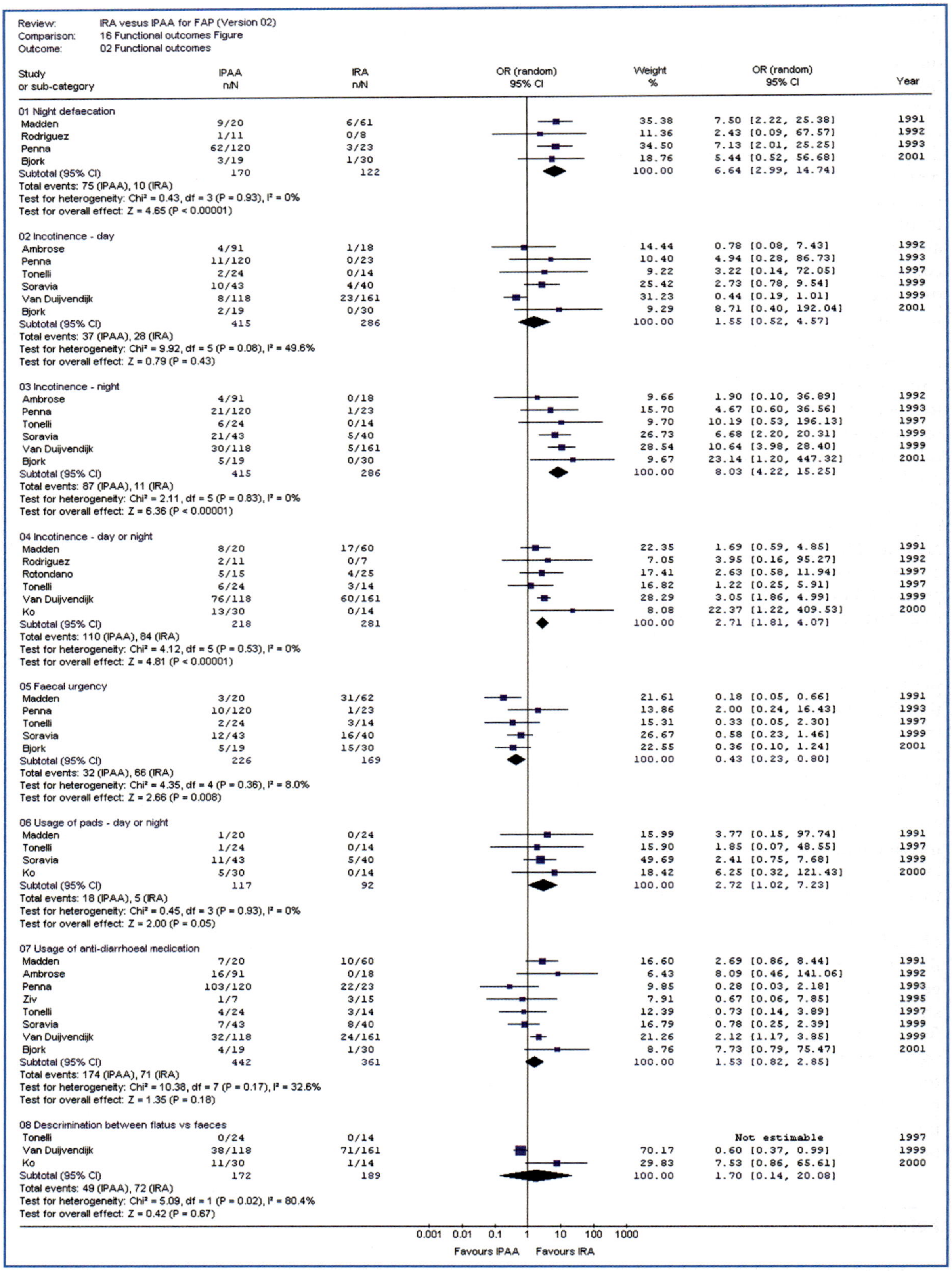

Fig. 6. Meta-analysis of functional outcomes

with mucosectomy. The decision to undertake IRA as the primary operation for FAP is therefore justified on the basis of post-operative morbidity and functional outcome (except for faecal urgency, which is greater than in IPAA), but at the expense of cancer recurrence. Whether regression of rectal polyps with drugs such as sundilac, a non-steroidal anti-inflammatory agent used to reduce rectal polyp size and number in FAP patients following IRA [49], remains to be seen. Whilst a selective COX-2 inhibitor has also recently been shown to reduce the number of colorectal polyps in patients with FAP [50], concerns over the long-term risks of this class of drug have made its role uncertain.

Molecular genetic testing may be useful in guiding the surgical management of patients with FAP, with authors suggesting that patients with APC mutations following codon 1250 are at higher risk of developing rectal cancer and should therefore undergo IPAA rather than IRA [51]. Other mutations that have been implicated include codons 1309 and 1328, again suggesting the need for IPAA in these patients [9]. It is important to consider, however, that these patients are also at higher risk of developing pouch adenomas, and will therefore require close follow-up of their pouch following IPAA. In the FAP patient where molecular genetic testing has not detected mutations predisposing to a higher risk of cancer, severity of polyposis must also be taken into account. For example IPAA may be the best primary surgical intervention for patients with over 20 rectal polyps and greater than 2 000 colonic polyps, whereas those with less than five rectal polyps and fewer than 1 000 colonic polyps would qualify for IRA and surveillance of the rectal stump as they may represent an attenuated FAP group. Careful patient selection is required in the intermediate group (those with more than five but less than twenty rectal polyps) before deciding on their primary surgical interventional strategy.

This chapter highlights the merits and weaknesses of both IPAA and IRA as the primary treatment of FAP, both of which require close follow-up after surgery. Although it highlights several factors that should be considered, it also highlights the need for further investigation of which patients benefit most from which operation depending on their risk factors. The age of the patient, their sex, lifestyle and preferences, occupation, and compliance to follow-up are all very important in deciding the operative outcome most appropriate for them.

References

1. Groden J, Thliveris A, Samowitz W et al (1991) Identification and characterization of the familial adenomatous polyposis coli gene. Cell 66:589–600
2. Ambrose WL Jr, Dozois RR, Pemberton JH et al (1992) Familial adenomatous polyposis: results following ileal pouch-anal anastomosis and ileorectostomy. Dis Colon Rectum 35:12–15
3. Jagelman DG (1991) Ileorectal anastomosis: familial adenomatous polyposis. Hepatogastroenterology 38:535-537
4. De Cosse JJ, Bulow S, Neale K et al (1991) Rectal cancer risk in patients treated for familial adenomatous polyposis: The Leeds Castle Polyposis Group. Br J Surg 79:1372–1375
5. Heiskanen I, Jarvinen HJ (1997) Fate of the rectal stump after colectomy and ileorectal anastomosis for familial adenomatous polyposis. Int J Colorectal Dis 12:9–13
6. Tekkis PP, Heriot A, Gallagher M et al (2005) Phenotypic factors can predict the risk of proctectomy after total colectomy and ileorectal anastomosis for patients with familial adenomatous polyposis (FAP): a multifactorial model. Dis Colon Rectum 48:613
7. Nugent KP, Phillips RKS (1991) Rectal cancer risk in older patients with familial adenomatous polyposis and an ileorectal anastomosis: a cause for concern. Br J Surg 79:1204–1206
8. Bertario L, Russo A, Radice P et al (2000) Genotype and phenotype factors as determinants for rectal stump cancer in patients with familial adenomatous polyposis: Hereditary Colorectal Tumors Registry. Ann Surg 231:538–543
9. Wu JS, Paul P, McGannon EA, Church JM (1998) APC genotype, polyp number, and surgical options in familial adenomatous polyposis. Ann Surg 227:57–62
10. Debinski HS, Love S, Spigelman AD, Phillips RKS (1996) Colorectal polyp counts and cancer risk in familial adenomatous polyposis. Gastroenterology 110:1028–1030
11. Slors JF, den Hartog Jager FC, Trum JW et al (1989) Long-term follow-up after colectomy and ileorectal anastomosis in familial adenomatous polyposis coli. Is there still a place for the procedure? Hepatogastroenterology 36:109–112
12. Gingold BS, Jagelman DG (1989) Sparing the rectum in familial polyposis: causes for failure. Surgery 89:314–318
13. Ziv Y, Church JM, Oakley JR et al (1995) Surgery for the teenager with familial adenomatous polyposis: ileo-rectal anastomosis or restorative proctocolectomy? Int J Colorectal Dis 10:6–9
14. Tonelli F, Valanzano R, Monaci I et al (1997) Restorative proctocolectomy or rectum-preserving surgery in patients with familial adenomatous polyposis: results of a prospective study. World J Surg 21:653–658, discussion 659
15. Church J, Burke C, McGannon E et al (2003) Risk of rectal cancer in patients after colectomy and ileorectal anastomosis for familial adenomatous polyposis: a function of available surgical options. Dis Colon Rectum 46:1175–1181
16. Shepherd NA, Jass JR, Duval I et al (1987) Restorative proctocolectomy with ileal reservoir: pathological and histochemical study of mucosal biopsy specimens. J Clin Pathol 40:601–607
17. Slors JF, Ponson AE, Taat CW, Bosma A (1995) Risk of residual rectal mucosa after proctocolectomy and ileal

pouch-anal reconstruction with the double-stapling technique. Postoperative endoscopic follow-up study. Dis Colon Rectum 38:207–210
18. Hoehner JC, Metcalf AM (1994) Development of invasive adenocarcinoma following colectomy with ileoanal anastomosis for familial polyposis coli. Dis Colon Rectum 37:824–828
19. Remzi FH, Church JM, Bast J et al (2001) Mucosectomy vs. stapled ileal pouch-anal anastomosis in patients with familial adenomatous polyposis: functional outcome and neoplasia control. Dis Colon Rectum 44:1590–1596
20. Soravia C, Klein L, Berk T et al (1999) Comparison of ileal pouch-anal anastomosis and ileorectal anastomosis in patients with familial adenomatous polyposis. Dis Colon Rectum 42:1028–1033, discussion 1033–1034
21. Pemberton JH, Kelly KA, Beart RW Jr et al (1987) Ileal pouch-anal anastomosis for chronic ulcerative colitis: long-term results. Ann Surg 206:504–513
22. Tuckson W, Lavery I, Fazio V et al (1991) Manometric and functional comparison of ileal pouch anal anastomosis with and without anal manipulation. Am J Surg 161:90–95, discussion 95–96
23. Dozois RR, Kelly KA, Welling DR et al (1989) Ileal pouch-anal anastomosis: comparison of results in familial adenomatous polyposis and chronic ulcerative colitis. Ann Surg 210:268–271, discussion 272–263
24. Soravia C, O'Connor BI, Berk T et al (1999) Functional outcome of conversion of ileorectal anastomosis to ileal pouch-anal anastomosis in patients with familial adenomatous polyposis and ulcerative colitis. Dis Colon Rectum 42:903–908
25. Kartheuser AH, Parc R, Penna CP et al (1996) Ileal pouch-anal anastomosis as the first choice operation in patients with familial adenomatous polyposis: a ten-year experience. Surgery 119:615–623
26. Tjandra JJ, Fazio VW, Milsom JW et al (1993) Omission of temporary diversion in restorative proctocolectomy: Is it safe? Dis Colon Rectum 36:1007–1014
27. Galandiuk S, Wolff BG, Dozois RR, Beart RW Jr (1991) Ileal pouch-anal anastomosis without ileostomy. Dis Colon Rectum 34:870–873
28. Everett WG, Pollard SG (1990) Restorative proctocolectomy without temporary ileostomy. Br J Surg 77:621–622
29. Penna C, Kartheuser A, Parc R et al (1993) Secondary proctectomy and ileal pouch-anal anastomosis after ileorectal anastomosis for familial adenomatous polyposis. Br J Surg 80:1621–1623
30. Zenilman ME, Soper NJ, Dunnegan D, Becker JM (1990) Previous abdominal colectomy affects functional results after ileal pouch-anal anastomosis. World J Surg 14:594–599
31. Bjork J, Akerbrant H, Iselius L et al (2001) Outcome of primary and secondary ileal pouch-anal anastomosis and ileorectal anastomosis in patients with familial adenomatous polyposis. Dis Colon Rectum 44:984–992
32. Clark SK, Phillips RK (1996) Desmoids in familial adenomatous polyposis. Br J Surg 83:1494–1504
33. Penna C, Tiret E, Parc R et al (1993) Operation and abdominal desmoid tumors in familial adenomatous polyposis. Surg Gynecol Obstet 177:263–268
34. Jones IT, Jagelman DG, Fazio VW et al (1986) Desmoid tumors in familial polyposis coli. Ann Surg 204:94–97
35. Madden MV, Neale KF, Nicholls RJ et al (1991) Comparison of morbidity and function after colectomy with ileorectal anastomosis or restorative proctocolectomy for familial adenomatous polyposis. Br J Surg 78:789–792
36. Van Duijvendijk P, Slors JF, Taat CW et al (2000) Quality of life after total colectomy with ileorectal anastomosis or proctocolectomy and ileal pouch-anal anastomosis for familial adenomatous polyposis. Br J Surg 87:590–596
37. Gunther K, Braunrieder G, Bittorf BR et al (2003) Patients with familial adenomatous polyposis experience better bowel function and quality of life after ileorectal anastomosis than after ileoanal pouch. Colorectal Dis 5:38–44
38. The Cochrane Collaboration (2001) Cochrane Reviewer's Handbook 4.1.3. Uk:Update Software, 2001, The Chochrane Library, Oxford
39. Moher D, Cook DJ, Eastwood S et al (2000) Improving the quality of reports of meta-analyses of randomised controlled trials: the QUOROM statement. Onkologie 23:597–602
40. DerSimonian R, Laird N (1986) Meta-analysis in clinical trials. Control Clin Trials 7:177–188
41. Ko CY, Rusin LC, Schoetz DJ Jr et al (2000) Does better functional result equate with better quality of life? Implications for surgical treatment in familial adenomatous polyposis. Dis Colon Rectum 43:829–835, discussion 835–837
42. Rodriguez SanJuan JC, Casanova Rituerto D, Martino Fernandez E et al (1992) Familial adenomatous polyposis: proctocolectomy with an ileal pouch versus rectal preservation (in Spanish). Rev Esp Enferm Dig 82:159–163
43. Rotondano G, Esposito P, Novi A et al (1997) Surgery for familial polyposis of the colon: a functional follow-up (in Spanish). Minerva Chir 52:1163–1167
44. Van Duijvendijk P, Slors JF, Taat CW et al (1999) Functional outcome after colectomy and ileorectal anastomosis compared with proctocolectomy and ileal pouch-anal anastomosis in familial adenomatous polyposis. Ann Surg 230:648–654
45. Malafosse M (2003) Familial adenomatous polyposis: long term follow-up of patients after surgical treatment. Prognostic factors (in French). Bull Acad Natl Med 187:103–114, discussion 114–116
46. Vasen HF, van Duijvendijk P, Buskens E et al (2001) Decision analysis in the surgical treatment of patients with familial adenomatous polyposis: a Dutch-Scandinavian collaborative study including 659 patients. Gut 49:231–235
47. Bruwer M, Stern J, Schmidt-Gayk H et al (1998) Effect of proctocolectomy on fluid balance: comparison of conventional ileostomy, ileorectal anastomosis and ileoanal pouch operation (in German). Z Gastroenterol 36:201–208
48. Penna CP, Tiret E, Kartheuser AH et al (1992) Comparison of functional results of ileorectal and ileo-anal anastomoses in familial adenomatous polyposis: conversions of ileorectal anastomoses into ileo-anal anastomoses (in French). Gastroenterol Clin Biol 16:401–405
49. Spagnesi MT, Tonelli F, Dolara P et al (1994) Rectal

proliferation and polyp occurrence in patients with familial adenomatous polyposis after sulindac treatment. Gastroenterology 106:362–366

50. Steinbach G, Lynch PM, Phillips RK et al (2000) The effect of celecoxib, a cyclooxygenase-2 inhibitor, in familial adenomatous polyposis. N Engl J Med 342:1946–1952
51. Vasen HF, van der Luijt RB, Slors JF et al (1996) Molecular genetic tests as a guide to surgical management of familial adenomatous polyposis. Lancet 348:433–435

Surgery and Surveillance in Colon Polyposis Syndrome

Tomáš Skřička

Introduction

Familial polyposis syndromes create a group of hereditary syndromes of gastrointestinal (GI) tumours. This chapter focuses on those primarily affecting the large bowel and which require radical surgery.

A GI polyp is defined as a mass of the mucosal surface protruding into the bowel lumen. Polyps can be neoplastic, non-neoplastic or submucosal. GI polyposis is characterised by multiple polyps within the GI tract (GIT). A variety of polyposis syndromes can affect the GIT. Familial polyposis syndromes can be classified as familial, inherited (autosomal dominant) or nonfamilial. Inherited polyposis syndromes can be further subdivided into two groups depending on whether the polyps are adenomas or hamartomas. Adenomatous polyposis syndromes include the classic familial adenomatous polyposis (FAP), Gardner's syndrome and Turcot syndrome. Hamartomatous familial polyposis syndromes include Peutz-Jeghers syndrome (PJS), juvenile polyposis syndrome (JPS), Cowden disease and Ruvalcaba-Myhre-Smith syndrome. The non-inherited polyposis syndromes include Cronkhite-Canada syndrome and a variety of miscellaneous non-familial polyposis.

From a prognostic viewpoint, these syndromes must be recognised, because adenomatous polyps are premalignant. These syndromes should be considered when an intestinal polyp is recognized in the young, when two or more polyps are seen in any patient, when colic carcinoma is discovered in patients younger than 40 years and when extraintestinal manifestations associated with these syndromes are discovered. GI polyps may be asymptomatic but may also occur with rectal bleeding and diarrhoea. The urgency of case tracing and genetic counseling is related not so much to symptoms of the disease but to the potential for development of a colic carcinoma. It is probable that patients with FAP, if untreated, will develop a colic carcinoma.

Familial Adenomatous Polyposis

FAP is also known as familial polyposis coli. The polyps are adenomatous and occur primarily in the colon. Carcinoma occurs mostly in the left colon and are often multiple. It is also possible, however, for polyps, adenomas and carcinomas to grow in the stomach, duodenum and small intestine. Connected with extraintestinal manifestation, it is known as Gardner's syndrome. Manifestations include osteomas, jaw cysts, dental anomalies, brain tumours, other skin and soft tissues tumours and congenital hypertrophy of the retinal pigmentary epithelium [1]. FAP shows autosomal dominant transmission. Frequency is one in 8,300-13,500 births. In Denmark, new mutations account for 25% of cases [2]. Average age at the time of diagnosis is 35 years, and average age at cancer diagnosis is 39 years [3]. About 50% of symptomatic and 10% of asymptomatic patients have carcinoma of the colon at the time of diagnosis. Carcinoma may be present in all cases by the age of 50 years. Penetrance is nearly completed by age 40 years [2].

Gardner's Syndrome

Gardner's syndrome was originally described in individuals with FAP-like polyps who had additional findings outside the GIT, including epidermal cysts and subcutaneous fibromas of the skin, desmoids of the skin and abdomen, osteomas, dental abnormalities, pigmented patches in the retina and tumours of other organs [4]. Gardner's syndrome includes a variety of manifestations:

Soft-tissue tumours:

- Epidermoid inclusion cysts of the skin
- Dermoid tumours
- Fibromas
- Lipomas
- Lipofibromas
- Neurofibromas
- Leiomyomas

- Mammary fibromatosis
- Intra-abdominal desmoid tumours and peritoneal fibromas

GI tumours:

- Colic polyposis (nearly 100% precancerosis)
- Gastric adenomatous polyps
- Gastric hamartomatous polyps
- Duodenal adenomatous polyps
- Periampullary carcinoma
- Hepatoblastoma
- Pancreatic carcinoma
- Lymphoid hyperplasia of the terminal ileum

Osseous abnormalities:

- Usually involving the membranous bones, mandible, calvaria, maxilla, ribs and long bones
- Self-limited benign exostosis
- Bone islands and periosteal thickening

Endocrine tumours:

- Thyroid carcinoma (papillary)
- Carcinoid tumours of the small bowel
- Parathyroid adenoma
- Adrenal adenoma/carcinoma
- Pituitary chromophobe adenoma

Central nervous system medulloblastoma;

Abnormal dentition:

- Supernumerary teeth
- Impacted teeth
- Odontoma
- Hypercementosis
- Teeth more prone to carries

The distinction between Gardner's syndrome and FAP was initially unclear, however, because some individuals diagnosed with FAP also had extraintestinal signs. Clinically, Gardner's syndrome and FAP can occur in the same kindred. It was subsequently found that both conditions can result from the same mutation in the APC gene. Thus, Gardner's syndrome and FAP are allelic. [Many genes show alterations in GIT neoplasia that do not, as yet, have an immunohistochemically detectable protein product. These genes include the APC (adenomatous polyposis coli) and the MCC (mutated in colon cancer) genes].

Other Hereditary Syndromes of GI Tumours

Turcot Syndrome

Turcot first described an association between colic polyps and tumours [5]. Turcot syndrome is characterized by the presence of a malignant brain tumour in patients with colic adenomatous polyps [5]. Recent advances [6] have clarified the relationship between Turcot syndrome and Gardner's syndrome, which may also be associated with brain tumours.

Cronkhite-Canada Syndrome

This syndrome includes generalized GI polyposis in association with neuroectodermal changes consisting of alopecia, hyperpigmentation and nail atrophy. Electron microscopic studies of the skin reveal increased numbers of melanin granules in keratocytes, increased number of melanosomes in melanocytes, increased melanocytes, compact hyperkeratosis, perivascular inflammation and exocytosis. A number of haematologic, neurologic and metabolic abnormalities are associated with Cronkhite-Canada syndrome.

Attenuated FAP

This is a less severe form of polyposis, with a low number of polyps (adenomas), usually less than 100, yet patients sustain a high risk for colorectal cancer. These cancers usually develop 15 years later than the classic FAP patient, but ten years earlier than sporadic cancer [7].

Hamartomatous Polyposis

Polyps in both PJS and familial JPS are hamartomatous, but the major tissue components are different. The Peutz-Jeghers polyp is composed of intestinal crypts and villi and smooth-muscle bundles in a disorganised fashion. Inflammatory cells are absent or scanty, and glandular structures are not excessively dilated. The juvenile polyp is composed of dilated intestinal glands and abundant connective tissue of the lamina propria. Smooth-muscle elements are usually absent; lymphoid cells are common. These features closely resemble those of inflammatory retention polyps in children, also known as juvenile polyps, as well as inflammatory polyps of Cronkhite-Canada syndrome, which occur among the elderly.

PJS is characterized by the presence of Peutz-Jeghers polyps throughout the entire GIT and melanin spots on the lip (96%), buccal mucosa (83%), face (36%) and extremities (32%) [8].The small bowel is the favoured site of polyposis and the number of polyps is small. Other associated abnormalities include polyps in the urinary bladder and nasal cavity, bone deformities, congenital heart disease and retarded development. The symptoms of PJS develop before the age of 20 in two-thirds of cases, with an average age at time of diagnosis of 22 years [3]. Symptoms are noted at a younger age than those associated with FAP. Peutz-Jeghers polyps are generally not prone to malignant change. However, carcinoma of the GIT has been reported in about 3% of cases, most commonly in the proximal small intestine [9]. In many reports, the relationship between polyp and carcinoma is unclear. When the origin of malignancy was carefully studied, the carcinoma was usually found to arise in the adenomatous or dysplastic epithelium in the polyp [10]. Malignancy can also occur outside of the GIT. The condition is linked to 19p chromosomes in at least some families.

Discrete Adenomas and Carcinomas of the Colon

Whereas polyposis syndromes are rare, discrete adenomas in small numbers occur in from 10% to 50% of the general population. Overall, colorectal cancer may affect 3% of the population. The inheritance pattern of these cases is largely unknown. Park et al. [11] studied a large groups with clusters of colorectal cancer. Extensive screening with flexible proctosigmoidoscopy revealed adenomas in 21% of the 191 pedigree members in contrast to 9% of controls. The excess of adenomas showed autosomal dominant inheritance. A subsequent expanded study of 670 persons in 34 kindreds revealed the estimated prevalence of adenoma at age 60 years in related family members was 24% whereas that in unrelated spouses was 12%. Such studies emphasise the importance of screening for colorectal tumours in first-degree relatives of patients with these lesions.

Hereditary Flat Adenoma Syndrome

Hereditary flat adenoma syndrome (HFAS) is presently thought to be a variant of FAP, with the genetic defect linked to 5q21-22. Signs of HFAS are:

- Multiple colorectal adenomas, but usually fewer than 100
- Polyps tend to occur at a later age than in classic FAP
- Adenomas tend to show a proximal location
- Onset of colorectal cancer is later than in hereditary non-polyposis colorectal cancer (HNPCC) and FAP
- These individuals have adenomas and cancers of the stomach and duodenum
- Fundic gland polyps of the stomach are also noted

In some patients fundic may be present in the absence of colorectal adenomas [12]. Lynch stressed that only about 1% of such adenomas have high-grade dysplasia, which is much lower than reported in patients with sporadic flat adenoma [12].

Muir Torre syndrome

Muir Torre syndrome was originally subclassified as a form of FAP. Muir Torre syndrome is a rare autosomal dominant disorder with fewer than 100 adenomas, typically present in the proximal colon. This syndrome is associated with skin lesions such as basal cell carcinoma, sebaceous carcinoma and squamous carcinoma. The genetics of this syndrome is not yet known.

Cowden Disease

Cowden disease is an uncommon autosomal dominant disorder and is the family name of the original report patient, Rachel Cowden. This syndrome is a rare disorder that is inherited in autosomal dominant manner with intrafamilial and interfamilial differences in symptom expression. In Cowden disease, one sees facial trichilemmomas, acral keratosis and oral mucosal papillomas. This disorder is also associated with breast and thyroid cancer. There are numerous colic and small-intestinal polyps. They have been described as hamartomatous lesions [13] consisting of mildly fibrotic, mildly disordered mucosa overlying a submucosa that display disorganisation and splaying of smooth-muscle fibres. These lesions show some similarities to the pathology seen in solitary rectal ulcer syndrome. Other authors reported polyps that they described as inflammatory lesions, lipomas and ganglioneuromas. There is no increased risk for GI cancers in this disorder [14].

Ruvalcaba-Myhre-Smith Syndrome

Ruvalcaba-Myhre-Smith syndrome is inherited in an autosomal dominant manner. There are also some sporadic cases. The syndrome is characterised by macrocephaly, pigmented genital lesions, subcutaneous and visceral lipomas, haemangiomas and GI hamartomatous polyps. Mesodermal hamartomas can affect the subcutaneous, intracranial, visceral, intestinal, thoracic and osseous tissues. Hydrocephalus and diffuse thickening of the corpus callosum have also been reported [15].

Intestinal Ganglioneuromatosis

Intestinal ganglioneuromatosis is a familial disorder that has been associated with multiple endocrine neoplasia syndrome type 2b and with the Recklinghausen's disease. There may be a diffuse proliferation of ganglioneuromatous elements, which at times may be polypoid. In some instances, the ganglioneuromatosis has been found in association with JP and adenomas [16].

Lymphoid Polyposis

Multiple benign lymphoid polyposis of the large bowel has been reported. Most cases occur in children. Histologically similar to solitary lymphoid polyps of the rectum, lymphoid polyposis consists of prominent active lymphoid nodules in the mucosa and submucosa [17]. Lesions are entirely benign and in some cases have been reported to disappear spontaneously. In patients with family histories of polyps, it is essential to determine the exact histologic nature of the lesions so that unnecessary surgery is not performed. Benign lymphoid polyposis of the terminal ileum has been reported in patients with Gardner's syndrome and FAP [18].

Hereditary Mixed Polyposis Syndrome

This is an autosomal dominant disorder that has been mapped to chromosome 6q. Five types of polyps have been described in individuals with this disorder:

- tubular adenomas
- Villous adenomas
- Flat adenomas
- Hyperplastic polyps
- Typical juvenile polyps.

Colorectal cancer is also seen in this disorder, which might be a variant of JP. But in JP, adenomas are uncommon (2%) while in hereditary mixed polyposis, the number of polyps are fewer than seen in JP [19]. JP usually presents one decade earlier than hereditary mixed polyposis.

Non-Surgical Treatment of FAP

There are reports [20] of attempts to treat FAP without operation, and even though the authors reported a decrease in the number of polyps to 44% a their size to 35% by means of sulindac (sulfoxide non-steroidal anti-inflammatory drug) in 18 patients, this method could not replace colectomy.

Surgical Treatment of FAP

As FAP is 100% precancerous, colectomy is recommended. Treatment of FAP is influenced by the natural history of the disease, which is variable. If patients are left long enough without colectomy, they will all develop carcinoma. The sooner is patient diagnosed, the better prognosis could be if colectomy is performed. There are three possibilities of surgical treatment. Each has its pros and cons:

- Total colectomy with permanent ileostomy (in cases of malignancy in the lower rectum)
- Total colectomy with ileoanal anastomosis (IAA) (poor functional results)
- Subtotal colectomy with ileorectal anastomosis (IRA) (good functional results but risk of recurrence in the rectal stump)

The procedure of choice is the subject of much debate, particularly since restorative proctocolectomy became feasible [21]. The other options are colectomy and IRA, proctocolectomy or colectomy and rectal mucosectomy without restoration of GI continuity. Conventional panproctocolectomy has the advantage of eliminating all colorectal polyps and virtually eliminating the risk of carcinoma of the large bowel. This operation does not protect against ampullary or small-bowel malignancy. In addition, there is the burden of an ileostomy in a condition where 50% of family members are at risk of disease, and the patient is exposed to the small risk of pelvic nerve damage with resulting bladder and sexual problems. Also, there is a perineal wound, which although less likely to break down than after proctocolectomy for inflammatory bowel disease, may leave the patient with a persistent sinus.

Intersphincteric excision of the rectum reduces risk of pelvic nerve injury, and rectal mucosectomy eliminates problems with the perineal wound. Risk associated with a long rectal mucosectomy is that all the diseased mucosa may not be removed, and there is then a slight risk of carcinoma developing in any remaining remnant. The overwhelming disadvantage, however, of any procedure that leaves a permanent ileostomy, is that it is a poor advertisement of treatment for other members of the family. Although a patient with an ileostomy can lead a full and active life, it is difficult to convince a young and active family member, who may well be asymptomatic, to undergo such a procedure. It is for this reason that sphincter-saving procedures such as colectomy with IRA or restorative proctocolectomy have become popular [22].

The procedure of colectomy and IRA has the advantage that GI continuity is restored and bowel function is reasonable. Its disadvantage is that polyps are left in the rectum, with the potential of malignant change. To prevent this unfortunate outcome, patient need to have repeated fulguration of residual or newly formed polyps [23]. Not only can this procedure be uncomfortable, it also requires the patient to return repeatedly for rectoscopic examination. In addition, although it would seem logical, if the adenoma-carcinoma sequence is accepted - that removal of polyps removes the risk of carcinoma - this does not necessarily follow. There is evidence to suggest that carcinoma can develop de novo in rectal mucosa not occupied by polyps.

Mucosal proctectomy and pelvic ileal reservoir, now generally termed restorative proctocolectomy, has the theoretical advantage that the disease is eradicated, GI continuity is restored and continence is maintained. It appears, unfortunately, from some results reported, that bowel function is not always as satisfactory as after IRA. However, these results have in the main been described in patients who have suffered from ulcerative colitis. There is now substantial evidence either from our own experience or from others that the clinical results of restorative proctocolectomy for polyposis are far superior to those reported in patients with colitis. Nevertheless, restorative proctocolectomy is a complex procedure and although mortality is very low, morbidity can be high. Although results are steadily improving, the procedure is still developing, and the long-term results in FAP are unknown, perhaps due to the small number of patients. Further modifications may be desirable before it can be categorically accepted as the operation of first choice for all patients with FAP.

The conventional policy in many units dealing with these patients is still to perform a colectomy and ileorectal anastomosis in the first instance, provided patients are likely to be reliable in attending for follow-up. Follow-up at regular 6-month intervals is usually necessary so that rectal polyps, if present, can be destroyed by fulguration. In order to determine if this is still a reasonable policy, it is necessary to access the risk of developing a rectal carcinoma after IRA.

Carcinoma Risk after Colectomy and Ileorectal Anastomosis

There is considerable controversy concerning the incidence of carcinoma following colectomy and IRA. The evidence against ileorectal anastomosis came mainly from the Mayo Clinic. Moertel et al. [24] found that in 145 patients treated by subtotal colectomy and IRA, there was a continuing risk of rectal cancer. This was 25% after 15 years of follow-up and 59% after 23 years. They found that women were at greater risk than men and that the incidence was markedly increased if the patient had carcinoma in the resected colon. Another factor with important clinical application was that the risk of carcinoma was considerably reduced if there were fewer than 20 polyps in the rectum compared with patients having more than 100. Some doubt has since been expressed about how many of these patients actually had a true IRA. It would appear that many underwent an ileosigmoid anastomosis, and it is unknown what influence the latter procedure might have had on the outcome, particularly since surveillance following this operation is more difficult than after a true IRA [25]. Fuel for the controversy was further supplied by reports from other centres [26]. They reported a series of 89 patients treated by a true IRA and 6-monthly surveillance. Included in this series were 47 patients followed for 10 years, 27 followed for 15 years and 13 followed for 20 years. Only two patients (2.2%) developed carcinoma, both of which were Duke's A lesions, and both patients survived. There are similar reports from other centres [27, 28] showing, that carcinoma develops in up to 6% of cases.

Making recommendations from these contradictory data, particularly at a time when restorative proctocolectomy is not fully tested, is clearly difficult. There is no doubt that there is a risk of developing carcinoma after colectomy and IRA, which relates to the number of polyps in the rectum and the presence of coexisting carcinoma. This may also be related to how much colorectum remains; there may be a geographic difference. Consequently, there has been general unease about performing colectomy and IRA in various countries.

Present Surgical Policy

At present, policy around the world is variable. Most surgeons still seem content to treat their patients with colectomy and IRA followed by regular surveillance. An increasing proportion, on the other hand, is performing restorative proctocolectomy in most of their patients and certainly on those with severe rectal polyposis. A more rational policy, perhaps, is the compromise advocated by some surgeons. If the number of polyps within 15 cm from the anal verge is less than 20, we perform a colectomy and IRA. Restorative proctocolectomy is used for patients with more than 100 rectal polyps. Patients with 20-100 polyps are treated by colectomy and IRA if the minimum time off school is desirable or if the patient can be relied upon to attend follow-up. All others in this intermediate group are advised to have a pouch. As the morbidity of restorative proctocolectomy falls and more centres gain expertise, we are sure that it will become the operation of first choice for all patients with the disease. Until then, operative treatment is likely to be governed by each surgeon's beliefs and experience coupled with the patient's attitude towards attending 6-monthly rectoscopy as well as the views of the patient's family.

In general, there are three options available to surgeon seeking to prevent patients with FAP from dying of colorectal cancer:

- proctocolectomy with ileostomy
- Colectomy with IRA
- Proctocolectomy with ileoanal reservoir.

The choice of operation should be based on clinical knowledge of the disease process and the fact that prophylactic colectomy does not necessarily cure the condition. Other considerations involve the patient's age and anatomy, the presence or absence of extracolic manifestations and the surgeon's expertise. Over the years, debate has centred on the value of proctocolectomy and ileostomy with colectomy and IRA. This debate was further compounded by the development of the ileal reservoir procedure. Today it seems obvious that proctocolectomy and ileostomy should rarely be necessary for patients with FAP and other polyposis syndromes. Therefore, the debate now centres on the value of IRA versus proctocolectomy with ileoanal reservoir or restorative proctocolectomy. It is up to surgeon and the institution as to whether the approach will be "traditional" (open surgery), laparoscopically assisted, hand assisted or completely laparoscopic. Recently [29], many authors refer to good experiences with the laparoscopic approach. It could be safe and effective treatment for selected patients with FAP. As techniques and instrumentation for laparoscopic colon surgery are perfected, this procedure will likely become an appealing option in the management of patients with FAP

Technique of Colectomy and Colorectal Anastomosis

This method seem recently mostly accepted

The major concern with colectomy and IRA as a prophylactic surgical option in patients with FAP is the subsequent risk of rectal cancer. It was easier to recommend IRA to patients, and many surgeons prefer this option after the advent of the ileoanal reservoir. The actual documented risk of dying of cancer of the rectum subsequent to colectomy and IRA is somewhat small [30]. The risk of developing polyps and cancer are, of course, higher. It would appear that proctoscopic surveillance and ablation of polyps that arise in the rectal segment are possible, but this does not eliminate fully the risk of rectal cancer. Long-term follow-up studies demonstrate that development of cancer does not always equate with death from that cancer. IRA is compatible with good functional results. It is a simpler procedure than the ileoanal reservoir and is usually a one-stage procedure as opposed to the two-stage procedure commonly used to construct an ileoanal reservoir. More recent improvements in surgical technique and skill suggest that a one-stage ileoanal reservoir without temporary ileostomy would be an appropriate option. Refinements in technique achieved in recent years have improved functional results and decreased surgical complications of proctocolectomy and ileoanal reservoir. The ability to perform the operation as a one-stage procedure makes it an appropriated option as a contemporary alternative to IRA. To support use of IRA, there are quality-of-life (QOL) studies [31]. The authors argue that there were no differences with respect to health status between patients in groups of IRA and IAA and that preference for either procedure cannot be based on QOL.

Rectal Stump Control after Subtotal Colectomy and Ileorectal Anastomosis

It is advised that a rectoscopy be conducted every 6 months and eventually to remove polyp remnants by means of laser, fulguration, photocoagulation or transanal microsurgery. Lifetime surveillance of the rectal stump is crucial, as showed in authors from Ankara [32]. They report a local recurrence 19 years after IRA. There are some optimistic reports [33] that colectomy with IRA in FAP is associated with a significant reduction in rectal mucosal cell proliferation. These findings claim reduced risk of rectal cancer following this procedure in FAP and are of relevance to the study of environmental versus genetic control of cell proliferation.

Conclusion

FAP and other polyposis syndromes are generalised disorders with ramifications throughout the body. Early diagnosis by recognition of at-risk individuals and proctoscopic surveillance is important in preventing cancer. Surgical options now available can eliminate the risk of colorectal cancer and provide a good functional outcome without a permanent ileostomy. Ongoing surveillance programmes are important because there is still a risk of dying of extra-colic manifestations of the disorder. Prophylactic colectomy of whatever type does not predict total cure of the disease. The two most frequent procedures (IRA and IAA) have been evaluated [34]. The long-term survival following either approach is similar: 87% for IRA and 83% for IAA.

Management of these families is best accomplished within the framework of a familial polyposis registry. In the Czech Republic, there are more than 80 families registered. This allows for better communication with individual patients and family members, for identification of those at risk and for education of family members. These family members must be encouraged to undergo surveillance examinations so that the condition can be diagnosed early, and surgical intervention can prevent the development of colorectal cancer.

Interesting developments in the management of desmoids with medical agents should be further pursued in a prospective fashion in an effort to determine their true role in management of the condition. The potential of similar therapeutic agents, such as Sundilac, to promote regression of colic polyps has been suggested and requires further prospective investigation. Sundilac suppositories for patients with polyps in the rectal stump after IRA also show some promise. Whether the disappearance of polyps with the use of Sundilac eliminates the risk of developing cancer or simply eliminates the polyps is still undetermined.

There is also uncertainty regarding the management of upper gastrointestinal polyps in FAP. Further investigation into the local factors that dictate the development of adenomas in the duodenum and the polyp-cancer sequence in this area is necessary. The effect of bile on that sequence of events remains an important area for further research. The possibility of medical management of GI polyps is obviously attractive, and there are some ongoing studies that are seeking to determine whether medical agents can influence the development of upper GI polyps in FAP patients. It is hoped that further research into the chromosomal abnormality and a distinct blood tests for this disease are truly forthcoming because these could eliminate the problem of the unavailability of blood samples from other family members. The growth in the number of familial polyposis registries and the addition of increasing numbers of patients to them are certainly helpful for patients, their families and their physicians. The registries give researchers more long-term follow-up information on the clinical manifestations of the disease and on the results of medical and surgical treatment.

References

1. Bosari S, Viale G, Roncalli M et al (1995) p53 gene mutations, p53 protein accumulation and compartmentalization in colorectal adenocarcinoma. Am J Pathol 19:790-798
2. Bisgaard ML, Fenger K, Bullow S et al (1994) Familial adenomatous polyposis (FAP): frequency, penetrance and mutation rate. Hum Mutat 3:121-125
3. Burt RW, Samowitz WS (1988) The adenomatous polyp and the hereditary polyposis syndromes. Gastroenterol Clin North Am 17:657-678
4. Gardner EJ, Plenk HP (1952) Hereditary pattern for multiple osteomas in a family group. Am J Hum Genet 5:139-147
5. Turcot J, Depres JP, St. Pierre F (1959) Malignant tumors of the central nervous system associated with familial polyposis of the colon. Dis Colon Rectum 2:465-468
6. Hamilton SR, Liu B, Parsons RE et al (1995) The molecular basis of Turcot's syndrome. N Eng J Med 332:839-847
7. Spirio L, Olschwang S, Groden J et al (1993) Alleles of the APC gene: an attenuated form of familial polyposis. Cell 75:951-957
8. Bartholomew LG, Moore CE, Dahlin DC et al (1962) Intestinal polyposis associated with mucocutaneous pigmentation. Surg Gynecol Obstet 115:1-11
9. Ried JD (1974) Intestinal carcinoma in the Peutz-Jeghers syndrome. JAMA 229:833-834
10. Perzin KH, Ridge MF (1982) Adenomatous and carcinomatous changes in hamartomatous polyps of the small intestine (Peutz-Jeghers syndrome). Cancer 49:971-983
11. Park JG, Han HJ, Kang MS et al (1994) Presymptomatic diagnosis of familial adenomatous polyposis coli. Dis Colon Rectum 37:700-707
12. Lynch HT, Smyrk CT, Lanspa SJ et al (1993) Upper gastrointestinal manifestation in families with hereditary flat adenoma syndrome. Cancer 71:2709-2714
13. Carlson GJ, Nivatvongs S, Snover DC (1984) Colorectal polyps in Cowden's disease. Am J Surg Pathol 8:763-770
14. Rustgi A (1994) Hereditary gastrointestinal polyposis and nonpolyposis syndrome. N Engl J Med 331:1694-1702
15. Khan AN, Macdonald S, Pankhania A (2006) Colon polyposis syndromes. Emedicine 2006:1-31
16. Weidner N, Flanders DJ, Mitros FA (1984) Mucosal ganglioneuromatosis associated with multiple colic polyps. Am J Surg Pathol 8:779-786
17. Louw JH (1968) Polypoid lesions of the large bowel in children with particular reference to benign lymphoid polyposis. J Pediatr Surg 3:195-209
18. Thomford NR, Greenberger NJ (1968) Lymphoid polyps of the ileum associated with Gardner's syndrome. Arch Surg 96:289-291
19. Thomas HJW, Whitelax SC, Cottrell SE et al (1996) Hereditary mixed polyposis syndrome: genetic mapping to chromosome 6q. Gastroenterology 110:89
20. Giardiello FM, Hamilton SR, Krush AJ et al (1993) Treatment of colic and rectal adenomas with Sulindac in familial adenomatous polyposis. N Eng J Med 328:1313-1316
21. Parks AG, Nicholls RJ (1978) Proctocolectomy without ileostomy for ulcerative colitis. Br Med J 2:85-88
22. Williams NS (1997) Polypoid disease and polypoid syndromes. In: Keighley MRB, Williams NS (eds) Surgery of the anus, rectum and colon. WB Saunders, London, pp 760-829
23. Williams CB (1973) Diathermy biopsy - technique for the endoscopic management of small polyps.

Endoscopy 5:215-218
24. Moertel CG, Hill JR, Adson MA (1970) Surgical management of multiple polyposis. The problem of cancer in retained bowel segment. Arch Surg 100:521-525
25. Jagelman DG (1983) Familial polyposis coli. Surg Clin North Am 63:117-128
26. Bussey HJR, Eyres AA, Ritchie SM et al (1985) The rectum in adenomatous polyposis: the St. Mark's policy. Br J Surg 72[Suppl]:529-531
27. Schaupp WC, Volpe PA (1972) Management of diffuse colic polyposis. Am J Surg 124:218-220
28. Gingold BS, Jagelman D, Turnbull RB (1979) Surgical management of familial polyposis and Gardner's syndrome. Am J Surg, 137:54-57
29. Milsom JW, Ludwig KA, Church JM et al (1997) Laparoscopic total abdominal colectomy with ileorectal anastomosis for familial adenomatous polyposis. Dis Colon Rectum 40:675-678
30. Sarre RG, Jagelman DC, Beck GT et al (1987) colectomy with ileorectal anastomosis for familial adenomatous polyposis: The risk of rectal cancer. Surgery 101:120-124
31. Duijvendijk P, Slors JFM, Taat CW et al (2000) Quality of life after total colectomy with ileorectal anastomosis or proctocolectomy and ileal pouch-anal anastomosis for familial adenomatous polyposis. Br J Surg 87:590-597
32. Ula M, Nessar G, Bostanoglu A et al (2006) Development of two cancers in the same patient after ileorectal and ileal pouch anal anastomosis for familial adenomatous polyposis. Med Principles Practice 15:83-86
33. Farmer KC, Phillips RKS (1993) Colectomy with ileorectal anastomosis lowers rectal mucosal cell proliferation in familial adenomatous polyposis. Dis Colon Rectum 36:167-171
34. Bertario L (2004) Survival of familial adenomatous polyposis patients after total colectomy: ileorectal anastomosis vs ileoanal pouch. Gastrointestinal Cancers Symposium, San Francisco (abstract 177)

SECTION IV

Special Topics

Psyche and Colitis: What the Surgeon Should Know

Mario Pescatori

Introduction: "To Cut is not to Cure"

The challenge of inflammatory bowel disease (IBD) is formidable. For the patient, there are the symptoms of the disease, causing personal suffering and interference with physical and social activities. For the clinician, the problems are just as challenging: the pathogenesis is yet obscure, and the diagnosis, especially for Crohn's disease, can prove frustrating, as the disease may be diffuse and latent in parts of the bowel that appears normal. The surgeon can be particularly frustrated by the knowledge that he or she can never claim to be able to cure the patient's problem.

The crude recurrence rate of Crohn's disease was 72% 1 year after surgery and 77% after more than 3 years in a large series of 114 patients reported by Rutgeerts et al. [1]. Unfortunately, there was a progressively more severe nature of the lesion at the longer follow-up intervals. Optimal therapy has been reported to embrace many possibilities: drugs, nutrition, psychology and surgery [1], but surgeons, due both to their heavy schedule and their "organic" approach, usually concentrate their efforts on the selection and execution of the best operative procedure rather than on the psychological and emotional patterns of patients. For example, restorative proctocolectomy is considered the gold standard in the surgical treatment of ulcerative colitis, but, surprisingly, having an ileostomy does not seem to affect patients' quality of life while having an ileoanal anastomosis may lead to more anxiety and depression [2].

Can a psychological approach be of any help to the surgeon in the management of patients with IBD? To find it out, the surgeon should know whether or not emotional distress plays a causative role in the onset of the disease and whether a stressful event may facilitate an acute attack. Moreover, the surgeon should be aware of the role of psychological support, if any, in the recovery of patients after surgery, especially considering the high recurrence rate of Crohn's disease.

The aim of the present chapter is to clarify these aspects and stimulate surgeons' interest to consider and improve the emotional state and psychological patterns of their patients.

The Sad Story of Angela F.

I was a young surgeon in September 1979 when Angela F., 28 years old, presented at our Department of Surgery in Rome with rectal bleeding, diarrhoea and a diagnosis of ulcerative colitis. As I had a special interest in colorectal diseases, I was told to take care of her. She had a course of Salazopyrin and prednisone, we spent hours talking and, fortunately, she rapidly improved. After a couple of weeks, I had to leave to attend my first congress in the USA, but I told her about that only the day before. Her discharge had been planned for the end of the week, and she was really better. Nevertheless, when she knew about my departure, she was very upset, cried and asked me not to leave her alone. "You will not be alone, Angela", I told her. "Older and more expert doctors will take care of you; don't worry". When I came back 10 days later, I called one of my colleagues from home "What about Angela?" I asked "A disaster", he said. "She was very depressed, did not talk any more had an attack of toxic megacolon the day after you left. We waited for a few days; then, as she worsened despite i.v. fluids and antibiotics, we took her to the theatre: her colon was perforated and she had diffuse faecal peritonitis. We did a colectomy with an ileostomy and sent her to the ICU. But she died after 24 hours".

That was my first sad, unforgettable experience with psyche and colitis. Since then, I always take special care of both the mental and emotional state of patients with IBD.

Do Stressful Events and Depressive Mood Exacerbate IBD?

The answer is: yes, according to many authors, but there is not a full agreement. North et al. carried out a prospective study on a consecutive sample of 32 patients with IBD who had at least one relapse in a 2-year period after entry into the study. A mean of 2.2 exacerbations was seen per subject during the study period. Mood changed concurrently with exacerbations of IBD, but no evidence indicated that stressful life events or depressed mood precipitated exacerbations in this study group [3]. Interestingly, in another investigation carried out on a larger series of 107 IBD patients and 60 controls, patients reported a lower amount of life-event stress than controls but listed more feelings of being under pressure [4]. Greene et al. found that psychosocial stress contributes to the clinical course of IBD [5] and, more recently, Mittermaier et al. reported that psychological factors such as a depressive mood associated with anxiety and impaired quality of life may exert a negative influence on the course of IBD. Therefore, assessment and management of psychological distress should be included in clinical treatment of patients with IBD [6].

According to my experience, very few patients easily accept being examined and managed by a psychotherapist; therefore, both surgeons and gastroenterologists should be prepared to assess the psychological pattern of their patients by means of appropriate tests, among them the Draw-the-Family test, which may well provide evidence of and objectively score latent psychodynamic disorders, mainly related to family life. This test may be useful in case of IBD patients and may be separately shown to the psychologist afterwards to obtain more useful comments on the personality and mood of the examined subject [7]. An indirect evaluation of psychological reactions of the IBD patient may be carried out by means of the so-called Balint group, i.e. periodical meetings among the clinicians and nurses in charge of the patient. In this case, staff report to a psychiatrist patient reactions to treatment and transfer to the psychiatrist their own emotional distress felt with the patients on some occasions. We used this method with satisfactory results when dealing with cancer and IBD stoma patients [8].

Neurosurgery for Ulcerative Colitis

Half a century ago, in the late 1950s, some neurosurgeons reported on the treatment of patients with ulcerative colitis and psychosis with a prefrontal lobotomy followed by an improvement of their abdominal symptoms [9]. As a few patients had profound psychological disturbances due to the undesired damage of cerebral pathways, some years later the technique was refined using a more selective electrocautery approach aimed at dividing part of the association fibres between the frontal cortex and the thalamic-hypothalamic system, with better results [10]. However, whether these results were due to a spontaneous remission or to the intervention remained unclear, so the procedure was abandoned.

The Psychosomatic Theory

Among the several hypothesised aetiologies of IBD (autoimmune, infective, etc.), there is also a psychosomatic theory. I report several cases that seem to support this theory.

I saw patients who started to suffer from ulcerative colitis after the death of the mother, or a divorce or a car accident as well as patients whose colitis disappeared after retirement from a stressful job. It may seem anecdotical, but it is well known that there are very close connections between the central nervous system (CNS), the autonomic nerves and the so-called "gut brain", represented by the intrinsic nervous system of the bowel devoted to motility, absorption, secretion, hormonal and immunological response to endogenous and external stimuli. The psycho-neuro-endocrine-immune system (PNEI) is an interactive cybernetic network that regulates activity of abdominopelvic viscera in health and disease [11]. As an example, the role of enterochromaffin cells in determining mucosal inflammation has been recently investigated in the large bowel; they may be involved in determining both appendicitis and ulcerative colitis [12].

The rationale of the psychosomatic theory is that, primarily due to incapacity to express their emotions, patients concentrate negative stressful energies towards a target organ. Therefore, a holistic (body and mind, the whole individual) approach is strongly suggested when dealing with patients with IBD. Should the surgeon just remove the segment of diseased intestine without considering the underlying disorders of the whole "brain-body" system [13], another target organ (e.g. the terminal small bowel that replaced the rectum as a reservoir after restorative proctocolectomy) might well become involved by the diseased PNEI and would cause further distress and illness to the patient due to infective, metabolic or immune disorders.

Role of the Family in IBD Patients

"Neuroticism", depression and anxiety are common complaints of colitic patients. It is known but not widely investigated that the family can influence both onset and course of IBD [14]. However, there is evidence that the patient's adjustment is more difficult if family relationships are unstable whereas it is easier in case of strong social support [15]. Family life itself is affected by the course of the IBD patient, as expressed emotions of family members play a major role in helping the patient adjust within the community [15]. Patients with hostile relatives are likely to have more recurrences of their colitis when compared with subjects whose family do not show these high emotional components [16, 17].

The mothers of 72 children and adolescents with IBD and the mothers of 44 controls with severe illness (cystic fibrosis) were interviewed. Fifty-one per cent of IBD mothers had a lifetime history of depression compared with 41% of controls. More IBD mothers than controls had a history of suicide attempts [18]. Twenty families who had children with IBD and 20 comparison families were studied concerning parental distress. Interestingly, mothers in the IBD group scored very high on parental distress whereas fathers did not differ from the comparison group [19].

Therefore, apparently the mother plays a major role when compared with the father in the illness of an IBD son or daughter. However, the following case report, even if anecdotical, might demonstrate that also the relationship between a son with IBD and his father might be important for the course of the disease.

The Impressive Story of the Peniform Foot of a Southern Father

Five years ago, I was seeing patients in a small hospital in the south of Italy, an area with some degree of social depression, where the father was still the undisputed chief in most families. In the outpatient department, I saw a nice young man, 22 years old, with diarrhoea and rectal bleeding. I thought he might have ulcerative colitis and, as a routine, I asked him to draw his family, which I new was quite numerous. Honestly, the patient looked like a quite relaxed chap, and I did not suspect any clear psychosomatic involvement. However, as the Draw-the-Family-test may help to provide evidence of some occult psychological disorder, I decided to ask the patient to do it. He drew the components of his family and put his father in first place, which, in that area of Italy, as I said, was not surprising at all. Moreover, the father appeared big and tall, with long feet. The patient drew himself just beside the father, on his left, very close to him. Well, nothing remarkable, I must say. Nevertheless, as I used to do when dealing with suspected IBD cases, I showed the drawing to our psychologist when I was back in Rome. She looked at it and, suddenly, her face changed expression, and she said: "Have you seen the father's left foot? It looks like a big penis!" Well, I must say that I was rather skeptical about that, and I thought, once again, that sometimes psychologists and psychiatrists are more crazy than their patients. "Did you ask him if he has been a victim of abuse, maybe when he was a child? Did you ask him deeply about the relationship with his father?" "Not too much", I said. "Well, OK, I will do it, even if I feel that this time you are wrong. It seems to me a rather happy family".

Needless to say, when I saw the patient again after a month, I talked to him for half an hour in the office, keeping his relatives (always numerous when you make consultations in the south) out of the door. Well, the patient, even though reluctant, admitted that he had been physically abused by his father for years and then developed the symptoms of colitis. Now he had left the family to work in another town and was feeling much better. So I had used the drawing to allow him to communicate a nonverbal message. I advised him to look for psychological support, and he markedly improved in a few months.

Do Patients with Crohn's Disease Differ Psychologically from Those with Ulcerative Colitis?

According to German authors, the psychological pattern of patients with ulcerative colitis is more uniform, older patients with Crohn's disease appeared more depressed whereas younger individuals look more active but have pronounced dependency conflicts [20]. North and Alpers reported that Crohn's disease, unlike ulcerative colitis, may be statistically associated with lifetime psychiatric disorders [21] whereas Porcelli et al. found no significant difference as far the capacity to express emotions between ulcerative colitis and Crohn's disease patients [22]. The same finding, i.e. no significant differences among the two types of IBD, was reported by others when looking at the of state anxiety and depression even if both Crohn's disease and ulcerative colitis patients looked more anxious and depressed than controls [23]. The degree of correlation between psychosocial stress and subsequent increased disease was found to be higher in patients with Crohn's disease than in those with ulcerative colitis [24] whereas the latter group did worse than Crohn's subjects when obsessive-compulsive symptoms were compared in 44 children [25].

Alpers, reviewing the published studies, found that Crohn's disease, unlike ulcerative colitis, may be statistically associated with lifetime psychiatric disorders [21]. In a more recent report, when looking at depression scores and health-related quality of life, Guthrie et al. found no difference between Crohn's disease and ulcerative colitis patients [26]. As to levels of anxiety, defensive strategies and self-image, patients with colonic Crohn's disease were more childishly concrete and more alexithymic, i.e. unable recognise and describe emotions, than patients with ileocolonic Crohn's disease.

Response to Stress

A close relationship has been found between ulcerative and Crohn's colitis and psychological distress. Patients with active colitis showed higher scores for psychological distress, obsessive-compulsive symptoms, depression, phobic anxiety and psychosis [27]. Why some patients with IBD have long periods of quiescence whereas others have frequent relapses remains an enigma: does major stress play a role in influencing clinical episodes? The results of a prospective study carried out in 124 IBD patients seem to support this hypothesis: stress-exposed subjects demonstrated increased risk of clinical episodes of disease when compared with unexposed subjects [28]. Therefore, psychological stress may favour recurrences, and surgeons should be aware of that when discharging their patients after an operation for Crohn's disease.

Generally speaking, psychosomatic disorders, i.e. the onset of a disease involving the "target" organ, in this respect colitis, is the most frequent response to a stressful event or situation, the others being pathological behaviours such as alcoholism or drug dependence, psychosis, anxiety, depression or, the most unlikely, a structured cognitive and sensitive response leading to recovery of bodily and mental health. The aim of the surgeon, aided by the psychologist and/or psychiatrist, and, of course, by the gastroenterologist, is to make the patient well aware of his/her "brain-body" global disorder and remove the "target "organ only when indicated while adequately treating and modifying the related PNEI pattern, if altered. Most IBD patients have alexithymia and do not dream during sleep, or at least they do not remember their dreams, thus showing that the unconscious emotions are not likely to be adequately felt, processed and cleared and therefore might perhaps trigger a pathological visceral response.

Cause or Just Association? Psychiatric Illness and IBD

Some confusion has occurred in the past decades on the psychosomatic aetiology or pathogenesis of IBD. There is enough evidence that depression or any psychiatric diagnosis is statistically more often associated with Crohn's disease than with diabetes, hypertension or cardiac diseases [29] and that emotional distress may cause exacerbation of IBD, as reported at the beginning of this chapter with the sad story of Angela F. Psychiatric illness may precede the onset of Crohn's disease, but no significant data have been reported to strongly support a causative relationship. Patients with ulcerative colitis have no unusual predisposing factors in the onset of their disease when compared with matched controls. Also colectomy is usually followed by a marked improvement in preexisting psychiatric illness. Whereas in European reports there is a tendency to consider psychoneurosis among the aetiological factors underlying IBD, most American authors feel that anxiety and depression, despite being frequent in IBD patients, should not be considered aetiopathogenetic factors but just psychological reactions to the disease [30]. However, there is a higher prevalence of psychiatric disorder in patients with Crohn's diseases compared with the normal population, and a small but significant percentage of individuals with Crohn's disease may have a psychiatric disturbance that predates their medical illness [31].

Should IBD Patients be Treated by Psychologists and Psychiatrists?

An Italian study reported that anxiety was significantly associated with a higher disease activity and that it should appropriately evaluated and treated with the exacerbated symptoms in IBD patients [32].

Depression: How Crohn's Disease Patients Defend Themselves

Depression itself is a mechanism of defence in a person whose quality of life is severely affected by Crohn's colitis. The more the patient interacts with people, deals with his/her job, enjoys – or tries to enjoy – social life, the more he/she gets frustrated and suffers, as routine daily activities are prevented by anal soiling, frequent diarrhoea or abdominal pain.. Therefore, depression, i.e. refusal to participate actively in life, introversion and self-confinement to a comfortable jail represented by his/her own dark bedroom, may represent an apparent provisional solution to "feel safe" and to avoid further conflicts, at least with the external environment.

This is especially true for patients classified as "very poor" or grade 4 in Helzer's and coworkers' grading scale of Crohn's activity index [28]. Instead of being criticised for clearly manifesting fear of people and work, the patient prefers to create a personal, inviolable safe shell, i.e. to be depressed. After all, depression represents a more quiet and respectable state than spending a day outside desperately looking for public toilets in which to change dirty sanitary pads when observed by unknown healthy people.

Is the Psychological Pattern of IBD Patients Underestimated by Colorectal Surgeons?

When Grace et al. [33], in 1951, found that emotional influences can produce changes in the colon mucosa up to frank ulcerations, both intrinsic nerves and neurotransmitters in the bowel were either poorly known or fully ignored. In the 1970, Paulley [34] claimed dramatic improvement of colitic patients by means of psychotherapy, but Latimer [35], reviewing 20 studies, found that only three of them had used consecutive cases and therefore criticized Paulley's and others' conclusions that psyche played key role in IBD. More recently, Kiss and Ferenci [36] reported that psychotherapy – regardless of how intensive it might be – has not been proven to cure the underlying biologic disturbance. Therefore, the hope of complete cure by psychotherapy is not warranted. While improvement and even freedom of all symptoms may take place, psychotherapy cannot prevent stress-related response. With increased skepticism regarding the psychological component, Goligher, in his book, the Bible of colorectal surgery, reported that only 14% of his patients considered the relapses of colitis due to emotional distresses or attended a psychiatrist, the immunologic theory being the more accredited to explain the etiology of IBD [37]. Keighley's and Williams' "Surgery of the Anus, Rectum and Colon" dedicate just a few lines to the topic of "psyche and colitis" in their extensive chapter on ulcerative colitis, even admitting that psychological factors play a role in the mechanism of relapse. Moreover, there is no mention of psychological involvement or psychosomatic aetiology in the modern *Beck's Handbook of Colorectal Surgery* [38].

Finally, the topic "psyche and colitis" does not appear in any issues of *Diseases of the Colon and Rectum* – the journal with the highest impact on the colorectal community – between 1985 and 2005. Therefore, it is not surprising at all that the role of psychological and emotional disorders may be either neglected or underestimated by surgeons when dealing with colitic patients.

The "PNEI-G" System: a Cybernetic Array is Closely Related to the Bowel

As mentioned above, the PNEI system is a network strictly related to the controlled organ (the large bowel in this case) and modulated with feed back by the effector organ (the large bowel), being itself a site of nervous, hormonal and immunological output, as represented in Figure 1. There are nervous, endocrine and immunologic cells in the intestine.

We may add a "G" to PNEI, as genetic makeup has been strongly hypothesised to play a pivotal role on some occasions in IBD patients, e.g. in determining, together with cytokine production from colonic T cells, the onset of primary sclerosing cholangitis in some patients with ulcerative colitis [39]. Moreover, gastrointestinal (GI) inflammation involves numerous genes, some of which directly modulate the expression pattern of inflammatory cells [40]. It is now well established that clinical manifestation of IBD is determined by a multigenic background: low-power immunogenic agents can be hyperactivated by the presence of sterile mycobacterial fragments, thus allowing sufficient immune response. A disorder of this mechanism may be an important aetiological factor in IBD [41]. There are strict connections among intestinal flora, genetic makeup and the immune system: the integrity of our "self" is guaranteed by the mucosal immune system, and enterocytes transport to the lumen immunoglobulin (Ig)A antibodies, which cover the bowel surface as a protective film against bacteria and viruses. Disruption of this balance may cause IBD. Therefore, the con-

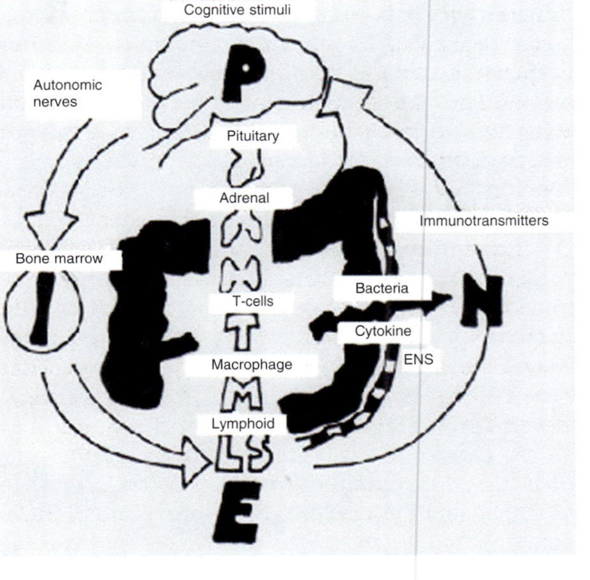

Fig. 1. The large bowel controls (and is controlled by) the *P* (psycho), *N* (neuro), *E* (endocrine) and *I* (immune) system. The altered balance between bacteria and cytokine may initiate the inflammatory bowel disease (IBD) process. IBD patients need a holistic approach, taking care of the whole psyche-body-enteric nervous system

nections between this protective system and the nervous system is of paramount importance in determining the role of psychiatric illness in the IBD process.

There is an impact of mind, central nervous system and neuromodulation on the overly active immune response in the intestinal mucosa, which may initiate IBD, and the degree to which mind–body influences and stress impact levels of local inflammation deserves closer attention by the clinician [42].

Enteric Nervous System: the Brain of the Gut

Our immune system is closely related to the axis gut-brain through the enteric nervous system (ENS). Nerves from both the brain and the spinal cord of our colitic or potentially colitic patients interact with structures and substances situated and produced in the bowel wall in both health and in disease. What we feel and what we think, what we hope and what we fear, is communicated to the above-mentioned enteric immune and nervous system and vice versa through the transport of cranial sensation. The ENS consists of hundreds of millions of neurons of four types , each with a specific function. Motor neurons, impinging the bowel muscular layers and the vessels; secretory neurons, triggering exocrine and endocrine functions; interneurons, deputed to the connection among nerve fibres; and sensory neurons, whose dendrites are in the bowel wall originating from neurons in the sacral ganglia and carrying cranial sensation. From a biochemical point of view, the intrinsic gut nerves are of five types: cholinergic, adrenergic, serotoninergic, gamma-amino-butyric-acid (GABA)ergic and peptidergic – the last being the larger group. A wide variety of peptides have been identified as neurotransmitters in the enteric nervous system [43].

John Furness is an Australian. He was rather young and enthusiastic, had a reddish curly hair, and when I met him in Adelaide, he took me to visit Flinders University, surrounded by olive trees, on the top of the hill close to the town, which was lying beautifully at the edge of the ocean, like most Australian cities. Marcello Costa left Turin and joined him to carry out outstanding research on intestinal peristalsis. I met him in Rome a few years later when he joined the editorial board of our journal, *Techniques in Coloproctology*. At that time, I was working with bioengineers and physiologists on a mathematical model of intestinal motor activity in the rabbit colon in vitro [44].

ENS plays a major role in regulation of secretion, motility, immune function and inflammation in the small and large bowel. Alterations of this regulation are likely to cause GI symptoms in various conditions, including IBD. The immune system and the ENS are integrated in the gut. Galen stated in the second century AD that the emotional state of an individual can cause and, in some case, relieve disease. Immune system alteration was documented in patients suffering from stress, and animals subjected to profound severe stress suffered from immune disturbances such atrophy of lymph nodes and consequently developed intestinal ulcers.

Psychological stress influence immune function, and it has been demonstrated that lymphoid tissue is directly innervated. Secretory products of the immune system, which include interleukins and neuropeptides, may also influence the neuroendocrine system. Communication between the two systems is therefore bidirectional [45]. Lymphocyte function is altered by ENS neuropeptides, such as somatostatin. Conversely, endocrine products of the immune system, such interleukin (IL)-1, have an effect on the gut. In IBD, vasoactive intestinal polypeptide (VIP)ergic neurons are prominent immunohistochemically, and concentrations of rectal mucosal VIP are elevated [46]. Patients with IBD have elevated circulating and mucosal cytokine production [47]. Lymphokines and immunotransmitters seem to transfer information from the immune centres to the brain [48].

Put together, these findings suggest, but do not prove, that the pathophysiology of IBD may be related to alterations in immune ENS and gut–brain interactions, resulting in inflammation and diarrhoea [49]. Further clarification of the underlying pathophysiologic derangements offer hope for specific therapeutic intervention focused on the PNEI-G system [50].

What the Surgeon Should Really Know

The large bowel of the IBD patient is not an isolated organ (as was our rabbit colon in vitro) but is strictly connected to the PNEI-G system via reciprocal interactions. Therefore, if the surgeon wants to cure the patients and not simply "repair" his/her colon and see him or her "broken" again after a short while, the surgeon must take into consideration this entire complex system. This is called a holistic approach, which usually is not taught at university. The harmonic balance among intrinsic and extrinsic nerves, brain, immunoendocrine system, intestinal flora and genetic pattern, all connected through neurotransmitters and other substances, maintain homeostasis of the patient. A localised failure of this complex system may favour the onset of IBD. The so-called brain–gut system, when altered, may trigger psychiatric illness, and vice versa.

Complete understanding of this system is difficult because it is based on a number of complex mechanisms involving both structures and substances, which are not yet well known. Among them are energy and emotions. A better understanding of such mechanisms may assist physicians in identifying particular subsets of patients who may respond to novel forms of adjunctive treatments for IBD, including hypnosis and meditation. At present, there is evidence to suggest that cognitive behavioural psychological group treatment for outpatients is a feasible and effective approach for the reduction of psychological distress in IBD patients [50]. In conclusion, trying to answer the questions asked in the introduction on the basis of scientific evidence:

- NO, it is unlikely that emotional distress causes IBD (the father with the penile foot might not himself have caused ulcerative colitis by abusing his son), but a significant proportion of Crohn's patients have psychiatric disturbances before the onset of their disease. On the other hand, IBD frequently causes major psychological disorders in the first year of the disease.
- YES, stressful events can exacerbate the course of IBD by precipitating an acute attack (the emotional distress due to my sudden departure to the US might have caused the toxic megacolon of poor Angela F.).
- YES, family and social problems may well worsen the prognosis of a patient with IBD. Therefore, clinicians should take care not only of the in-hospital postoperative course but also of the patient's social and family life after discharge from the hospital.
- YES, depression is more likely to affect a patient with Crohn's disease rather than a patient with another medical disease. Patients with Crohn's disease, unlike those with ulcerative colitis, have lifetime psychiatric disorders, and stress may influence their recurrence rate.

And finally:

- YES, the psychotherapist may well help the surgeon to improve the prognosis of patients with IBD.

As quite a few patients refuse psychiatric consultation, the surgeon needs to know how to approach the IBD patient from a psychological and emotional point of view, if he or she is keen to improve the results of surgery.

Acknowledgements. The author wishes to thank Dr. G. Tornusciolo, psychiatrist, and Dr. C. Miliacca and Dr. A.M. Lombardi, psychologists, who kindly revised the manuscript, and Dr. M. Fiorino, who helped with references.

References

1. McManus J (1985) Comment in: Rutgeerts P, Geboes K, Vantrappen G et al (eds) Natural history or recurrent Crohn's disease of the ileo-colonic anastomosis after curative surgery. Gut, pp 665–672
2. Nordin K, Pahlman L, Larsson K et al (2002) Health-related quality of life and psychological distress in a population-based sample of Swedish patients with inflammatory bowel disease. Scand J Gastroenterol 37:450–457
3. North CS, Alpers DH, Helzer JF et al (1991) Do life events or depression exacerbate inflammatory bowel disease? A prospective study. Ann Intern Med 114:381–386
4. von Wieterstein J, Kohler T, Feiereis H (1992) Relapse-precipitating life events and feelings in patients with inflammatory bowel disease. Psychother Psycosom 58:103–112
5. Greene BR, Blanchard EB, Wan CK (1994) Long-term monitoring of psychosocial stress and symptomatology in inflammatory bowel disease. Behav Res Ther 32:217–226
6. Mittermaier C, Dejaco C, Waldhoer T et al (2004) Impact of depressive mood on relapse in patients with inflammatory bowel disease: a prospective 18-month follow-up study. Psychosom Med 66:79–84
7. Renzi C, Pescatori M (2002) Family drawing with clinical approach to patients with chronic constipation: preliminary data. Neurogastroenterologia 8:56–58
8. Nesci DA, Pescatori M, Ferro FM (1983) Unconscious dynamics in the care of stoma patients. Acta Med Rom 21:389–396
9. Levy R, Wilkins H, Herrmann J et al (1956) Experiences with prefrontal lobotomy for intractable ulcerative colitis. J Am Med Assoc 160:1277–1280
10. Blalock JE (1992) Neuroimmunoendocrinology, 2nd edn. Karger, Basilea
11. Bucaille M (1962) Selective frontal lobe operation for treatment of some disease of the digestive tract with special reference to ulcerative colitis. Surgery 52:690–692
12. Crowell MD, Shetzolone MA, Moses PL et al (2004) Enterochromaffin cells and SHT signaling in the pathophysiology of disorders of gastrointestinal function. Curr Opin Investig Drugs 5:55–60
13. Chopra D (1997) Guarirsi da dentro. Sperling & Kupfer
14. Vaughan CE, Leff J, Sarner M (1999) Relatives' expressed emotion and the course and the inflammatory bowel disease. J Psychosom Res 47:461–469
15. McMahon AW, Schmitt P, Patterson JF, Rothman E (1973) Personality differences between inflammatory bowel disease patients and their healthy siblings. Psychosom Med 35:35–91
16. Brown GW, Birley JLT (1976) Influence of family and social factors on the course schizophrenic disorders: a replication. Br J Psychiatry 121:241–258
17. Vaughan CE, Leff J (1976) The influence of family and social factors on the course of psychiatric illness: a comparison of schizophrenic and depressed neurotic patients. Br J Psychiatry 129:125–137
18. Burke PM, Kochoshis S, Neigut D (1994) Maternal psychiatric disorders in pediatric inflammatory bowel

disease and cystic fibrosis. Child Psychiatry Hum Dev 25:45–52
19. Engstrom I (1991) Parental distress and social interaction in families with children with inflammatory bowel disease. J Am Acad Child Adolesc Psychiatry 30(6):904–912
20. Reindell A, Ferner H, Gmelin K (1981) Psychosomatic differentiation between colitis ulcerosa and ileitis terminalis (Crohn disease). Z Psychosom Med Psychoanal 27:358–371
21. North CS, Alpers DH (1994) A review of studies of psychiatric factors in Crohn's disease: etiologic implication. Ann Clin Psychiatry 6:117–124
22. Porcelli P, Zaka S, Leoci C (1995) Alexithymia in inflammatory bowel disease. A case-control study. Psychother Psychosom 64:49–53
23. Addolorato G, Capristo E, Stefanini GF, Gasbarrini G (1997) Inflammatory bowel disease: a study of the association between anxiety and depression, physical morbidity, and nutritional status. Scand J Gastroenterol 32:1013–1021
24. Paar GH, Bezzenberger U, Lorenz-Meyer H (1988) The correlation of psychosocial stress and disease activity in patients with Crohn's disease and ulcerative colitis. Z Gastroenterol 26:648–657
25. Burke P, Meyer V, Kochoshis S et al (1989) Obsessive-compulsive symptoms in childhood inflammatory bowel disease and cystic fibrosis. J Am Acad Child Adolesc Psychiatry 28:525–527
26. Guthrie E, Jackson J, Shaffer J et al (2002) Psychological disorders and severity of inflammatory bowel disease predict health-related quality of life in ulcerative colitis and Crohn' disease. Am J Gastroenterol 97:1994–1999
27. Sewitch MJ, Abrahamowicz M, Bitton A (2001) Psychological support and disease activity in patients with inflammatory bowel disease. Am J Gastroenterol 96:1340–1349
28. Duffy LC, Zielezny MA, Marshall JR et al (1991) Relevance of major stress in events as an indicator of disease activity prevalence in inflammatory bowel disease. Behav Med 17:101–102
29. Helzer JE, Chammas S, Norland CC (1984) A study of the association between Crohn's disease and psychiatric illness. Gastroenterology 86:324–330
30. Biondi M (1998) Al confine tra psichiatria, psicologia e gastroenterologia. Aspetti psicologici come cofattori patogenetici in alcune patologie gastrointestinali. Neurogastroenterologia 2:47–52
31. Tarter RE, Switala J, Carra J et al (1987) Inflammatory bowel disease: psychiatric status of patients before and after disease onset. Int J Psychiatry Med 17:173–181
32. Porcelli P, Zaka S, Centone S, Sisto G (1994) Psychological di stress and level of disease activity in inflammatory bowel disease. Ital J Gastroenterol 26:111–115
33. Grace WJ, Wolf S, Wolff HG (1951) The human colon. Heinemann, London
34. Paulley JW (1956) The emotional factors in ulcerative colitis. Gastroenterology 86:709–712
35. Latimer PR (1978) Crohn's disease: a review of the psychological and social outcome. Psychol Med 8:649–656
36. Kiss A, Ferenci P (1991) [Phychosomatic treatment of patients with Crohn's disease]. Schweiz Rundsch Med Prax 80(5):85-89
37. Goligher JC (1984) Surgery of the anus rectum and colon, 5th edn. Bailliere Tindall, London
38. Beck DE (2003) Handbook of colorectal surgery (2nd ed) Marcel Dekker Inc., New York
39. Broomé U, Hultcrantz MD, Lefvert AK, Yi Q (1998) Cytokine production from colonic T cells in patients with ulcerative colitis with and without primary sclerosing cholangitis. Dis Colon Rectum 41:1543–1549
40. van Montfrans C, Velde AA, van Deventer AJH, Rodriguez Pena MS (2004) Gene therapy in the treatment of intestinal inflammation. Int J Colorectal Dis 19:79–86
41. Raedler A (2001) Etiology of inflammatory bowel syndrome. Int J Colorectal Dis 16:269–270
42. Anton PA (1999) Stress and mind-body impact on the course inflammatory bowel diseases. Semin Gastrointest Dis 10:14–19
43. Furness JB, Costa M (1987) The enteric nervous z-system. Churchill Livingstone, New York, pp 55–89
44. Pescatori M, Grassetti F, Ronzoni G et al (1979) Peristalsis in distal colon of the rabbit: an analysis of mechanical events. Am J Physiol 236:E464–E472
45. Shanahan F, Anton P (1988) Neuroendocrine modulation of the immune system. Possible implications for inflammatory bowel disease. Dig Dis Sci 33:S41–S49
46. O'Morain C, Bishop AE, McGregor GP (1984) Vasoactive intestinal peptide concentration and immunocytochemical studies in rectal biopsies from patients with inflammatory bowel disease. Gut 25:57–61
47. Gross V, Andus T, Caesar I et al (1988) Evidence for continuos stimulation of interleukin-6 production in Crohn's disease. Gastroenterology 102:514–519
48. Hall NR, McGillis JP, Spangello BL, Goldstein AL (1985) Evidence that thymosins and other biological response modifiers can function as neuroactive immunotransmitters. J Immunol 135:806–813
49. Pullman WE, Elsebury S, Kobayashi M et al (1992) Evidence for continuous stimulation of interleukin. Gastroenterology 102:514–519
50. Mulvihill SJ, Debas HT (1992) Neuroendocrine regulation of intestinal function. Enhanced mucosal cytokine production in inflammatory bowel disease. Gastroenterology 102:529–537
51. Mussell M, Bocker U, Nagel N et al (2003) Reducing psychological distress in patients with inflammatory bowel disease by cognitive-behavioural treatment: exploratory study of effectiveness. Scand J Gastroenterol 38:755–762

Interdisciplinary Management of Inflammatory Bowel Diseases

Michele Comberlato, Federico Martin

Introduction

Inflammatory bowel diseases (IBD), which appear mainly in the form of ulcerative colitis (UC) and Crohn's disease (CD), represent complex disorders as documented by the wide variations found in clinical practice. IBD has an impressive impact on patients and society because the presentation of the disease occurs in the majority of cases at a young age and, depending on its chronic evolution, has the potential of causing lifelong ill health.

Patients suffering from this disease present symptoms and clinical situations often embarrassing and having deep impact on their quality of life. Considering the young age of this patient population and the long duration of the disease, the problem of adequate medical management has crucial relevance. Consequently, we realised an interdisciplinary IBD Unit in our hospital with the aim of improving our clinical results and developing closer and stronger contact with the patients.

The medical strategy should always take in account some critical points such as the type of the disease, the severity and extent, the clinical response and tolerance of drugs and the follow-up in terms of monitoring the quality of life and preventing possible complications.

Diagnosis of IBD

This is often not a simple issue. The classical clinical pattern is well known, but the symptoms are not so clear and the differential diagnosis includes infective diarrhoeas, drugs intolerance, haematological diseases and neoplasia. Once the diagnosis of IBD is clear, we have to remember, before starting with therapy, that 50% of relapses are associated with pathogens. Moreover, the radiologist, the endoscopist and the pathologist should have detailed information about the clinical situation, so that they can make every effort to get the right diagnosis. That means that special attention and training in this disease is required for any specialist involved in the diagnostic process.

Ulcerative Colitis

Proctitis affects approximately 30% of patients at presentation and later spreading to a more proximal extent is possible in about 40% of cases. The mainstay of treatment is topical administration of mesalazine or steroids. The topical or oral route is sometimes insufficient with the frustrating problem of a proctitis unresponsive to medical therapy. In the non-responders, rectal bismuth preparations [1] and arsenical suppositories [2] seem to be effective and safe, but about 5% of the cases need total colectomy because of impaired quality of life [3].

Left-sided and pan-colitis are usually well managed with the standard regimens of steroids and mesalazine, but attention has to be paid to the patients who develop resistance or dependence of steroids. The gastroenterologist and the surgeon should very carefully consider the possible options, particularly in cases of severe, unresponsive or fulminant colitis in which the lack of clinical improvement within the first week of medical therapy represents an indication for colectomy. This observation is even stronger in patients with toxic dilation of the colon-in this case colectomy is mandatory in the absence of response within 24 h [4].

In all these situations we should always bear in mind a comprehensive view of the life of our patients in terms of severity of symptoms, safety of the current therapy, drug toxicity, safety of surgical procedure and quality of life expectancy. As David Sachar said some years ago "we too readily accept as a criterion of success the ability to keep patients out of surgery. Somehow the internists tend to view surgery as a last resort or as indication of failure of medical therapy. In adopting such an attitude we render our patients a terrible disservice."

Crohn's Disease

Given the complexity and heterogeneity of the disease and the different options for combining therapy, it is unlikely that sufficient controlled trials will ever be conducted to provide evidence for the best treatment for every clinical scenario. In many patients, several therapeutic options may represent valid alternatives. In this field, as in many others, patient preference should be an important factor in determining the choice of therapy. All physicians need to be aware that smoking is the most important risk factor statistically associated with Crohn's disease, with higher relapse rates following surgical resections and a greater risk of perforating disease [5, 6]. In a patient with a classical clinical ileal/colonic manifestation, there are many valid options including antibiotics, steroids, immunosuppressives, enteral nutrition and surgery.

A typical ileitis with poor response to medical therapy, and consequently poor quality of life for the patient, is a clear and unquestionable indication for surgery. On the other hand, a patient with multiple ileal localisations of the disease has to be conservatively managed for as long as possible.

In any severe situation, we should consider the great impact of the quality of nutrition on the state of the intestinal wall. Enteral nutrition employed as the only source of feeding is an effective therapy for Crohn's disease and its mechanism of action, although poorly understood, consists of an immunomodulatory procedure on the bowel mucosa, which consequently effects the bacterial flora. An elemental or polymeric diet is equally effective [7, 8].

Perineal disease occurs in up to one third of patients with Crohn's disease, impacting differently according to the different clinical phenotypes: ileal CD 12%, ileo-cecal CD 15%, colonic CD 41%, colorectal CD 92% [9]. The medical management of perineal disease has been absolutely unsatisfactory with poor results in the short as well as in the long term. The availability of infliximab made it possible to greatly improve our results, which were even better when infliximab was associated with local non-invasive surgery such as drainage of fluid collection, fistulotomy or application of setons [10].

Topics on IBD

Fecundity and Pregnancy

Women with UC and CD are known to have fecundity and pregnancy equal to that of the general population [11, 12], but they are worried about the risks to the newborn in terms of damage by drugs or by the illness itself. The medical staff plays a very crucial role in informing and encouraging women with IBD, explaining the safety of the drugs employed and the general risks regarding pregnancy for healthy women.

In comparison with the general population, women in remission under azatioprine have no impairment, either in fecundity or in the capability of having a regular pregnancy without particular risks. In women who underwent restorative proctocolectomy with ileo pouch-anal anastomosis (IPAA), parturition is normal and IPAA function is not damaged [13]. However, there are reports in the literature that give advice about the critical risk of infertility after IPAA including a decrease of potential fertility up to 80% [14, 15]. Our female patients should be correctly and tactfully informed about this possible complication, due in most cases to a tubal occlusion from adhesive disease. Would a more diffuse laparoscopic approach ameliorate this data?

Pouchitis

Pouchitis seldom occurs after IPAA and is usually easily resolved with topical therapy and antibiotics, but doubts should arise in case of poor response and a tendency to chronicity. IPAA fails in 8% of patients with evident differences in the different groups: 6.5–19% in indeterminate colitis, 15–43% in CD and 1.4–8% in UC [16–18]. Only close collaboration between the gastroenterologist and the surgeon during the follow-up of pouchitis can evaluate the results of conservative therapy and decide the right time for revision of the pouch, which shows good clinical outcome in up to two thirds of patients [19, 20].

Surveillance for Dysplasia and Cancer

The clinical heterogeneity of IBD is reflected in the heterogeneity in the macro and microscopic feature and makes cancer surveillance in this population much more challenging than in the general population. IBD associated risk factors for colorectal cancer are well known and this is the reason why any patient with a history of extensive disease, whether UC or CD, of more than 10 years must undergo a complete colonoscopy with multiple biopsies every 2 years. Any dubious situation should be carefully discussed by the gastroenterologist, the surgeon and the pathologist and the maximal alert in case of dysplasia or cancer on flat inflamed mucosa should be given.

In the past, the more crucial issue was the significance of dysplasia in endoscopically visible lesions (Dysplasia Associated Lesion or Mass) with high rates of carcinoma when these patients underwent colectomy. In more recent data, about 10 surveillance programs reported findings of carcinoma in 17 out of 40 (43%) colectomies performed with an indication of DALM [21]. However, not all polypoid lesions with dysplasia carry the same significance for IBD patients. Some polyps can be snared like adenomas unrelated to colitis, particularly if they arise in a segment of the colon not involved in inflammation, and can be managed like polyps in the general population [22].

The dysplasia encountered in an adenoma or in chronic inflammation is quite identical and so we have no reliable means of differentiating between them in regards to our decision. A well-conducted study tried to answer this question and concluded that no adverse outcomes resulted after endoscopic removal of 70 polyps (three with high-grade non-invasive dysplasia) from 48 IBD patients in a mean follow-up time of 4.1 years [23].

The best way to manage dysplasia and colorectal cancer is via a surveillance program; however, in this case the patients have to be correctly and clearly informed that dysplasia and cancer can still arise despite the program of close observation and the skilfulness of the medical staff [24]. In our opinion, the development of dysplasia itself in a surveillance program is not enough in itself to advise patients to undergo colectomy. Situations are different and, as mentioned before, even a severe dysplasia in an adenomatous polyp not related to inflammatory disease, could be optimally managed with a radical polypectomy. As always in this context, such a decision of course requires that the gastroenterologist, surgeon and pathologist develop a decision-making protocol through which information about the patient, specific literature data, personal experience and skills are clearly shared and accepted.

Intestinal Strictures

Intestinal fibrostenosis is a debilitating complication; even in this era of potent biologic therapies, the mechanisms promoting the underlying fibrosis in IBD are still misunderstood. From a conservative point of view, the target of therapy in this field is TGFb and its intracellular mediators (SMAD proteins) and, theoretically, interleukin 10 could be the ideal cytokine to be used in IBD, since it has been proven to be a potent anti-inflammatory and anti-fibrogenic agent. Nevertheless, clinical data about IL-10, antibodies against TGFb and SMAD proteins, Ca^{2+} blocking and cyclic nucleotides to modulate collagen production gave no results.

Drugs are useful in reducing the inflammatory component of the stricture, but once the fibrosis has scared the lumen, there are only two options: endoscopic balloon dilation or surgical intervention, which means either strictureplasty or resection.

Endoscopic balloon dilation has been proven to be very effective, safe and repeatable when used in short and anastomotic strictures. A recent trial on endoscopic management of CD upper and lower strictures in association with local steroid injection had very good results: technical success (ability of the scope to pass the stenosis) of 29 dilations on 17 patients was 96.5%, the long-term success (mean follow-up 18.8 months, 5–50) was 70% if the dilation was<15 mm and 68.4% for dilations >15 mm. The recurrence rate in the group with steroid injection was 10 and 31.3% in patients who only received dilation. The long-term success rate was 76.5% with a 10% complication rate, with no mortality [25].

As in other critical situations, the decision of what to do should be shared with the patient; repeat endoscopic dilation is of course a valid and safe option and the length of the symptom-free interval will be the main parameter used to decide between conservative management and surgery.

Prevention of Post-Operative Relapse

The 5-aminosalicylates remain the most controversial agents in the maintenance of remission of Crohn's disease. Several studies and a recent meta-analysis have shown no significant benefit in comparison to placebo, but the meta-analysis suggested a potential role in patients with surgically induced remission, where mesalazine lowered the risk of relapse by 13% [26]. These general data were better clarified in a randomised study in which 5-ASA gained a significant reduction in relapse rate in post-operative prophylaxis in a subgroup of patients with limited ileal disease [27]. Therefore, while waiting for confirmation data, our team routinely treats resected patients for ileal CD.

The Patient's Point of View

The patient's point of view is a very crucial issue in regard to patients who suffer from IBD. The majority of newly diagnosed cases are between 18 and 35 years of age and, considering the peculiar characteristics of the disease, it is fundamental that any doctors involved in the management of the patient establish, maintain and improve on a long-term doctor–patient relationship.

The diagnosis of IBD has a profound impact on the

lives of patients, so any physician notifying the patient should be aware of this impact, be able to handle a variety of reactions of the patient, and be sure to leave the patient with a sense that they are not going to have to go through the challenges of IBD alone [28].

The characteristics of the disease must be explained as well as the medical options and even the chance of possible surgery. A recent UK study outlined the key issues that concern IBD patients:

- Fear of incontinence when using public transport, shopping, vacationing and when at work.
- Fear of hospitals and treatment.
- Fear of cancer.
- Effects on employment including limitations in regards to types of jobs and promotion prospects
- Effects on holiday medical and life insurance.
- Guilt because of the effects of the above problems on the family.
- Anxiety and sense of isolation.

Regarding these considerations, the multidisciplinarity organisation of the management program should be made clear to the patient. Previously healthy young patients who seldom saw a physician find themselves in a situation where they are surrounded by many doctors and, therefore, they absolutely need a primary care figure who can mediate with others, discuss and explain any proposal offered by different specialists and coordinate the work of the entire group.

IBD group support services are very helpful for patients with severe disease in providing practical information, sharing concerns and personal fears and acquiring, step by step, the balance necessary to enjoy a good life in spite of IBD.

References

1. Ryder SP, Walker RJ, Rhodes JM et al (1990) Rectal bismuth subsalicylate therapy for ulcerative colitis. Aliment Pharmacol Ther 4:333–338
2. Forbes A, Britton TC, Gazzard BG (1989) Safety and efficacy of acetarsol suppositories in unresponsive proctitis. Aliment Pharmacol Ther 3:553–556
3. Nayar M, Rhodes JM (2004) Management of inflammatory bowel disease. Postgrad Med J 80:206–213
4. Jewell DP, Caprilli R, Mortensen N et al (1991) Indication and timing for surgery for severe ulcerative colitis. Gastroenterol Int 4:161–164
5. Cosnes J, Beaugerie L, Carbonnel F et al (2001) Smoking cessation and the course of Crohn's disease: an intervention study. Gastroenterology 120:1093–1099
6. Louis E, Michel V, Hugot JP et al (2003) Early development of stricturing or penetrating pattern in Crohn's disease is influenced by disease location, number of flares and smoking, but not by NOD2/CARD15 genotype. Gut 52:552–557
7. Verma S, Brown S, Kirkwood B et al (2000) Polymeric versus elemental diet as primary treatment in active Crohn's disease: a randomised double blind trial. Am J Gastroenterol 95:735–739
8. Fell JM, Paintin M, Arnaud-Battandier F et al (2000) Mucosal healing and a fall in mucosal pro-inflammatory cytokine mRNA induced by a specific oral polymeric diet in paediatric Crohn's disease. Aliment Pharmacol Ther 14:281–289
9. Hellers G, Bergstrand O, Ewerth S et al (1980) Occurrence and outcome after primary treatment of anal fistulae in Crohn's disease. Gut 21:525–527
10. Regueiro M, Mardini H (2003) Treatment of perianal fistulizing Crohn's disease with infliximab alone or as an adjunct to exam under anesthesia with seton placement. Infamm Bowel Dis 9(2):98–103
11. Fonager K, Sorensen HAT, Olsen J et al (1998) Pregnancy outcome for women with Crohn's disease: a follow up study based on linkage between national registries. Am J Gastroenterol 93:2426–2430
12. Woolfson K, Cohen Z, McLeod RS (1990) Crohn's disease and pregnancy. Dis Colon Rectum 33:869–873
13. Hahnloser D, Pemberton JH, Wolff BG et al (2004) Pregnancy and delivery before and after ileal pouch-anal anastomosis (IPAA) for inflammatory bowel disease: immediate and long-term consequences and outcomes. Dis Colon Rectum 47:1127–1135
14. Ording OK, Juul S, Berndtsson I et al (2002) Ulcerative colitis: female fecundity before diagnosis, during disease and after surgery compared with a population sample. Gastroenterology 122:15–19
15. Sagar PM, Dozois RR, Wolff BG et al (1996) Disconnection, pouch revision and reconnection of the ileal pouch-anal anastomosis. Br J Surgery 83:1401–1405
16. Breen EM, Schoetz DJ Jr, Marcello PW et al (1998) Functional results after perineal complications of ileal pouch-anal anastomosis. Dis Colon Rectum 41:691–695
17. Marcello PW, Schoetz DJ Jr, Roberts PL et al (1997) Evolutionary changes in the pathologic diagnosis after the ileoanal pouch procedure. Dis Colon Rectum 40:263–269
18. Foley EF, Schoetz DJ Jr, Roberts PL et al (1995) Rediversion after ileal pouch-anal anastomosis: causes of failures and predictors of subsequent pouch salvage. Dis Colon Rectum 38:793–798
19. Zmora O, Efron JE, Nogueras JJ et al (2001) Reoperative abdominal and perineal surgery in ileoanal pouch patients. Dis Colon Rectum 44:1310–1314
20. Fonkalsrud EW, Bustorff-Silva J (1999) Reconstruction for chronic dysfunction of ileoanal pouches. Ann Surg 229:197–204
21. Bernstein CN, Shanahan F, Weinstein WM (1994) Are we telling patients the truth about surveillance colonoscopy in ulcerative colitis? Lancet 343:71–74
22. Torres C, Antonioli D, Odze RD (1998) Polypoid dysplasia and adenomas in inflammatory bowel disease: a clinical, pathologic and follow up study of 89 polyps from 59 patients. Am J Surg Pathol 22:275–284
23. Rubin PH, Friedman S, Harpaz N et al (1999) Colonoscopic polypectomy in chronic colitis: conservative management after endoscopic resection of dysplastic polyps. Gastroenterology 117:1295–1300
24. Connell WR, Lennard-Jones JE, Williams CB et al

(1994) Factors affecting the outcome of endoscopic surveillance for cancer in ulcerative colitis. Gastroenterology 107:934–944

25. Singh VV, Draganov P, Valentine J (2005) Efficacy and safety of endoscopic balloon dilation of symptomatic upper and lower gastrointestinal Crohn's disease strictures. J Clin Gastroenterol 39(4):284–290
26. Camma C, Giunta M, Rosselli M et al (1997) 5-Aminosalicylic acid in the maintenance treatment of Crohn's disease: a meta-analysis adjusted for confounding variables. Gastroenterology 113:1465–1473
27. Lochs H, Mayer M, Fleig WE et al (2000) Prophylaxis of post-operative relapse in Crohn's disease with mesalamine: European Cooperative Crohn's Disease Study VI. Gastroenterology 118:264–273
28. Fallowfield LJ, Clark AW (1997) Delivering bad news in gastroenterology. Am J Gastroenterol 92:457–460

Interdisciplinary Management of Familial Adenomatous Polyposis

Michele Comberlato, Federico Martin

Introduction

Colorectal carcinoma (CRC) represents a clinical and epidemiological relevant illness due to problems of acquiring an early diagnosis and the fact that it is a major cause of mortality worldwide and accounts for nearly 4% of all deaths in Western countries [1, 2]. Nearly 90% of CRC is the final result of a step-by-step progression from the normal mucosa to adenomatous polyps and finally to dysplasia and adenocarcinoma. The biological evolution takes many years and should allow enough time for early diagnosis and therapy, as it is widely accepted that endoscopic/surgical polypectomy prevents the otherwise natural progression to carcinoma.

The two major forms of hereditary CRC, which are quite different, include the hereditary non-polyposis colorectal cancer (HNPCC) and the familial adenomatous polyposis (FAP), which represents 5–10% of the total number of cases of CRC. Familial adenomatous polyposis is a troublesome autosomal dominant disease that evolves quietly until clinical manifestations appear, which means that the development of innumerable adenomatous polyps start to develop at puberty and gradually increase their growth to involve the whole colon at adulthood. The management of FAP represents a challenge for gastroenterologists and surgeons in terms of history of the disease, evaluation of the clinical pattern, therapeutic options, follow up and chemoprevention of relapses.

History of the Disease

As mentioned before, FAP is a hereditary autosomal dominant disease and the responsible gene is the APC gene, a quite large gene located on chromosome 5q21, of which there are more than 1400 described mutations [3, 4]. The APC mutation is inherited as a germline mutation from the affected parent, but adenomas start their uncontrolled growth only when the second allele has mutated or is inactivated. The coded APC protein plays a critical role in the difficult balance between healthy and diseased cells, since it is responsible for tumour suppression, cellular proliferation, regular differentiation, migration and apoptosis [5].

This multifactorial regulation produces many extremely different clinical features and the main difficulty lies in relating a peculiar disease to a multifactorial genetic disease. Most likely, before the APC gene was identified, many syndromes were known: Turcot's syndrome (FAP, neoplasia of central nervous system); Gardner's syndrome (intestinal polyps, multiple osteomata, cysts, desmoid tumours, gastroduodenal polyps, mesenteric fibromatosis, lymphoid hyperplasia of the distal ileum, ileal adenomas and dental abnormalities); Cronkite-Canada syndrome (gastrointestinal polyps, skin hyperpigmentation, nail dystrophy and alopecia) and attenuated FAP (<100 intestinal polyps, primarily located in the right colon) [6, 7], which now simply reflect different locations of mutations along the gene.

A recent study in the UK examined 614 families recorded in six regional registries regarding polyposis and identified 111 family clusters as having neither the dominant transmission nor evidence of APC mutation. Molecular genetic tests showed the presence of a biallelic mutation in the MYH gene [8] in 25 families.

The MYH gene is responsible for base excision repair mechanisms and its mutations have been shown to produce an autosomal recessive trait expressed by multiple colorectal adenomas and related high risk of colorectal cancer [9,10]. Now we know that FAP can be transmitted not only as an autosomal dominant disease but also as an autosomal recessive trait, a situation that requires a change in how the physicians regard FAP, in genetic counselling, testing and surveillance.

Clinical Features

The core of the clinical and diagnostic problem is the nature of APC gene itself. The APC gene is a germline mutation, which means there is a wide possibility that the mutation will find expression not only in intestinal but also in extra-intestinal sites including the thyroid, pancreas and duodenum, adrenal glands and liver. Such variability in clinical manifestation of the same genetic disorder represents real problems for physicians in terms of the right initial diagnosis, therapeutic options, follow-up and need for accurate clinical surveillance of the relatives.

The classical intestinal syndrome has a specific and more or less severe pattern including intestinal bleeding, abdominal pain, diarrhoea, mucous discharge. A patient reporting these symptoms usually refers to the family doctor and then will be sent to a gastrointestinal unit for a visit or colonoscopy. What a surprise for the endoscopist and for the patient as well in discovering hundreds of polyps along the colon.

The presence of a hypercatabolic balance with weight loss, anaemia and intestinal obstruction makes the development of a neoplasia suspicious and approximately 25% of patients present colorectal cancer at first diagnosis [11]. Moreover, the risk of developing a CRC is directly related to the number of polyps [12]. The first point at this time is to be aware of the peculiar genetic pathology and of the wide display of clinical features and to create a task force involving all the needed specialists–the pathologist, the gastroenterologist, the surgeon, the radiologist and the geneticist–in the management of the patient.

While waiting for molecular genetic tests, which need months to be completed, the patient should undergo a full diagnostic program to detect or exclude other clinical relevant diseases, due to the wide clinical expression of the genetic alteration. Genetic testing is the sole and most efficient procedure for discovering gene carriers in a suspected FAP patient and in the relatives. Once a distinct mutation is recognised in a subject, the linkage analysis on chromosome 5 has an accuracy of 70–90% [13].

Screening colonoscopy in patients known as carriers of an APC mutation should start at the age of 10–12 years and in the risk population of 15 years of age, with colonoscopic follow up every year between 15–26 years of age, every second year from 26–35 years of age and then every 3 years [14]. In spite of the lack of a clear, validated diagnostic protocol, all patients should undergo an upper tract endoscopy with forward- and side-viewing instruments.

Duodenal polyps are found in the majority of polyposis patients and may lead to carcinoma development. An endoscopic and histological classification for the evaluation of the severity of duodenal adenomatosis was published in 1998 and has become the gold standard in several subsequent studies [15]. As in the colon, duodenal and ampullary polyps have to be resected, either endoscopically or surgically, and then regular scheduled follow-ups have to start, based on the histology of the removed polyps. Carcinoma of the duodenum, ampulla of Vater or pancreas have been strongly associated with Gardner's syndrome and a research at St. Mark's Hospital documented a 12% incidence of periampullary cancer in a series of patients 5 years after colonoscopy [16]. That means that every patient should undergo frequent upper gastrointestinal endoscopies yearly, a full clinical examination and many other examinations because of the risk of developing diseases in extra-colonic sites.

Mesenteric fibrosis and desmoid tumours are often severe complications of FAP with a reported incidence of 3.5–5.7% between 1 and 3 years after colectomy [17]. Desmoid tumours usually arise in the abdominal cavity, in the retroperitoneum or in the abdominal incision; extensive small bowel and urinary resections are often needed to resolve complications usually secondary to intestinal or vascular occlusion [18, 19]. Epidermal cysts are common benign findings, but seldom appear before puberty, so an early diagnosis could represent a warning for the physician to proceed with further evaluations for gastrointestinal polyps [20].

Sites for osteomas are typically found in the mandibula and skull and may be the only extracolonic manifestation of the disease [21, 22]. Annual examinations should screen the thyroid and liver because of the risk of neoplasia. Lastly, the presence of ocular alteration as asymptomatic pigmented fundic lesions are reported in more than 90% of FAP and Gardner's patients. The congenital hypertrophy of the retinal pigmented epithelium, when present in the relatives, is almost 100% predictive of FAP (Table 1) [6, 7].

So the familial adenomatous polyposis is much more than a disease of the bowel and a very close cooperation between different physicians is necessary to ensure that our patients receive the best chances for an early and correct diagnosis, the best possible management and an optimal follow-up.

Management

Up to now, surgery is the only effective therapy for removing all the polyps and preventing the inevitable progression to cancer. The general recommendation is that prophylactic colectomy is advisable by the late teens in patients with a sure diagnosis of FAP [5]. There are currently three surgical options including: (1) restorative proctocolectomy with ileal pouch anal anastomosis (RPC/IPAA) with mucosectomy, (2)

Table 1. FAP: associated benign and malign lesions (modified from [5])

Neoplastic lesions	Non-neoplastic lesions
Duodenal polyps/tumour (5–11%)	Osteomas
Pancreatic tumour (2%)	Desmoid tumours
Thyroid cancer (2%)	Duodenal, jejunal, ileal polyps
Brain, medulloblastoma (<1%)	Gastric adenomas
Hepatoblastoma (0.7% of children <5 years)	Ocular fundic lesions
	Epidermoid cysts
	Radiopaque jaw lesions

RPC/IPAA using the double staple technique and (3) colectomy with ileo-rectal anastomosis (IRA). A fourth option, a proctocolectomy with permanent ileostomy, can only be considered in the few cases in which an RPC/IPAA or an IRA is contraindicated.

An RPC/IPAA with mucosectomy has the advantage of removing the entire colon, that means all the polyps, and taking away the anal mucosa with minimal remaining risk of developing colorectal cancer. In spite of the obvious technical problems, restorative proctocolectomy with IPAA and mucosectomy has been the preferred approach at the Mayo Clinic with a low reported post-operative complication rate and satisfactory functional results [23, 24].

As a critical comment on these results, some authors argue that islands of rectal mucosa might be retained even with mucosectomy, in other words the risk of developing new polyps is reduced, but not eliminated [25, 26]. The alterative double-stapling technique performed at the Cleveland Clinic offers a better functional outcome, but also presents a 28% increase in the development of adenomas in the transitional zone [27].

A total colectomy with ileo-rectal anastomosis could offer better compliance, but needs a very careful surveillance program. It is usually offered to young patients with partial rectal sparing and less than 20 rectal polyps. As in other critical patient populations, like the IBD patients, surgical management should be tailored to the different patients.

A review at Mount Sinai Medical Center documented the rise of rectal cancer at a mean follow-up of 13 years in 25% of patients with ileo-rectal anastomosis. They concluded that proctocolectomy with ileo-anal pouch should be the preferred surgical option, which is in agreement with other authors [28, 29].

Medical Management

Prophylactic resection of target organs is usually performed as treatment for familial tumours. However, it should be preferable in preventing the development of tumours thereby ensuring a better functional result for the patient and a better quality of life. Although cancer prevention has been a matter of debate for many years, an effective and safe strategy has not yet been established. Since the first report by Kudo about the ability of indomethacin in preventing chemically induced colon cancer in rats [30], many authors reported the low incidence of CRC in people taking aspirin for a long time [31, 32]. In 1983, Waddell and Loughry observed a significant reduction in rectal polyps in four patients with FAP who took NSAIDs on a regular basis for pain relief [33].

Successive studies reported that sulindac decreases polyps in FAP and that cyclooxygenase 2 (COX-2), which is not expressed in normal mucosa, is largely expressed in colonic adenomas and cancerous tissue [34, 35] with a large amount of proneoplastic effects such as resistance to apoptosis via an increased level of the Bcl-2 protein [36], increased cell migration and invasion due to an over-expression of metalloproteinases [37] and increased levels of angiogenic factors [38].

This data promoted a lot of interest about the therapeutic use of the new generation of the COX-2 inhibitors, which are more effective and clinically safer in comparison with other NSAIDS. Recent studies have noted the role of the COX-2 inhibitors presenting evidence of its abilities in reducing the amount and size of polyps, preventing the occurrence/recurrence of colorectal adenomas and cancer and counter-regulating angiogenesis in CRC liver metastases [39-41]. Therefore, once the efficacy of the COX-2 inhibitors is verified, what then should be the role of medical therapy in this complex disease?

There is no doubt about the supremacy of surgery as the only effective option for treating patients with FAP in a radical way. However, considering the risk of tumour should the relatives be diagnosed as carriers of a high-risk mutation, and the risk of new adenomas in the rectum should an ileo-rectal anastomoses be performed, anti-COX-2 drugs represent a good therapeutic option, but clinical data do not authorise their wide use outside of clinical trials.

In spite of all that, the efficacy shown in previous studies using sulindac was not confirmed and the National Cancer Institute in the United States is currently enrolling patients with FAP for a new clinical study of a combination therapy with celecoxib, eflorinithine (an ornithine decarboxylase inhibitor) or a placebo [42].

Surveillance Protocol

As far as the post-surgical surveillance program is concerned, there are no approved guide lines, so the following considerations are based on data taken from the literature.

Ileo-Rectal Anastomosis

In patients not protected by prophylactic therapy or by a surveillance program, the incidence of cancer is 7% and 23–37% after 10 and 20 years respectively, with a risk of secondary proctectomy at 70% 40 years after initial surgery [43]. An endoscopy should be performed 6 months after surgery and then every year, and every single polyp should be resected or destroyed with laser or APC coagulation.

Ileo-Anal Anastomosis

Data from literature report a 13 and 50% persistence of residual rectal mucosa in manual and mechanical anastomosis, respectively [44], with an ongoing risk for new adenomas and cancer also in the pouch where polyps can arise in 30–60% of patients, in relation to the endoscopic technique with or without staining [45]. As in other fields, the literature in this field also lacks validated data and in our opinion we confirm the above recommendations about ileo-rectal anastomosis.

Upper Digestive Tract and Small Bowel

As mentioned before, adenomas can also develop in the upper digestive tract and the general risk of an adenocarcinoma developing in these sites is 300 times higher than in the general population. Surveillance should start very early in life at 20 years, and full endoscopic examination has to be performed at an interval of 6 months to 1 year, depending on the amount of polyposis. Exams should be performed with forward and side-view instruments in an attempt to enhance the diagnostic power, and with a liberal use of endoscopic staining.

The Spiegelman's classification has defined four stages according to the number of polyps, size, histological pattern (tubular or villous) and degree of dysplasia [15]. The presence of multiple small adenomas is not an indication for therapy, but the development of invasive cancer in the submucosa indicates a clear need for surgical resection. Because of the variety of clinical patterns of the disease, which causes over 500 000 deaths annually all over the world, looking at FAP is like looking in a kaleidoscope. The key to the problem is to better understand the complex mechanisms that promote colon carcinogenesis so that we can better target the diagnostic and therapeutic protocols.

References

1. Peek RM Jr (2004) Prevention of colorectal cancer through the use of COX-2 selective inhibitors. Cancer Chemoter Pharmacol 54(S1):S50–S56
2. Micheli A, Mugno E, Krogh V et al (2002) Cancer prevalence in European registry areas. Ann Oncol 13:840–845
3. Kinzler KW, Nilbert MC, Su LK et al (1991) Identification of FAP locus genes from chromosome 5q21. Science 253(5020):661–665
4. Nishisho I, Nakamura Y, Miyoshi Y et al (1991) Mutations of chromosome 5q21 genes in FAP and colorectal cancer patients. Science 253(5020):665–669
5. Nandakumar G, Morgan JA, Silverberg D et al (2004) Familial polyposis coli: clinical manifestations, evaluation, management and treatment. Mount Sinai J Med 71(6):384–391
6. Boardman LA (2002) Heritable colorectal cancer syndromes: recognition and preventive management. Gastroenterol Clin North Am 31(4):1107–1131
7. Cruz-Correa M, Giardiello FM (2002) Diagnosis and management of hereditary colon cancer. Gastroenterol Clin North Am 31(2):537–549
8. Sampson JR, Dolwani S, Jones S et al (2003) Autosomal recessive colorectal adenomatous polyposis due to inherited mutations of MYH. Lancet 362(9377):39–41
9. Al-Tassan N, Chmiel NH, Maynard J et al (2002) Inherited variants of MYH associated with somatic G:C→T:A mutations in colorectal tumors. Nature Genet 30:227–232
10. Jones S, Emmerson P, Maynard J et al (2002) Biallelic germline mutations in MYH predispose to multiple colorectal adenomas and somatic G:C→T:A mutations. Hum Mol Genet 11:2961–2967
11. Lynch HT, de la Chapelle A (2003) Hereditary colorectal cancer. NEJM 348(10):919–932
12. Debinsky HS, Love S, Spigelman AD et al (1996) Colorectal polyp counts and cancer risk in familial adenomatous polyposis. Gastroenterology 110(4):1028–1030
13. Cromwell DM, Moore RD, Brensinger JD et al (1998) Cost analysis of alternative approaches to colorectal screening in familial adenomatous polyposis. Gastroenterology 114:893–901
14. Powell SM, Petersen GM, Krush AJ et al (1993) Molec-

ular diagnosis of familial adenomatous polyposis. NEJM 329:1982–1987
15. Spigelman AD, Williams CB, Talbot IC et al (1989) Upper gastrointestinal cancer in patients with familial adenomatous polyposis. Lancet 2:783–785
16. Corman LM (1998) Colon and rectal surgery. Lippincott-Raven, Philadelphia, PA, USA
17. Smith WG (1959) Desmoid tumors in familial multiple polyposis. Mayo Clinic Proc 34:31–38
18. Gurbuz AK, Giardiello FM, Petersen GM et al (1994) Desmoid tumors in familial adenomatous polyposis. Gut 35(3):377–381
19. Jones IT, Jagelman DG, Fazio VW et al (1986) Desmoid tumors in familial polyposis coli. Ann Surg 204(1): 94–97
20. Leppard B (1974) Epidermoid cysts and polyposis coli. Proc R Soc Med 67:1036–1037
21. Utsunomiya J, Nakamura T (1975) The occult osteomatous changes in the mandible in patients with familial polyposis coli. Br J Surg 62:45–51
22. Watne AL, Core SK, Carrier JM (1975) Gardner's syndrome. Surg Gynecol Obstet 141:53–56
23. Nyam DC, Brillant PT, Dozois RR et al (1997) Ileal pouch-anal canal anastomosis for familial adenomatous polyposis: early and late results. Ann Surg 226(4):514–521
24. Parc YR, Moslein G, Dozois RR et al (2000) Familial adenomatous polyposis: results following ileal pouch-anal anastomosis in teenagers. Dis Colon Rectum 43(7):893–902
25. Church J, Simmang C (2003) Practice parameters for the treatment of patients with dominantly inherited colorectal cancer (familial adenomatous polyposis and hereditary nonpolyposis colorectal cancer). Dis Colon Rectum 46:1001–1012
26. Remzi FH, Church JM, Bast J et al (2001) Mucosectomy vs. stapled ileal pouch-anal anastomosis in patients with familial adenomatous polyposis: functional outcome and neoplasia control. Dis Colon Rectum 44:1590–1596
27. Fazio VW, Tjandra JJ (1994) Transanal mucosectomy: ileal pouch advancement for anorectal dysplasia or inflammation after restorative proctocolectomy. Dis Colon Rectum 37:1008–1011
28. Yang YS, Steinhagen RM, Heimann TM (1997) Colorectal cancer in familial adenomatous polyposis. Dis Colon Rectum 40:312–316
29. Tonelli F, Valanzano R, Monaci I et al (1997) Restorative proctocolectomy or rectum preserving surgery in patients with familial adenomatous polyposis: results of a prospective study. World J Surg 21(6):653–659
30. Kudo T, Narisawa T, Abo S (1980) Antitumor activity of indomethacin on ethylazoxymethanol-induced large bowel tumors in rats. Gann 71:260–264
31. Suh O, Mettlin C, Petrelli NJ (1993) Aspirin use, cancer and polyps of the large bowel. Cancer 72:1171–1177
32. Giovannucci E, Rimm EB, Stampfer MJ et al (1994) Aspirin use and the risk for colorectal cancer and adenoma in male health professionals. Ann Intern Med 121:241–246
33. Waddell WR, Loughry RW (1983) Sulindac for polyposis of the colon. J Surg Oncol 24:83–87
34. Kargman SL, O'Neil GP, Vickers PJ et al (1995) Expression of prostaglandin G/H synthase-1 and -2 protein in human colon cancer. Cancer Res 55:25–56
35. Sano H, Kawahito Y, Wilder RL et al (1995) Expression of cycloxygenase-1 and -2 in human colorectal cancer. Cancer Res 55:3785
36. Tsujii M, DuBois RN (1995) Alterations in cellular adhesion and apoptosis in epithelial cells overexpressing prostaglandin endoperoxide synthase 2. Cell 83:493
37. Tsujii M, Kawano S, DuBois RN (1997) Cyclooxygenase-2 expression in human colon cancer cells increases metastatic potential. Proc Natl Acad Sci USA 94:3336
38. Tsujii M, Kawano Tsujii S et val (1998) Cyclooxygenase regulates angiogenesis induced by colon cancer calls. Cell 93:705
39. Fenwick SW, Toogood GJ Lodge JP et al (2003) The effect of the selective cyclooxygenase-2 inhibitor rofecoxib on human colorectal cancer liver metastases. Gastroeterology 125:716–720
40. Rahme E, Barkun AN, Toubouti Y et al (2003) The cyclooxygenase-2 selective inhibitors rofecoxib and celecoxib prevent colorectal neoplasia occurrence and recurrence. Gastroenterology 125:404–408
41. Steinbach G, Lynch PM, Phillips RK et al (2000) The effect of celecoxib, a cyclooxygenase-2 inhibitor in familial adenomatous polyposis. NEJM 342:1946–1950
42. Lynch P (2004) Colorectal cancer prevention study in people with familial adenomatous polyposis. http://cancer.gov/clinicaltrials/ft-MDA-ID-0091
43. Saurin JC, Napoleon B, Gay G et al (2005) Endoscopic management of patients with familial adenomatous polyposis (FAP) following a colectomy. Endoscopy 37(5):499–501
44. O'Connell PR, Pemberton JH, Kelly KA (1987) Motor function of the ileal J pouch and its relation to clinical outcome after ileal pouch-anal anastomosis. World J Surg 11:735–741
45. Nugent KP, Spigelman AD, Nicholls RJ et al (1993) Pouch adenomas in patients with familial adenomatous polyposis. Br J Surg 80:1620–1624

Ileoanal Pouches and Indeterminate Colitis

Gilberto Poggioli, Silvio Laureti, Filippo Pierangeli, Federica Ugolini, Maurizio Coscia, Lorenzo Gentilini, Piero Bazzi

Introduction

Indeterminate colitis (IC) is a definition first proposed by Kent in 1970 [1] for some features of both ulcerative colitis (UC) and Crohn's Disease (CD) found in patients' colonic surgical specimen. Some years later, Morson [2] proposed the term "unclassified colitis", describing surgical specimen of patients operated for acute fulminant colitis with suspicion of CD or UC but equivocal pathology. Thus, originally, the term IC was a pure histopathologic diagnosis. It would still probably represent a strictly academic argument if total proctocolectomy with ileal pouch-anal anastomosis (IPAA) did not obtain such a wide popularity for the treatment of UC.

The need for preoperative differential diagnosis between UC and CD is essential to the surgeon since different surgical procedures are indicated in the two entities. In fact, patients with CD submitted to IPAA appear to have a significantly higher rate of pouch failure and long-term complications than those with UC. In recent years, the term IC has become a clinicopathologic diagnosis, and it has been applied to include all those cases with endoscopic, radiographic and histologic signs of inflammatory bowel disease (IBD) confined to the colon but "without fulfillment of diagnostic criteria for UC and CD" [3]. Many reports show how, despite many clinical investigations performed by expert teams, a considerable rate of IC patients continue to be classified as IC after long-term follow-up [4–7]. It is still not clear, then, whether IC is only a temporary diagnosis, a kind of "colitis in evolution" [8], or represents itself a disease entity.

Incidence

Stewenius et al. [9] found an annual incidence of 1.6 cases per 100,000 population compared with 7.3 of cases of UC. Another recent epidemiological study [10], considering patients submitted or not to surgical treatment, showed an annual incidence of IC of up to 2.4 per 100,000 population, which means about a 20% incidence. This rate seems to be too high and confirms how assessment depends on diagnostic accuracy and the parameters on which it is measured. In fact, Price [11], who considered only pathological features of the resected specimens in patients submitted to colectomy and identifying IC when a firm diagnosis of either UC or CD could not be made, found a 10% incidence of IC. Similarly, Lee [12] found IC in 16% of urgent colectomy specimens. However, this number decreases by half when clinical features, serologic data, radiologic and endoscopic features are taken into account [8]. In addition, other factors may contribute to the variation in the incidence of IC, such as interobserver variation in histological interpretation, making diagnosis on the surgical specimen with or without follow-up, basing diagnosis on endoscopic biopsy and not on the colectomy specimen.

Diagnosis

Histology

There are a number of exceptions to the classic principles of IBD pathology that may lead to diagnostic confusion [13]. Difficulty in distinguishing UC from CD, which leads to a diagnosis of IC, can be related to the presence of fulminant or refractory colitis, chronic colitis, prolonged medical treatment and earliest stages of colitis. The most frequent scenario is fulminant or refractory colitis requiring urgent colectomy. In this case, the histologic distinction of UC from CD is difficult because of histologic feature overlap. Granulomas and transmural lymphoid hyperplasia are the two most specific indicators of CD in specimens from patients with fulminant colitis. Relative rectal sparing, intermittent ulceration, regular glandular pattern and lack of mucin depletion [3], which are usually typical of CD, can be found in IC cases subsequently proved to be UC [11]. Even superficial fissuring-type ulcers may be present in patients with fulminant colitis and should not lead to a diagnosis of IC or CD [14].

Medical treatment can deeply modify the mucosal histology with a variable effect depending on time and type of treatment and disease severity. Usually, patchiness of disease can be found in patients treated with long-term oral or topical therapy (i.e. sulphasalazine) [13, 15]. Focal healing, including rectal healing, can be observed in all forms of treatment. Finally, patchiness of the disease or rectal sparing can be present in the early stages of the disease, especially in children [16, 17].

Clinical Features

Data in the literature on clinical features of IC are scarce. The ratio of male to female patients is usually close to 1 while in UC there is a prevalence of males [18]. Geboes [3] reports a more severe clinical course in patients with IC, with pronounced need for immunosuppressives and higher risk of colectomy and colon cancer compared with definite UC. Different data are reported by Meucci et al. [6], who examined symptoms of 50 patients with IC at disease onset and found no specific feature. Specifically, diarrhoea, abdominal cramps and hematochesia were similar to other IBDs while incidence of weight loss and fever resulted more frequently in IC than UC. Gender, age, smoking and extraintestinal manifestations were similar and not significantly different between patients with UC and CD. However, multivariate analysis showed how some features, specifically fever, segmental colitis, presence of extraintestinal disease, rectal sparing and smoking habitus was significantly predictive for final diagnosis of CD. Finally, the occurrence of pouch-anal fistulae, which represents the most important issue, will be discussed below, describing how this scenario can determine failure or success of surgical treatment.

Serological Markers

Identification of perinuclear antineutrophil cytoplasmic antibodies (pANCA) and anti-Saccharomyces cerevisiae antibodies (ASCA) antibodies, which present quite good specificity for UC and CD, initially suggested how their combined screening could better characterise patients with IC [19, 20]. However, their sensitivity is limited to 40–60% so that their value in the clinical practice is still controversial. Peeters et al. [21] found in 28 patients with IC an intermediate frequency of pANCA and ASCA. In these patients with high prevalence of both antibodies, combination of results showed and high predictive value, and the authors concluded that ASCA+/pANCA- predicts CD in 80% of patients with IC and that ASCA-/pANCA+ predicts UC in 63.6%. Interestingly, 48.5% of patients do not show antibodies against ASCA or pANCA. Most of these patients remain diagnosed with IC during their further clinical course, "perhaps reflecting a distinct clinicoserological entity". Similar results have been reported by a large prospective study [7]. Recently, Hui et al. [22] showed a significant relation between high expression of antibodies [defined as positive antibody reactivity profile (ARP)] before ileal pouch-anal anastomosis and chronic pouchitis after surgery. The authors suggest that in patients with positive ARP, aggressive traditional or experimental medication should be considered to avoid surgery due to the higher risk of chronic pouchitis or CD postsurgical development

Imaging

Unfortunately, there are no particular diagnostic radiological features of IC. In fact, even if the classic radiographic features of CD and UC are well known, some cases cannot be diagnosed since usually they present a combination of features found both in UC and CD. Recently, magnetic resonance spectroscopy (1H MR) has been showed to have a strong potential for diagnosis of IC [23]. The procedure was used on 76 colon mucosal biopsies, and only one case of CD was misclassified. However, since other studies failed to show the same encouraging results, further studies are needed for substantiation. Wireless capsule endoscopy could be a valuable diagnostic tool in patients with suspected CD that has not been confirmed using standard imaging techniques [24]. Mow et al. [25], in a recent study, reported that 18 out of 22 patients evaluated for medically refractory UC or IC were found to have small-bowel lesions and ultimately diagnosed with CD. However, as reported above, the significance of finding few small bowel lesions in patients with UC is still not clear.

Treatment

Treatment of IC is still controversial; in fact, due to its relative infrequency, there are no controlled prospective studies based on large series that could indicate the most appropriate therapeutic options.

Medical Treatment

The current medical therapy for IC is substantially the same, which is usually utilised for UC and CD. In particular, therapy utilises anti-inflammatories drugs (mostly mesalazine with selective colonic release), steroids and immunosuppressives and varies on the basis of disease activity. Black et al. [26] recently evaluated the effectiveness of infliximab in 20 patients with severe, medically refractory IC. Fourteen patients showed complete response, two partial response and four no response. Non-responders underwent ileal pouch-anal anastomosis, and in all cases, surgical specimen was consistent with UC even if two were subsequently reclassified as having CD. Among the remaining patients, eight were diagnosed as having CD and eight UC after long-term follow-up. No significant differences were reported in terms of response to therapy based on diagnosis. Treatment with infliximab could then represent an effective option for patients with refractory IC who are likely to undergo surgery, offering prolonged follow-up time in order to obtain a more definite diagnosis.

Surgical Treatment

Accurate diagnosis of UC and CD has major implications on the choice of surgical treatment and long-term prognosis. The controversial issue of IC has become fundamental in the so-called pouch era. The need to obtain a differential diagnosis rises from the data widely accepted that ileoanal anastomosis should be contraindicated in patients with Crohn's colitis. Panis et al. [27] reported a 10% rate of pouch failure in highly selected patients with confirmed preoperative diagnosis of CD. It has to be highlighted that none of these patients had a history of anal lesions or small-bowel involvement. However, most series reported in the literature show poor outcomes after IPAA in CD patients [28–30]. Keighley [31] found a 52% rate of pouch failure in patients with CD. Mylonakis [32], analysing patients with CD submitted to IPAA and IRA, reported 47.8% of pouch excision compared with 8% of rectal excision, respectively. Similarly, Brown et al. [33] reported a 56% rate of pouch failure in CD patients compared with 6% UC and 10% IC patients. Fazio et al. [34] reported that more than 50% of patients who developed late perianal fistulas after IPAA suffer from CD. On the other hand, Sagar et al. [29] found a 53% failure rate in patients with preoperative diagnosis of CD versus 41% in those with postoperative diagnosis.

Concerns are raised based on the assumption, not widely accepted, that IC might present with a clinical course comparable with Crohn's colitis or, at least, imply a significant risk of evolution of Crohn's colitis. In fact, many Authors describe significantly higher rates of complications and failure in IC patients compared with UC so that, in their opinion, IPAA should be contraindicated in cases without a firm preoperative diagnosis. Considering IC as an evolutionary diagnosis with a significant risk of change into CD, Marcello et al. [35] advise some caution in offering IPAA procedure in patient with IC until a certain diagnosis is obtained. They reported an incidence of perianal complications and pouch failure of 23% and 2%, respectively, in patients with UC; 44% and 12%, respectively, in IC patients and 63% and 37% in patients with CD. In addition, only 3% of UC patients where successively diagnosed as having CD compared with 13% of IC patients. Other reports confirm these data [36–39], with rates of perianal complications significantly higher in IC (30–50% vs 3–20%) and consequent higher risk of failure (19–28% vs 0.4–8%, respectively). Gramlich et al. [40] found a ten-times more frequent incidence of pelvic sepsis after IPAA in IC versus UC patients. Odze [13] reported that about 20% of IC patients develop severe septic pouch complications compared with 10% in UC and 40% in CD. On the other hand, many authors [8, 28, 30, 41–43] do not confirm these trends and suggest that there is no significantly increased risk in constructing a pouch-anal anastomosis in IC patients compared with UC patients. Yu et al. [44], from the Mayo Clinic group, in a large series of 1,437 patients with UC and 82 with IC, reported higher rates of pouch-related complications in the IC group; however, 15% of IC patients, after long-term follow-up, had their diagnosis changed to CD. When CD patients where considered in a separate group, complication rates and functional outcome were similar in the remaining IC and UC patients.

The presence of these conflicting results in the literature could be related to how IC is defined. In fact, when diagnosis of IC is founded only on the pathological appearance of the colectomy specimen, the incidence of complications is increased in IC compared with UC. Otherwise, if diagnosis is made taking into account all available clinical data, incidence of complications and failure rates are similar in the two groups. Since the surgeon might face this controversial dilemma at different times during the patient's clinical history, it is important to select the safest surgical approach. From the practical point of view, the problem is relatively insignificant in patients with fulminant colitis. In fact, these patients must be treated similarly to UC patients, with total abdominal colectomy and Hartmann's pouch. Histologic examination of the specimen will probably provide more accurate information.

Another favourable scenario occurs when suspicion of IC or CD is raised prior to surgical procedure, after mucosal biopsy or due to the occurrence of perianal lesions. The latter, although up to 5% of UC patients present with perianal disease, should be considered an alarming sign since it might represent a revealing symptom of CD. In this condition, it seems more appropriate to submit patients to repeated biopsies (endoscopic and of the fistula tract), small-bowel instrumental evaluation and careful inspection of intestinal loops at surgery. If the suspicion is consistent with CD, it is indicated to proceed to total abdominal colectomy only. Moreover, some authors observed a significantly higher risk of postoperative anastomotic leak in patients with perianal lesions (21% vs 11.4%, respectively) [45].

The most important scenario is represented by long-term follow-up of pouch-anal anastomosis in IC patients. As highlighted above, data reported in the literature are still controversial. Our experience consist of 514 patients submitted to IPAA: 427(83%) had UC, 34 (7%) IC and 51 (10%) familial adenomatous polyposis (FAP). Among patients with IC, ten (29.4%) were successively diagnosed as having CD. Incidence of pelvic sepsis was 8.7% in UC patients and 3.8% in IC patients. Incidence of abdominal sepsis was 3.0% in UC and 7.7% in IC. Five out of ten patients (50%) with subsequent diagnosis of CD had their pouch excised for multiple pouch fistulae compared with UC patients (1.8%) who were submitted to pouch excision for postsurgical chronic sepsis. Two patients refused excision, but their loop ileostomy has to be considered as definitive (Fig. 1).

Among late complications, the cumulative incidence of pouchitis was 28% and resulted in an increase in patients with IC (52.7%) and CD (50%). Late pouch-anal or pouch-vaginal fistulae occurred in 31 cases (6.0%). Only two of the 19 patients with pouch-anal fistula had CD while four among 12 with pouch-vaginal fistulae had IC (Table 1).

We then classified idiopathic colitis submitted to IPAA as UC, CD and IC. Among the last group, we classified three different subgroups (modified from Wells) [8]. The first group consisted of all cases in which diagnosis was impossible: IC "tout court". Another group consisted of colitises not clearly definable as UC but more easily assimilable to them: IC "probable UC". The last group consisted of indeterminate "probable CD", including colitises not clearly identifiable as CD but presenting features that could resemble it. Therefore, the original 34 IC cases resulted in 23 cases of IC not ulteriorly specified, which we called "true" IC. Five cases resulted IC "probable UC" and six cases IC "probable CD". Finally, a careful retrospective examination of the surgical specimen combined with clinical history of the 23 patients with "true" IC allowed us to extrapolate four more cases of confirmed CD.

Clinical outcome of patients with IC varies. IC and the indeterminate forms "probable UC" have an absolutely similar outcome to UC. Out of the ten patients with sure CD, five were submitted to demolition of the reservoir for disease recurrence. The other five are in good health although one reported recurrent episodes of pouchitis. Finally, patients with IC "probable CD" have an acceptable outcome although the incidence of pouchitis seems to be higher. Dayton et al. [41] reported that patients with IC "probable CD" present a significantly higher risk of pouch excision compared with those with "true" IC and IC "probable UC". Similarly, Tekkis et al. [46] found an increased risk of failure in CD or IC favouring CD patients (57.5% vs 11.5% in UC or IC favouring UC).

We can conclude that "true" IC and IC "probable UC" can be treated similarly to patients with certain

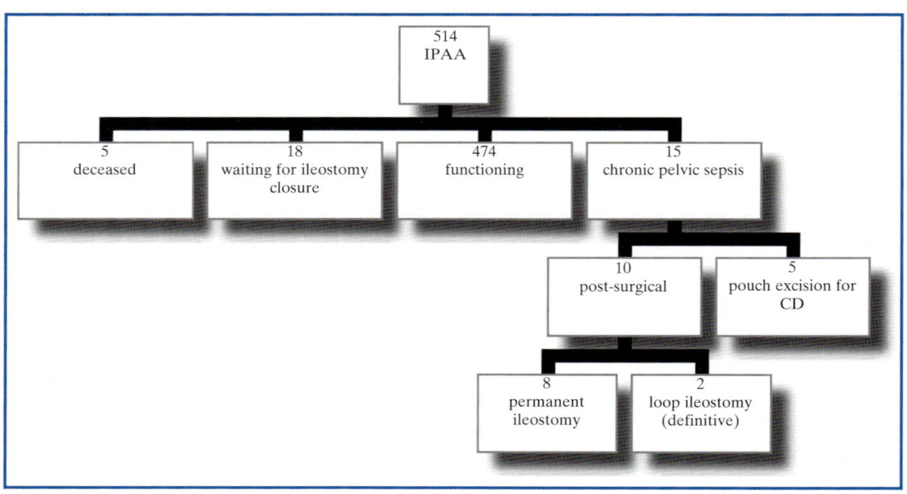

Fig. 1. Long-term follow-up

Table 1. Late complications

	Ulcerative colitis	Indeterminate colitis	Crohn's disease
Pouchitis	32%	52.7%	50%
Pouch excision	1.8%	0	50%
Pelvic sepsis	8.7%	3.8%	
Abdominal sepsis	3.0%	7.7%	

UC diagnosis. Moreover, preoperative diagnosis of CD represents in our opinion a contraindication to IPAA although long-term results in our series are satisfactory in almost 50% of these cases. Finally, when preoperative diagnosis of IC "probable CD" is made, total abdominal colectomy is advisable, and if the histologic evaluation of the specimen confirms such diagnosis, it is worthwhile to wait at least 2 years then proceed to IPAA only in those cases where no signs of small-bowel disease occurred during the follow-up.

Analysis of our personal experience leads us to some considerations:

We believe that the development of late pouch-anal or pouch-vaginal fistulae does not necessarily indicate CD, unlike some authors who believe it is reasonable to classify patients with pouch fistula as CD [35, 47, 48].

The diagnosis of IC does not necessarily mean evolution to CD and worse outcome.

Conclusions

Correct diagnosis of IC has become essential in the "pouch era" for the good outcome of patients submitted to IPAA.

Patients with IC have an increased risk of emergency colectomy. It is still not clear whether this is related to a more aggressive natural history of IC or if the certain diagnosis of IC is more difficult in case of emergency colectomy.

From the practical point of view, one of the most important issues is represented by diagnosis of IC in the surgical specimen; the pathologists should provide a "likelihood" diagnosis in order to help the surgeon's decision-making process. Moreover, this "likelihood" diagnosis is confirmed in many papers by the long-term follow-up in many series.

Late complications of IPAA are represented mainly by small-bowel stenosis or fistula and pouch-anal or pouch-vaginal fistulae. Only the first are pathognomonic of mislead CD while the occurrence of anal fistulae not necessarily indicate evolution to CD.

References

1. Kent Th, Ammon Rk, Den Besten L (1970) Differentiation of ulcerative colitis and regional enteritis. Arch Pathol 89:20–29
2. Morson BC (1974) Colitis unclassified. In: Morson BC, Dawson IMP (eds) Gastrointestinal pathology. Blackwell, Oxford, pp 485–486
3. Geboes K, De Hertogh G (2003) Indeterminate colitis. Inflamm Bowel Dis 9:324–331
4. Hildebrand H, Brydolf M, Holmquist L et al (1994) Incidence and prevalence of IBD in children in South Western Sweden. Acta Pediatr 83:640–645
5. Moum B, Vatn MH, Ekbom A et al (1996) Incidence of Ulcerative Colitis and indeterminate colitis in four counties of South Western Norway. 1990–93: a prospective population-based study. Scand J Gastroenterol 31:362–366
6. Meucci G, Bortoli A, Riccioli FA et al (1999) Frequency and clinical evolution of indeterminate colitis: a retrospective multicenter study in Northern Italy. Eur J Gastroenterol Hepatol 11:909–913
7. Joossens S, Reinish W, Vermeire S et al (2002) The value of anti-saccharomyces cerevisiae antibodies (ASCA) and perinuclear anti-neutrophil cytoplasmic antibodies in indeterminate colitis: a prospective follow-up study. Gastroentrology 122:1242–1247
8. Wells Ad, Mcmillan I, Price Ab et al (1991) Natural history of indeterminate colitis. Br J Surg 78:179–181
9. Stewenius J, Adnerhill I, Ekelund G et al (1995) Ulcerative colitis and indeterminate colitis in the city of Malmo, Sweden. A 25-year incidence study. Scand J Gastroenterol 30(1):38–43
10. Burakoff R (2004) Indeterminate colitis: clinical spectrum of disease. J Clin Gastroenterol 38(Suppl 5):41–43
11. Price AB (1978) Overlap in the spectrum of non-specific inflammatory bowel diseases – "colitis indeterminate". J Clin Pathol 31:567–577
12. Lee KS, Medline A, Shockey S et al (1979) Indeterminate colitis in the spectrum of inflammatory bowel disease. Arch Pathol Lab Med 103:173–176
13. Odze R (2003) Diagnostic problems and advances in inflammatory bowel disease. Mod Pathol 16:347–358
14. Yantiss RK, Farraye FA, O'Brien MJ et al (2006) Prognostic significance of superficial fissuring ulceration in patients with severe "indeterminate" colitis. Am J Surg Pathol 30:165–170
15. Robert ME, Skacel M, Ullman T et al (2004) Patterns of

colonic involvement at initial presentation in ulcerative colitis: a retrospective study of 46 newly diagnosed cases. Am J Clin Pathol 122(1):94–99
16. Washington K, Greenson JK, Montgomery E et al (2002) Histopathology of Ulcerative COlitis in initial rectal biopsy in children. Am J Surg Pathos 26:1441–1449
17. Tang LH, Reyes-Mugica M, Hao L et al (2000) Histologic difference between children and adults presenting with ulcerative colitis. Mod Pathol 14:96A
18. Ekbom A (2000) Indeterminate IBD: the magnitude of the problem. Inflamm Bowel Dis 6:S14–S15
19. Quinton JF, Sendid B, Reumaux D et al (1998) Anti-saccharomyces cerevisiae mannan antibodies combined with anti-neutrophil cytoplasmic auto-antibodies in inflammatory bowel disease: prevalence and diagnostic role. Gut 42:788–791
20. Zachos M, Reumaux D, Critch J et al (2001) utility of ASCA and ANCA in pediatric colitis. J Pediatr Gastroenterol Nutr 33:378–381
21. Peeters M, Joossens S, Vermeire S et al (2001) Diagnostic value of anti-saccharomyces cerevisiae and anti-neutrophil cytoplasmic antibodies in inflammatory bowel disease. Am J Gastroenterol 96:730–734
22. Hui T, Landers C, Vasiliauskas E et al (2005) Serologic responses in indeterminate colitis patients before ileal pouch-anal anastomosis may determine those at risk for continuous pouch inflammation. Dis Colon Rectum 48:1254–1262
23. Bezabeh T, Somoryai RL, Smith IC et al (2001) The use of 1 H magnetic resonance spectroscopy in inflammatory bowel diseases: distinguishing ulcerative colitis from Crohn's disease. Am J Gastroenterol 96:442–448
24. Costamagna G, Shah SK, Riccioni ME et al (2002) A prospective trial comparing small bowel radiographs and video capsule endoscopy for suspected small bowel disease. Gastroenterol 123:999–1005
25. Mow WS, LO SK, Targan SR et al (2004) Initial experience with wireless capsule enteroscopy in the diagnosis and management of inflammatory bowel disease. Clin Gastroenterol Hepathol 2:31–40
26. Black APB, Bhayani H, Ryder CAJ et al (2004) Infliximab in the treatment of medically refractory indeterminate colitis. Aliment Pharmacol Ther 18:741–748
27. Panis Y, Poupard B, Nemeth J et al (1996) Ileal pouch/anal anastomosis for Crohn's disease. Lancet 347:854–857
28. Deutsch AA, Mc Leod RS, Cullen J et al (1991) Results of the pelvic pouch procedure in patients with Crohn's disease. Dis Colon Rectum 34:475–477
29. Sagar PM, Dozois RR, Wolff BG (1996) Long-term results of ileal pouch-anal anastomosis in patients with Crohn's disease. Dis Colon Rectum 39:893–898
30. Hyman NH, Fazio VW, Tuckson WB et al (1991) Consequences of ileal pouch-anal anastomosis for Crohn's Disease. Dis Colon Rectum 34:653–657
31. Keighley MR (2000) The final diagnosis in pouch patients for presumed Ulcerative Colitis may change to Crohn's disease: patients should be warned of the consequences. Acta Chir Jugosl 47:27–31
32. Mylonakis E, Allan RN, Keighley MR (2001) How does pouch construction for a final diagnosis of Crohn's disease compare with ileoproctostomy for established Crohn's proctocolitis? Dis Colon Rectum 44(8):1137–1142; discussion 1142–1143
33. Brown CJ, MacLean AR, Cohen Z et al (2005) Crohn's disease and indeterminate colitis and the ileal pouch-anal anastomosis: outcome and patterns of failure. Dis Colon Rectum 48:1542–1549
34. Fazio VW, Wu JS, Lavery IC (1998) Repeat ileal pouch-anal anastomosis to salvage septic complications of pelvic pouches: clinical outcome and quality of life assessment. Ann Surg 228:588–597
35. Marcello P, Schoetz DJ Jr, Roberts PL et al (1997) Evolutionary changes in the pathologic diagnosis after the ileoanal pouch procedure. Dis Colon Rectum 40:263–269
36. Koltun WA, Schoetz DJ Jr, Roberts PL et al (1991) Indeterminate colitis predisposes to perineal complications after ileal pouch-anal anastomosis. Dis Colon Rectum 34:857–860
37. Mc Intyre PB, Pemberton JH, Wolff BG et al (1995) Indeterminate colitis: long-term in patients after ileal pouch-anal anastomosis. Dis Colon Rectum 38:51–54
38. Atkinson KG, Owen DA, Wankling G (1994) Restorative proctocolectomy and indeterminate colitis. Am J Surg 167:516–518
39. Grobler SP, Hosie KB, Affie E et al (1993) Outcome of restorative proctocolectomy when the diagnosis is suggestive of Crohn's disease. Gut 34(10):1384–1388
40. Gramlich T, Delaney CP, Lynch AC et al (2003) Pathological subgroups may predict complications but not late failure after ileal pouch-anal anastomosis for indeterminate colitis. Colorectal Dis 5:315–319
41. Dayton MT, Larsen KR, Christiansen DD (2002) Similar functional results and complications after ileal pouch-anal anastomosis in patients with indeterminate vs ulcerative colitis. Arch Surg 137:690–695
42. Rudolph WG, Uthoff SMS, McAuliffe TL et al (2002) Indeterminate colitis: the real story. Dis Colon Rectum 45:1528–1534
43. Pishori T, Dinnewitzer A, Zmora O et al (2004) Outcome of patients with indeterminate colitis undergoing a double-stapled ileal pouch-anal anastomosis. Dis Colon Rectum 47:717–721
44. Yu CS, Pemberton JH, Larson MS (1999) Ileal pouch-anal anastomosis in patients with indeterminate colitis: long-term results. Oral Presentation at the 85th ACS Clinical Congress, San Francisco, CA
45. Richard CS, Cohen Z, Stern HS et al (1997) Outcome of the pelvic pouch procedure in patients with prior perianal disease. Dis Colon Rectum 40:647–652
46. Tekkis PP, Heriot AG, Smith O et al (2005) Long-term outcomes of restorative proctocolectomy for Crohn's disease and indeterminate colitis. Colorectal Dis 7:218–223
47. Colombel JF, Ricart E, Loftus EV et al (2003) Management of Crohn's disease of the ileo-anal pouch with Infliximab. Am J Gastroenterol 98:2239–2244
48. Ozuner G, Hull T, Lee P et al (1997) What happens to a pelvic pouch when a fistula develops? Dis Colon Rectum 40:543–547

Quality of Life in the Pouch Patient

Gian Gaetano Delaini, Gianluca Colucci, Monica Fontana, Filippo Nifosì

Introduction

Restorative proctocolectomy (RPC) with ileal pouch-anal anastomosis (IPAA) has become the surgical procedure of choice for patients with ulcerative colitis (UC) and familial adenomatous polyposis (FAP). This high level of satisfaction has led to the referral of patients who would not have otherwise considered a procedure requiring permanent ileostomy [1, 2].

In the past, total proctocolectomy with terminal ileostomy was the most radical and oncologically safest procedure. Alternatively, when the rectum contained only a few polyps, total colectomy with ileorectal anastomosis was the preferred treatment [3].

The advantage of obviating the need for a stoma while preserving sexual and voiding function was offset by the disadvantage of close and lifelong follow-up with the aim of removing new rectal polyps, or excising the rectum before cancer develops.

Nowadays, restorative proctocolectomy with the formation of (IPAA), which preserves the sphincters as well as sexual and bladder function while nevertheless completely removing colorectal mucosa, is the procedure of choice in the elective treatment of patients affected by (UC) [4].

Amelioration of the technique reduced procedure morbidity; nevertheless, some unsatisfactory functional results led several authors to consider the importance of quality of life [9, 10].

Health-related quality of life (HRQL) is defined as the patient's' own appraisal of their current physical and mental health, social interactions, and general well- being . Knowledge of postoperative health status is important in decision- making about the type of operation necessary in patients with FAP and inflammatory bowel disease (IBD). Although long-term functional results, described by some authors, are excellent, there is a relevant incidence of complications related to the ileal pouch [11].

The difficulty of quantifying such dysfunction, and its impact on HRQL, make it necessary to use an investigative instrument that not only explores clinical parameters of each patient but also his/ or her emotional and social function.

Several authors reported a. high level of satisfaction in patients submitted to colectomy in general [[15, 16] and in particular to RPC [10, 12, 16]. However, despite the dramatic improvement of patients' general condition, functional results are not always perfect. In fact, some patient complains of occasional episodes of soiling or urgency, elevated number of daily bowel movements, difficulties in pouch emptying or dietary restrictions. And even more, without such complications, patients with IPAA may refer to a conspicuous number of daily stool, and a certain degree of incontinence or urgency [16, 18].

The difficulty quantifying such dysfunction, and its impact on HRQL make it necessary to use an investigative instrument, that not only explores clinical parameters, especially bowel function (BF) of each patient but also his/ or her emotional and social function.

Many studies provide evidence that there is a statistically significant association between HRQL levels and BF [10]

Of the numerous BF characteristics, five appear to be of greater importance with regard to certain HRQL domains [18, 19, 38]. The physical function domain is improved with the ability to pass flatus independent of stool, physical role and mental health domains are improved with decreased stool frequency, social function domain is improved with increased stool retention time while perception of general health is improved with less diaper usage and less sexual dysfunction [18, 20].

RPC is generally considered to achieve better functional results and therefore HRQL in patients with than in those with UC.

Patients with UC usually have a higher overall complication rate and more pouch-related septic complications. Functional results are similar for daytime and nighttime stool frequency and the median duration that defecation could take.The use of antidiarrhoeal medications does not differ between patient with RPC affected by FAP and UC. Even though pouchitis is more common in UC than FAP, many studies suggest that the functional outcome, quality of life and health and satisfaction with outcome is identical between the groups [19, 20].

HRQL after RPC in FAP Patients

The latest treatment of choice in FAP in the past two decades, has been RCP with IPAA, which preserves the sphincters as well as sexual and bladder function while nevertheless completely removing colorectal mucosa [19, 21].

However, increasing experience with long-term postoperative care of FAP patients has raised doubts as to whether - apart from its well-known elevated rate of complications [22, 23]

- IPAA really offers as much comfort as was initially thought. Indeed, ileorectal anastomosis (IRA) in the upper third of the rectum is again being discussed as an alternative procedure, and proposals have been made to base the choice between IPAA and IRA on an assessment of rectal cancer risk as defined by either the type of APC gene mutation, i.e. genotype-phenotype correlation-based surgery or the number of rectal polyps found, or a combination of the two [24-27] and pouch polyposis may even occur [27, 28].

At the same time, increasing experience with the postoperative care of FAP patients has provided evidence that IPAA might not be as comfortable as originally assumed [28-32].

Many studies comparing functional results of FAP patients with IPAA with patients with IRA point out that results for patients with IPAA were poorer regarding the number of bowel movements per day, leakage, pad usage, perianal skin problems, food avoidance and inability to distinguish gas. Results of the HRQL surveys, however, demonstrate no difference between the IPAA and IRA groups. The Physical and Mental Summary Scales for IPAA and IRA groups are not significantly different, and none of the eight dimensions of the SF-36 Health Survey demonstrated statistical differences between IPAA and IRA groups. Therefore, better functional results are not equated with better HRQL.

Although patients with the IRA have better functional results than those with IPAA, the measured HRQL as determined by a validated generic HRQL instrument is the same for both groups. These results suggest that all patients with FAP might be optimally treated with an IPAA. More importantly, they evidence that HRQL should play a greater role in the evaluation of care and treatment in colon rectal surgery [33]

For the most part, studies focusing on quality of life [18, 32, 35] are difficult to interpret and compare, since different methods were used to measure function and quality of life. In summary, the main results of these studies show that both IRA and IPAA can be performed without postoperative mortality [21, 23, 32, 33]. However, subsequent complications are more common after IPAA [24, 26], with the lack of significance possibly due to the small number of patients, and IRA provides better overall continence function [24, 25, 28, 29, 33].

Nocturnal soiling and incontinence, in particular, as well as a significantly higher frequency of night-time bowel movements, are responsible for this observation. Interestingly, IPAA does not inevitably lead to a lower quality of life compared with IRA. Ko et al. [17] observed no difference, while two reports judged IRA to be better, although statistical significance was lacking [28, 29, 34, 36].

Thus, the undoubtedly better function provided by IRA does not necessarily translate as improved quality of life, which is in good accord with other studies specifically investigating the relationship between continence function and quality of life [17, 33, 35 , 37].

Continence function, which is the main factor influencing patient comfort after rectal surgery, is also related to age and gender. Older and female patients are more likely to suffer from incontinence, especially after rectal surgery.

A major unresolved problem is the relationship between continence function and quality of life. It is still a moot point whether and to what extent, disordered continence inevitably leads to impaired quality of life.

Nor is the patient's ability to psychologically compensate for reduced function and, as it were, restore previous quality of life well understood. Many studies found no significant correlation between function and quality of life [17, 33]. In contrast, many others showed that continence function in otherwise healthy patients does affect quality of life [37].

HRQL after RPC in UC Patients

Total proctocolectomy and IPAA is often advocated as the definitive treatment for UC [36, 4]. In fact, RPC with IPAA guarantees complete excision of the diseased bowel, reduction of cancer risk and preserves the natural route of defecation, so it can be fully considered as the first choice for the elective treatment of patients affected by UC who need surgical therapy [38, 39].

Amelioration of the technique and the increased surgical experience reduced procedure morbidity; nevertheless, some unsatisfactory functional results may affect quality of life, which has led several authors to consider the importance of quality of life [39, 40] after this treatment.

The relatively young age of such patients and their subsequent life expectancy imposed an accurate analysis of quality of life that became the measure of thefor efficiency of the procedure. .

In fact the relatively young age of such patients and their subsequent life expectancy imposed an accurate analysis of quality of life that became the measure for efficiency of the procedure. So HRQL questionnaires are the indispensable instruments to assess the quality of surgery.

Although long-term functional results described by some authors, are excellent, there is a relevant incidence of complications related to ileal pouch [41]. Several authors reported a high level of satisfaction in patients submitted to colectomy in general [42-44] and in particular to RPC [44-47].

However, despite dramatic improvement of patients' general conditions, functional results are not always perfect. In fact, some patients complains of occasional episodes of soiling or urgency, elevated number of daily bowel movements, difficulties in pouch emptying or dietary restrictions. And even more, also without such complications, patients with IPAA may refer a conspicuous number of daily stool and a certain degree of incontinence or urgency [47].

The difficulty of quantifying such dysfunction, and its impact on HRQL, make it necessary to use an investigative instrument, that not only explores clinical parameters of each patient but also his/ or her emotional and social function [48, 49].

Several authors report excellent long-term functional results of RPC with IPAA and HRQL comparable to those of healthy subjects, probably for the different consideration given to the emotional function, which is among the least important components of the Cleveland Global Quality of Life Score (CGQL), which is one of the most affirmed instrument used for HRQL analysis in RPC patients [44] .

On the contrary, according to some other authors , patients submitted to RPC for UC experience a long-term quality of life similar to those of UC patients, with mild or remission of disease activity because of long-term pouch complications, conspicuous number of daily stool or a certain degree of incontinence or urgency [42-44].

In particular, RPC patients reported HRQL scores similar to to those with moderate UC for intestinal and systemic symptoms and similar to those with mild remission UC for emotional and social function. The global scores indicate that RPC patients obtained similar scores to those with mild/ remission UC, so once again, we emphasise the role and weight of emotional and social function for HRQL [44]. RPC patients have similar scores to healthy controls for actual quality of life and for energy levels as well as to moderate UC for actual quality of life to patients with mild/remission UC for quality of health and to mild/remission UC for energy levels.

Once again, this result emphasises the role and the weight of the emotional and social function for HRQL [44, 49].

Age, gender, marriage status, education, job, fertility after the operation, type of anastomosis, elective or urgent surgery, 3two- or three-stage surgery, number of operations, age at stoma closure and duration of UC have not anyno actual role in predicting long-term HRQL outcome. There are some other critical factors for a good HRQL outcome: use of drugs, number of daily bowel movements, presence of pouchitis, rectal stenosis, sinus tracts or occasional incontinence, and age at UC diagnosis or at ileostomy closure.

The subjective perception of being ill is still present in many patients, and it may be reinforced, in part, by the medical follow-up that patients undergo but even more by the use of drugs that some patients still must take. Furthermore, the emotional function of patients who had their UC diagnosed and were operated in late childhood did not improve even 10.3 ± 7.0 years after their last operation. Only this item gives them a lower HRQL outcome (even if in the group of younger operated patients the difference is not statistically significant, probably because of the small number). Probably, this is not only due to more severe or fulminating onset of UC and higher incidence of pancolitis or postoperative pouchitis in childhood [50, 51] but also to the psychological trauma they suffered at this particularly fragile age.

So it is possible that they have grown up with the idea of being ill. These results should be considered by physicians when they are preparing a patient for the impact of RPC.

HRQL after RPC in Crohn's Disease Patients

IPAA has come to represent the procedure of choice for patients requiring surgery for mucosal UC [36]. In contrast, a proven diagnosis of Crohn's disease is generally held to preclude IPAA. However, patients with IPAA for apparent mucosal UC who are subsequently found to have Crohn's disease have a variable course.

In fact, up to 15% of cases of UC are mistakenly diagnosed in patients with Crohn's disease because of overlap in the clinical, endoscopic and histologic findings [52-54]. Even the classic histologic abnormality of Crohn's disease, noncaseating granuloma, is found in only 50-60% of resected specimens [54].

As a result, as many as 3.5-9% of patients who undergo total proctocolectomy and IPAA are found to develop recurrent Crohn's disease in the ileal pouch [55, 56] so that, in retrospect, these individuals presumably had surgery for Crohn's disease involving the colon rather than for UC.

In general, patients with Crohn's disease are not usually offered IPAA because recurrence, refractory fistulase, abscesses and strictures, extraintestinal manifestation and the high morbidity in these patients [57, 58,] may lead to a higher incidence of pouch failure. Neoplastic transformation of the pelvic pouch has also been reported, particularly in patients with chronic pouchitis.

Moreover, when total proctocolectomy is required for patients with intractable Crohn's colitis (i.e. granulomatous colitis), some surgeons advocate an IPAA in select cases to avoid the need for a permanent end ileostomy [59, 60].

However, surgery for Crohn's disease is only a temporary intervention in most cases because of the high rate of recurrencet: the reported prevalence of radiographic or endoscopic recurrence of Crohn's disease in the small bowel at or near surgical anastomoses is as high as 18-55% at 5 years and 40-76% at 10 years [61].

Most colorectal surgeons therefore do not recommend an IPAA for Crohn's colitis because of the high risk of developing recurrent Crohn's disease in the ileal pouch and the high morbidity in these patients [62-66].

Nevertheless the secondary diagnosis of Crohn's disease after IPAA is associated with protracted freedom from clinically evident Crohn's disease, low pouch-loss rate and good functional outcome. Such results can only be improved by the continued development of medical strategies for long-term suppression of Crohn's disease. These data support a prospective evaluation of IPAA in selected patients with Crohn's disease. [62-64].

Despite the fact that a diagnosis of Crohn's disease is currently considered a contraindication for an IPAA, some patients with secondary diagnosis of Crohn's disease have good functional outcome and quality of life after restorative proctocolectomy. [65, 66].

References

1. Robb B, Pritts T, Gang G et al (2002) Quality of life in patients undergoing ileal pouch-anal anastomosis at the University of Cincinnati. Am J Surg 183:353–360
2. Metzger U, Schnider A (2001) Prophylactic surgery in families with familial adenomatous polyposis (FAP) and in colitis. Swiss Surg 7:278–280
3. Lockhart-Mummery JP (1934) The causation and treatment of multiple adenomatosis of the colon. Ann Surg 99:178–184
4. Onaitis MW, Mantyh C (2003) Ileal pouch-anal anastomosis for ulcerative colitis and familial adenomatous polyposis: historical development and current status. Ann Surg 238:S42–S48
5. Robb B, Pritts T, Gang G et al (2002) Quality of life in patients undergoing ileal pouch anal anastomosis at the University of Cincinnati. Am J Surg; 183:343–360
6. Utsunomiya J. (1997) Development of ileal J-pouch anal anastomosis. Nippon Geka Gakkai Zasshi 98:443–448
7. Delaini GG, Scaglia M, Colucci G, Hulten L (2005) The ileoanal pouch procedure in the long-term perspective: a critical review Tech Coloproctol 9:187–192
8. Robb B, Pritts T, Gang G et al (2002) Quality of life in patients undergoing ileal pouch anal anastomosis at the University of Cincinnati. Am J Surg 183:343–360
9. Pemberton JH, Phillips SF, Ready RR et al (1989) Quality of life after Brooke ileostomy and ileal pouch-anal anastomosis. Comparison of performance status. Ann Surg 209:620–628
10. Karlbolm U, Raab Y, Ejerblad S et al (2000)Factors influencing the functional outcome of restorative proctocolectomy in ulcerative colitis. Br J Surg 87:1401–1408
11. Dayton MT (2000) Redo ileal pouch anal anastomosis for malfunctioning pouch acceptable alternative to permanent ileostomy? Am J Surg 180:561–565
12. Delaney CP, Dadvand B, Remzi FH et al (2002) Functional outcome, quality of life and complication after ileal pouch-anal anastomosis in selected septuagenarians. Dis Colon Rectum 45:890–894
13. Coffey JC, Winter DC, Neary P et al (2002) Quality of life after ileal pouch-anal anastomosis: an evaluation of diet and other factors using the Cleveland Global Quality of Life Instrument. Dis Colon Rectum 45:30–38
14. Delaney CP, Remzi FH, Gramlich T et al (2002) Equivalent function, quality of life and pouch survival rates after ileal pouch-anal anastomosis for indeterminate and ulcerative colitis. Ann Surg 236:43–48
15. Delaney CP, Fazio VW, Remzi FH et al (2003) Prospective, age related analysis of surgical results functional outcome and quality of life after ileal pouch-anal anastomosis. Ann Surg 238:221–228
16. Ko CY, Rusin LC, Schoetz DJ et al (2000) Does better functional result equate with better quality of life? Implications for surgical treatment in familial adenomatous polyposis. Dis Colon Rectum 43:829–835
17. Ko CY, Rusin LC, Schoetz DJ Jr et al (2001) Long-term outcomes of the ileal pouch anal anastomosis: the association of bowel function and quality of life 5 years after surgery. J Surg Res 98:102–107
18. Seidel SA, Newman M, Sharp KW (2000) Ileoanal pouch versus ileostomy: is there a difference in quality of life? Am Surg 66:540-546; discussion 546–547
19. Tjandra JJ, Fazio VW, Church JM et al (1993) Similar functional results after restorative proctocolectomy in patients with familial adenomatous polyposis and mucosal ulcerative colitis. Am J Surg 165:322–325
20. Utsunomiya J (1997) Development of ileal J-pouch

anal anastomosis. Nippon Geka Gakkai Zasshi 98:443–448
21. Ambroze WL Jr, Dozois RR, Pemberton JH et al (1992) Familial adenomatous polyposis. Results following ileal pouch-anal anastomosis and ileorectostomy. Dis Colon Rectum 35:12–15
22. Gunther K, Braunrieder G, Bittorf BR et al (2003) Patients with familial adenomatous polyposis experience better bowel function and quality of life after ileo rectal anastomosis than after ileo anal pouch. Colorectal Dis 5:38–44
23. Tonelli F, Valanzano R, Monaci I et al (1997)Restorative proctocolectomy or rectum-preserving surgery in patients with familial adenomatous polyposis. results of a prospective study. World J Surg 21:653–659.
24. Barton JG, Paden MA, Lane M, Postier RG (2001) Comparison of postoperative outcomes in ulcerative colitis and familial polyposis patients after ileoanal pouch operations. Am J Surg 182:616–620
25. Heuschen UA, Heuschen G, Lucas M et al (1998) Pre- and postoperative quality of life of patients with ulcerative colitis and familial adenomatous polyposis with ileoanal pouch operation. Chirurg 69:1329–1333
26. Ficari F (1997) Restorative proctocolectomy or rectum-preserving surgery in patients with familial adenomatous polyposis. Results of a prospective study. World J Surg 21:653–659
27. Beveridge IG, Groves CJ, Swain DJW et al (2001) Incidence, nature and aetiology of pouch adenomas in patients with familial adenomatous polyposis (oral presentation). Third joint meeting of the Leeds Castle Polyposis Group, Venice
28. Van Duijvendijk P, Slors JF, Taat CW et al (1999) Functional outcome after colectomy and ileorectal anastomosis compared with proctocolectomy and ileal pouch-anal anastomosis in familial adenomatous polyposis. Ann Surg 230:648–654
29. Soravia C, Klein L, Berk T et al (1999) Comparison of ileal pouch-anal anastomosis and ileorectal anastomosis in patients with familial adenomatous polyposis. Dis Colon Rectum 42:1028–1034
30. Madden MV, Neale KF, Nicholls RJ et al (1991) Comparison of morbidity and function after colectomy with ileorectal anastomosis or restorative proctocolectomy for familial adenomatous polyposis. Br J Surg 78:789–792
31. Wu JS, McGannon EA, Church JM (1998) Incidence of neoplastic polyps in the ileal pouch of patients with familial adenomatous polyposis after restorative proctocolectomy. Dis Colon Rectum 41:552–557
32. Reilly WT, Pemberton JH, Wolff BG et al. (1997) Randomized prospective trial comparing ileal pouch-anal anastomosis performed by excising the anal mucosa to ileal pouch-anal anastomosis performed by preserving the anal mucosa. Ann Surg 225:666–667
33. Ko CY, Rusin LC, Schoetz DJ Jr et al (2000) Does better functional result equate with better quality of life? Implications for surgical treatment in familial adenomatous polyposis. Dis Colon Rectum. 43:829–835; discussion 835–837
34. Van Duijvendijk P, Slors JF, Taat CW et al (2000) Quality of life after total colectomy with ileorectal anastomosis or proctocolectomy and ileal pouch-anal anastomosis for familial adenomatous polyposis. Br J Surg 87:590–596
35. Steens J, Meijerink WJ, Masclee AA et al (2000) Limited influence of pouch function on quality of life after ileal pouch-anal anastomosis. Hepatogastroenterology 47:746–750
36. Williams NS (1989) Restorative proctocolectomy is the first choice elective surgical treatment for ulcerative colitis. Br J Surg 76:1109–1110
37. Rothbarth J, Bemelman WA, Meijerink WJ et al. (2001) What is the impact of fecal incontinence on quality of life? Dis Colon Rectum 44:76–81
38. Fazio VW, Ziv Y, Church JM et al (1995) Ileal pouch-anal anastomoses complications and function in 1005 patients. Ann Surg 222:120–127
39. Pemberton JH, Phillips SF, Ready RR et al (1989) Quality of life after Brooke ileostomy and ileal pouch-anal anastomosis. Comparison of performance status. Ann Surg 209:620–628
40. Karlbolm U, Raab Y, Ejerblad S et al (2000) Factors influencing the functional outcome of restorative proctocolectomy in ulcerative colitis. Br J Surg 87:1401–1408
41. Dayton MT (2000) Redo ileal pouch anal anastomosis for malfunctioning pouch acceptable alternative to permanent ileostomy? Am J Surg 180:561–565
42. McLeod RS, Fazio VW (1984). Quality of life with the continent ileostomy. World J Surg 8:90–95
43. McLeod RS, Lavery IC, Leatherman JR et al (1986) Factors affecting quality of life with a conventional ileostomy. World J Surg 10:474–480
44. Fazio VW, O'Riordain MG, Lavery IC et al (1999) Long term functional outcome and quality of life after stapled restorative proctocolectomy. Ann Surg 1230:575–586
45. Robb B, Pritts T, Gang G et al (2002) Quality of life in patients undergoing ileal pouch anal anastomosis at the University of Cincinnati. Am J Surg 183:343–360
46. Karlbolm U, Raab Y, Ejerblad S et al (2000) Factors influencing the functional outcome of restorative proctocolectomy in ulcerative colitis. Br J Surg 87:1401–1408
47. McLeod RS, Baxter NN (1998) Quality of life of patients with inflammatory bowel disease after surgery. World J Surg 28:375–381
48. Caselas F, Lopez-Vivancos J, Vergara M et al (1999) Impact of inflammatory bowel disease on health-related quality of life. Dig Dis 17:208–218
49. Scarpa M, Angriman I, Ruffolo C et al (2004) Health related quality of life after restorative proctocolectomy for ulcerative colitis:long-term results. World J Surg 58:122–126
50. Fonkalsrud EW, Thakur A, Beanes S. (2001) Ileo-anal pouch procedures in children. J Ped Surg; 36:1689–1692
51. Rintala RJ, Lindahl HG. (2002) Proctocolectomy and J pouch ileo-anal anastomosis in children. J Ped Surg 37:66–70
52. Achkar JP, Shen B (2001) Medical management of postoperative complications of inflammatory bowel disease: pouchitis and Crohn's disease recurrence. Curr Gastroenterol Rep 3:484–490
53. Price AB (1978) Overlap in the spectrum of non-specific inflammatory bowel disease—"colitis indetermi-

nate" J Clin Pathol 31:567–577
54. Lewin KJ, Riddell RH, Weinstein WF. (1992) Inflammatory bowel diseases. In: Lewin KJ, Riddell RH, Weinstein WF (eds.) Gastrointestinal pathology and its clinical implications. Igaku-Shoin, New York, pp 812–989
55. Deutsch AA, McLeod RS, Cullen J, Cohen Z (1991) Results of the pelvic-pouch procedure in patients with Crohn's disease. Dis Colon Rectum 34:475–477
56. Keighley MR. (2000) The final diagnosis in pouch patients for presumed ulcerative colitis may change to Crohn's disease: patients should be warned of the consequences. Act Chir Iugosl 47:27–31
57. Hyman NH, Fazio VW, Tuckson WB, Lavery IC. (1991) Consequences of ileal pouch-anal anastomosis for Crohn's colitis. Dis Colon Rectum 34:653–657
58. Grobler SP, Hosie KB, Affie E et al (1993) Outcome of restorative proctocolectomy when the diagnosis is suggestive of Crohn's disease. Gut 34:1384–1388
59. Panis Y, Poupard B, Nemeth J et al (1996) Ileal pouch/anal anastomosis for Crohn's disease. Lancet 347:854–857
60. Regimbeau JM, Panis Y, Pocard Met al (2001) Long-term results of ileal pouch-anal anastomosis for colorectal Crohn's disease. Dis Colon Rectum 44:769 –778
61. Borley NR, Mortensen NJ, Jewell DP. (1997) Preventing postoperative recurrence of Crohn's disease. Br J Surg 84:1493–1502
62. Hartley JE, Fazio VW, Remzi FH et al (2004) Analysis of the outcome of ileal pouch-anal anastomosis in patients with Crohn's disease. Dis Colon Rectum 47:1808–1815
63. Peyregne V, Francois Y, Gilly FN et al (2000) Outcome of ileal pouch after secondary diagnosis of Crohn's disease. Int J Colorectal Dis 15:49–53
64. Braveman JM, Schoetz DJ Jr, Marcello PW et al (2004) The fate of the ileal pouch in patients developing Crohn's disease. Dis Colon Rectum 47:1613–1619
65. De Oca J, Sanchez-Santos R, Rague JM et al (2003) Long-term results of ileal pouch-anal anastomosis in Crohn's disease. Inflamm Bowel Dis 9:171–175
66. Thirlby RC, Sobrino MA, Randall JB. The long-term benefit of surgery on health-related quality of life in patients with inflammatory bowel disease. Arch Surg 136:521–527

The Place of Proctocolectomy with Ileostomy in the Era of Restorative Proctocolectomy

Giovanni Romano, Francesco Bianco, Vittorio D'Onofrio

Introduction

Over the second half of the last century, proctocolectomy in regards to terminal ileostomy has played an important role in the management of inflammatory diseases affecting the colon and rectum. For a long time it has been considered the gold-standard operation and all the results of alternative procedures have been compared with it. Before the era of restorative proctocolectomy, the possibility of removing all the diseased tissue in a one-stage procedure while avoiding the risk of cancer made this technique very successful. However, although this procedure has a low rate of morbidity and mortality and allows the patients an early return to normal activities [1], there are some important drawbacks that have spurred surgeons on to develop restorative proctocolectomy. First of all, the patients perceive the ileostomy as an unnatural condition which impairs their relationships and social life. Although modern stoma care allows an easier management of the stoma appliance, the unpredictable faecal and noisy gaseous discharge may be of such an extent that they restrict patient activities to the point of becoming a psychological barrier. Sexual complaints of the patients depend on both the functional and psychological impairment. Permanent impotence is rare with the intersphinteric technique and some authors have reported no permanent male dysfunction, either partial or complete, when using a perimuscular rectal excision during the proctocolectomy [2]. Women often complain of vaginal discharge and dyspareunia because of the perineal scar. However, psychological lability and the perception of the self-image are the factors that mainly affect sexual intercourse and the relationship of the patient. Moreover, some bladder dysfunctions may occur [3] and the perineal wound healing may take a long time, particularly in patients with undetected Crohn's disease [4]. Finally, the cost of the management of the ileostomy should be considered.

Indications

The choice of the ideal surgical procedure for treating these patients is based upon the following considerations:

- the need of definitive treatment with a one-stage procedure that allows a complete removal of the diseased tissue and avoids the risk of cancer.
- The possibility of restoring the anatomy as well as the bowel function and the faecal continence.
- The outcome and the complications of different surgical procedures.
- The patient's skills in managing the new condition and coping with the possible complications.
- And, above all, the possibility of improving the quality of life of the patient, which implies the evaluation of multiple functional and psychological factors.

Nowadays, restorative proctocolectomy is certainly the gold-standard technique for treating patients with ulcerative colitis or familial adenomatous polyposis [5, 6]. Nevertheless, there are still a few patients in which the proctocolectomy along with definitive ileostomy may be considered a good indication. The proctocolectomy with perineal excision and definitive ileostomy may be an indication of necessity in patients presenting with cancer or severe dysplasia of the very low rectum or anus [7]. In these cases, the choice of this surgical procedure should be based on the tumour stage and the need for radiotherapy. In other cases, the indications are more controversial and are still being debated. Provided that all the alternatives are discussed with the patient, the decision of the surgeon should be drawn from a sort of balance between the factors mentioned above. In elderly patients with a longstanding disease and a weak sphincter, a one-stage procedure with definitive ileostomy could be beneficial and better accepted by the patient. Similarly, all the patients with sphincter damage, particularly women with post-obstetric neuropathic sphincter trauma, might be good candidates for a definitive ileostomy. In these patients, the excision of the rectum to the level of the perineal muscles and the removal of the diseased anal mucosa could lead to disappointing results in terms of continence with much more discomfort and distress symptoms for the patient than a well-managed ileostomy. All the patients should be correctly informed about the outcome and the possible complications after restorative proctocolectomy such as diarrhoea, nocturnal soiling and recurrent pouchitis, so that patients who refuse to take these risks can be candidates for a proctocolectomy with a definitive ileostomy. Other patients are too psychologically weak and unstable to cope with the uncertainties of the outcome of a restorative procedure or are not available to attend the strict follow-up that is mandatory when an ileal pouch-anal anastomosis has been performed [8]. Furthermore, the definitive ileostomy, as salvage surgery, constitutes the last option for patients who previously underwent a restorative proctocolectomy in which the ileal pelvic pouch had to be removed [9]. The emergency operations are a particular problem. In patients with a previously detected severe inflammatory anorectal involvement, continuous bleeding from the ultra-low rectum or a perforation at this site may occasionally constitute an indication for a radical proctocolectomy without anastomotic reconstruction. Nevertheless, some authors suggest that even in these cases the rectum should be mobilised at the level of the levator ani and transected at the anorectal junction so that a pelvic pouch might be subsequently performed [4]. However, it should be stressed that, recently, many authors have reported that, in emergency, the primary procedure is more frequently a total colectomy with an ileostomy. They suggest that in these circumstances the surgeon should do a minimal intervention, and subsequently the patient may undergo a restorative proctectomy or an ileo-rectal anastomosis [10]. Emergency operations certainly have more complications such as a higher risk of fistula and pelvic nerve damage, and in these cases the surgeon's experience plays an important role in the choice of surgical options [11].

The surgeon and the stoma care nurse should arrange a pre-operative meeting with the patients whenever an elective procedure is performed. In order to make the right choice, the patient and the partner have to be aware of the alternative procedures such as restorative proctocolectomy with an ileal pelvic pouch and total colectomy with ileo-rectal anastomosis. The procedures have to be carefully described to the patients with particular attention to technical details, drawings and literature data. Moreover, they should be correctly informed about the quality of life and the possible implications of these operations. Particularly, some aspects of both the procedures have to be discussed such as complications, continence, soiling, diarrhoea, dietary restrictions, social restrictions and the necessity of long-term follow-up. The patient should be reassured that a stoma care unit is always available for all his needs. However, above all, the information given to the patients must be as objective as possible since, patients potentially unsuitable for the restorative operation may be persuaded by the excessive enthusiasm of the surgeons for the pouch procedure [8].

Once a decision to perform a definitive ileostomy has been taken, the surgeon is requested to make a second choice: whether or not to perform a continent reservoir ileostomy according to a modified Kock technique instead of a conventional Brooke ileostomy [12, 13]. Nowadays, the Kock ileostomy is rarely used as the primary treatment for ulcerative colitis or familial adenomatous polyposis due to the other alternative surgical options that are available and the surgical and metabolic complications associated with the reservoir ileostomy [14]. Nevertheless, besides the above-mentioned indications for conventional ileostomy, patients who have a poorly functioning ileoanal pouch and who are unsatisfied with their continence and quality of life, may be suitable for a conversion to a continent reservoir ileostomy [9, 15]. Similarly, the continent reservoir may be proposed to a limited cohort of selected and strongly motivated patients who have previously had a terminal conventional ileostomy. However, it is necessary to stress that there is an important learning curve for this operation and, just because nowadays the indications are rare, only a few centres have acquired sufficient experience with the procedure.

Even in this case, a detailed description of the procedure and its aims should be given to the patient, since a failure of the reservoir exposes the patient to the risk of a reoperation, a further loss of 50–60 cm of the ileum along with consequent metabolic derangement and, finally, the need for wearing a conventional appliance for the stoma. Therefore, it is obvious that the possibility of evaluating whether or not the procedure will be successful depends on a clear and objective definition of the aims of the reservoir ileostomy. Some authors have described these aims as the possibility of achieving a pouch completely continent to the gas and faeces with a capacity of 800–1 000 ml. This pouch should be emptied by a catheter no more than two or three times a day, without the urgency of draining at night, and the catheterisation should take no longer than 15 min. The exit conduit of the stoma should be invisible under the clothes and there should be no need of wearing a stoma bag as the mucous discharge should be minimal and there is complete control achieved by the application of a disposable dressing over the stoma. Finally, there should be no restrictions of food intake, sexual activities, work or any other social functions [8].

A careful selection of these patients is of paramount importance. A psychological assessment should be made in order to verify the real motivation of the patient and the psychological profile, thus excluding psychologically unstable patients who are seeking attention. The social environment should be evaluated as well as the physical skill of the patient to manage the pouch. Some patients have been described as having badly managed and perforated the pouch during catheterisation, others, with psychological lability, manipulate and deteriorate the pouch themselves; likewise, the elderly patients should not be considered for this procedure. Patients with pathological and psychological dietary disturbances such as the alcoholic, the anorexic, the bulimic, the obese and the very thin should be excluded. Particular attention should be paid to the patients who have previously undergone abdominal surgery, because the presence of thick adhesions may be a contraindication. Moreover, previous small-bowel resections, gastrectomy or pancreatic insufficiency are criteria for exclusion since in these cases there is an increased risk of electrolyte deficiency and metabolic complications. Finally, the emergency operation may be considered a contraindication for this procedure.

In 1997, Williams reported ten cases of Kock pouch construction. Four patients had a primary conventional proctocolectomy with a Kock pouch for ulcerative colitis with good long-term results. Six patients who had previously undergone restorative proctocolectomy for ulcerative colitis were converted to reservoir ileostomy. Among these latter, the reservoir was successful in four patients and failed in two: one due to sepsis and one due to obesity [8].

Although many authors consider a diagnosis of Crohn's disease as an absolute contraindication for a Kock pouch construction, this particular topic is still being debated [16]. In most of the reported cases, the patients with Crohn's disease who had a reservoir ileostomy as the primary operation, had a diagnosis of ulcerative colitis at the time of the first operation and, only subsequently, was the underlying diagnosis of Crohn's disease confirmed. In these patients, the diagnosis is usually achieved by the histological examination of the colon specimen in the early post-operative period or, later—via the analysis of the removed ileal pouch as a consequence of complications. In these latter cases, the histological examination of the colon, at the time of the first operation, has features similar to those of the ulcerative colitis, but the subsequent pouch complications reveals Crohn's disease. Some of these patients with Crohn's disease develop complications in the early post-operative period such as sepsis, fistula, bleeding and poor functional results requiring pouch excision; others, after years of good functional results, begin to have the typical symptoms of pouchitis. These patients complain of abdominal pain, fever, diarrhoea with high volume of fluid discharge and loss of electrolytes, bleeding, obstruction and difficult catheterisation. Frequently, they are classified as having chronic pouchitis and only the endoscopic biopsy allows the correct diagnosis of the underlying Crohn's disease. In these recurrent forms of Crohn's disease, medical treatment rarely achieves good results and, often, the patients end up with the removal of the pouch and a conventional ileostomy. Myrvold and Kock, in their important study that was a milestone in this specific area, reported only 27% of complications out of a total of 52 patients with Crohn's disease who underwent a reservoir ileostomy. The same incidence of complications was found in patients operated on for ulcerative colitis or familial adenomatous polyposis [17]. Other authors reported similar results in a small subset of patients with Crohn's disease. These authors suggested that patients with Crohn's disease confined to the colon and no evidence of disease to the small bowel, after a minimum follow-up of 5 years might be candidates for a reservoir ileostomy. Similarly patients with indeterminate colitis without evidence of disease to the ileum might be suitable for the Kock ileostomy [18]. On the contrary, Handelsman reported four pouch excisions out of eight patients operated on with Crohn's disease compared to only two pouch excisions in 87 patients with ulcerative colitis, so that he concluded that the suspicion of Crohn's disease is a contraindication to continent reservoir ileostomy.

Management, Outcome and Complications

The management of a conventional Brooke ileostomy is quite easy, both for the surgeon and the patient. As soon as possible, the patient is allowed to drink to easily achieve a correct balance of fluid intake. Beginning in the early post-operative period, a stoma care nurse should instruct the patient and his partner to empty and change the bag and to apply the flange. Although the rehabilitation mainly depends on patient motivation, the availability of a stoma care unit greatly helps the patient. They have to be informed about the correct volume of fluid intake, the need of wound dressing until complete healing is achieved and the risk of intestinal obstruction due to stoma impairment or post-operative adhesions.

Mortality is related to the proctocolectomy and

ranges between 2 and 3%, but for emergency procedures, a mortality of 23% has been reported. A depression may occur in the first period probably due to the new perception of the self-image and to the suspension of steroids medication. The most frequent complications in the early post-operative period are perineal sepsis and bleeding from the perineal wound, which are conservatively treated; a persistent sepsis or bleeding from the abdomen or the pelvis may require a second laparotomy. The loss of a large volume of fluid and electrolytes through the ileostomy may represent a serious problem, particularly in the first days after the post-operative ileus has resolved; therefore, it may be necessary to continue intravenous infusion to replace fluid loss. In some cases, chronic ileostomy diarrhoea occurs and the patients need to increase the volume of fluid and electrolyte intake. As the follow-up lengthens, an increased incidence of urolithiasis is reported, probably related to the extent of bowel excision. As in all, the patient who undergoes a bowel resection, an intestinal obstruction due to adhesions may complicate the early and late post-operative course; it must be remarked that this occurrence may be disastrous for these patients since a reoperation may lead to a further loss of bowel.

What is more difficult, is the management of a reservoir ileostomy in the early and late post-operative periods; however, the selected patients are usually very strongly motivated to actively cope with the new condition. At the end of the operation, and as long as the ileus has completely resolved, a permanent catheter is placed in the reservoir in order to drain the pouch and avoid disruption, leakage and nipple valve desusception. Subsequently, the catheter is periodically occluded and the time of drainage is progressively reduced. Some irrigation may be necessary to avoid faeces and food particles obstructing the catheter both in the early post-operative period, when the patient starts eating, and then at the time when the pouch is functioning. After a few weeks, the patient becomes aware of the necessity of emptying the reservoir and, usually, this manoeuvre is easily accomplished three or four times a day. Besides the complications already mentioned as being associated with any ileostomy and major laparotomy, there are a few others that are specific to a stoma reservoir construction. Some patients complain of continuous abdominal bloating and pain and others need to spend too much time in frequent catheterisations and irrigations to wash out the pouch from smelly particulate contents. These complaints are likely to be more frequent in patients with slow small-bowel transit. Accordingly, some authors consider that patients having a chronic constipation with a slow bowel transit, for which a conventional total proctocolectomy has been indicated as the last option, should have a Brooke ileostomy rather than a reservoir ileostomy [8, 19]. In the past years, valve slippage was reported as the most common complication, up to 44% of incidence, but this problem has been almost completely solved by using stapling machines. More important complications are the ischaemia or the fistula of a part of the ileostomy such as the exit conduit, the nipple valve or, at worst, the pouch. The fistula may be a consequence of an ischaemic tract, a suture line dehiscence or a perforation subsequent to catheterisation. Obviously, the most serious complication is the leakage in the abdomen of bowel contents particularly from the pouch since, if the fistula is not immediately recognised, the life of the patient may be threatened. In such circumstances, salvage surgery is mandatory. In case of a simple slippage of the valve, a new nipple valve can be refashioned [20]. When the valve or the exit conduit are ischaemic with a possible fistula, or the bowel tract is not sufficient, a reconstruction procedure is needed such as a rotational procedure or an interposed loop, in which a new bowel segment is adopted for the new valve and conduit. However, in the worst cases, the pouch cannot be saved. In these circumstances the reservoir must be entirely removed, and a completely new pouch ileostomy may be performed or, in some cases, a conversion to a Brooke ileostomy. Failes reported a 21% of reoperation rate and most of the revisions were undertaken within 1 year from the first operation [21]. In order to improve the functional results and reduce the early and late complications, over the last years a series of novel techniques for performing a continent ileostomy have been described such as the Barnett reservoir, the T pouch, and the ileocecal valve-preserving ileostomy [14, 22, 23, 24]. These new procedures are reported as improving the continence and the quality of life of the patients. However, although the preliminary reports are encouraging, a long-term follow-up is not yet available for correctly comparing the results.

The incidence of pouchitis has been reported to range between 4 and 40% in patients with a Kock reservoir for ulcerative colitis [25, 26]. The diagnosis is based on the typical above-mentioned symptoms and on an endoscopic biopsy that reveals diffuse bleeding inflammation and/or a villous atrophy. However, the histological features are often non-specific and may hide Crohn's disease. It is likely that this pouchitis rate is higher in patients who underwent the same operation for Crohn's disease than in those with ulcerative colitis, and much lower in patients operated on for familial adenomatous polyposis; besides, the more the follow-up lengthens, the more the incidence of pouchitis increases. In 1993, the group from Göteborg University compared the pouchitis rate after a long-lasting follow-up of patients with a Kock reservoir to that of patients with a pelvic reservoir. Pouchitis was found to be more frequent in the pelvic pouches as it occurred in 34% of the Kock procedures and 51% of the pelvic pouches; and in 64 and 76% of the cases there was only a single episode or a slight and short form of disease [26]. Nevertheless, patients with a Kock reservoir more frequently developed a chronic form of pouchitis than those with a pelvic pouch: 18 *vs.* 6%. Pouchitis is likely to be due to a bacterial overgrowth and a delayed small-bowel transit, and thus in most of the cases it quickly responds to conservative treatment with metronidazole and pouch catheterisation. Some metabolic disturbances such as fluid and electrolyte deficiencies, megaloblastic anaemia due to the depletion of vitamin B_{12}, fat or bile-salt malabsorption, as well as villous atrophy, may occur both in patients with pouchitis and those with a normal functioning reservoir. Moreover, the same metabolic complications have been found in patients with a conventional Brooke ileostomy, so it is likely that these metabolic imbalances depend on the volume of the ileostomy output, regardless of the type of ileostomy.

Many authors have reported a better quality of life in patients who underwent a restorative proctocolectomy than those who underwent a conventional proctocolectomy with ileostomy [5, 6]. In 1991, in order to assess whether the improvement of the quality of life in patients with restorative proctocolectomy was due to the absence of a stoma or to a better faecal continence, Kohler and Pemberton examined functional and performance activities in 406 patients with Brooke ileostomies (stoma present, incontinent), 313 with Kock pouches (stoma present, continent), and 298 with ileal pouch-anal anastomoses (stoma absent, continent). All the patients had been operated on for ulcerative colitis or familial adenomatous polyposis. Patients with ileal pouch-anal anastomoses had fewer restrictions in sports and sexual activities than those with Kock pouch, whereas those with Kock pouches, in turn, had fewer restrictions in these activities but more restrictions in travel than those with Brooke ileostomies. Performance in the categories of family, work and social life were similar between the groups. They concluded that both the presence of a stoma and faecal incontinence impair the quality of life after proctectomy, so therefore the ileal pouch-anal anastomosis allows the best quality of life [6]. On the contrary, more recently, some other authors reached more controversial conclusions. Mikkola evaluated the clinical differences between conventional and restorative proctocolectomy among 240 patients, the reoperation rate was 38 and 36% respectively; but as major complications were more frequent in the pouch group, he therefore concluded that ulcerative colitis can safely be managed with either conventional or restorative proctocolectomy, and more remarkable, in most cases the patient's preference should dictate the choice of procedure [27]. Likewise, in 2003, Camilleri-Brennan [28] analysed morbidity and quality of life in two matched groups of patients who underwent a restorative proctocolectomy or a conventional proctocolectomy with a Brooke ileostomy. The restorative proctocolectomy was found to be associated with a significantly better perception of body image than a permanent stoma, although the quality of life in general was similar in both groups and the patients with the pelvic pouch had more long-term complications than patients with ileostomy: 52.6 *vs.* 26.3% respectively. Therefore, because of the higher complication rate and the relatively small advantage in terms of quality of life associated with the restorative proctocolectomy, patients should be thoroughly advised before agreeing to this operation [28]. Moreover, conventional ileostomy usually represents the ultimate procedure after unsuccessful salvage surgery for patients who have experienced the failure of an ileal anal-pouch. As an alternative, the group from Göteborg University converted 13 patients with a failed previous restorative proctocolectomy to a continent ileostomy with reservoir. Subsequent revisional surgery was required in eight patients but, after a follow-up of 6 years, ten patients with intact ileostomy were fully continent and none had to use a stoma appliance. Provided that this operation should certainly be done in specialised units, it may be considered as an alternative salvage surgery to the Brooke ileostomy in motivated patients [29].

Closing Remarks

Although in the era of restorative proctocolectomy it is hard to accept that a reservoir ileostomy may be a satisfactory alternative to the ileal anal-pouch, it cannot be denied that, recently, many have reported rewarding results with the continent ileostomy even after a long-term follow-up. In 2004, Berndtsson et al. analysed data from 68 patients operated on with continent ileostomy between 1967 and 1974 to assess the long-term pouch durability and the health-related quality of life. The median follow-up was 31 years. The majority of patients reported good physical condition and satisfactory pouch function. Patients emptied the pouch a median of four times every day and 65% of patients had at least one post-operative revision to restore continence. The quality of life scores were compared to those of a control group. Seventy-eight percent of the patients rated their overall health as good, very good or excellent and the scores were comparable to the reference values [30]. Likewise, in 2005, Castillo reported a retrospective study in which the results of 24 patients operated on with a modified Kock pouch between 1993 and 2003 were evaluated. The median follow-up was 66 months. The underlying disease was ulcerative colitis in 71% of the patients, 20 patients had already been operated on: 13 patients were converted from a Brooke ileostomy to a continent ileostomy and 7 patients were operated on for a failure of a previous ileal anal-pouch. Revisional operations were performed in 58% of patients. The failure rate with reconversion to conventional ileostomy was only 8.3%, and 90% of the patients were satisfied with the continent pouch [31].

Although a high rate of reoperations may be needed to restore continence, continent ileostomy has good durability, satisfactory pouch function or quality of life, which are, in most cases, similar to that of the normal population. Therefore, the results reported make this procedure a viable option for patients with a previous restorative proctocolectomy that has failed, or whenever a restorative proctocolectomy is not likely to be advisable for the reasons discussed above. However, the patients must be carefully selected and before performing a reservoir ileostomy, they should always be advised of the high risk of revisional operations. Moreover, despite the high reoperation rate, most patients are reported to be pleased with continent ileostomy and, even in the case of reservoir failure or dysfunction, when they are asked to choose, most of them prefer to cope with revision operations rather than manage a conventional ileostomy for their entire lifetime [8].

References

1. Kettlewell MGW (1990) Proctocolectomy for ulcerative colitis. In: Allan MR, Keighley MRB, Alexander-Williams J, Hawkins C (eds) Inflammatory bowel disease (2nd edn) Churchill Livingstone, Edinburgh, pp 439–445
2. Berry AR, De Campos R, Lee ECG (1986) Perineal and pelvic morbidity following perimuscolar excision of the rectum for inflammatory bowel disease. Br J Surg 73:675–677
3. Asztely M, Palmblad S, Wikland M, Hulten L (1991) Radiological study of changes following proctocolectomy. Int J Colorect Dis 6:103–107
4. Frizelle A, Pemberton JH (1997) Removal of the anus during proctectomy. Br J Surg 84:68
5. Pemberton JH, Phillips SF, Ready RR et al (1989) Quality of life after Brooke ileostomy and ileal pouch-anal anastomosis: comparison of performance status. Ann Surg 209:626–628
6. Kohler LW, Pemberton JH, Zinsmeister AR, Kelly KA (1991) Quality of life after proctocolectomy: a comparison of Brooke ileostomy, Kock pouch, and ileal pouch-anal anastomosis. Gastroenterology 101:679–684
7. Rotholtz NA, Pikarsky AJ, Singh JJ, Wexner SD (2001) Adenocarcinoma arising from along the rectal stump after double-stapled ileorectal J-pouch in a patient with ulcerative colitis: the need to perform a distal anastomosis: report of a case. Dis Colon Rectum 44:1214–1217
8. Williams NS (1997) Conventional proctocolectomy with ileostomy and proctectomy alone in ulcerative colitis. In: Keighley MRB, Williams NS (eds) Surgery of the anus rectum and colon (2nd edn) Saunders, London, pp 1677–1706
9. Borjesson L, Oresland T, Hulten L (2004) The failed pelvic pouch: conversion to a continent ileostomy. Tech Coloproctol 8:102–1055
10. Marion JF, Present DH (1997) The modern medical management of acute, severe ulcerative colitis. Eur J Gastroenterol Hepatol 9:831–835
11. Melville DM, Ritchie JK, Nicholls RJ, Hawley PR (1994) Surgery of ulcerative colitis in the era of the pouch: the St Mark's hospital experience. Gut 35:1076–1080
12. Kock NG, Myrvold HE, Nilsson LO, Philipson BM (1981) Continent ileostomy: an account of 314 patients. Acta Chir Scand 147:67–72
13. Brooke BN (1956) The outcome of surgery for ulcerative colitis. Lancet 7:532–536
14. Mullen P, Beherens D, Chalmers T (1995) Barnett continent intestinal reservoir: multicentre experience with an alternative to the Brooke ileostomy. Dis Colon Rectum 36:573–582
15. Ecker KW, Haberer M, Feifel G (1996) Conversion of the failing ileoanal pouch to reservoir-ileostomy rather than to ileostomy alone. Dis Colon Rectum 39:977–980
16. Handelsman JC, Gottlieb LM, Hamilton SR (1993) Crohn's disease as a contraindication to Kock pouch (continent ileostomy). Dis Colon Rectum 36:840–843
17. Myrvold HR, Kock NG (1981) Continent ileostomy in patients with Crohn's disease. Gastroenterology 80:1237
18. Bloom RJ, Larsen CP, Watt R, Oberhelman HA (1986) A reappraisal of the continent Kock ileostomy in patients with Crohn's disease. Surg Gynecol Obstet 162:105–108
19. Ecker KW, Haberer M, Feifel G (1996) Conversion of failing ileoanal pouch to reservoir-ileostomy rather than to ileostomy alone. Dis Colon Rectum 39:977–890
20. Fazio VW, Tjandra JJ (1992) Technique for nipple valve fixation to prevent valve slippage in continent ileostomy. Dis Colon Rectum 35:1177–1179
21. Failes DG (1984) The continent ileostomy: an 11-year experience. Aust NZJ Surg 54:345–352
22. Behrens DT, Paris M, Luttrell JM (1999) Conversion of failed ileal pouch-anal anastomosis to continent ileostomy. Dis Colon Rectum 42:490–495
23. Kaiser AM, Stein JP, Beart RW (2002) T-pouch: a new valve design for a continent ileostomy. Dis Colon Rectum 45:411–415
24. Nyo Y, Itakura M, Yamaguchi K, Hirahara N (2004) Ileocecal valve-preserving ileostomy after total proctocolectomy: a novel technique for ileostomy. Dig Surg 21:7–9

25. Ojerskog B, Kock NG, Nilsson LO et al (1990) Long-term follow up of patients with continent ileostomies. Dis Colon Rectum 33:184–189
26. Svaninger G, Nordgren S, Oresland T, Hulten L (1993) Incidence and characteristics of pouchitis in the Kock continent ileostomy and the pelvic pouch. Scand J Gastroenterol 28:695–700
27. Mikkola K, Luukkonen P, Jarvinen HJ (1996) Restorative compared with conventional proctocolectomy for the treatment of ulcerative colitis. Eur J Surg 162:315–319
28. Camilleri-Brennan J, Munro A, Steele RJ (2003) Does an ileoanal pouch offer a better quality of life than a permanent ileostomy for patients with ulcerative colitis? Gastrointest Surg 7:814–819
29. Borjesson L, Oresland T, Hulten L (2004) The failed pelvic pouch: conversion to a continent ileostomy. Tech Coloproctol 8:102–105
30. Berndtsson IE, Lindholm E, Oresland T, Hulten L (2004) Health related quality of life and pouch function in continent ileostomy patients: a 30-year perspective. Dis Colon Rectum 47:2131–2137
31. Castillo E, Thomassie LM, Whitlow CB et al (2005) Continent ileostomy: current experience. Dis Colon Rectum 48:1263–1268

Surgical Management of IBD Emergencies: the Approach in a Peripheral Hospital

Walter Thaler, Hansjörg Marsoner, Gianluca Colucci, Barbara Mahlknecht, Umberto Pandini, Anke Gutweniger, Monika Niederkofler, Emanuela Dapunt, Alex Wiegele, Hans Dejaco, Siegfried Jesacher

Introduction

The most common complications of inflammatory bowel disease (IBD) requiring emergency treatment are toxic colitis, perforation, toxic megacolon, bleeding, sepsis and intestinal occlusion [1]. Admittedly, our experience with these situations is limited. Our gastroenterologist treats about 50 patients with IBD and an incidence rate of 5–6 newly detected patients per year per 70 000 habitants in our area, which corresponds to the nationwide population-based study in Italy (Table 1) [2]. Whereas most of these patients are amenable to medical treatment, some of them sooner or later present with intestinal emergencies. Furthermore, septic, hemorrhagic or perforative complications may be the first clinical manifestations of IBD. A transfer of these patients to specialized centres may be hazardous. This contribution gives true insight into the surgical management of IBD emergencies in a peripheral hospital based on 7 years of experience.

Patients and Methods

In a 7-year period, from 1997 to 2004, 13 patients were referred to our surgical department for management of IBD emergencies (Table 2). Most of them had to be operated on more than once. Patients with ulcerative colitis (UC) or Crohn's disease (CD) admitted for elective surgical procedures as well as those suitable for an ileal pouch-anal anastomosis are not included. The mean age of women (n=6) was 32.5 years, while the mean age of men (n=7) was 46.3 years. Ten patients had CD-associated emergencies, only three had ulcerative colitis. Abscess and fistula formation, associated with sepsis (n=7), were the most frequent emergencies regarding our IBD patients. We emphasise that these patients had to be operated on under general anaesthesia and that those with superficial lesions treated in local anaesthesia and in an ambulatory setting are not included in this group. As a rare occurrence, one patient presented with ulcerative colitis and a giant subhepatic abscess, which could be successfully drained by a transcutaneous echoguided approach. Another patient presented with a right multiloculated psoas abscess. After successful drainage of the abscess, diagnosis of Crohn's disease of terminal ileum was established. Despite adequate medical therapy, the patient developed another psoas abscess. Therefore, besides abscess drainage, an ileocecal resection was performed. Since then, the patient is doing well. Four patients with CD underwent urgent ileocecal resection for intestinal obstruction. In three of them the obstruction was associated with the abscess formation; in one it was associated with an enteroenteric fistula. In a patient with a descendent colon obstruction due to CD, only a cecostomy was carried out; after 1 year of medical treatment the obstruction resolved and the cecostomy could be closed. Two patients with ileal CD underwent appendectomy without complications. The patient with toxic megacolon underwent colectomy and an ileal pouch-anal anastomosis in another hospital where he was known as an UC patient. Some months later, when the specimen was re-examined by a famous pathologist, the diagnosis of UC was changed to CD. The patient, indeed, developed severe complications caused by the ileal pouch such as diarrhoea, incontinence and perianal fistula.

Table 1. Incidence of inflammatory bowel disease in Italy [39]

	UC	CD
Age adjusted incidence rates per 100 000 per year	5.2	2.3
Rates computed after correcting underestimation	6.8	2.8
Sex ratio M/F	1.7	1.0
Highest age specific incidence rates	30-39 years	20-29 years

Table 2. Emergencies in IBD: our experience

Gender	Age of patient	Diagnosis	Treatment	Results
Male	60	1990: intestinal bleeding (UC) 1993: toxic megacolon Histological diagnosis revisited: Crohn's disease Increasing perianal problems	Colectomy, end-ileostomy and mucous fistula. Some months later ileo-anal-pouch Several operations for perianal- and abdominal-wall fistula 2000: end-ileostomy	Has mild symptoms of perianal CD and lastly a low output enterocutaneous fistula has developed. General state of health is good
Female	29	1998: diagnosis of CD 2000: acute appendicitis	Laparoscopic appendectomy	Histologically severe inflamed appendix without specific signs of CD No further surgical treatment until now
Female	38	1989: diagnosis of CD 1997: fulminant colitis 1999: development of a rectovaginal fistula. Severe perianal CD 2001: duodenal CD	Subtotal colectomy, ileorectal anastomosis 2001: end-ileostomy	Azothioprin-induced pancreatitis Improvement of perineal CD, no evidence for rectovaginal fistula and duodenal CD today
Male	36	1990: diagnosis of CD 1998: perianal fistula	Fistulectomy	No recurrence of perianal CD
Female	25	1995: diagnosis of CD of the small bowel 2000: bowel obstruction	Ileal resection and end-to-anastomosis	No further surgical therapy
Female	32	1998: diagnosis of CD 1999: acute appendicitis	Appendectomy	No further surgical therapy
Male	30	1997: diagnosis of CD 2002: anorectal fistula 2004: abscess with bowel obstruction	Ileocecal resection, abscess drainage relaparotomy for multiple intraperitoneal abscesses 7 days later	Enterocutaneous fistula for 5 months. Actually on medical treatment without complaints
Female	43	1989: diagnosis of CD 1998: abscess, enteroenteric fistula and bowel obstruction	1998: ileocecal resection	Good state of health without medical treatment, 2 childbirths
Female	44	2002: psoas abscess (diagnosis of CD) 2002: bowel obstruction 2005: psoas abscess	Drainage, ileocecal resection, re-resection of terminal ileum, abscess drainage	Actually on medical therapy without complaints
Male	63	1999: diagnosis of Crohn's colitis 2003: colonic obstruction	Cecostomy, medical treatment 2004: closure of cecostomy	Actually on medical therapy without complaints
Male	73	1987: diagnosis of UC 1998: acute colitis 2003: free sigmoid colon perforation	Left hemicolectomy, end transversostomy, closure of the rectum	No evidence for IBD in the right colon and in the rectum Abdominal wall rupture, stomal problems, rectal stump failure, sepsis, death after two months of intensive care
Male	65	1987 diagnosis of UC 2004: subhepatic abscess	Percutaneous drainage	Actually on medical therapy without complaints
Male	52	2004: cecal perforation in ileocecal CD and cecal carcinoma	Laparoscopic closure of the perforation and biopsy, which revealed carcinoma	Died after right hemicolectomy in his reference hospital

These symptoms could be successfully managed by an ileostomy. Another patient underwent subtotal colectomy and ileo-rectal anastomosis for Crohn's disease. One year later, severe anal CD developed postoperatively with perianal und rectovaginal fistula formation. Additionally, an azathioprine associated pancreatitis and a duodenal manifestation of Crohn's disease impaired the state of health of this young woman. Four years after colectomy, an end-ileostomy was performed and since that time the patient is doing well: she has regained her normal body weight, she is on medical treatment without evidence of duodenal CD and the disastrous perianal situation has improved dramatically showing a disappearance of the rectovaginal fistula. Two patients had free intestinal perforation. The first, a 73-year-old man with UC for 16 years, was referred to our department with free sigmoid colon perforation. The patient was on medical treatment for acute colitis at the medical department of our hospital when he developed multiorgan failure. Interestingly, there was no evidence of toxic megacolon, and free air evidenced on the abdominal plain X-ray was not associated with a classical appearance of acute abdominal pain. The patient was immediately referred to the operating theatre where a large perforation of the sigmoid colon with advanced signs of general peritonitis was found. The right colon, however, and the rectum were free of disease. Therefore, a modified Hartmann's procedure was carried out with resection of the sigmoid colon, closure of the rectal stump and construction of an end-transverse colostomy. After an uneventful postoperative phase of 5 days, a rectal stump insufficiency and an abdominal wall dehiscence had to be repaired twice. Finally, the patient died after 2 months of intensive care treatment. The other patient, a 56-year-old man with CD for more than 10 years, was referred for acute abdomen. This patient also had a long history of duodenal ulcer disease and therefore he underwent laparoscopic exploration. A small perforation of the cecum was found, biopsied, and, because of the absence of typical signs of peritonitis, closed by direct suture. A drain was placed near to the perforation and the postoperative phase was uneventful. Histologic examination of biopsies revealed a carcinoma. The patient underwent a right hemicolectomy some weeks later in his reference hospital, and he died due to anastomotic leakage.

Discussion

Perianal Abscesses and Fistulae

Perianal abscesses and fistulae were the most frequent complications of IBD of patients who required emergency treatment in our series. Many of them underwent more than one operation for fistulae. When cases of Crohn's disease are described as "fistulising", one has to distinguish between perianal and intestinal fistulation. The question, however, remains open as to whether or not there is truly an association between perianal fistulisation and intra-abdominal intestinal fistulisation in CD. There is a statistically significant association between perianal CD and intestinal fistulisation, which is much stronger and more consistent in cases of Crohn's colitis than in cases limited to the small bowel [3]. The management of perianal CD continues to be challenging. Roughly half of patients require permanent faecal diversion, which is even more frequently true for patients with colonic CD and anal stenosis. Recognising these tendencies will assist both patients and surgeons in planning optimal treatment [4]. If it is indeed a superficial fistula, the correct course of action for most patients would be a fistulotomy and perhaps a short course of antibiotics. Failing this, most patients would receive a non-cutting seton [5]. Long-term indwelling seton is an effective management modality for complex perianal Crohn's fistulas which do not negatively impact faecal continence [6].

Endoanal ultrasound has been suggested for the evaluation of rectal abscesses and fistulas [7]. The insertion of rectal probes can, however, still be painful. The use of a rigid endoanal ultrasound probe can even be impossible in patients with inflammatory perianal disease due to anal stenosis. This limitation is obviated by the use of perineal ultrasonography, which is a simple, painless, feasible, real-time method that can be performed without specific patient preparation and which is comparable in its sensitivity to pelvic MRI in the detection of perianal fistulae and/or abscesses [8]. The combination of MRI and endoanal ultrasound is capable of detecting perianal fistulae with a sensitivity of 100% [9]. We have little experience with perineal ultrasonography. In our opinion, transrectal ultrasonography is an excellent method in cases of newly diagnosed perianal disease, but it is less exact in cases of recurrent fistulae.

Rectovaginal fistulae are a well-recognized complication of Crohn's disease, occurring in 5–10% of women [10]. The management of rectovaginal fistulae complicating Crohn's disease is often unsatisfactory. Faecal diversion has been used to achieve remission in colonic Crohn's disease [11]. Most patients with rectovaginal fistulae secondary to rectal disease, even if it is quiescent, eventually require a proctectomy due to progressive rectal disease or unmanageable incontinence [12, 13]. The role of faecal diversion applied on its own in perianal Crohn's disease remains unclear. Many perianal lesions, particularly ulcers and fistulae, heal completely without any specific therapy [14]. The advantage of fecal diversion is that it is a relatively minor procedure, and it may promote healing of an anal ulcer and some fistulae. It would be helpful if we could predict which patients with perianal disease might respond to faecal diversion. No predictive factors could be found by Yamamoto et al. [15]. Patients have to be warned that the ileostomy is closed in only a few cases, but that the severe sepsis or anal pain is usually alleviated. Our two patients who underwent ileostomy for intractable perianal CD didn't ask for a closure of ileostomy until now.

Infliximab is an efficacious treatment for fistulae in patients with Crohn's disease [16]. The perianal disease process should first be fully delineated with endoscopy and either MRI or EUS before treatment is begun. Although the initial response to infliximab is dramatic, the median duration of fistula closure is approximately 3 months, and repeated infusions are required [16]. Patients with fistulising CD treated with infliximab are more likely to maintain fistula closure if the treatment is preceded by an evaluation under anaesthesia and seton placement [17]. Complex fistulae first require surgical intervention prior to medical treatment. A combination of antibiotics, immunosuppressive therapy and infliximab are then initiated to facilitate fistula healing [18]. Two of our patients have been treated with infliximab; both of them, finally, required an ileostomy for permanent improvement of their perianal disease.

Intra-Abdominal Abscesses

Intra-abdominal abscesses can be successfully drained by an echoguided mini-invasive access like that described in regards to our patient with ulcerative colitis and a subhepatic abscess. In many cases, however, fistula formation and intestinal obstruction is associated with intra-abdominal abscesses, and abscess drainage does not improve the situation in the long term. More than 25% of patients undergoing surgery for Crohn's disease will have either an intra-abdominal mass or abscess. Of these masses, 40% will have an associated fistula [19, 20]. Traditionally, the majority of abscesses associated with Crohn's disease have been approached with operative drainage; however, improved interventional radiological techniques have resulted in an increased use of percutaneous drainage. Doing so will facilitate an improvement in the patients general condition prior to definitive surgical repair [20]. Non-operative therapy prevented subsequent surgery in half of the patients and may be a reasonable treatment option [21]. In cases with no associated abscess primary reconstruction can be proposed.

Psoas Abscesses

As for psoas abscesses, Crohn's disease is today the most common cause of this entity. Nevertheless, it is a rare event as it develops in less than 1% of patients with CD [22]. An occasional patient will require multiple operations [23].

Acute Appendicitis

Acute appendicitis and appendectomy in patients with CD is a matter of debate. Crohn's disease confined to the appendix is rare but has been well described in the literature [24]. Crohn's disease of the appendix can mimic acute appendicitis, although often with a more indolent course. It has been suggested that appendectomy in patients with CD may be complicated by fistula formation. Interestingly, in patients with abdominal pain for less than 1 week, appendectomy was followed by minimal problems, whereas in those with pain for longer than a week, incidental appendectomy was followed by an 83% incidence of fistulae, arising not from the appendiceal stump but from the terminal ileum [25]. The disease may be treated successfully by laparoscopic appendectomy with good long-term results [26]. A laparoscopic approach may be advantageous since the trocars are inserted far away from the diseased ileocecal region and scar formation is reduced in comparison with an open access.

Toxic Colitis

Toxic colitis, with or without megacolon, is an emergent life-threatening complication of inflammatory bowel disease. Its overall incidence in patients with ulcerative colitis is about 10% [27]. Although in the past, toxic colitis was thought to be a rare complication of Crohn's disease compared with ulcerative colitis, recent studies have shown that Crohn's colitis is the etiology in approximately 50% of the cases [28]. The overall incidence of complicated Crohn's disease is about 6%, with an increasing number occurring in Crohn's colitis [29]. The presentation of toxic "fulminant" colitis includes fever, an abrupt onset of bloody diarrhoea, abdominal tenderness, colicky pain, and anorexia [30]. Toxic megacolon is present if, in addition to toxic colitis, either total or segmental dilatation of the colon occurs [31, 32]. Once the diagnosis of toxic colitis is suspected, aggressive medical therapy is initiated. A team approach is required involving both gastroenterologists and surgeons. Prompt surgery is indicated for patients with toxic colitis or megacolon if there is evidence of free perforation, peritonitis, or massive haemorrhage. Surgery may also be indicated to avoid perforation if no clinical improvement occurs with aggressive medical management within 48–72 h. A persistently dilated colon on plain films is also often an indication for operative intervention. The optimal operation involves subtotal colectomy with end ileostomy. This allows removal of the majority of the bowel and avoids an anastomosis in a critically ill patient [30]. Total colectomy was at one time the procedure of choice, but has fallen out of favour due to increased morbidity and mortality. An endoscopic decompression by sigmoido- or colonoscopy can be achieved [33, 34], but it cannot be recommended unless used in a non-surgical candidate. Computed tomography scans should be performed on all patients for whom the diagnosis of toxic megacolon is suspected, as several complications can be identified before clinical or plain film findings. Diffuse colonic wall thickening, submucosal edema and pericolic stranding are all indicative of severe colitis [35]. Timing of surgery regarding toxic megacolon may be crucial, and delay in surgical management can result in perforation and the poor prognosis that accompanies it. The long-term prognosis of medically managed, ulcerative colitis-related toxic megacolon is poor [36].

Intestinal Obstruction

Intestinal obstruction most commonly occurs in patients with Crohn's disease. Small bowel obstruction is the most common complication requiring surgical correction in Crohn's disease and affects 35–54% of patients [37, 38]. It is important to rule out a malignancy whenever a stricture, especially colonic, is present. The initial management of intestinal obstruction in Crohn's disease is medical therapy. Obstruction that is unresponsive to medical treatment requires resection or possible strictureplasty [39]. Septic problems or phlegmon, a stricture close to a planned resection and extensive ulceration or bleeding are contraindications for strictureplasty. Ileocecal resection is a very satisfactory procedure since most patients enjoy longstanding good health after this procedure. "Don't operate until a patient gets a complication from Crohn's disease; but don't wait for a complication to become further complicated" [40]. Extended resection margins confer no advantage to patients in reducing cumulative recurrence rates. The presence of residual microscopic Crohn's disease at resection margins does not increase recurrence rates *vs.* normal margins. Resection margins of 2 or 12 cm after a median follow-up of 56 months had the same recurrence rate [41].

Haemorrhage

Although we had no patients with massive bleeding in our hospital in the last 7 years to treat, this issue is worth mentioning. Severe bleeding occurs in 0–6% of patients with inflammatory bowel disease with most series quoting a 2–3% incidence [42–44]. As compared with ulcerative colitis, where bleeding may diffuse from large areas of ulcerated mucosa, in Crohn's disease the bleeding is often from a localised source. It is important to rule out a gastroduodenal source prior to bowel resection. Robert et al. [43] found that nearly 30% of patients with Crohn's disease treated for significant gastrointestinal bleeding had a bleeding duodenal ulcer as its source. In Crohn's disease, it is important to localise the source of bleeding preoperatively. If gastroscopy and colonoscopy are not successful, the use of angiography may be considered, but only if patient stability is obtained. Other methods include the use of a nuclear medicine known as red cell scan.

Life-threatening haemorrhage and exsanguination from Crohn's disease in four patients were described in 1995, when 34 cases similar to the medical literature were reviewed [45]. Five patients died, in 30 (90%) surgery was necessary to cease haemorrhage and ileocolectomy was the most frequently performed procedure. Mesenteric arteriography was positive in 17 patients, providing precise preoperative localisation, resulting in no mortality in this group [45]. A retrospective study of 34 patients with acute lower gastrointestinal bleeding in Crohn's disease, the largest to date, shows a more favourable result [46]. Acute haemorrhage was defined as acute rectal bleeding originating in diseased bowel, requiring a transfusion of at least 2 units of red blood cells within 24 h. Upper gastrointestinal tract haemorrhage or anal lesions and postoperative bleeding were excluded. Recently, several promising studies have been published that describe transcatheter embolization for the treatment of massive lower gastrointestinal bleeding in cases of bleeding colonic diverticular disease and angiodysplasia. This approach may be useful for bleeding in Crohn's disease as well.

Perforation

Crohn stated in a 1957 paper: "Free perforation of ileitis into the peritoneal cavity never occurs or at least I have not seen it" [47]. In 1965 however, he reported seven cases of free perforation [48]. Free perforation occurs in approximately 2% of patients with ulcerative colitis and is usually associated with toxic colitis or megacolon [28]. Its occurrence without megacolon is rare [49]. The diagnosis may be delayed, as high-dose steroids may mask the signs of peritonitis. In Crohn's disease, free perforation is a rare but severe complication occurring in 1–3% of cases [50, 51]. Holzheimer et al. [52] reported an incidence of 13% in 1995. Such different incidence rates are due to the fact that in some reports, abscess formation is included and in others it is not. A large series of free perforation in Crohn's disease has been published by Greenstein et al. [53] in 1985 and by Ikeuchi et al. [54] in 2003; it seems that the incidence of free perforation in Japan is higher than in Western countries. The procedure of choice for a patient with ulcerative colitis and free perforation is a subtotal colectomy and end ileostomy. Gastroduodenal perforations in Crohn's patients are best managed with debridement and primary repair. Perforated Crohn's colitis, which is often in the setting of toxic colitis, requires subtotal colectomy with rectal preservation and end ileostomy [51]. If the perforation occurs in a diseased small-bowel segment, this segment along with the perforation is resected. In a recent study, Nissan et al. [55], who advocated a more liberal approach to surgical treatment, found free perforation in only 3.8% of their study group. Intensive medical treatment resulted in a 6.2-year delay from diagnosis until surgery, in contrast to 3.3 years in the study by Greenstein et al. [56]. It is possible that a serious complication such as free perforation resulted from a conservative medical approach. Perforative Crohn's disease is accompanied by more postoperative complications, anastomotic healing is poor, and recurrent disease is more frequent in the short-term (up to 5 years) follow-up than in obstructive Crohn's disease [57]. Based on the results of many authors [55, 56, 58], early surgery in Crohn's disease patients depending on the clinical presentation, intensity and duration of medical treatment, and life quality impairment, is recommended. It is generally accepted that 1–3 % of patients with CD will present with a free perforation—initially or eventually in the course of their disease [53, 58, 59]. Operative mortality in case of perforation is 20–40% [31, 60], whereas it is 4% in patients with toxic megacolon operated on before perforation has taken place. In half of patients, perforation is not associated with toxic megacolon. Free perforation of the bowel due to cancer in Crohn's disease is very rare [61].

Perforated Cancer in IBD

People with ulcerative colitis and Crohn's disease are at greater risk for colon cancer than the general population. Four patients with bowel perforation because of carcinoma in Crohn's disease are described in the literature [61, 62]. In case of a conservative procedure such as suture of perforated intestine or drainage only or strictureplasty, stenting, biopsies of the perforated area are recommended. Prognosis of carcinoma in IBD, according to Fraschini [61], is good. His patient underwent a right hemicolectomy and was alive without recurrence or metastases at the 31-months follow-up. Prognosis of carcinoma in IBD, according to Greenstein [62], is bad. Two of his patients died because of operative complications. Our patient, who underwent laparoscopic closure of the cecal perforation, was discharged 6 days postoperatively, but, as mentioned above, he died after a planned right hemicolectomy in his reference hospital.

Laparoscopy

The final role of laparoscopic surgery for the management of inflammatory bowel disease is still under evaluation, but it is attractive. Since it is well known that development of laparoscopic techniques is not reserved for university centres or high volume hospitals, minimal invasive procedures can also be applied in peripheral hospitals. Certainly, laparoscopy is not the first choice approach in the emergency treatment of our patients with inflammatory bowel disease, but we do not hesitate to perform a diagnostic laparoscopy in patients with known inflammatory bowel disease which present with unclear acute abdominal complaints. In this way, we managed a cecal perforation in a patient with Crohn's disease and cecal carcinoma by direct closure of the perforation and peritoneal lavage and drainage. Laparoscopic ileocolic resection is a feasible procedure for skilled surgeons. When compared with an open approach, laparoscopic ileocolic resection led to lower 5-year small-bowel obstruction rates in selected patients with ileocecal Crohn's disease, whereas the 5-year recurrence rates did not differ [63].

Conclusion

Treatment of inflammatory bowel disease is a challenge. Many surgeons are not enthusiastic about treatment of patients with Crohn's disease or ulcerative colitis. During recent decades, specialised centres have been created where a team of skilled surgeons, gastroenterologists, radiologists, pathologists, and psychologists guarantee an optimal management of patients with IBD. This opportunity should be offered to IBD patients whenever possible. However, in case of emergencies such as toxic megacolon, bowel perforation, bleeding, and intestinal obstruction, treatment In Loco is unavoidable. Transfer to a specialised centre, which doesn't always mean the next closest hospital, may be very dangerous for patients with IBD emergencies. An immediate surgical intervention is required, and the surgeon has to know what to do. This is expecially true for patients presenting with acute abdominal pain as a first manifestation of IBD, a rare event nowadays.

Since ulcerative colitis and Crohn's disease are not extremely rare, doctors in peripheral hospitals are familiar with them. Surgical management of patients with IBD is not extremely difficult from the technical point of view. The question is when and how to choose the right approach. Decisions made in emergency situations, or better, before these develop, are made in an interdisciplinary way. For instance, every patient with IBD should be evaluated by the gastroenterologist and the surgeon together at the time of the initial hospital admission and at every readmission thereafter.

Histologic examination of biopsies may be hazardous. A proven diagnosis of Crohn's disease is generally seen as precluding ileal pouch-anal anastomosis. This problem exists in peripheral hospitals as well as in big institutions.

In a peripheral hospital such as ours, there is a surgeon, a gastroenterologist and endoscopist, a radiologist, a blood bank, an intensive care unit, and a CT-scan available. Using these resources, we have treated patients with IBD emergencies with the results reported above (Table 2). If we have to resolve emergency situations regarding IBD patients, some planned operations should also be done. Treatment of IBD patients in our department is performed in accordance and in synchronisation with our gastroenterologist and specialised centres. We do not carry out ileal pouch-anal anastomoses because of the low number of patients requiring this operation at our hospital.

References

1. Cheung OR (2003) Inflammatory bowel disease emergencies. Gastroenterol Clin North Am 32:1269–1288
2. Tragnone A, Corrao G, Miglio F et al (1997) Incidence of inflammatory bowel disease in Italy: a nationwide population-based study. Gruppo Italiano per lo Studio del Colon e del Retto (GISC). Int J Epidemiol 26:904–906
3. Sachar DB, Bodian CA, Goldstein ES et al (2005) Is perianal Crohn's disease associated with intestinal fistulization? Am J Gastroenterol 100:1547–1549
4. Galandiuk S, Kimberling J, Al Mishlab T et al (2005) Perianal Crohn's disease: predictors of need for permanent diversion. Ann Surg 241:796–802
5. Sangwan YP, Schoetz DJ Jr, Murray JJ et al (1996) Perianal Crohn's disease. results of local surgical treatment. Dis Colon Rectum 39:529–535
6. Thornton M, Solomon MJ (2005) Long-term indwelling seton for complex anal fistulas in Crohn's disease. Dis Colon Rectum 48:459–463
7. Cataldo PA, Senagore A, Luchtefeld MA (1993) Intrarectal ultrasound in the evaluation of perirectal abscesses. Dis Colon Rectum 36:554–558
8. Wedemeyer J, Kirchhoff T, Sellge G et al (2004) Transcutaneous perianal sonography: a sensitive method for the detection of perianal inflammatory lesions in Crohn's disease. World J Gastroenterol 10:2859–2863
9. Schwartz DA, Wiersema DJ, Dudiak KM et al (2001) A comparison of endoscopic ultrasound, magnetic resonance imaging, and exam under anethesia for evaluation of Crohn's perianal fistulas. Gastroenterology 121:1064–1072
10. Radcliffe AG, Ritchie JK, Hawley PR et al (1988) Anovaginal and rectovaginal fistulas in Crohn's disease. Dis Colon Rectum 31:94
11. Winslet MC, Andrews H, Allan RN et al (1993) Fecal diversion in the management of Crohn's disease of the colon. Dis Colon Rectum 36:757
12. Heyen F, Winslet MC, Andrews H et al (1989) Vaginal fistulas in Crohn's disease. Dis Colon Rectum 32:379
13. Person B, Wexner SD (2005) Management of perianal Crohn's disease. Curr Treat Options Gastroenterol 8:197–209
14. Keighley MRB, Allan RN (1986) Current status and influence of operation on perianal Crohn's disease. Int J Colorectal Dis 1:104
15. Yamamoto T, Allan R, Keighley MRB (2000) Effect of fecal diversion alone on perianal Crohn's disease. World J Surg 24:1258–1263
16. Present DH, Ruutgerts P, Targan S et al (1999) Infliximab for the treatment of fistulas in patients with Crohn's disease. N Engl J Med 340:1398–1405
17. Regueiro M, Mardini H (2003) Treatment of perianal fistulizing Crohn's disease with infliximab alone or as an adjunct to exam under anesthesia with seton placement. Inflamm Bowel Dis 9:98–103
18. Schwartz DA, Herdman CR (2004) The medical treatment of Crohn's perianal fistulas. Aliment Pharmacol Ther 19:953–967
19. Nagler SM, Poticha SM (1979) Intraabdominal abscess in regional enteritis. Am J Surg 137:350–354
20. Nichols RJ (1999) Intraabdominal mass and/or abscess. In: Michelassi F, Milsom JW (eds) Operative strategies in inflammatory bowel disease. Springer, Berlin Heidelberg New York, pp 360–368
21. Garcia JC, Persky SE, Bonis PAL et al (2001) Abscesses in Crohn's disease: outcome of medical versus surgical treatment. J Clin Gastroenterol 32:409–412
22. Agha FP, Woolsey EJ, Amendola MA (1985) Psoas abscess in inflammatory bowel disease. Am J Gastroenterol 80:924–928
23. Procaccio JA, Lavery IC, Fazio VW et al (1991) Psoas abscess: difficulties encountered. Dis Colon Rectum 34:784–789
24. Roth T, Zimmer G, Tschanz P (2000) Crohn's disease of the appendix. Ann Chir 7:665–667
25. Simonowitz DA, Rusch VW, Stevenson JK (1982) Natural history of incidental appendectomy in patients

with Crohn's disease who required subsequent bowel resection. Am J Surg 143:171–173
26. Zager JS, Gusani NJ, Derubertis BG et al (2001) Laparoscopic appendectomy for Crohn's disease of the appendix presenting as acute appendicitis. J Laparoendosc Adv Surg Tech A 4:255–258
27. Marion JF, Present DH (1997) The modern medical management of acute, severe ulcerative colitis. Eur J Gastroenterol Hepatol 9:831–835
28. Keighley MRB (1993) Acute fulminating colitis and emergency colectomy In: Keighley MRB, Williams NS (eds) Surgery of the anus, rectum and colon. Saunders, London, pp 1379–1397
29. Reddy SB, Jeejeebhoy KN (1988) Acute complications of Crohn's disease. Crit Care Med 16:557–561
30. Tjandra JJ (1999) Toxic colitis and perforation. In: Michelassi F, Milsom JW (eds) Operative strategies in inflammatory bowel disease. Springer, Berlin Heidelberg New York, pp 234–245
31. Sheth SG, LaMont JT (1998) Toxic megacolon. Lancet 351:509–512
32. Present DH (1993) Toxic megacolon. Med Clin North Am 77:1129–1148
33. Banez AV, Yamanishi F, Crans CA (1987) Endoscopic colonic decompression of toxic megacolon, placement of colonic tube, and steroid colonclysis. Am J Gastroenterol 82:692–694
34. Riedler L, Wohlgenannt D, Thaler W et al (1989) Endoscopic decompression in "toxic megacolon". Surg Endosc 3:51–53
35. Imbriaco M, Balthazar EJ (2001) Toxic megacolon: role of CT in evaluation and detection of complications. Clin Imaging 25:349–354
36. Gan SI, Beck PL (2003) A new look at toxic megacolon: an update and review of incidence, etiology, pathogenesis, and management. Am J Gastroenterol 98:2363–2371
37. Stone W, Veidenheimer MC, Corman ML et al (1977) The dilemma of Crohn's disease: long term follow-up of Crohn's disease of the small intestine. Dis Colon Rectum 20:372–376
38. Platell C, Mackay J, Collopy B et al (1995) Crohn's disease: a colon and rectal department experience. Aust NZ J Surg 65:570–575
39. Yamamoto T, Bain IM, Allan RN et al (1999) An audit of stricturoplasty for small bowel Crohn's disease. Dis Colon Rectum 42:797–803
40. Kumar D, JA Williams (1993) Crohn's disease und ulcerative colitis: surgical management. Springer, Berlin Heidelberg New York, pp 188
41. Fazio VW, Marchetti F, Church J et al (1996) Effect of resection margins on the recurrence of Crohn's disease in the small bowel: a randomized controlled trial. Ann Surg 224:563–573
42. Park R, Roger V, Penna C (1999) Management of hemorrhage. In: Michelassi F, Milsom JW (eds) Operative strategies in inflammatory bowel disease. Springer, Berlin Heidelberg New York, pp 229–233
43. Robert JR, Sachar DB, Greenstein AJ (1991) Severe gastrointestinal hemorrhage in Crohn's disease. Ann Surg 213:207–211
44. Robert JH, Sachar DB, Aufses AH et al (1990) Management of severe hemorrhage in ulcerative colitis. Am J Surg 159:550–555
45. Cirocco WC, Reilly JC, Rusin LC (1995) Life-threatening hemorrhage and exsanguinations from Crohn's disease: report of four cases. Dis Colon Rectum 38:85–95
46. Belaiche J, Louis E, D'Haens G et al (1999) Acute lower gastrointestinal bleeding in Crohn's disease: characteristics of a unique series of 34 patients. Am J Gastroenterol 94:2178–2181
47. Crohn BB (1957) Indication for surgical intervention in regional enteritis. Arch Surg 74:305–311
48. Crohn BB (1965) Acute regional enteritis: clinical aspects and follow-up studies. NY State J Med 65:641–644
49. Greenstein AJ, Barth JA, Sachar DB et al (1986) Free colonic perforation without dilatation in ulcerative colitis. Am J Surg 152:272–275
50. Bundred NJ, Dixon JM, Lumsden AB et al (1985) Free perforation in Crohn's colitis: a ten year review. Dis Colon Rectum 28:35–37
51. Nordlinger B, Saint-Marc O (1999) Free perforation. In: Michelassi F, Milsom JW (eds) Operative strategies in inflammatory bowel disease. Springer, Berlin Heidelberg New York, pp 369–373
52. Holzheimer RG, Molloy RG, Wittmann DH (1995) Postoperative complications predict recurrence of Crohn's disease. Eur J Surg 161:129–135
53. Greenstein AJ, Mann D, Sachar B et al (1985) Free perforation in Crohn's disease: a survey of 99 cases. Am J Gastroenterol 80:682–689
54. Ikeuchi H, Yamamura T (2002) Free perforation in Crohn's disease: review of the Japanese literature. J Gastroenterol 37:1020–1027
55. Nissan A, Zamir O, Spira M et al (1997) A more liberal approach to the surgical treatment of Crohn's disease. Am J Surg 174:339–341
56. Greenstein AJ, Sachar D, Mann D et al (1986) Spontaneous free perforation and perforated abscess in 30 patients with Crohn's disease. Ann Surg 205:72–76
57. Werbin N, Haddad R, Greenberg R et al (2003) Free perforation in Crohn's disease. Is Med Assoc J 5:175–177
58. Voeller G, Britt L (1990) Surgical management of perforated Crohn's disease. Am Surg 56:100–103
59. Katz S, Schulman N, Levin L (1986) Free perforation in Crohn's disease: a report of 33 cases and review of literature. Am J Gastroenterol 81:38–43
60. Nicholls RJ (2002) Ulcerative colitis: surgical indications and treatment. Aliment Pharmacol Ther 4 [Suppl 16]:25–28
61. Fraschini A, Sella D, Gullotta R et al (1989) Free perforation due to colonic adenocarcinoma in Crohn's disease. Ital J Surg Sci 19:85–88
62. Greenstein AJ, Gennuso R, Sachar DB et al (1987) Free perforation due to cancer in Crohn's disease. Int J Colorectal Dis 2:201–202
63. Bergamaschi R, Pessaux P, Arnaud JP (2003) Comparison of conventional and laparoscopic ileocolic resection for Crohn's disease. Dis Colon Rectum 46:1129–1133

Management of the Unhealed Perineal Wound

Diego Segre, Herbert M. Dal Corso, Marino Landra, Maria C. Giuffrida

Introduction

Since the introduction of the abdominoperineal resection of the rectum (APR) for cancer or IBD [1], an increasing number of perineal complications have been reported. Delayed wound healing and local infection are in fact common complications. Healing depends on the patient's general and nutritional status, the nature of the underlying disease, the technique used for perineal reconstruction (primary closure or healing by secondary intention) and the development of perineal infection. Simple primary skin closure has been used in the past with poor results, mainly from insufficient control of local infection [2]. For some decades, frequent dressing of the perineal wound with swabs has been considered the treatment of choice, although healing by secondary intention involves prolonged hospital stay and persistent wound drainage, usually requiring frequent dressings and occasionally the development of a persistent perineal sinus (PPS). In the seventies, the introduction of closed suction drainage brought new interest to primary perineal closure techniques. McLeod et al. [3] evaluated the results of primary closure and suction drainage on 57 APRs (40 ulcerative colitis, 4 Crohn's disease, 10 carcinoma of the rectum, 2 had carcinoma of the anus and 1 had anal incontinence), reporting an overall 72% closure rate and concluding that primary healing can be achieved in a large proportion of patients operated on for cancer or IBD. More recently, the introduction of neoadjuvant radiotherapy seems to have greatly increased the risk of perineal wound complication after APR with direct primary closure.

Common experience shows that when the perineum is left open, healing by secondary intention is accompanied by a significant morbidity, prolonged hospitalisation, discomfort, protracted postoperative drainage and higher risk of PPS. The patient usually requires daily care of the perineum for 2–12 months. The wound heals more slowly in patients with inflammatory disease of the colon.

The presence of a persistent perineal sinus is certainly a disabling complication for the patient as it is usually accompanied by foul secretions, perineal pain, chronic pelvic pain, local dermatitis, infections and dyspareunia. It represents the most frequent late complication of APR and it is a challenging condition for the surgeon. According to Eftaiha and Abcarian [4], after a 4-month period from APR, the perineal wound completely healed in 78% of patients. For this reason it is important to monitor the perineal wound at 4 months. If the repair process has failed, it is important to differentiate unhealed perineal wound (UPW), those wounds still open at 6 months from initial surgery, from persistent perineal sinus (PPS), those steady fibrous wounds still present 1 year after surgery and probably unable to heal by themselves. According to some authors, a small shallow UPW can be successfully treated with curettage and local treatments, while long and complex UPW as well as PPS usually require a more extended surgical approach [5–7]. As reported by Opelka, after 6 months from radical proctectomy, the perineum heals in 58% of the patients with IBD and 70% of the patients with carcinoma. After 1 year, the wound is completely closed in 98% of the patients [8]. In all cases, especially when cancer is involved, an evaluation under anaesthesia with multiple-site biopsies is mandatory.

The anatomical limits of a perineal sinus largely depend upon the operation performed. When the rectum and the anal canal are removed, the anterior aspect of the sinus is usually formed in the female by the posterior aspect of the uterus and the posterior vaginal wall, and by the bladder, the seminal vesicles and the prostate gland in the male. These organs are rather fix, but they can nevertheless slide down to some extent with the loops of the small bowel, contributing to the closure of the pelvic defect. The lateral and the posterior aspect of the small pelvis are formed by the pelvic sidewalls and by the anterior aspect of the sacrum and coccyx covered by the presacral fascia. These structures do not take part in the process that finally leads to the closure of the pelvic wound. When APR is performed, the levator ani muscle is partially removed with the specimen so that its margins are very seldom useful for primary closure. Lubbers et al. [9] have reported a reduced number of perineal wound dehiscence and PPS after intersphincteric or perimuscular dissection of the rectum compared to wide APR.

Pathophysiology

Healing is a complex process not yet completely understood. Soon after tissue damage, the inflammation phase takes place with subsequent migration and proliferation of macrophages, lymphocytes and fibroblasts; thereafter, neoangiogenesis and fibroplasias lead to wound closure, and finally, contraction of the scar tissue and remodelling complete the healing process. This organised sequence of events can be retarded by many endogenous factors such as ischaemia or poor blood supply, and nutritional deficiencies (common in IBD patients) as well as exogenous ones such as infection, trauma and the use of anti-inflammatory drugs.

Inadequate perfusion or low haemoglobin level, metabolic diseases (e.g. diabetes mellitus) and connective tissue disorders are all systemic factors that contribute to alterations in the healing process. Before focusing on local treatment of an unhealed perineal wound, the surgeon has to correct possible nutritional and circulatory deficiencies, maintain blood glucose within the normal range and control high blood pressure. Radiotherapy, usually performed preoperatively in patients with rectal or anal cancer, represent a further factor that may delay healing and lead to PPS. Microangiosclerosis related to ionising radiation may alter the perfusion at the wound margins, while oedema and subsequent fibrosis of the pelvic tissues prevent an adequate closure of the pelvic dead space.

Patients with IBD have shown more complications in healing perineal wounds in respect to patients undergoing proctectomy for cancer. In fact, as shown by Manjoney et al. [10] in their report, at 6 weeks 39% of patients in the IBD group had completely healed in comparison to 64% in the cancer group. Patients affected by Crohn's disease are at higher risk for PPS compared to those with ulcerative rectocolitis. The frequent involvement of the small bowel in Crohn's disease and the constant hypovitaminosis with malabsorption of ascorbate and zinc, both key elements in enzyme activation, involved in the healing process are possible explanations. Furthermore, the inflamed small bowel usually becomes rigid and does not descend to occupy the empty pelvis, leading to a persistent pelvic dead space. The risk of pelvic infection is then very much increased and fistulisation of the remaining bowel is always of great concern. Finally, at the time of operation, the rectal wall, hardened by chronic inflammation, may easily tear with spillage of content into the pelvis. Under these circumstances infection is very likely to occur [11].

Yamamoto et al. [12] reviewed the records of 145 patients who underwent proctocolectomy for Crohn's disease between 1970 and 1997 and found that PPS was present in 33 (23%) of the cases. The factors indicated by the authors as contributing to the significantly increased risk included the younger age, the presence of rectal inflammation, perianal sepsis, high fistulous tracts, extra-sphincteric excision of the rectum and fecal contamination of the pelvis. In their experience, the surgical eradication of the perineal sinus gave such poor results as to make them question the usefulness of any aggressive surgical approach for perineal sinus after proctocolectomy for Crohn's disease. In any case, patients should be thoroughly informed about the possibility that perineal complication may frequently occur [13]. Whitlow et al. [14] evaluated a series of 195 patients all undergoing proctectomy at the Ochsner Clinic in New Orleans from 1980 to 1996. They reported minor wound complications in 45 (23%) patients and major complications in 13 (7%). Diagnosis of Crohn's disease, neoadjuvant full course radiotherapy, the presence of perineal fistulae or abscesses preoperatively and the direct closure of the peritoneum were all factors that significantly increased the risk of wound complication.

A persistent perineal sinus was the most common late complication in a series of 67 patients who underwent pouch removal after failed restorative proctocolectomy at St. Mark's Hospital between 1977 and 2002 [15]. After 6 months from pouch excision, 40 patients had completely healed while 27 had a PPS that required at least another operation; at 1 year 7 patients were still unhealed.

In order to reduce the risk of perineal wound infection and finally PPS, it is mandatory to avoid any contamination of the pelvis during surgery. Nevertheless, should any spillage of bowel content occur, a generous washing of the pelvic cavity is not a reliable remedy, in this case the perineal wound should be better dressed open. During APR, the laceration of the rectum is more frequent when two surgical teams are operating at the same time; for this reason Keighley [16] recommends performing the abdominal part of the operation first, and then, while the assistant completes the colostomy, the same surgeon carries out the perineal dissection. The control of haemorrhage is essential as a careful haemostasis prevents the formation of a pelvic haematoma and subsequent infections. Blood pressure needs to be checked throughout the procedure as bleeding or oozing can be difficult to detect if the patient's blood pressure is too low. The obliteration of the pelvic dead space may be useful in preventing later infection. For this reason, an intersphincteric dissection should be considered whenever possible, and the pelvic peritoneum should not be sutured in order to allow the descent of the bowel loops into the pelvis. A suction drainage is useful for preventing the collection of blood and the formation of an haematoma, thus reducing the risk of infection. The drainage is best delivered through the abdominal wall [16]. Primary closure is certainly a choice, provided that pelvic contamination has not occurred and suction drainage has been put in place. Packing should be reserved for those patients in whom contamination has occurred or when intraoperative haemostasis has not been satisfactorily accomplished. According to Jalen et al. [17], an unhealed perineal wound was present at 6 months after operation in 40% of patients with primary closure and in 60% of patients with perineal packing.

Treatment Options

Conservative Treatment

Spontaneous healing can occur in about half of all patients who still have an unhealed wound 12 months after rectal excision, if the diagnosis is ulcerative colitis; almost all persistently discharging wounds will have healed in 18–24 months. Even in Crohn's disease some perineal sinuses can heal spontaneously up to 12 months after proctocolectomy [16]. The patient should be advised and instructed to take an active part in the daily care of the wound. Simple sitz baths are rarely sufficient, and a regular use of a small shower-like "Water Pik" (Water Pik Technologies Inc., CA, USA) will favour a correct wound cleansing. The dressing should not be too tight to deter mechanical delay of the healing process. Topical antibiotic agents are sometimes useful to alleviate symptoms such as pain, pruritus and local inflammation while systemic antibiotics cannot usually reach therapeutic tissue concentrations [18] and are generally less helpful.

Adequate debridement of the perineal wound with surgical removal of all devitalised and infected tissue is of great importance. Unfortunately, the presence of multiple tracks or abscess on the buttocks or surrounding perineal skin often interferes with the above-mentioned local procedures. It is usually advisable to examine all fistulae under anaesthesia in order to define its exact position, dilate any strictures present and collect some samples for histology and cultures [16]. A daily irrigation of the cavity with antiseptic solution is effective in reducing purulent discharge [20]. In selected cases, oral metronidazole and low doses of steroids may be confidently used to reduce inflammation.

Special and complex dressings have been empirically used over the years to help closure. Among the many different types of advanced dressings, subatmospheric pressure dressings (SPD) are safe and easy to manage. The wound is filled with a sterile sponge, a silastic drain tube is placed on top and the system is sealed with airtight plastic drape. The tube is connected to a vacuum device or a vacuum bottle to maintain the wound bed at subatmospheric pressure. A vacuum allows higher blood flow in the wound bed favouring granulation tissue formation and absorbs exudates thus reducing bacterial contamination. This method has been adopted in many cases with good results [8, 21, 22].

Curettage

According to Keighley [16], curettage alone brings poor results and often requires many repeated treatments. Corman et al. [23] achieved closure in all the patients with ulcerative colitis and in 10 of 11 patients with Crohn's disease after repeated sessions of curettage of the wound (mean 3 treatments/patient).

Excision and Primary Closure

Wide excision and primary closure with removal of all fibrous tracks can be a very difficult procedure to carry out, especially in high presacral tracks. Quite often the wound cannot be sutured directly, and resulting the dead space is likely to become infected. As a matter of fact, Scammel and Keighley [24], in a group of 17 patients with Crohn's disease, obtained primary closure in three cases only. Neoadjuvant RT increases the risk of perineal wound complications after APR [25]. Bullard et al. [26] have recently reported the results of primary perineal closure after APR in a series of 117 patients who received neoadjuvant radiotherapy to downstage rectal cancer and decrease the risk of local recurrence. Major perineal wound complications were reported in 35%. Delayed healing was the most common complication with a mean healing time of 3.8±2.7 months (range 1–12). Five patients developed a PPS: four in the RT group, one in the control group. The authors concluded that in patients undergoing neoadjuvant radiotherapy, primary closure of the perineum should not be considered the option of choice.

Skin Grafting

This rather easy approach may be indicated in patients with very superficial tracks or with small cavities. Unfortunately, the majority of perineal sinuses are quite long and tortuous and after the complete excision of the cavity a complex reconstruction is often required [16].

Cutaneous and Myocutaneous Flaps

Many techniques of muscle transposition have been described for the treatment of PPS. The procedure can be carried out soon after the excision of the sinus, usually involving parts of the coccyx and lower sacrum, or a few days later, when the walls of the cavity are covered with granulation tissue [16]. Marti et al. [27] used a wide V-Y full-thickness flap to cover large perineal defects in six cases (Fig. 1). The authors used this technique in two cases of giant condyloma of the perineum without the involvement of the anal canal, two cases of hidradenitis suppurativa and two cases of salvage total rectal excision after failed radiotherapy for anal carcinoma. All wounds healed primarily without infection even in the last two patients who, as reported, had signs of perineal radiodermitis. In persistent perineal sinus after proctectomy for Crohn's disease, Bascom et al. [28] suggest an easy technique, using a skin flap 1 cm thick, whose healing is favoured when an asymmetric suture line is placed to one side of the repair.

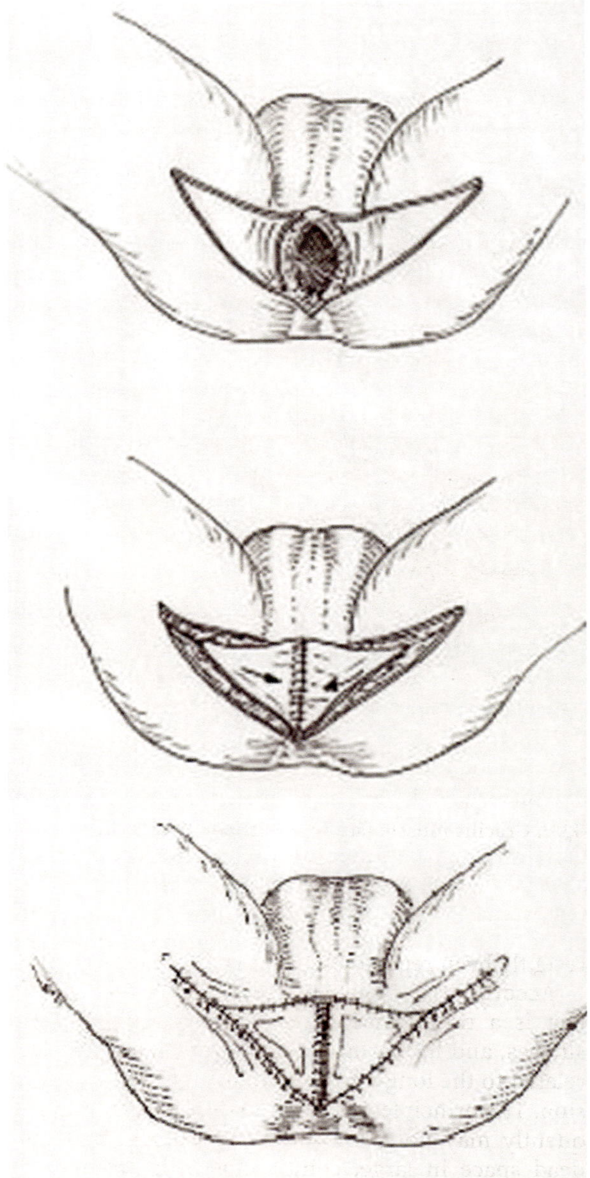

Fig. 1. V-Y fasciocutaneous flap. Two large triangular flaps extending to the inner aspects of the thighs are marked (*top*). The skin, subcutaneous fat and deep fascia are incised (*middle*). The flaps are mobilised 4–6 cm medially on each side and sutured (*bottom*)

Gracilis Muscle Flap

Bartholdson and Hulten described the gracilis muscle flap for perineal reconstruction in 1975 [29]. This fusiform muscle lies along the medial side of the thigh and knee and serves to adduct the thigh, and to flex and medially rotate the leg. It attaches proximally at the body and inferior ramus of the pubic bone and distally to the superior part of the medial surface of the tibia. The dominant vascular pedicle of this flap is the medial femoral circumflex artery and vein that branches off the profunda femoris artery and vein [18]. The muscle is exposed through a longitudinal thigh incision and the distal end is divided near the knee (Fig. 2). It may be rotated as a muscle or as a myocutaneous unit. Usually the muscle alone is used for rotation as the overlying skin has a rather uncertain blood supply. Moreover, the inclusion of the skin tends to limit the degree of muscle transposition into the perineal wound. Furthermore, the donor site may be difficult to close [16].

This flap can be used as a pedicle graft for filling the cavity created after excision of a long perineal sinus. Some authors consider the gracilis muscle flap the technique of choice for many perineal wounds. Ryan [30] reported a successful healing in 12 of 15 patients [80%), including 9 with ulcerative colitis and 6 with Crohn's disease. The same good results have

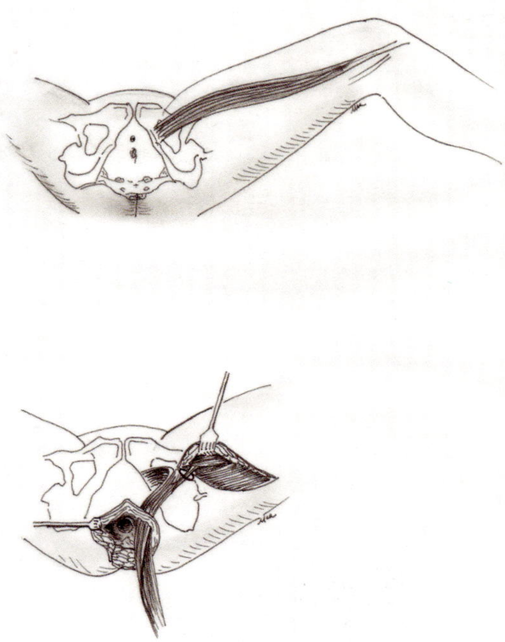

Fig. 2. Gracilis muscle flap reconstruction for PPS

recently been reported by Rius et al. [31].

According to Keighley [16], the gracilis muscle flap is a useful option in postirradiation perineal sinuses, and he warns about the risk of sensory loss related to the long and potentially painful thigh incision. The principle drawback to this flap is that it frequently may not provide sufficient bulk to fill the dead space in large, complex perineal wounds. In addition, the proximal two thirds of the gracilis muscle, which represents the main bulk of the flap, may not reach the deepest point of the perineal wound due to its low axis of rotation [18]. Finally the vascularity of the distal third of the flap may be unreliable. For these reasons many reconstructive surgeons are actually cautious in utilising this flap.

Gluteal Thigh Flap

This fasciocutaneous flap, based on the descending branch of the inferior gluteal artery, includes the skin and subcutaneous tissue of the proximal posterior thigh. The posterior cutaneous nerve of the thigh is intimately associated with the vascular pedicle and provides the opportunity of transferring a flap that maintains a certain skin sensitivity. The point of rotation of the flap is 5 cm above the ischial tuberosity which overlies the emergence of the inferior gluteal artery from underneath the piriformis muscle. The central axis of the flap is midway between the greater trochanter and the ischial tuberosity, running perpendicularly to the gluteal crease.

The donor site can be usually sutured straightforwardly. To facilitate donor site closure, the flap should be designed to be less than 12 cm in width. It may be extended to within 8 cm from the popliteal fossa. In a series of 19 patients with 21 buttock and perineal wounds closed in a single stage, Hurtwitz et al. demonstrated the reliability, versatility and low morbidity of the gluteal thigh flap [18, 32]. It provides excellent soft tissue bulk and usually little to no functional deficit is noted postoperatively [19]. Many authors consider it to be the gold standard for the chronic, deep midline perineal defect, while others feel that de-epithelialised fasciocutaneous flaps have a limited capability in filling completely dead spaces, especially in complex sinuses [18].

Gluteus Maximus Muscle and Musculocutaneous Flap

The gluteus maximus muscle is one of the largest muscles in the body. Its principle actions are to extend the thigh and assist in its lateral rotation, steady the thigh and assist in raising the trunk from the flexed position. It has a dual blood supply from the superior and inferior gluteal vessels. The inferior gluteal artery and posterior cutaneous nerve of the thigh supply the inferior portion of gluteus maximus and the skin of the posterior thigh. Excision of the lower aspect of the gluteus maximus results in no functional deficit; the donor site can be closed primarily and the muscle is sufficiently bulky to fill the cavity [16]. Baird et al. reported a series of 16 patients in which the inferior gluteal myocutaneous flap was employed to close large perineal wounds [33], all but one patient achieved complete healing of the perineal wound. In addition, Gottlieb and Jejurikar [18] prefer the inferior gluteus maximus muscle. To facilitate exposure, dissection and elevation of the lateral distal aspect of the inferior gluteus maximus muscle from the ileotibial tract, a counter-incision is made in the upper lateral posterior thigh. By detaching the origin and insertion of the inferior portion of the gluteus maximus muscle, leaving it attached only by its vascular pedicle, the flap will be able to fill the dead space of very large and deep perineal and pelvic

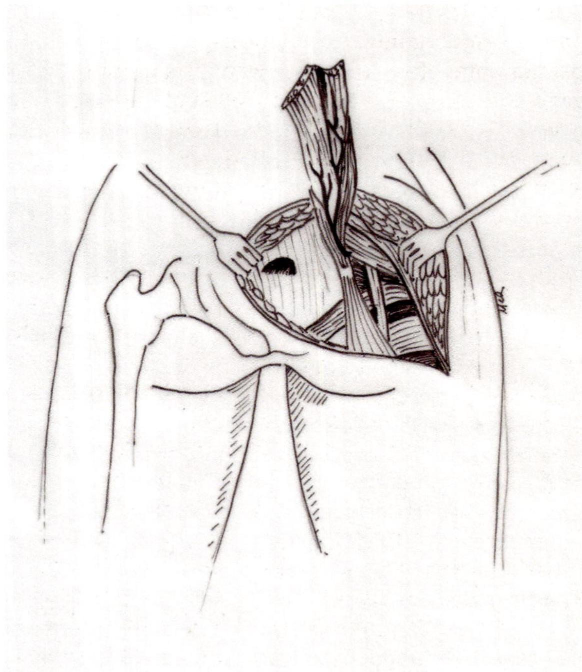

Fig. 3. The gluteus maximus musculocutaneous flap

wounds (Fig. 3). Bell et al. [34] think that this flap cannot fill the pelvis deeply and reserve this technique for patients in whom a chronic sinus occurs after primary simple closure of the perineal wound. This has the important advantage of avoiding reentering the pelvic cavity from the abdomen.

Gluteus Maximus V-Y Advancement Flaps

Shallow perineal defects may be closed utilising single or bilateral gluteus maximus V-Y flaps. The origins of the gluteal muscles are detached from their attachment to the sacrum, advanced medially and secured to each other in the midline. A V-shaped incision is made in the posterior/lateral buttock skin down to the gluteal muscle. The musculocutaneous unit is advanced medially and a midline closure is performed without tension. The donor site is closed as a V-Y plasty [18]. Hurst et al. [19] utilised this flap in 4 of 12 patients (12.4% of 97 patients submitted to proctectomy for Crohn's disease) achieving primary closure.

Gluteal Posterior Thigh Chimera Flap

If additional skin is required to accomplish perineal wound closure without tension, the gluteal thigh flap may be elevated in combination with a gluteal muscle flap based on the same pedicle. The pedicle of the gluteal thigh flap, the descending branch of the inferior gluteal artery can be separated from beneath the gluteal muscle and dissected to its take-off from the inferior gluteal artery as it emerges from underneath the piriformis muscle, allowing independent placement of the muscle in the cavity and the skin paddle on the surface [18]. This technique allows two separate tissue transfers in a single flap procedure and is well suited for patients that require a wider pelvic dissection in addition to an extensive resection of the perineal skin [19].

Rectus Abdominis Myocutaneous Flap

This technique was described by Taylor et al. in 1983 [35]. It is an excellent method for closing a large perineal defect. Based on the inferior epigastric artery and vein, it may be passed into the pelvis to close the pelvic floor and fill the dead space. It is best employed prophylactically in high risk patients at the time of proctectomy when potential perineal wound problems are anticipated [17], or at the time of abdominoperineal excision for a large neoplasm [34] when extensive perineal excision is needed in Crohn's disease [36], or, finally, when the combined approach is used to excise a large perineal sinus in Crohn's disease or after radiotherapy [16]. As a delayed or secondary procedure, the advantages of this flap must be weighed against the potential difficulties and morbidity of having to reenter the lower abdomen and mobilise the bowel to provide space to pass this flap into the pelvis, which is often severely fibrotic. Moreover, in very large pelvic wounds, the bulk of a single rectus abdominis muscle is inadequate to entirely obliterate the dead space [17]. In cases in which a completion proctectomy is performed solely by a perineal approach or for closure of a chronic perineal sinus gluteus maximus, posterior thigh or even gracilis, flaps are often adequate and do not require laparotomy [19].

A rectus abdominis myocutaneous flap has to be designed opposite to the site of the stoma provided that the muscle on that side has not been damaged by repeated laparotomies or by a previous stoma. It is important to assess the vascular supply of the flap preoperatively and, if necessary, an angiogram can be performed, particularly if the patient has received groin irradiation [34]. The abdomen is opened and a synchronous combined excision of the rectum and the perineal sinus is completed. A disc of skin slightly larger than the perineal defect is cut over one rectus muscle, 3–4 cm below the costal margin, to reconstruct the perineum and occasionally the posterior aspect of the vagina.

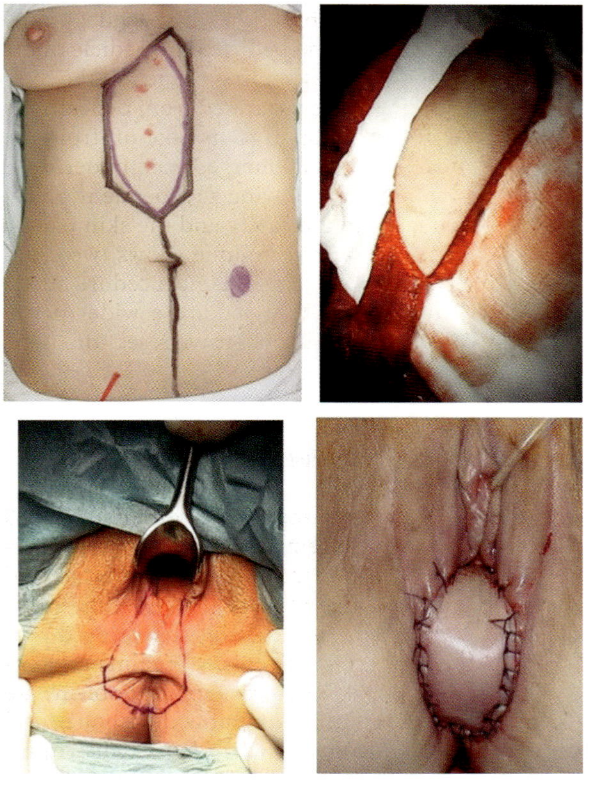

Fig. 4. Vertically oriented rectus abdominis myocutaneous (VRAM) flap. The skin paddle is designed to match the size of the defect (*top left*). The myocutaneous flap is raised and includes the anterior fascia of the rectus sheath (*top right*). Marking the line of perineal resection including posterior vaginal wall (*bottom left*). The skin paddle is secured with interrupted sutures (*bottom right*)

Traditionally, the two main types of flap are described by the orientation of the skin paddle, i.e. the vertical rectus abdominis flap (VRAM] or the transverse rectus abdominis flap (TRAM) [37]. The subcutaneous tissue is divided with the skin to the rectus. The segment of rectus above the flap is divided, ligating the superior epigastric vessels. The inferior epigastric vessels are then dissected free, dividing branches or tributaries which do not supply the inferior aspect of the rectus muscle. An adequate length of vascular pedicle is needed to rotate the skin disc and underlying muscle through the pelvis and on to the perineum. The defect in the rectus sheath is closed over suction drainage and the skin flap is sutured to the perineal skin over suction drainage with the muscle filling the dead space above (Fig. 4) [16]. Undoubtedly this technique may compromise the strength of the abdominal incision and may compromise management of stoma complications or recurrent ileal disease, particularly if the stoma needs to be resited [12].

Smith et al. [38] published the results of 22 patients undergoing the Taylor flap, 21 at the time of primary operation, but these were predominantly for vaginal reconstruction alone. Bell et al. [34] reported a series of 31 consecutive patients undergoing one-stage rectus abdominis myocutaneous flap reconstruction of extensive perineal wounds expected to generate substantial morbidity: 26 had surgery for recurrent or persistent epidermoid anal cancer or low rectal cancer and 21 had high-dose preoperative radiotherapy.

The authors modified the original Taylor's technique using an oblique skin paddle over the longitudinal rectus muscle, mainly because the oblique flap showed many advantages compared to the vertical one. In fact, the laxity of the abdominal skin is more significant in the oblique direction than in the vertical direction, allowing a larger paddle and minimising tension at the donor site [34]. Three weeks after operation, complete healing of the perineal wound was seen in 27 of the 31 patients and none developed a chronic sinus. At the completion of follow-up (median 9 months) there were no unhealed wounds.

Collie et al. [36] reviewed a series of 15 patients who received proctectomy for Crohn's disease, five of which had a gracilis interposition and 11 a rectus abdominis flap (one that had failed after gracilis interposition). All 11 patients with a rectus abdominis flap had a healed perineum at 3 months after surgery and no donor-site complications. The perineum healed in only one of those who had gracilis interposition.

Loessin et al. [39] employed an inferiorly based transpelvic rectus abdominis muscle or musculocutaneous flap to treat persistent sacral and perineal defects secondary to radiation and abdominoperineal resection with or without sacrectomy-14 of the 15 patients achieved healing and 7 had no complications. The remaining eight patients required one or more operative debridement or prolonged wound care to accomplish healing of the wound. Many authors think that reconstruction with a VRAM flap represents the best chance for facilitating healing in irradiated pelvises and they recommend its use for locally advanced rectal cancers requiring intense preoperative and intraoperative chemoradiation [40, 41]. In Table 1, the results of VRAM flap repair used for primary perineal repair soon after APR and for repair after PPS wide excision are reported.

Omentoplasty

In patients who have undergone proctectomy for inflammatory bowel disease, the main problem may be a deep presacral cavity with only a small skin

Table 1. Comparison of VRAM flap use for perineal primary closure and for PPS repair

Author	Primary perineal repair with VRAM	PPS repair with VRAM	Major flap-related complications	Healed at 3 months
Brough [45]	0	7	0	7
Loessin [39]	0	7	4	3
Smith [38]	21	1	2	– [*]
Radice [41]	13	0	1	12
Hurst [19]	5	0	1	5
D'Souza [40]	12	0	2	12
Bell [34]	31	0	9	27
Collie [36]	10	1	0	11

[*], unreported date

defect. Use of a pedicled omental graft to fill this cavity is a simple solution which does not compromise skeletal muscle bulk or function and can be more readily applied by general and colorectal surgeons than the more specialised myocutaneous flap [42, 43]. It is particularly appropriate in Crohn's disease where the rectus muscle may already have been damaged because of multiple stoma sites. The omentum may be based on the right gastroepiploic artery, in which case the left gastroepiploic close to the short gastric vessels is divided and the left side of the omentum is mobilised in order to bring the apex down to the perineum (Fig. 5).

In some cases, to allow a longer pedicle, the omental flap can be obtained on the left gastroepiploic artery, dividing the right gastroepiploic at the level of the second portion of the duodenum [16]. For Bell et al. [34], primary closure over a pedicled omentoplasty is the standard practice for perineal wound repair following APR. Radice et al. [41] employed primary perineal wound closure with or without an omental pedicle graft for pelvic space obliteration, followed by delayed myocutaneous flap advancement as required for wound complications, after resection of locally advanced pelvic malignancies. Pujol [44], in a multicentre study, reported 100% success utilising epiploonplasty in 28 abdominoperineal resections and 32 pelvectomies. Brough et al. [45], in a series of ten cases with a persistent sinus after previous proctectomy, used a plug of greater omentum (two cases), a muscle plug using the rectus abdominis muscle (two cases) and a full myocutaneous flap based on the rectus abdominis muscle where there was considerable loss of perineal skin (six cases). Complications of omentoplasty include haemorrhage, infarction, causing peritonism, intestinal obstruction and perineal hernia. Reoperation for omentoplasty-related complications is required in 0–7% of patients [42, 43, 46].

Conclusion

The unhealed perineal wound is a complication that is disabling for the patient, causing a significant amount of morbidity and anxiety, and is difficult and

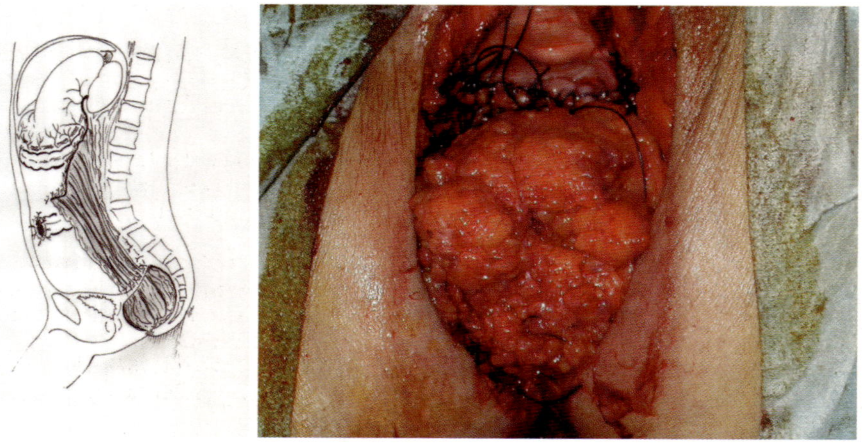

Fig. 5. Omentoplasty. The right portion of the great omentum is transposed in the sacral cavity after APR (*left*). View of the perineum after omentoplasty is completed and before skin suturing (*right*)

challenging for the colorectal surgeon. Fortunately, in the last few decades treatment options have progressed from repeated unreliable procedures to successful one-stage closure, considering modern principles of wound management.

References

1. Miles WE (1908) A method of performing abdomino-perineal excision for carcinoma of the rectum and of the terminal portion of the pelvic colon. Lancet 2:1812–1813
2. Saha SK, Robinson AF (1976) A study of wound healing after abdominoperineal resection. Br J Surg 63:555
3. McLeod R, Cohen Z, Langer B, Taylor B (1983) Primary perineal wound closure following excision of the rectum. Can J Surg 26:122–124
4. Eftaiha M, Abcarian H (1978) Management of perineal wounds after proctocolectomy: a retrospective study of 50 cases in which treatment by the open technique was used. Dis Colon Rectum 21:287–291
5. Watts JM, DeDombal FT, Goligher JC (1966) Long term complications and prognosis following major surgery for ulcerative colitis. Br J Surg 53:1014
6. Silen W, Glotzer DJ T (1974) The prevention and treatment of the persistent perineal sinus. Surgery 75:535–542
7. Ferrari BT, Den Besten L (1980) The prevention and treatment of the persistent perineal sinus. World J Surg 4:167–172
8. Opelka FG (2001) Unhealed perineal wound. Clinic Colon Rectal Surg 14(1):65–68
9. Lubbers EJC (1982) Healing of the perineal wound after proctectomy for nonmalignant conditions. Dis Colon Rectum 25:351–357
10. Manjoney DL, Koplewitz MJ, Abrams JS (1983) Factors influencing perineal wound healing after proctectomy. Am J Surg 145:183–189
11. The American Society of Colon and Rectal Surgeons (2005) Practice parameters for the surgical treatment of ulcerative colitis. Dis Colon Rectum 48:1997–2009
12. Yamamoto T, Bain I A, Allan R N, Keighley MRB (1999) Persistent perineal sinus after proctocolectomy for Crohn's disease. Dis Colon Rectum 42:96–101
13. Yamamoto T, Allan RN, Keighley MRB (2000) Audit of single-stage proctocolectomy for Crohn's disease. Dis Colon Rectum 43:249–256
14. Whitlow CB, Opelka FG, Terrel CH et al (2000) Perineal wounds complications following proctectomy. Perspect Colon Rectal Surg 13:69–77
15. Karoui M, Cohen R, Nicholls J (2004) Results of surgical removal of the pouch after failed restorative proctocolectomy. Dis Colon Rectum 47:869–875
16. Keighley MRB (1999) Persistent perineal sinus. In: Keighley MRB, Williams NS (eds) Surgery of the anus, rectum and colon. Saunders, London, pp 308–331
17. Jalen AN, Smith CV, Ruckley CW et al (1969) Perineal wound healing in ulcerative colitis. Br J Surg 56:749
18. Gottlieb LJ, Jejurikar SS (1999) Management of the persistent perineal wound. In: Michelassi F, Milsom JW (eds) Operative strategies in inflammatory bowel disease Springer, Berlin Heidelberg NewYork, pp 445–457
19. Hurst RD, Gottlieb LJ, Crucitti P et al (2001) Primary closure of complicated perineal wounds with myocutaneous and fasciocutaneous flaps after proctectomy for Crohn's disease. Surgery 130:767–73
20. Galandiuk S, Fazio VW (1991) Postoperative irrigation-suction drainage after pelvic colonic surgery: prospective randomized trial. Dis Colon Rectum 34:223–228
21. Argenta LC, Morykwas MJ (1997) Vacuum assisted closure: a new method for wound control and treatment: clinical experience 38:563–577
22. Moykwas MJ, Argenta LC, Shelton-Brown EI, McGuirt W (1997) Vacuum assisted closure: a new method for wound control and treatment: animal studies and basic foundation. Ann Plast Surg 38:553–562
23. Corman ML, Veidenheimer MC, Collet JA, Ross VH (1978) Perineal wound healing after proctectomy for IBD. Dis Colon Rectum 21:155–159
24. Scammel B, Keighley MRB (1986) Delayed perineal wound healing after proctectomy for Crohn's colitis. Br J Surg 73:150–152
25. Janjan N, KhooV, Rich T et al (1998) Locally advanced rectal cancer: surgical complications after infusional chemotherapy and radiation therapy. Radiology 206:131–136
26. Bullard K, Trudel JL, Baxter NN, Rothenberger DA (2005) Primary perineal wound closure after preoperative radiotherapy and abdominoperineal resection has a high incidence of wound failure. Dis Colon Rectum 48:438–443
27. Marti MC, Roche B, Gumener RG (1994) Skin cover of perineal defects using V-Y flaps. Int J Colorectal Dis 9:163–164
28. Bascom T, Bascom JU (2002) Persistent perineal sinus after proctectomy for Crohn's disease: simplified repair using skin flap. Am J Surg 184:84
29. Bartholdson L, Hulten L (1975) Repair of persistent perineal sinuses by means of a pedicle flap of musculus gracilis. Scand J Plast Reconstr Surg 9:74–76
30. Ryan JA (1984) Gracilis muscle flap for the persistent perineal sinus in inflammatory bowel disease. Am J Surg 148:64–70
31. Rius J, Nessim A, Nogueras JJ, Wexner SD (2000) Gracilis transposition in complicated perianal fistula and unhealed perineal wounds in Crohn's disease. Eur J Surg 166:218–222
32. Hurtwitz DJ, Swartz WM, Mathes SJ (1981) The gluteal thigh flap: a reliable, sensate flap for the closure of buttock and perineal wounds. Plast Reconstr Surg 68:521–530
33. Baird WL,Hester TR, Nahai F et al (1990) Management of perineal wounds following abdominoperineal resection with inferior gluteal flaps. Arch Surg 125:1486–1489
34. Bell SW, Dehni N, Chaouat M et al (2005) Primary rectus abdominis myocutaneous flap for repair of perineal and vaginal defects after extended abdominoperineal resection. Br J Surg 92:482–486
35. Taylor GI, Corlett R, Boyd JB (1983) The extended deep inferior epigastric flap: a clinical technique. Plast Reconstr Surg 72:751–765

36. Collie MHS, Potter MA, Bartolo DCC (2005) Myocutaneous flaps promote perineal healing in inflammatory bowel disease. Br J Surg 92:740–741
37. Waterhouse N, Northover JMA (1993) Reconstructive surgery of the groin and perineum. In: Phillips RKS, Northover J (eds) Modern coloproctology. Arnold, London, pp 10–22
38. Smith HO, Genesen MC, Runowicz CD, Goldberg GL (1998) The rectus abdominis myocutaneous flap: modifications, complications and sexual function. Cancer 83:510–520
39. Loessin SJ, Bradly Meland N, Devine RM et al (1995) Management of sacral and perineal defects following abdominoperineal resection and radiation with transpelvic muscle flaps. Dis Colon Rectum 38:940–945
40. D'Souza DN, Pera M, Nelson H et al (2003) Vaginal reconstruction following resection of primary locally advanced and recurrent colorectal malignancies. Arch Surg 138:1340–1343
41. Radice E, Nelson H, Mercill S et al (1999) Primary myocutaneous flap closure following resection of locally advanced pelvic malignancies. Br J Surg 86:349–354
42. O'Leary DP (1999) Use of the greater omentum in colorectal surgery. Dis Colon Rectum 42:533–539
43. Hay J-M, Fingerhut A, Paquet J-C et al (1997) Management of the pelvic space with or without omentoplasty after abdominoperineal resection for carcinoma of the rectum: a prospective multicenter study. Eur Surg Res 163:199–206
44. Pujol H (1981) De l'utilisation du grand épiploon en cancérologie: a propos de 297 cas. Travail du Groupe des Chirurgiens du Centre Francais de Lutte contre le Cancer. Chirurgie 107:292–298
45. Brough WA, Schofield PF (1991) The value of the rectus abdominis myocutaneous flap in the treatment of complex perineal fistula. Dis Colon Rectum 34:148–150
46. van Garderen JA, Wiggers TH, van Geel AN (1991) Complications of pedicled omentoplasty. Neth J Surg 43:171–174

Rehabilitation in Patients with Inflammatory Bowel Disease and Familial Adenomatous Polyposis

Federica Lipanje, Gianluca Colucci, Gian Gaetano Delaini

Introduction

Rehabilitation medicine can be defined as the multidisciplinary and interdisciplinary science that aims at attaining the complete functionality and health of a person by reducing the disability and its correlated symptoms. Rehabilitation is a both a process that involves finding solutions to given problems and also a process of education whereby a person is helped to achieve the best possible level of life in its physical, functional, social and emotional dimensions with the least possible limitation to their operative choices. The process also requires the involvement of the patients' family and those around them. Consequently, "the rehabilitation process concerns not only strictly clinical aspects" but also "encompasses psychological and social dimensions. To achieve a good level of efficacy, each patient's rehabilitation project must have rationally planned, multiple objectives so that the autonomy to be attained in various areas can be translated into the personal independence of the patient as a whole being, with enhanced quality of life for the patient" [1].

In patients affected by inflammatory bowel disease (IBD) and familial adenomatous polyposis (FAP), the rehabilitation process aims at attaining, recovering and maintaining an increased level of autonomy by relying on: (1) surgical intervention, and (2) study of the disability problems associated with these pathologies.

Surgery for IBD and FAP

The rehabilitation process takes into account surgical intervention and its technical aspects, as well as the probable quality of life of the patient after therapeutic treatment. Whenever possible, the rehabilitation process will begin before surgery by informing and educating the patient about the therapeutic strategy to be adopted. After surgery, all efforts will concentrate on maintaining and/or recovering the patient's autonomy and functionality.

On this subject, attention will be paid to both the recovery of basic functions, that is to say, those linked to vegetative life (such as correct breathing, blood circulation and the tegumentary function) and to functions related to social life. The main objectives are to:

- improve overall functionality.
- Reduce or to keep in check all postoperative symptoms and/or complications.
- Reduce the level of disability.
- Promote rehabilitation to social and working life.
- Help the patient become aware of the disability and actual functionality and to support that new awareness.

Diagnostic evaluation and planning an appropriate therapeutic intervention are needed in order to realise these objectives.

Among the existing colic surgery protocols, one that certainly deserves to be mentioned is the protocol developed by Kehlet and his Danish team [2]: with their concept of "accelerated rehabilitation", they developed a series of perioperative treatments that allow speedy recovery and an early dismissal. This treatment concept preserves bodily organ functions and avoids the usual postoperative deterioration in pulmonary function, body composition and cardiovascular response to exercise [3]. (See Table 1 for a comparison of this protocol with the Conventional Care and Multimodal Rehabilitation programmes.) The multimodal rehabilitation programme, with epidural analgesia, early oral nutrition and mobilisation, besides application after open colonic surgery for noninflammatory bowel disease, is also used after ileocolic resections for Crohn's disease [4]. Andersen and Kehlet, at the end of this prospective, nonrandomized study, observed that open ileocolic resections for Crohn's disease combined with fast-track multimodal rehabilitation with continuos epidural analgesia and enforced early oral feeding and mobilisation enhanced recovery and decreased median hospital stay to 3 days with a low morbidity and readmission rate. Moreover, they suggested that "prospective studies using multimodal

Table 1. Protocol for anaesthesia, surgery and rehabilitation programme after colonic resection with conventional care (group 1) and multimodal rehabilitation (group 2) [3]

	Group 1	Group 2
Anaesthesia	Premedication: oral diazepam 10 mg Epidural catheter: T8-T10 Carbocaine 2% (4+4) ml with epinephrine Carbocaine 2% 4 ml with epinephrine hourly General anesthesia: Fentanyl 0.1 mg Thiomebumal 3-5 mg/kg Rocuronium O_2-N_2O-sevoflurane Dextran 70 (Macrodex) 500 ml Saline 3,000 ml (max)	Premedication: none Epidural catheter Right hemicolectomy: T6-T7 Sigmoid resection: T9-T10 Test: lidocaine 2% 3 ml with epinephrine Bupivacaine 0.5% (6+6) ml Bupivacaine 0.25% 5 ml 2 h intraoperatively Morphine 2 mg if <70 years Morphine 1 mg ≥70 years General anaesthesia: Remifentanil 1 mg/kg/min Propofol 2-4 mg/kg/h Cicatriceum 0.15 mg/kg Hydroxyethyl starch (HAES) 500 ml Saline 1500 ml (max) Ondansetron 4 mg Ketorolac 30 mg Bupivacaine 0.25% 20 ml (incision)
Surgery	Median laparotomy	Transverse or curved incision
Postoperatively	Continuous epidural analgesia (3 days): Bupivacaine 0.25% 4 ml and morphine 0.2 mg/h Breakthrough pain: morphine IM or IV After removal of epidural catheter: morphine 10 mg orally No standard care program: fluid, food, mobilization and discharge depending on the attending surgeon Postoperative nasogastric tube depending on surgeon who performed the operation Physiotherapy: breathing exercise 10 min per day during the first 2 postoperative days and only on working days	Continuous epidural analgesia (2 days): Bupivacaine 0.25% 4 ml and morphine 0.2 mg/h Breakthrough pain: ibuprofen 600 mg orally Bupivacaine 0.125% 6 ml epidurally Morphine 10 mg orally (last choice) Food, protein drink 60–80 g protein per day and mobilization from the day of surgery following a well-defined nursing care programme Day of surgery start: acetaminophen (slow release) 2 g/12 hourly Cisapride 20 mg/12 hourly 1st postoperative day: remove bladder catheter in the morning 2nd postoperative day: remove epidural catheter in the morning; discharge after lunch

rehabilitation are indicated to evaluate the role of laparoscopic assisted vs open resection for ileo-colic Crohn's disease".

Fundamentals of Rehabilitation

The definition of a rehabilitation program is based upon four areas of intervention:

- physical training and the development of a physical training programme.
- A programme of health education in order to eliminate or reduce all risk factors that may affect clinical condition.
- Evaluation of the patient's psychological condition and social and working environment and the development of a program of topical intervention.
- Evaluation and treatment of possible surgical or internal complications.

Physical Training and the Development of Physical Training Programs

A physical training programme is developed in three phases: preoperative, acute postoperative and long term.

Pre-operative Phase

During this phase, patients learn all the exercises they will have to practise also in the postoperative phase, including the best strategies to counteract the main postoperative problems, thus developing a greater awareness of their condition. However, depending on the urgency of the patient's condition, this rehabilitative intervention may not always be possible, particularly if patient is affected by Crohn's disease. During the preoperative phase, a preventive functional evaluation is established. Patients are trained in breathing induction and relaxation techniques. Moreover, they learn the different types of cough, to be mainly performed using their intercostal muscles, and breathing techniques. They are also trained to adopt the correct posture when forced to bed for certain periods.

Acute Post-operative Phase

The rehabilitation process includes pain treatment, breathing re-education, as well as functional, motor and sphincterial re-education.

The main objectives of breathing rehabilitation are to:
- achieve optimal blood oxygen levels.
- Promote the dissolving of and then elimination of bronchial secretions.
- Train the patient how to best face and overcome physical efforts.

Motor re-education aims at:
- Promoting autonomy in moving to and from the bed, allowing the patient to slowly reach a correct standing and walking position.
- Helping the patient adopt the correct posture when lying, sitting or standing.
- Promoting progressive tolerance of physical efforts.

Exercises in this phase are designed to:
- Re-establish good general muscular tone.
- Counteract the effects of long periods of immobilisation on the metabolism of bones, muscles and articulations so as to prevent muscle contractures, osteoporosis and thromboembolic complications.

Attention is also paid to the patient's posture in order to avoid the development of skin breakdown. It must be stressed how beneficial training is from a psychological point of view: in fact, it helps reduce and manage anxiety and stress, contributes to higher morale and promotes greater self-esteem.

Sphincterial re-education consists of early removal of bladder catheters (usually within 1–2 days). Functional re-education aims at attaining autonomy in carrying out daily activities and achieving early oral nutrition. Patients also learn the correct use of stomas.

Long-Term Rehabilitation

Exercises learnt during the hospital stay must also be practised once the patient has returned home. Parameters such as frequency, intensity, duration, mode and time progression of physical training may vary after hospitalisation. As to long-term rehabilitation, at the moment, there are no definite guidelines or parameters suggesting exercises and follow-up schedules.

Specific Health Training

Health education refers to the patients' knowledge of their medical condition and the critical factors that may affect it. Patients are therefore instructed to recognise early possible signs of complications and are made aware of the importance of following constantly the therapeutic physical and pharmacological programme designed for them. In particular, patients are checked for and informed about:
- pain management.
- Colonic carcinoma.
- Metabolism and nutritional balance.
- Specific training techniques to use stomas correctly.

Psychosocial Evaluation

A psychological evaluation is performed to determine:
- The kind of social/family environment the patient comes from and the kind of support he/she can receive from it.
- The patient's engagement in free-time/recreational activities.
- The patient's job and physical and emotional work involvement.

Evaluation and Treatment of Possible Surgical or Internal Complications

Faecal Incontinence

Faecal incontinence is defined as either involuntary passage or inability to control the discharge of faecal matter through the anus. Three subtypes of faecal incontinence have been identified [5]:
1. Passive incontinence: involuntary discharge of stool or gas without the patient's awareness.
2. Urge incontinence: discharge of faecal matter despite the patient's active attempts to retain bowel contents.

3. Faecal seepage: leakage of stool that follows otherwise normal evacuation.

The severity of incontinence can range from unintentional elimination of flatus to seepage of liquid faecal matter or, sometimes, to the complete evacuation of bowel contents. These events can be a cause of considerable embarrassment for patients, affecting in the long run their self-esteem and causing in turn social isolation and a poorer quality of life [6]. To maintain normal faecal continence, it is important to preserve the neuromuscular integrity of the rectum, anus and adjoining pelvic floor musculature. It follows that incontinence occurs when there is disruption of one or more mechanisms that maintain continence; the disruption is to such an extent that other mechanisms are unable to compensate. Incontinence in patients affected by IBD and by FAP is caused by [5]:

- Decrease in rectal compliance and accommodation.
- Disruption of the external anal sphincter complex due to (a) anorectal surgery for fistulas, hemorrhoids or fissure; (b) anal dilation of lateral sphincterotomy.

The aim of the treatment is to restore continence and improve quality of life.

Conservative Therapy

Habit training involves a regular schedule for defaecation, usually after breakfast, and often including the use of extra fibre. Hygienic measures are also taken, such as changing undergarments and cleaning the perianal skin immediately after a soiling episode. Other supportive measures can include modifications in diet, such as reducing caffeine or fibre consumption.

Specific Treatment

1. Pharmacologic therapy: antidiarrhoeal agents, such as Loperamide, suppositories or enemas are usually prescribed [5].
2. Biofeedback: this is a "non-surgical, non-invasive, and relatively inexpensive method of treating faecal incontinence on an outpatient basis" [7]. Biofeedback has proven effective in the strengthening of "the external sphincter and anorectal sensation" [8], providing "immediate and long-term improvement of faecal incontinence" and "restoring a normal quality of life" [9]. The patient is trained to recognise small volumes of rectal distension and contract the external anal sphincter while simultaneously keeping intraabdominal pressure low. This is accomplished by measuring anal canal pressure, showing this on a visual display to the patient, and providing verbal feedback. Usually, better results are observed with motivated, mentally capable patients. Patients should also have some degree of rectal sensation and be able to contract the external anal sphincter [10]. Among other approaches, the augmented biofeedback program is also to be mentioned. This programme includes electrical stimulation of the anal sphincter with electromyogram (EMG) feedback. To achieve a sustained improvement of bowel function, however, these neuromuscular conditioning techniques must be used together with pelvic muscle strengthening or other supportive measures.
3. Plugs, sphincter bulkers and electrical stimulation: At present, these devices should be considered as experimental and deserve further controlled clinical trials [5, 11].

Surgery

Surgery should only be considered for patients who fail conservative measures or biofeedback therapy [5].

Extraintestinal Symptoms Located in the Articulations

It has been observed that patients affected by IBD frequently experience complications of joints complaints, with prevalence that varies between 30% and 36%. IBD-related arthropathy may be expressed as peripheral or axial arthritis, frequently indistinguishable from the classical ankylosing spondylitis [12].

Ankylosing Spondylitis

This chronic inflammatory disease is characterised by a progressive ligament calcification with hardening of the spine that reduces the function of the spine and therefore causes disability [13]. Although at present there are few clinical trials to confirm the benefits of therapeutic exercise in treating ankylosing spondylitis [14], it is firmly believed that a rehabilitative program for patients with IBD should include:

1. Pain control treatment.
2. Achieving and maintaining correct posture.
3. Maintaining correct breathing function.
4. Maintaining quality of life.

Osteoporosis

Osteoporosis is common in patients with IBD [15, 16], which is confirmed using dual-energy X-ray absorptiometry that measures bone mineral density (BMD). Further studies and debates need to be undertaken to determine the absolute fracture risk, the contribution of steroids and the role of prophylaxis in treating osteoporosis. Population-based data on fracture incidence suggest only a small increased risk of fracture amongst patients with IBD compared with the general population [16]. A comparative study has evaluated, through the use of bone biopsy, microarchitecture and bone reshaping both in menopause patients and subjects being treated with corticosteroids (7.5 mg per day of prednisone for at least 6 months). This study revealed that patients treated with corticosteroids presented bones with smaller volume (bone volume/tissue volume) and reduced thickness of both trabecular and cortical bone as well as a smaller number of osteoids [17].

If therapy using corticosteroids is undertaken, it is recommended that the minimum effective dose be taken and that therapy be periodically interrupted. Use of calcium and vitamin D may be helpful to contrast the effects of corticosteroids, which can cause secondary hyperparathyroidism, a reduction in osteoblastic activity and have a negative effect on kidney and bowel calcium transport [18].

"For patients with IBD and low BMD, it is possible that calcium and Vitamin D supplementation alone may be sufficient unless the patient is also receiving corticosteroids or has a history of fragility fractures. . . . Combination antiresorptive therapy (typically a bisphosphonate combined with oestrogen or raloxifene) may produce greater gains in bone mass than either agent alone, but the use of two antiresorptive agents is not recommended because the benefit on fracture risk has not been demonstrated and there is increased cost and side effects" [16]. Bernstein and Leslie suggested that "to date, there remains no therapy proven to be efficacious in inflammatory bowel disease-related osteoporosis: however, calcium and vitamin D supplementation and bisphosphonates have their roles" [16].

References

1. Italian Society of Physical Medicine and Rehabilitation (2005) Guidelines for rehabilitation services in Italy. Eur Med Phys 41:95–109
2. Kehlet H (1997) Multimodal approach to control postoperative pathophysiology and rehabilitation. Br J Anaesth 78:506–517
3. Basse L, Raskow H, Jakobsen DH et al (2002) Accelerated postoperative recovery program after colonic resection improves physical performance, pulmonary function and body composition. Br J Surg 8:1–10
4. Andersen J, Kehlet H (2005) Fast track open ileo-colic resections for Crohn's disease. Colorectal Dis 7:394–397
5. Rao SSC (2004) Practice guidelines. Diagnosis and management of fecal incontinence. Am J Gastroenterol 99:1586–1604
6. Sailer M, Bussen D, Debus ES et al (1998) Quality of life in patients with benign anorectal disorders. Br J Surg 85:1716–1719
7. Wald A (1981) Biofeedback therapy for fecal incontinence. Ann Intern Med 95:146–149
8. Whitehead WE, Burgio KL, Engel BT (1985) Biofeedback treatment of fecal incontinence in geriatric patients. J Am Geriatr Soc 33:320–324
9. Enck P, Daublin G, Lubke HJ, Strohmeyer G (1994) Long-term efficacy of biofeedback training for fecal incontinence. Dis Colon Rectum 37:997–1001
10. Latimer PR, Campbell D, Kasperski J (1984) A components analysis of biofeedback in the treatment of fecal incontinence. Biofeedback Self Regul 9:311–324
11. Norton C, Hosker G, Brazzelli M (2004) Biofeedback and/or sphincter exercises for the treatment of faecal incontinence in adults (Cochrane Review). In: The Cochrane Library, Issue 2. John Wiley, Chichester
12. Podswiadek M, Punzi L, Stramare R et al (2004) The prevalence of radiographic sacroiliitis in patients affected by inflammatory bowel disease with inflammatory low back pain. Reumatismo 56(2):110–113
13. Brophy S, Mackay K, Al-Saidi A et al (2002) The natural history of ankylosing spondylitis as defined by radiological progression. J Rheumatol 29:1236–1243
14. Dagfinder H, Hagen K, Kvien TK (2005) Physiotherapy interventions for ankylosing spondylitis (2005) (Cochrane Review). In: The Cochrane Library, Issue 2, John Wiley, Chichester
15. Scott EM, Gaywood I, Scott BB (2000) Guidelines for osteoporosis in coeliac disease and inflammatory bowel disease. Gut 46(Suppl 1):1–8
16. Bernstein CN, Leslie WD (2004) Review article: osteoporosis and inflammatory bowel disease. Aliment Pharmacol Ther 19:941–952
17. Carbonare LD, Arlot ME (2001) Comparison of trabecular bone microarchitecture and remodelling in glucorticoid and postmenopausal osteoporosis. J Bone Mineral Res 16(1):97–103
18. Adachi JD, Bensen WG, Bianchi F et al (1996) Vitamin D and calcium in the prevention of corticosteroid induced osteoporosis : a 3 year follow-up. J Rheumat 23:995–1000

Subject Index

T

U